NURSING 2

NURSING 2

D. MIDDLETON
SRN RNT HospAdminCert
Tutor, Charles Frears
School of Nursing, Leicester

Blackwell Scientific Publications
OXFORD LONDON EDINBURGH
BOSTON PALO ALTO MELBOURNE

Editorial offices:
Osney Mead, Oxford, OX2 0EL
8 John Street, London, WC1N 2ES
23 Ainslie Place, Edinburgh, EH3 6AJ
52 Beacon Street, Boston
Massachusetts 02108, USA
667 Lytton Avenue, Palo Alto
California 94301, USA
107 Barry Street, Carlton
Victoria 3053, Australia

First published 1986

Printed in Great Britain
at the University Press, Cambridge

DISTRIBUTORS

USA
Blackwell Mosby Book Distributors
11830 Westline Industrial Drive
St Louis, Missouri 63141

Canada
The C. V. Mosby Company
5240 Finch Avenue East,
Scarborough, Ontario

Australia
Blackwell Scientific Publications (Australia) Pty Ltd
107 Barry Street
Carlton, Victoria 3053

British Library Cataloguing in Publication Data

Middleton, Douglas
Nursing 2.
1. Nursing—Problems, exercises, etc.
I. Title
610.73'076 RT55

ISBN 0-632-01009-6

Contents

Preface

As the title suggests, *Nursing 2* is the second text designed to meet the needs of student and pupil nurses in the second half of their training leading to registration (RGN) or enrolment (EN(G)).

The contents of the book are so arranged that they roughly parallel the syllabus of training current in Schools of Nursing. Equally important, the material is arranged in modular form. This implies that the learner can make reference to the text during a specific study block or during a clinical allocation.

In this second of two texts the material deals with aspects of nursing care merged with some clinical detail related to gynaecology, obstetrics, venereology, urology, endocrinology, oncology, trauma, the special senses, neurology, dermatology and the operating department. A brief resumé is given of the primary health care team and the professional responsibility which should be developed once the learner has achieved statutory qualification.

A considerable amount of thought has been given to the depth of knowledge and material required by the senior nurse learner to enable her or him to make a positive contribution to patient care, and at the same time learn essential aspects of clinical conditions. There is an obvious shift towards specialisation linked to an appropriate nursing model, but in a basic training there remains a need to explore general concepts which govern all types of illness and patient groups. While attempting to explain various aspects of disease the theme of nursing care constantly returns. The concept of 'total care' requires repeated reference to the psychological and social implications of acute and chronic illness to expand the learner's approach in 'management' as well as in the giving of expert clinical care.

Accompanying *Nursing 2* is a companion text of multiple choice questions, *Nursing 2: Multiple Choice Questions*. This companion text should enable the learner to test her or his understanding of the theory in this book and help on those occasions where multiple choice is used as an examination method.

Acknowledgements

My sincere thanks and appreciation are extended to the following friends and colleagues without whose help and cooperation this book would not have been completed:

Mr D. Shaw, SRN, RMN, RNT, Director of Nurse Education, for his permission to consult and utilise District Nursing Procedures and Policies in current use in the Leicestershire Health Authority

Mr C. Haynes, Audiovisual Aids Technician, for his cooperation in the use of photographs and slides used in the book

Mrs H. Lycett and Mrs R. Skelton, Librarians at the Charles Frears School of Nursing for their unstinting help and enthusiasm in tracing resource and research material

The Nursing and Paramedical Staff of the Hospitals within the Leicester Health Authority who patiently answered queries which arose during the compiling of this text.

Finally and not least, to the students and pupils whose enthusiasm for learning and understanding is the main pivot and motivation for many nursing authors.

Introduction

Having reached the half way stage of the training for RGN/EN(G) qualification, the nurse should have proven competency in many basic skills and an essential grasp of nursing theory. The latter half of training should be used to refine and consolidate clinical skills and, equally important, to begin the deeper studies to achieve professionalism.

The senior student or pupil nurse has to handle personal stress levels brought about by increasing responsibility in the clinical situation and studies for the final examinations. Gradually the nurse will find that the perception of self alters as personal coping strategies improve. Those who assess the senior student are also comparing the change between junior and senior learner and are looking for evidence of embryonic professionalism. How to cope with and relieve personal stress in the later stages of training should be included in the nurse's studies.

Each nursing specialty which is explored in this text tends to fall in the last 18 months of training. The nurse will find that greater flexibility in thought and approach is needed, the earlier training being the foundation on which to build. To help cope with increasing responsibility and demands the nurse should have as a mainstay a thorough grasp of 'Nursing Models', e.g., The Nursing Process. Many other models of care are emerging to meet the patient's needs in each specialty. Whichever nursing model the nurse has to use, it should prove the cornerstone for creative nursing care, give personal job satisfaction, as well as being a useful research technique.

Extending from the correct use of a Nursing Model is the added advantage that a senior learner should be adjusting more quickly to the 'role' expected by patients in hospital, clients in the community, and senior nurse managers. In the last few months of training the nurse should also have explored the elements of the 'qualified' nurse's role. The opportunity to participate in nurse team discussion and clinical care should already have been tested. This participative aspect will be an early preparation for the future role of team leadership, albeit at a junior level, in the ward situation. Leadership and Management are only words unless they are prefixed by the term *effective*. It is this element *effectiveness* which should be a proven competency immediately before qualification.

All nurse teachers have a strong motivation in preparing their students to achieve the ultimate goal, that the learner has become a competent, professional individual who has developed a strong caring attitude, is competent in a chosen clinical field and whose motivation remains as strong and obvious as it did on the first day of the Introductory Course.

Part I
Genitourinary Nursing

Chapter 1
Overview of the Genitourinary System

Essentially the renal system plays a major role in maintaining homeostasis of the body's internal environment. The structures and organs belonging to this system include 2 kidneys, 2 ureters, the bladder and urethra (Fig. 1.1). The formation and secretion of urine by the kidneys and its excretion from the bladder, via the urethra, ensures the body maintains its normal blood pH and is able to excrete many waste products of metabolism, thereby regulating the internal homeostasis of the body.

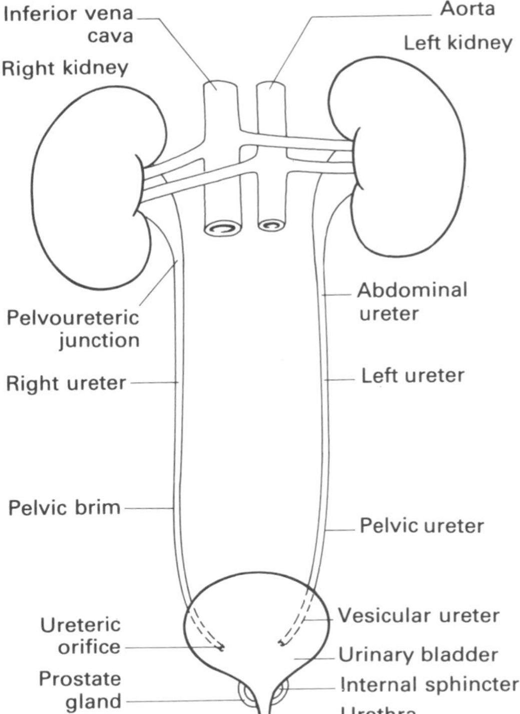

Fig. 1.1 Male renal system.

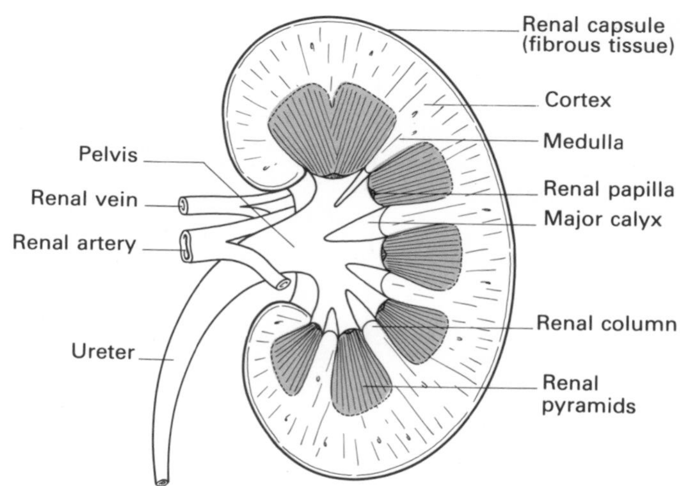

Fig. 1.2 Gross structure of a kidney.

THE KIDNEYS

The kidneys are 2 bean-shaped organs lying either side of the vertebral column between the twelfth thoracic and third lumbar vertebra. They measure approximately 11 cm in length, 7.5 cm in width and 2.5 cm in depth. They are relatively small structures for the amount of work they actually do. They lie retroperitoneally which means that all surgical approaches to the kidneys are via incisions made dorsally and parallel with the waist-line. Each kidney is surrounded by a dense layer of fat which is partly protective but also helps to keep the kidney in its correct anatomical position. Other connective tissues attach the kidney to surrounding structures (Fig. 1.2).

Structures between and around the kidneys include 2 major blood vessels: the aorta and the inferior vena cava lie between the kidneys, while behind and between the kidneys lies the vertebral column. Mounted on the upper pole of each kidney is an adrenal gland. The right kidney is immediately below the liver which may explain why the right kidney is placed lower than the left one.

The Nephrons

Within each kidney there are between 1 and 2 million nephrons. These structures are the basic functional units of the kidney. The nephrons possess distinct anatomical regions each having a unique function in the formation and secretion of urine (Fig. 1.3). Each part, therefore, has a different type of cell enabling the nephron to carry out its function. The *glomerulus* is a convoluted tuft of capillaries encapsulated by a 2 layered cellular envelope, the Bowman's capsule. Blood brought to the glomerulus is filtrated at this capsule so that only molecules of a small size will pass through. This filtration is continuous and is carried out under great pressure which forces a considerable amount of water, electrolytes and waste products to cross the Bowman's capsule into the proximal convoluted tubule. The substances forced through the capsule are referred to as the *filtrate* and this is composed of water, glucose, amino acids, salts, urea, creatinine, potassium and phosphates. The majority of these substances are reabsorbed by other parts of the nephron, with only urea, creatinine and some water being excreted as urine.

In a healthy kidney the antidiuretic hormone released from the posterior pituitary gland will exert its influence on the nephron to ensure that most of the water is reabsorbed. The majority of glucose is passively absorbed as the kidney only has a threshold of 180 mg %. *Aldosterone*, a hormone released from the adrenal cortex, aids the reabsorption of the majority of the salts to maintain the body's

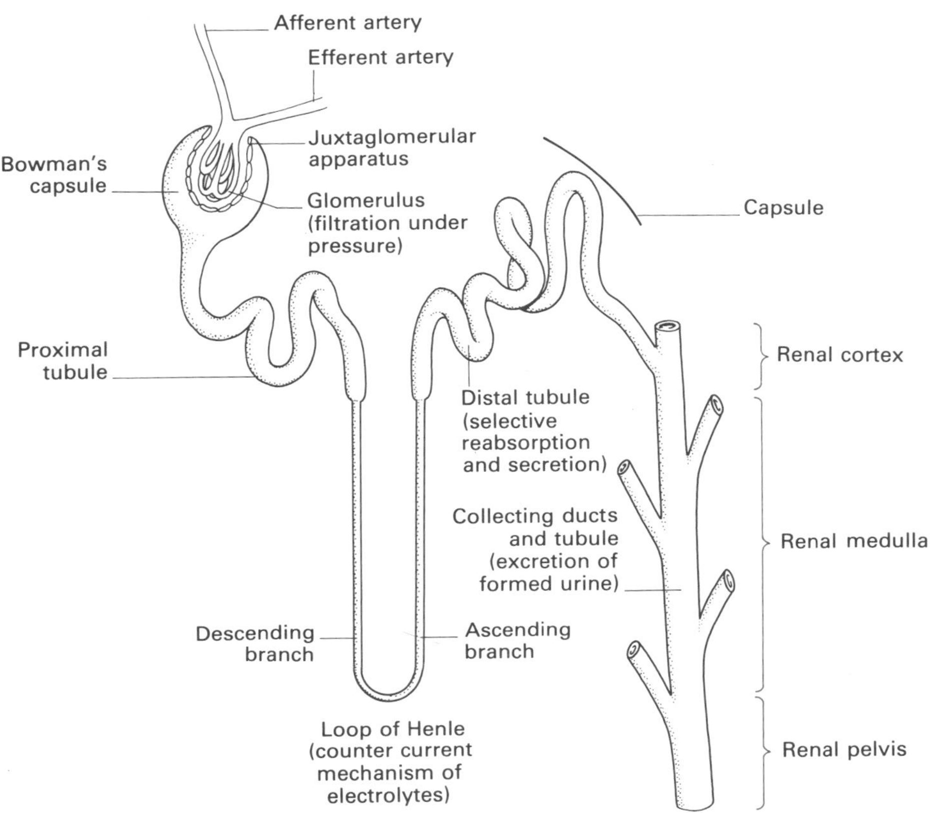

Fig. 1.3 Structure of a nephron.

electrolyte balance. The parathyroid hormone, *parathormone*, will also influence the kidney nephrons to absorb the amount of phosphate required. In addition to these hormonal influences the tubules absorb sodium by a process known as the counter current mechanism at the loop of Henle.

Blood Supply

The blood flow to the kidneys is quite unique. About 25% of the cardiac output is despatched directly to the kidneys at each heart beat.

For an average-sized adult with a circulation of 5 litres of blood and a heart beat of 72 beats per minute, the kidneys will receive 1000 ml of blood every minute. Each kidney will then filter the blood to produce 120 ml of filtrate of which 119 ml will be reabsorbed leaving 1 ml of urine formed each minute. Normally the kidneys filter 120 litres of blood every 24 hours.

The blood vessels enter and leave via the hilum of the kidney and follow an unusual course. The renal artery branches from the aorta and divides into interlobular arteries which penetrate the cortex of the kidney. These in turn subdivide into arcuate arteries before they reach the glomerulus. At the entrance to the glomerulus the afferent artery further subdivides into a tuft of capillaries which then rejoin to form the efferent arteriole. This then subdivides into capillaries before it forms a venule. The venules then join up to form the renal vein which drains into the inferior vena cava.

Functions

The kidney has 6 main functions:

1. Filtration of the blood at the glomerulus.
2. Selective reabsorption from the filtrate along the tubules under the influence of various hormones.
3. Concentration of the filtrate as reabsorption takes place.
4. Secretion of toxins along the length of the tubule, e.g., harmful bacteria, excess hydrogen ions. The latter is important in maintaining blood pH between 7.35 and 7.45 (the normal range).
5. Excretion of formed urine takes place at the collecting duct at about the rate of 1 ml of urine every minute.
6. The release of 2 hormones from the juxtaglomerular apparatus which is in the glomerulus. These are: renal *renin* which influences the diameter of the blood vessels and therefore the blood pressure, and *erythropoietin* which stimulates the formation of erythrocytes in the extremities of long bones.

These functions subserve to maintain the acid base balance of the body, i.e., the blood pH, to regulate the haemoglobin level by the action of erythropoietin, and to rid the body of waste products.

Urine Composition

Normal urine is pale in colour, has a pH between 5 and 8, and is odourless unless allowed to stand and decompose. In composition its constituents are mainly water, urea, which is deaminated amino acids, creatinine, the end product metabolite of muscular energy, and excess salts to the body's needs such as sodium, chloride, sulphate, phosphates, and oxalates. It should be noted that the healthy kidney cannot filter out the larger molecules such as the plasma proteins. When albumin, globulin or blood appears in the urine this should be **considered suspect** until other investigations rule out any need for further concern.

THE URETERS

The ureters are 2 narrow muscular hollow tubes approximately 25 cm in length. They leave the hilum of the kidney descending through the abdomen to enter the bladder at an oblique angle. The principal and middle layer is composed of involuntary muscle which permits the formed urine to be propelled downwards from the pelvis of the kidney to the bladder by peristalsis. The inner wall of the ureter is composed of a smooth mucous membrane while its outer wall is made of fibrous tissue.

The ureters are anatomically divided into 3 regions: the abdominal, the pelvic and the vesicular ureter. The ureters are found following a course downwards behind the peritoneum, over the tips of the transverse processes of the lumbar vertebrae and across towards the bladder at the pelvic brim.

Small renal stones often become trapped in the ureters because they narrow at 3 distinct points: at the pelviureteric junction, at the pelvic brim where they abruptly alter course, and at the cystoureteric orifice which is the narrowest point of the ureter. If the stone is trapped at these points it causes intense irritation of the ureteric mucosa inducing spasm of the involuntary muscle which the patient will describe as colic. The nerve supply to the ureters arises from the tenth lumbar nerve and it ensures that the urine is massaged down the ureter by peristalsis at roughly the rate of a drop of urine every 1.5 seconds from kidney pelvis to bladder. With an oblique entry into the bladder there are two advantages: firstly urine should not reflux back up the ureters and secondly the muscular arrangement of the bladder wall closes over the ureteric orifice like a sphincter.

THE BLADDER

In the adult the bladder, a hollow muscular bag, has an average capacity of between 600 and 800 ml of urine but the complex arrangement of its muscle walls allows it to stretch to a capacity of over 1000 ml (Fig. 1.4). The inner coat of mucous mem-

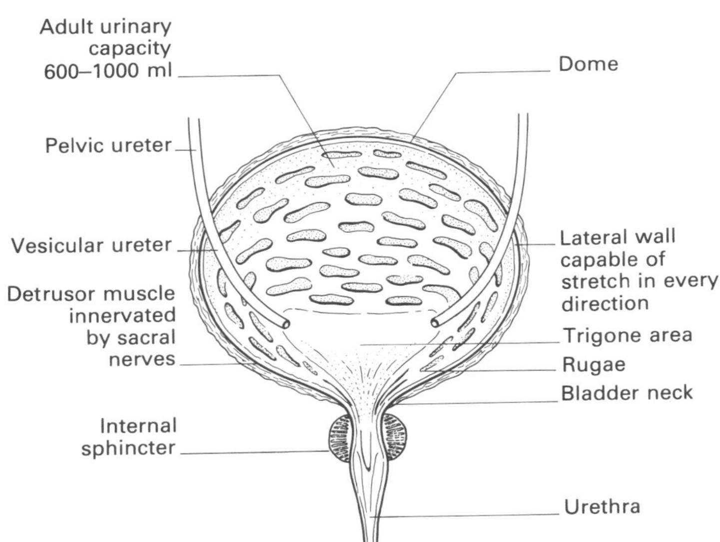

Fig. 1.4 The urinary bladder.

brane lies in folds called *rugae* and as the bladder fills these folds straighten. They permit considerable distension allowing for a greater capacity. The muscle layers are arranged in a criss-cross pattern and these stretch in unison with the mucous membrane. Overstretching of these muscle layers can cause *trabeculation* and this leads to weakness of the muscle coat which may induce bladder diverticulum.

The bladder lies behind the symphysis pubis and can be described as having a dome or roof over which lies the peritoneum and colon. Irritation from an impacted colon can cause urinary incontinence or frequency. The lateral walls and dome are capable of stretching. Lying on the base and posterior wall of the bladder is an area of tissue within which there are nerve cells sensitive to stretch. This is the *trigone area*. This triangular region is found between the ureteric orifices and the urethral opening. Although sensitive to stretch it is not capable of stretch.

The bladder neck leads towards the urethral opening and it is here that the powerful internal sphincter is located. Like the kidney the bladder is a highly vascular organ deriving its blood supply from the internal iliac artery. Any incision on or near the bladder implies serious bleeding both during and after surgery.

The control of micturition is at first glance quite complex. Basically, stretching of the bladder wall is a sensation received by the spinal cord from the trigone area producing a motor response which will relax the internal sphincter, i.e., completing a reflex arc. This is what happens in infants. This simple arrangement is somewhat altered by social training of toileting habits. The frontal lobes of the brain exert a powerful inhibition upon this reflex arc until it is socially convenient to void urine. Damage to the brain implies incontinence because the reflex arc remains intact. Damage to the spinal cord, however, implies retention of urine since the reflex arc may be totally inhibited from giving a motor response thus preventing the sphincter from relaxing.

THE URETHRA

The female urethra is relatively short in length (2.5–3 cm) while the male urethra is much longer (16–20 cm). The female urethra is solely concerned with conveying urine from the bladder, its likeness to the male urethra ending with a similar mucous membrane lining, secretory mucus ducts and a meatal opening.

The male urethra is divided into 3 portions:

Prostatic urethra (also known as the posterior urethra)

Membranous urethra
Spongy urethra (also known as the anterior urethra)

Prostatic Urethra

The prostatic urethra is about 3 cm in length and its inner membrane is continuous with the inner coat of the bladder, i.e., the transitional epithelium. This inner tissue gives way to columnar epithelium which is continuous with the surrounding prostate gland and the ejaculatory ducts. Surrounding the prostatic urethra is the prostate gland which is located immediately below the base of the bladder. Prostatic fluid enters the urethra via 15–20 ducts and is necessary for the motility of sperm when semen is ejaculated. The ejaculatory ducts enter the urethra at the base of the prostatic gland and are short muscular tubes linking the seminal vesicles to the prostatic urethra.

Membranous Urethra

The membranous urethra passes through an external sphincter. From this sphincter extends a ligament which is attached to the symphysis pubis providing both attachment and support for the male urethra. Situated either side of the external sphincter are the *bulbourethral glands* (Cowper's glands) which are mucus-secreting to lubricate the mucosa of the urethra.

Anterior Urethra

The anterior urethra extends from the membranous portion and is about 15 cm in length. It is *S* shaped and its structure is frequently interrupted with mucus-secreting glands, i.e., Littré's, Morgagni's and Tyson's glands. The spongy tissue of which it is composed is richly supplied with blood vessels which on sexual excitement fill and cause the penile shaft to erect.

Urinary Meatus

The urinary meatus is the most distal and narrowest portion of the male urethra and often becomes blocked by debris, e.g., blood clots and calculi. The walls of the urethra remain collapsed except during micturition, and it is for this reason that any attempt at catheterisation must always be done **gently** to avoid unnecessary trauma to the inner lining. Ascending infections in the urethra are more common with the shorter female urethra. Once a catheter has been introduced into the bladder of either a male or female, ascending infections become common.

Chapter 2 Examinations, Investigations and Procedures

For ease of reference the examinations, investigations, and procedures related to renal nursing are grouped under:

Physical examination
Haematology tests
Radiological examinations
Urinalysis
Endoscopic examination
Tissue biopsy
Renal function tests
Isotopic tests
Ultrasound

PHYSICAL EXAMINATION

A general physical examination by the doctor will assess the relevance of certain classical signs which are usually present if there is a disease of the genitourinary system. The nursing role while assisting the doctor and comforting the patient is to **assess** the patient's problems arising from these signs and consider their relevance when creating a plan of care.

Abdominal distension, if present, will embarrass respiratory function and the correct positioning of the patient should relieve the worst features of this discomfort.

Abnormal urinary flow is quite common and detailed questioning is required to note its exact nature. It is one of the more obvious signs of which the patient will complain.

Terminology

The meaning of terms likely to be employed by the doctor will help the nurse to understand the terminology.

Anuria absence of adequate urinary excretion.

Dysuria difficulty in starting or straining to start the urinary flow. This may occur in prostatic enlargement or in urethral obstruction from strictures, fibrosis, or urethral inflammation.

Nocturia an increased number of visits to the toilet to empty the bladder, especially at night, and may indicate urinary frequency from an irritation of the bladder or urethra.

Polyuria an excess of urinary secretion and excretion which is usually very dilute. It is normally a classical sign of diabetes mellitus and diabetes insipidus but may bring the patient to the doctor thinking it is a renal or bladder problem.

Haematuria blood in the urine. However slight, this may indicate internal problems arising from renal calculi, infection or inflammation which is damaging the capillaries of the genitourinary structure.

Incontinence the inability to control urinary flow. This may be due to many reasons, e.g., stress, bladder neck abnormality, prostatic enlargement, spinal injury, bladder calculi. It is a psychologically distressing feature requiring a great deal of sympathy until the further investigations establish its true cause. A detailed nursing plan will be needed to minimise the discomforts from urinary accidents.

Albuminuria presence of albumin in the urine. This should not normally be present in the urine. Being a plasma protein, it should not filtrate into the renal tubule. When it does escape it suggests damage to the glomerular apparatus within the cortex of the kidney.

Retention of urine the inability to pass urine. This is usually due to prostatic enlargement. It may be acute, occurring over a period of hours during which the distension of the bladder increases, causing severe lower abdominal pain. In the chronic form, the nature of the retention occurs over a period of weeks or months, with persistent urinary dribbling and problems of dysuria. Occasionally the chronic form suddenly becomes a complete urinary obstruction and then it is known as *acute upon chronic retention*. If the term is followed by *overflow*, it implies the urine is overflowing the maximum capacity of the bladder and is refluxing up into the ureter.

Urinary Tract Pain

The doctor will note the type and frequency of any pain. There are 3 forms of urinary tract pain: renal colic, ureteric and urethral pain.

Renal colic pain is localised around the loin and may spasmodically and painfully radiate to the groin or the umbilicus. Such pain is usually due to stones, trapped in the pelvis of the kidney, trying to escape down into the ureter propelled by peristaltic action. Such violent peristalsis causes the severe and crippling pain.

Ureteric pain involves the ureter only and travels from loin to groin. It is caused by a small renal stone passing down the ureter by strong peristaltic propulsion.

Urethral pain arises from infection or inflammation of the urethra, and is often described by the patient as scalding and accompanied by dysuria.

Palpation of the Kidney

Included in the examination of the abdomen is palpation of the kidney to ensure that it is not enlarged and retains its usual bean shape. If an enlarged prostate gland is suspected the doctor may request assistance to do a rectal examination. An expert diagnostician may be able to distinguish, by digital pressure, if the outer shell of the prostate gland is of a smooth contour or if it is irregular and knobbly. If it is the latter, the enlargement of the prostate gland may be malignant.

Patient Care

In general terms the majority of patients with renal disorders are tired, lethargic and irritable. This is invariably due to insomnia arising from the many symptoms of the disease, especially if the patient has had difficulty in passing urine. The skin colour may appear grey and its normal elasticity may be gone, most probably due to dehydration. From a behavioural point of view many patients deprive themselves of liquids in some attempt to lessen the severity of their symptoms. The nurse must realise that once any dehydration has been corrected the patient may still be reluctant to drink because of a very natural fear that the symptoms will recur. The patient will require persistent reassurance and encouragement to drink normal volumes.

HAEMATOLOGY TESTS

There are 5 standard haematology tests that are repeatedly completed on all patients with any form of renal disease. These are: haemoglobin estimation, leucocyte count, erythrocyte sedimentation rate, and estimation of blood urea and serum electrolytes. Apart from these main tests many others may be completed to confirm a suspected diagnosis or reappraise the progress of a particular disease.

Haemoglobin normal values: male 7.4–11.2 mmol/litre (13.5–18 g/l); female 7.4–10 mmol/litre (12–16 g/l).
In renal disease there is usually a reduced secretion of the hormone erythropoietin. This hormone is essential to stimulate the bone marrow to produce the precursor cells which develop into mature erythrocytes. Hence the relationship between anaemia and renal disease.

Leucocyte count normal value: $4–11 \times 10^9$/litre.
Although not diagnostic, a raised leucocyte count may indicate that an infection is present within the renal system and highlights the need for further investigations. Equally important the leucocyte count may be reduced if immunosuppressive drugs are prescribed following a renal transplant.

Erythrocyte sedimentation rate normal values: male 0.20 mm/hour; female 0.30 mm/hour.
A raised erythrocyte sedimentation level would indicate inflammation somewhere within the body and when the result is combined with presenting clinical features it may lead to a positive diagnosis. It also indicates the need for further investigations.

Blood urea normal values: 2.5–6.6 mmol/litre (15–40 g/litre).
Urea is the waste product of the deamination of excess protein which takes place in the liver. In healthy circumstances the waste product is conveyed to the kidney and is firstly secreted into the renal tubules and then excreted in the urine. Deamination is the removal of the nitrogen from excess amino acids; once this has been done the amino acid becomes a waste product. Since there are many different amino acids there is a correspondingly wide variety of protein waste products, e.g.,

Blood uric acid 0.18–0.47 mmol/litre (20–40 mg %)
Ammonia 22–44 μmol/litre (0.01–0.05 mg %).
Creatinine 60–120 μmol/litre (0.6–1.1 mg %)

In normal health all these substances are excreted. When there is a fall in the glomerular filtration rate, which happens in renal disease, the waste products are retained with a subsequent rise in the serum levels. They then act as toxins producing many of the symptoms of illness.

Serum electrolytes commonly assessed are:

Sodium (Na) normal values 134–144 mmol/litre
Potassium (K) normal values 3.5–5.3 mmol/litre
Chloride (Cl) normal values 94–104 mmol/litre

The results can be at great variance, e.g., in oedema the sodium is usually raised, in dehydration it is much reduced. A reduction or excess of potassium may have adverse effects on the conduction rhythm of the heart causing arrhythmia. If exceptionally low or high it may cause a cardiac arrest.

Other blood tests which are frequently completed include estimation of: serum and phosphatase, serum alkaline phosphatase, serum calcium and serum bilirubin.

Serum acid phosphatase normal values: 0.0–0.13 μ/ml King-Armstrong Units.
Serum acid phosphatase functions at a pH of 5.6 and is related to the function of spermatozoa. The enzyme is produced by the prostate gland and if this gland is affected by cancer the levels of the enzyme become raised.

Serum alkaline phosphatase normal values: 4–13 μ/ml King-Armstrong Units.
Serum alkaline phosphatase is manufactured in the liver and is active at a pH of 8.5. Its main function is concerned with the deposition of calcium phosphate in the bone. Its level is raised in diseases of either liver or bone, but it is taken as a contrast measure against serum acid phosphatase. It is useful should a patient be presenting with renal calculi but in fact have a primary disease of bone or liver.

Serum calcium normal values: 2.25– 2.60 mmol/litre.
Calcium is essential for the formation of bone, muscle contraction, heart function, nerve conduction, and blood coagulation. If for any reason the serum levels are raised it can precipitate the formation of renal calculi. About 12% of renal stones are formed from calcium deposits in the kidneys.

Serum bilirubin normal values: 5–17 μmol/litre (van den Bergh's test).
Bilirubin is the normal end product of haemoglobin breakdown. This pigment is the colouring material in the faeces and urine. In some circumstances, e.g., a mismatched blood transfusion or haemolytic anaemia, the volume of bilirubin increases and affects renal function. This test would indicate if any renal distortion is due to a primary renal disease or a secondary disease such as haemolytic anaemia.

RADIOLOGICAL EXAMINATIONS

Apart from a straightforward abdominal X-ray which will demonstrate gas and fluid levels in the abdomen, the majority of renal X-rays are invasive.

Preparing the Patient

The nursing role in preparing the patient may involve several stages.

An explanation of the procedure is essential before written consent is obtained. Many renal X-rays require the use of general anaesthesia or heavy sedation so written consent **must** be given by the patient. Note should be made of any written instructions received from the radiology department and such instructions attached to the patient's care plan or Kardex.

Having had a bath or shower, the patient will be gowned in a cotton theatre gown which ties at the back. Wherever possible a nurse should escort the patient to the X-ray department, but **must** do so under certain circumstances:

If the patient is to be given a general anaesthetic

If intravenous therapy or a blood transfusion is in progress

If the patient is elderly, confused, distressed, or obviously anxious

If the patient is having continuous oxygen therapy

Immediately before the procedure the patient is normally advised that the intravenous injection tends to cause hot sensations over the needling site, with feelings of flushes, and sometimes nausea, but that these discomforts will pass. If the patient is for general anaesthesia then the preoperative routine is carried out.

On return from the X-ray department any special instructions from the radiologist should be noted on the Kardex or care plan. If there has been a fasting period the patient should be offered a drink and food if it is not contraindicated, and then made comfortable in their own bedwear.

Intravenous Pyelography

For the patient about to undergo an intravenous pyelography the lower colon must be completely empty of faeces and gas. To achieve this the patient should have a low residue diet for the previous 24 hours. Aperients, e.g., Dulcolax or Senokot granules, may be prescribed the night before and their effectiveness noted. Fluid intake is restricted for 6–8 hours prior to the procedure. If, however, it is timed for late in the day a light breakfast should be offered to the patient. If the patient has a raised blood urea then the aperients, restricted fluids, or enemas are not allowed and the radiologist may cancel standard preparations. A radioopaque dye is injected intravenously and then X-rays are taken at 5-, 15- and 30-minute intervals. The resulting films will demonstrate any lesion which alters either the expected normal structure or the surfaces of the renal pelvis and ureters, and will indicate the location of any renal calculi.

Retrograde Pyelography

The aim of the retrograde pyelography X-ray is similar to that of intravenous pyelography, except that the dye is introduced into the pelvis of the kidney via a ureteric catheter. This procedure is invariably completed under a general anaesthetic. On recovery from the anaesthesia, permission will be required to remove the ureteric catheter; it is not usually removed until the films have been checked for clarity.

Micturating Cystogram

The micturating cystogram may be an unpleasant and embarrassing procedure for the patient, who will, most likely, require a great deal of reassurance during the taking of the films. It is usual to sedate the patient mildly 30 minutes before the procedure begins. A urinary catheter is passed into the bladder and a measured amount of a radioopaque substance is then injected into the bladder. After a few minutes the patient adopts the normal posture for micturition and as the dye is excreted serial films are taken. This test should demonstrate if there is any reflux from the bladder up into the ureter.

Cystourethrogram

While similar to a micturating cystogram, the cystourethrogram is usually combined with a cystoscopy. This double investigation is to try to determine if there is bladder neck abnormality or a urethral disorder which would account for stress incontinence.

Renal Arteriography

To demonstrate the presence of cysts, tumours, or emboli within the renal blood vessels renal arteriography is carried out. It requires the patient to be prepared either for general anaesthesia or for heavy sedation. Since the opaque dye is usually injected into the femoral artery, the selected limb will have to be shaved. Following the procedure, careful and frequent observation of the needling site should be made. Recordings of both pulse and blood pressure are made at 30-minute intervals until the risk of haemorrhage from the femoral artery has receded. Further invasive techniques are used to outline the renal artery as it branches from the aorta (aortography). A renal lymphangiography could be done to outline the lymph glands and lymph vessels located at the hilum of the kidney.

URINALYSIS

All patients admitted to hospital have a urinary sample routinely tested on the ward. The nurse must advise the patient of why this is necessary, the reason mainly being to exclude any relevant signs which should be pursued with further tests if necessary. The urine sample must be tested when it is fresh to avoid discrepancies in the results. Apart from the reagents' chemical reactions, the nurse should also note the colour, smell, pH, specific gravity and odd deposits and make note of the results in the patient's care plan or Kardex.

Collecting Specimens

Samples of urine required for culture and sensitivity, i.e., bacteriological culture and their sensitivity to a range of antibiotics, are requested in one of three ways:

Early morning urine (EMU)
Midstream specimen of urine (MSU)
Catheter specimen of urine (CSU)

An *early morning sample* of urine is collected as would be any routine sample and is used mainly to detect the presence of tubercle bacillus. It is increasingly rare to be asked for this specimen.

A *midstream specimen* of urine is as it suggests the middle part of the urinary stream. Prior to the sample being collected into a sterile container, the genitalia and urethral orifice have to be cleansed and dried. It is usual to collect the sample in a sterile tinfoil disposable tray and carefully transfer the sample into a specimen bottle.

A *catheter specimen* of urine is literally what it says. The catheter once passed should be clamped off 30 minutes before the urinary sample is collected. On some styles of urinary catheter there is an exit portal from which a sample of urine can be aspirated by needle and syringe. This is the preferred method and avoids disturbing a closed urinary drainage system and reduces the risk of introducing infection. The collected sample is despatched in the same way as a midstream specimen.

All urine specimens should be taken within the shortest time-span before their collection from the ward by the pathology department. The request forms must be complete in every detail and signed by the doctor requesting the test. These details are checked off by the nursing staff before the sample is taken from the ward.

Diagnosis

While acute infections of the urinary tract are relatively easy to diagnose and treat, greater difficulty is experienced with infections of a chronic nature. A definitive diagnosis of chronic urinary tract infection is said to be present when more than 100 000 organisms/ml of urine are present in 3 consecutive urine specimens, preferably being early morning specimens (Kass method).

The common bacteria found are:

Escherichia coli
Streptococcus faecalis
Staphylococcus albus and *S. aureus*
Klebsiella pneumoniae
Pseudomonas pyocyanae
Proteus vulgaris
Proteus mirabilis

Eighty percent of all cases of urinary tract infection are due to infection by *E. coli*. The last 4 micro-organisms mentioned are more commonly found in patients with structural abnormalities of the urinary tract.

24-hour Urinary Collection

The nurse may be requested to obtain a 24-hour urinary collection from a patient. There are several reasons for such a test, mainly to assay the volume of catecholamines and the quantity of albumin, urobilinogen, androgens, 17-corticosteroids and electrolytes. After explaining the procedure to the patient and if possible making him or her responsible for his or her own collection, it is a wise precaution to label the patient's bed to advise other members of staff and visitors.

Depending on the reason for the collection, the pathology department will provide a special container usually clearly labelled and normally with a preservative in it. The nurse is responsible for collecting and providing the patient with this container.

It is best to start this collection at 08.00 hours on any working day except Saturdays, as the pathology department is usually closed on Sundays for tests of this nature. The first specimen passed is discarded, and then all urine passed in the next 24 hours is collected into the provided container. It is essential to emphasise to the patient that *all* urine must be saved otherwise the test must be repeated. It is also important to finish the collection at the stated time.

If the 24-hour collection is to assess urea and creatinine clearance within the kidney then concurrent blood specimens are collected at several points during the 24-hour period.

ENDOSCOPIC EXAMINATION

An endoscopy or visual examination may be an isolated test such as a *cystoscopy* (visualisation of the bladder only) or be a total inspection of the bladder, bladder neck, ureteric orifices and urethra, in which case it may be referred to as a *panendoscopy*. Endoscopy is often complementary to a retrograde pyelogram, i.e., they are done together. The examination is routinely done in all cases of haematuria. It may be part of the investigations if there is a suspected bladder tumour, and cystoscopy is often combined with *cystometry*, i.e., measuring the volume capacity of the bladder. Lastly, cystoscopy is a prerequisite of any treatment given via the urethra, e.g., dilatation of urethral strictures, crushing of bladder stones and transurethral prostatectomy.

Since total relaxation of the patient is essential, endoscopy examinations are completed with the patient under a general anaesthetic. This is particularly important with children.

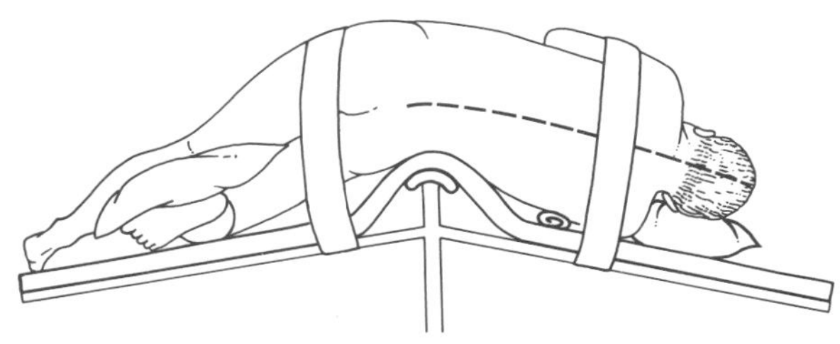

Fig. 2.1 Lateral position for renal surgery

Preoperative Care

Prior to preparation of the patient for an endoscopy the nurse must ascertain if the surgeon has any particular instructions, e.g., does he or she wish the patient to come to theatre with a full bladder. Previous investigations and their results should be on hand including X-ray films if previously taken. These should be available to the surgeon at the time of examination. A general anaesthetic is usually administered so the written consent of the patient should be obtained by the doctor who will have given an explanation of the procedure. This will need to be reinforced by the nurse in terms the patient will understand.

The perineal and pubic area may require to be shaved depending on the local policy and the surgeon's wishes. In addition to these basic essentials, the patient will be prepared as for theatre, i.e., identity, urinalysis, bath, gown, cap, sedation or premedication, and nurse escort to the theatre reception area.

The Patient in Theatre

Following anaesthesia the patient is placed on the theatre table in the dorsal position. It is relevant to note this as occasionally patients complain of backache following this procedure. Reassurance is given by explaining it is due to the position they are placed in during the investigation (Fig. 2.1).

The modern cystoscope incorporates a fibre-optic mechanism as well as additional parts which enable the surgeon to do a series of operations as well as inspecting structure. The ureters can be catheterised, small tumours may be coagulated, bladder stones can be crushed, tumours can be resected (*resectoscopy*), biopsy of the bladder tissue can be taken and the prostate gland can also be resected via the cystoscope.

Postoperative Care

On completion of the cystoscopy, the escorting ward nurse must ensure that she or he has clear instructions from the surgeon regarding any postoperative orders. If the patient is being returned to the ward with an indwelling catheter, this must be noted, and only when the patient has recovered the swallowing reflex should the nurse return to the ward.

On recovery from the anaesthesia, the patient will usually complain of urethral discomfort, and possibly pain. This can be minimised by the administration of prescribed analgesia. In male patients it is of some comfort to offer a scrotal sac support if there is any evidence of swelling or tenderness of the scrotum. Unless otherwise instructed, encourage the patient to drink copious volumes of clear fluids which will aid urinary output. In female patients it may prove necessary to apply a vaginal pad to absorb any discharge.

TISSUE BIOPSY

A biopsy of the kidney implies that a piece of tissue is taken from the renal cortex which will enable a histological study to be made of the glomerulus and proximal tubule. The main reasons for renal biopsy include:

Assessing the progress of renal failure
Determining if dialysis is necessary
Noting if treatment of nephrotic syndrome is effective
Confirming a functioning transplanted kidney following renal transplant

Precautions

Since a renal biopsy carries serious risks for the patient, certain precautions are taken, mainly to reduce the hazard of haemorrhage into or around the kidney. Such precautions include:

1. An intravenous pyelogram, or, if this is not possible, an X-ray of the renal area to demonstrate the position of the kidneys in relationship to surrounding structures.
2. Grouping and cross-matching of 2 units of blood which are held in reserve in case of haemorrhage.
3. Assessment of the clotting and prothrombin time of blood to exclude any existing tendency to haemorrhagic disorder.
4. Teaching the patient the correct method of breathing, especially the technique of breath-holding. This will be essential during the procedure when the needle is advanced through the tissues.
5. Assessment of the patient's physical and psychological state to decide on the technique of anaesthesia. The majority of adults, having been given a clear outline of the procedure, will be able to consent to local anaesthesia. Children, however, will require general anaesthesia.

Procedure

If available, a biopsy table should be used for the patient to lie on. If a standard bed is used, it must be of a reasonable height and capable of being braked, and needs to be screened to ensure privacy. A small dose of sedation should be administered to the patient 30 minutes prior to the procedure and the patient requested to empty the bladder. Previous X-rays and the results of all investigations must be available to the surgeon before the procedure begins. The patient should have had a shower or bath before being dressed in an open-backed cotton gown. The escorting nurse remains with the patient until after the procedure has been completed.

The preferred position is for the patient to lie prone on a firm base with either a hard pillow or large sandbag placed under the abdomen to tilt the renal area upwards and outwards. Some doctors may prefer that the patient sits upright on a firm chair leaning forward over a low level bedtable. Whichever position is adopted the nurse should request the patient to take several deep breaths and then to test if one breath can be held with reasonable comfort for a count of 20–30 seconds. The pulse and blood pressure should also be recorded and noted at this time and will be used as a contrast for the observations following the procedure.

The assembled equipment, determined by local policy, should not be brought to the bedside until the last moment and then positioned to be out of the patient's view. A second nurse will assist the doctor in the skills of preparing the trolley and handling the equipment in an aseptic manner. The needling site is usually the right kidney since it is lower than the left and not so hampered by the lower ribs. Its position is carefully measured from the existing X-rays and calculated from the lumbar spine outwards and the iliac crest upwards. The site is marked with a skin pencil over the lower pole of the kidney.

Following skin cleansing with an antiseptic, the skin site is injected with a local anaesthetic which should infiltrate down to the perirenal fat. Once the area is insensitive to pain a Vim-Silverman biopsy needle is advanced through the tissues towards the kidney. It is during this time that the patient must hold the breath. The reason for breath-holding is to avoid the kidney capsule being torn by the needle, since the kidney moves with each respiration. The doctor and nurse will know when the needle is safely ensconced in the renal cortex since it gently swings with each respiration.

When the stylette of the needle is withdrawn it will bring with it a small piece of tissue between its pincers, and this is immediately transferred to a prelabelled specimen jar containing a preservative. On removal of the Vim-Silverman needle, pressure is applied to the needling site to control any local bleeding from the tissues. An occlusive dressing is applied to the skin after it has been sealed with collodion solution. During the following 15 minutes the patient is asked to remain at rest and relax. After this the patient may be allowed to move into a more comfortable position.

The pulse and blood pressure are vital observations for the next 12 hours. The usual regimen which is recommended is: pulse and blood pressure recordings every 15 minutes for 2 hours, then every 30 minutes for 4 hours, and then every hour for 6 hours. Any variation from the normal expected values must be reported immediately to a senior colleague since an increasing pulse and falling blood pressure would perhaps indicate intrarenal or perirenal haemorrhage. To minimise this risk even further a period of bedrest from 12–24 hours is recommended and during this time sedation or analgesia may prove necessary to help the patient. At frequent intervals the occlusive dressing is checked for any blood staining, and all urine passed is tested for haematuria.

In the following 24 hours the nurse should observe for any complications:

Perirenal haematoma noted by localised pain and increasing shock

Retroperitoneal haemorrhage noted by rapid pulse and falling blood pressure

Urinary retention no urine passed within 12 hours of procedure

Infection of needling site skin appears red with localised heat

Hydronephrosis a longer-term complication and preceded by urinary retention.

RENAL FUNCTION TESTS

In addition to chemical or microscopic examination of urine specimens it is possible to assess renal function by directly testing if the renal tubules can clear a given substance, concentrate tubular water and excrete toxic substances. These 3 tests of renal function, i.e., clearance, concentration and excretion, can be used to investigate the severity or progress of renal function in renal disease.

Urinary Urea Concentration Test

Blood urea normal values: 2.5–6.6 mmol/litre.

After the patient is advised of the purpose of the test, the intake of fluids is restricted from the afternoon prior to the test and no breakfast is allowed on the morning of the test. Before the test begins a blood sample is collected to measure the blood urea levels. The patient then empties the bladder, and the sample of urine obtained is poured into a specimen jar labelled 1. A solution of 15 g of urea dissolved in 60 ml of water is then given to the patient to drink. At hourly intervals for the next 3 hours the patient is asked to void urine which is collected into specimen jars clearly labelled **2**, **3** and **4**. After measurement and testing in the laboratory a figure of 2% (2 g in 100 ml of urine) indicates that the kidney is competently concentrating the urea. The reason for collecting 4 specimens is that the first is used for comparison with any of the other 3, one of which should reach 2% to show a normal renal function. If the test is performed in children then the amount of urea is adjusted according to weight and age.

Urea Clearance test

Ideally, the urea clearance test is started at about 08.00 hours on any weekday, and commenced before breakfast has been eaten. The patient empties the bladder and this specimen of urine is discarded. A solution of 15 g of urea in 60 ml of water is given to the patient to drink. An hour later the patient empties the bladder again and this specimen of urine is also discarded. During the next hour a specimen of blood is collected for blood urea estimation and at the end of the 2 hours the patient once again voids urine and this specimen is collected into a clean bottle for despatch to the laboratory. The accuracy of timing is extremely important if the test results are to prove reliable. A healthy kidney will be able to clear over 75% of the urea within 2 hours of its being given, any value below 10% indicates a grossly diseased kidney.

Urine Concentration Test

To prove whether the kidneys can concentrate water in the tubules the patient has fluid restricted from 16.00 hours of one day until 08.00 hours on the following day. On each of the following 3 hours the patient is asked to empty the bladder and each specimen of urine is carefully measured and tested for its specific gravity. At least one of these specimens should have a specific gravity of 1025 or more if the tubules are concentrating normally.

For these tests patients will be admitted only if they are unreliable, or are already in hospital seriously ill. It is more usual for the patient to have these tests completed as an outpatient.

ISOTOPE RENOGRAPHY

The principle employed in isotope renography is that radioactive isotopes are attracted to heat generating areas within the tissues. It is abnormal for localised areas to generate heat above that of normal body temperature and therefore certain disorders can be specifically localised by this technique. These include:

Renal infection
Renal inflammation
Carcinoma
Obstruction within the renal system

The isotope commonly used is Iodine hippuran and a measured amount is injected intravenously. If the body is healthy the isotope should be totally excreted within 24 hours. The evening before the test the patient may be prescribed an oral dose of potassium iodide to saturate the thyroid gland with iodine and so remove the main source of local body heat.

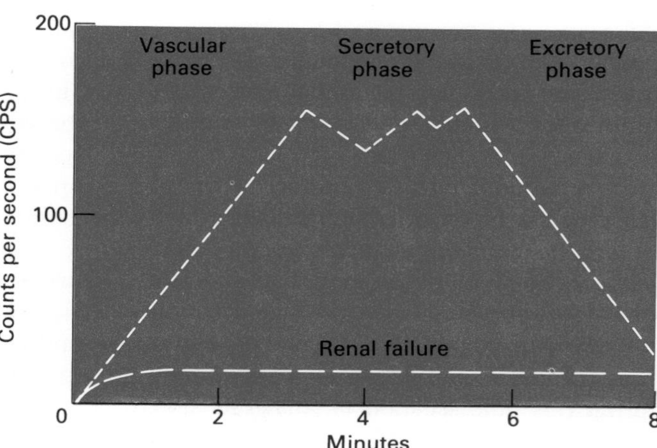

Fig. 2.2 Renal radioisotope uptake and output. The spikes are proportional to renal blood flow.

After the injection is given a Geiger counter is used to trace the progress of the isotope and Fig. 2.2 shows the 3 phases expected of a healthy individual contrasted with the flat trace of a patient in renal failure.

This test is often combined with a 24-hour urinary collection (see p. 14). The essential difference here is that the container used to collect the urine will be marked *radioactive*, it may be coloured red, and the patient's bed may be labelled with a warning sign to avoid unauthorised people handling the container. This is more of a precautionary measure, however, since the half-life of this particular isotope is extremely short.

ULTRASOUND

As a noninvasive investigation, ultrasound requires the minimal amount of patient preparation. High frequency sound waves are emitted from a transducer over and through the soft tissues of the renal area. If these sound waves strike anything solid in the tissues they echo against the density, and such echoes are traced on an oscilloscope. The denser the substance the more frequent the echoes of the sound waves. They may prove useful in distinguishing between a fluid-filled cyst or a fleshy tumour but are of limited value in precise diagnosis.

Chapter 3
Inflammation of the Kidney

Electron microscopic studies of the glomerulus and tubules are increasing the fund of knowledge about nephritis. While this is to be welcomed, it does create difficulties with international agreement on a system of classifying the disease entities related to the kidney.

Inflammatory conditions of the kidney may be either acute or chronic in type. Principally, the glomerulus is only affected in acute inflammation. It is realised, however, that the tubules also are ultimately affected which may eventually lead to a chronic type of inflammation. Histological studies show that there are 4 basic reasons why the glomerulus can become inflamed:

1. Antibodies destroy the basement membrane of the glomerulus.
2. Antigen-antibody complexes saturate the basement membrane causing the complex to become fixed. This in turn attracts platelets to the site which causes localised coagulation. This is then digested by leucocytes which result in an inflammatory process.
3. Vascular damage of the afferent arteries of the glomerulus, in particular, may lead to an infarction of the tuft of capillaries within the glomerulus.
4. Infiltration of the glomerular apparatus by hyaline tissue may arise from several disorders, e.g., diabetes or amyloid disease.

Disease Progress

The progress of any one of the 4 irregularities outlined can either lead to an inflammation of short duration with spontaneous resolution or cause scarring of the glomeruli with some irreversible loss. Should there be infarctions within the glomerular capillary tuft there will be more severe irreversible loss.

The progress of a renal lesion can be expressed as:

Minimal lesion which involves an excessive loss of protein across the filter mechanism of the glomerulus due to damage of Bowman's capsule.

Membranous glomerulonephritis when the whole of the glomerular apparatus is damaged with a resulting scarring and fibrosis, and there is loss to the body of the plasma proteins, albumin and globulin.

Proliferative glomerulonephritis when there is no effective filter mechanism due to both inflammation and fibrosis of the renal parenchyma.

From these changes and the damage to the glomerulus several disease entities emerge:

Acute nephritis
Nephrotic syndrome
Acute glomerulonephritis
Chronic glomerulonephritis
End stage sclerosing glomerulonephritis
Acute renal failure
Chronic renal failure

There is a great deal of overlap and similarity in the signs and symptoms and the specific diagnosis depends on the clinical findings or the patient's body biochemistry, and a definitive history. Equally the causes of many renal diseases are legion and this text can only deal with a few.

ACUTE NEPHRITIS

This inflammatory process, *acute nephritis*, has an insidious almost sinister development, the principal cause being a streptococcal throat infection several weeks before the renal signs or symptoms emerge. Oliguria or total anuria occurs indicating a complete renal failure. Any urine that is excreted may contain blood (*haematuria*). During the oliguric phase the patient develops serious hypertension. Several days or weeks after the oliguria or anuria the patient has a sudden diuresis, indicating a spontaneous resolution of the inflammation of the glomeruli, If, however, severe scarring or fibrosis occurs the patient may progress to chronic renal failure.

NEPHROTIC SYNDROME

Nephrotic syndrome is defined as the insidious onset of oedema, albuminuria and excess globulin in the urine (over 5 g in 24 hours). Lipids are also excreted in the urine. This loss of plasma proteins across the glomerulus alters the osmotic pressure throughout the body causing plasma fluid to remain within the tissue causing a widespread oedema. The waste products of metabolism, particularly urea, cannot escape and hence the blood urea levels rise. There are other important waste products but urea is the one used to monitor the patient's progress. The damaged glomerulus also releases the hormone renin in greater than normal amounts, causing hypertension, i.e., a persistent high blood pressure. The continuing loss of protein from the body reduces the patient's resistance to infection. Coupled to the renal disease is the liver's compensating mechanism of producing more albumin. The liver also manufactures more lipids and cholesterol, giving rise to hyperlipidaemia. The outcome of nephrotic syndrome is always uncertain; there may be a spontaneous recovery or it can develop into chronic renal failure.

ACUTE GLOMERULONEPHRITIS

The causes of the inflammation, *pyelonephritis*, are legion and women are affected more than men. Although a female can suffer an acute infection at any time during her lifespan there do seem to be peak periods when its incidence is more prone. Such peaks tend to occur when the young girl starts school, at the onset of menstruation, with the beginning of sexual relations, i.e., honeymoon cystitis, after childbirth, and after the menopause when any infection can prove to be intractable.

(2) Obstruction of the ureters, e.g., renal calculi

Urinary reflux

Indiscriminate use of commercially available analgesics

Diabetes mellitus

Drug addiction, especially if the drugs are self-administered by injection

Debility from any cause

Immunosuppressive therapy

The causative organisms of bacterial inflammation mainly arise from the perineum where commensal organisms of the bowel are to be found. The bacteria may gain entry via the urethra. Instrumentation of any kind into the bladder via the urethra carries the risk of introducing infection unless strict aseptic precautions are employed, e.g., catheterisation, cystoscopy, retrograde pyelogram. The organisms most frequently found to be the cause of bacterial inflammation include:

Escherichia coli *Klebsiella species* *Streptococcus faecalis*	Commensal to the gut
Proteus morganii	Related to renal stones
Pseudomonas pyocyanae	Related to the use of antibiotics

Treatment

Treatment centres on bedrest until the pyrexia, lethargy, and loin pain have subsided. A course of antibiotic therapy which may be either combined sulphonamide and ampicillin, or a course of trimethoprim sulphonamide, and nitrofurantoin is also commonly used. Once the patient is feeling better a series of investigations will be completed to establish the cause. These investigations usually consist of:

1. An intravenous pyelogram to establish if there is any damage to the kidney.
2. A micturating cystogram to note if there is any ureteric reflux.
3. Blood cultures to exclude bacteraemia.
4. Cystoscopy if the patient has haematuria.
5. A midstream specimen of urine to enable identification of the causative organism.

Repeated attacks of acute pyelonephritis are not uncommon in women and while investigations continue and the progress is monitored, it may be decided to commence a prolonged course of antibiotic low-dose therapy for between 6 and 12 months. Advice that may help those with these acute repeated attacks will be given by a genitourinary consultant. There are factors which may help patients combat repeated infections. They can increase their oral intake of fluids so that they void urine frequently, as often as every 2 hours, during the daytime. Following intercourse the female should try and remember to void the bladder. A female should also consider if she may be allergic to any contraceptive device being used.

Acute inflammation of the kidney, i.e., acute pyelonephritis, or acute glomerulonephritis, may suppurate giving rise to renal abscesses, scarring of the glomeruli, papillary necrosis and calculus formation.

Table 3.1. Causes of chronic nephritis

Cause	Agent
Infection	bacterial leptospirosis tuberculosis
Mechanical obstruction	calculi urinary reflux hydronephrosis ectopic ureter polycystic kidney pregnancy
Therapeutic	radiotherapy
Metabolic disorders	choline deficiency diabetes mellitus hyperuricaemia hyperphosphataemia sickle cell anaemia potassium depletion
Toxicity	drugs sulphonamides aspirin phenacetin codeine anticonvulsants chemicals lead cadmium

Table 3.2. Signs and symptoms of chronic renal failure

System affected	Signs and symptoms
Alimentary	Anorexia, nausea, vomiting Hiccoughs, thirst, parotitis Diarrhoea
Cardiovascular	Chest pain, oedema, hypertension, left ventricular failure or hypertrophy Raised jugular venous pressure Pericardial effusion or pericardial rub Anaemia, epistaxis Raised blood pH, i.e. acidosis Raised blood urea, electrolyte imbalance
Endocrine	Amenorrhoea, menorrhagia, impotence
Integumentary	Pruritis, pigmentation, purpura
Locomotor	Muscular cramp and weakness Myopathy, arthritis Rickets in children, osteomalacia in adults
Neurological	Lack of concentration and poor memory Delusions or depression and drowsiness Paraesthesia, tremor, peripheral neuropathy Hallucinations, mania Convulsions, coma
Ophthalmic	Corneal and conjunctival inflammation Hypertensive retinopathy, detached retina
Renal	Polyuria, nocturia Unable to concentrate urine
Respiratory	Dyspnoea, orthopnoea, ammoniacal breath Oral ulceration

CHRONIC GLOMERULONEPHRITIS

Chronic glomerulonephritis is currently defined as an insidious progressive inflammation of the interstitial structure of the renal parenchyma. This results in a 50% loss of renal function proven by excretion tests and intravenous pyelogram. The main causes are listed in Table 3.1. The term chronic nephritis refers to one of 3 possible disease entities:

Chronic pyelonephritis which is a persistent pyogenic infection

Interstitial nephritis in which there is excessive scarring and fibrosis

Papillary necrosis usually caused by indiscriminate indulgence in analgesic drugs

Once scarring of the renal tissue occurs it obstructs, distorts, and obliterates part or whole of the nephron. This implies that selective reabsorption, secretion, and excretion of waste products in the urine are over 50% ineffective. Combined with this destruction there is the ever present risk of infection and the likely formation of stones. The accumulative effect spares no body system (see Table 3.2) and the discomforts and distress of the patient are serious but variable in their intensity in each individual.

Once the investigations have established if the inflammatory process is irreversible the doctor will decide on one of 3 possible options:

Peritoneal dialysis
Haemodialysis
Renal transplant

END STAGE SCLEROSING NEPHRITIS

Severe fibrosis and scarring extends to involve the whole kidney, which becomes shrunken and contracted. There is excessive loss of protein and a marked hypertension. Several diseases which bring this about are:

1. Henoch's and Schonlein's purpura. Combined with the joint pains, gastrointestinal bleeding and purpura which are typical of this disease there may be an acute nephritis. In children the disease has a promising outlook but in adults the prognosis is very poor.
2. Goodpasture's syndrome. This is a rapidly occurring glomerulonephritis following upon a pulmonary infection. The antigen released by the damaged lung sensitises the glomerulus which then becomes inflamed.
3. Systemic lupus erythematosus (SLE). The patient's system produces antibodies against his or her own cellular DNA. This is more common in women, and in about 50% of patients, the SLE will progress to nephrotic syndrome.

ACUTE RENAL FAILURE

Acute renal failure is a sudden fall in the glomerular filtration rate resulting in an oliguria and an imbalance of the electrolytes. With the accumulation of the waste products of metabolism increasing in the blood stream there will be a temporary failure of renal function. Renal failure can be subdivided into 3 groups each being dependent on the primary cause.

Pre-renal Causes

Pre-renal causes include any condition which reduces cardiac output thereby resulting in a reduced renal blood flow, e.g., hypovolaemia from burns and haemorrhage, cardiogenic shock arising from severe cardiac arrythmias, and bacteraemic shock arising from blood-borne infections. Hypovolaemia is reversible in most of these situations.

Renal Causes

Renal causes may be due to: ischaemia of the kidney itself due to local emboli or thrombi; toxins arising from drugs; infections causing a temporary tubular failure which may extend to a necrosis. Inflammation of any part of the kidney structure may cause a temporary renal failure, e.g., pyelonephritis or glomerulonephritis. Incompatible blood transfusions, and jaundice have an immediate effect on the renal structure. Pregnancy may cause serious pressure on both the ureters and kidneys.

Stages

Renal causes are further subdivided into stages of acute renal failure:

Stage 1 Oliguric phase: this may last for several days or weeks, but if lasting for more than 30 days a renal biopsy is performed to ensure that it is not a chronic loss of function.

Stage 2 Diuretic phase: a dilute but increasing urinary volume accompanied by a decrease in plasma volume, urea, and creatinine levels.

Stage 3 Recovery phase: follows about 10 days after stage 2 with the urine composition back to normal. The electrolytes may remain unstable and require careful assessment.

Post-renal Causes

Post-renal causes are more likely to result in anuria than oliguria, and are invariably due to complete obstruction to the urinary flow from the pelvis of the kidney. Likely causes tend to be: large calculi, e.g., a staghorn calculus; prostatic enlargement which completely occludes the urethra; and either benign or malignant tumours occluding urinary flow anywhere along the genitourinary tract.

If the cause is either pre-renal or post-renal, the underlying problem will be treated if at all possible. The tendency now is to proceed with dialysis therapy and the classical picture of acute renal failure is rarely seen today.

CHRONIC RENAL FAILURE

See chronic glomerulonephritis p. 23.

NURSING CARE PLAN

The wide variety of symptoms and their tendency to overlap means that the nursing plan of care must be carefully structured to meet the needs of the individual. Assessment of problems is done on a daily basis. Trained members of staff should know when any proposed nursing action fails to resolve a given problem and be able to intervene with alternative proposals. Close liaison with medical staff, the dietician, and laboratory staff is essential so that the overall aims of therapy are achieved.

Diet Modifications

The main alterations to diet revolve upon modifying:

1. Protein intake which is reduced if the patient is uraemic and increased if there is proteinuria.
2. Sodium intake if there is either oedema or hypertension.
3. Potassium intake if there is hyperkalaemia.
4. Fluid intake if there is oedema and to compensate for insensible loss of fluids.
5. Food intake to meet the required energy needs although carbohydrates are restricted.

Protein

The protein intake, if reduced, will usually be to either a 20, 40, or 60 g protein intake per day, depending on the level of blood urea. At least 75% of the protein offered must be of first class protein and in addition protein foods which contain potassium will be restricted. Alternatively if the patient has excess loss of plasma proteins from the urine, *proteinuria*, a high protein diet will be offered. This will be to at least a 100 g protein intake per day or more, plus any supplements, e.g., Complan, Carnation feeds or build-up drinks.

Sodium

In the majority of renal diseases the patient's sodium intake is reduced to alleviate either oedema or hypertension. One of 3 possible approaches may be taken, which will depend on the level of sodium in the blood. A *salt free diet* (22 mmol) where no salt is added to either the cooking or at table. A *low salt diet* (30–50 mmol) where a wider range of foods may be selected but no salt added to either cooking or at table. An *added salt diet* (60–100 mmol) where a little salt is added to the cooking but not at table.

The result of such a diet is that any food offered can be bland and without flavour. It is possible to compensate for this with a few herbs or spices being added during the preparation and cooking of the meal.

Potassium

As with sodium, the potassium levels of the blood will be assessed very frequently to ensure that normal levels are being maintained. To help achieve this, all potassium-containing foods are restricted from the diet. Not only does this apply to the patient in hospital but also once the patient has been established on conservative and palliative therapy and is discharged home on independent care. It therefore becomes essential that the patients and their relatives are involved in any educational programme and their attention should be brought to bear on foods which they purchase or eat in restaurants. Examples of potassium-containing foods which are restricted include: instant coffee, chocolate drinks, citrus fruit juices, pickles, sauces, chutneys, nuts, crisps, whole wheat cereals, beers, ciders, wines, salt substitutes, meat extracts, mushrooms, and potatoes. If fruit or vegetables are offered in the diet they have first to be leached to remove their potassium content.

Fluid Intake

Fluid restriction is based on calculating the urinary output over a period of 24 hours.

Once this is established a further 500 ml is added which compensates for insensible loss which cannot under normal circumstances be calculated. The resulting total is the fluid intake permitted to the patient in the following 24 hours. It can therefore be appreciated that strict fluid balance recording is required. In specialised units, if the patient is severely oedematous, he or she could be nursed on a bed which monitors changes in the patient's body weight each day. This is the more accurate method of noting if the oedema is being contained by fluid restriction.

Food Intake

In any form of renal disease the patient will have depleted protein reserves and yet diet is restricted on carbohydrates. To prevent the patient utilising protein for energy purposes, high energy-yielding drinks are included in the total volume of fluids permitted per day, e.g., Hycal or Caloreen. Glucose is permitted as are jam, honey, marmalade, boiled sweets, and syrup. The ideal would be for the diet to achieve an intake of 8400–12 600 kJ (2000–3000 cal).

Additional to these modifications, vitamin supplements and iron medications are usually added to correct anaemia (normocytic hypochromic type usually). Blood transfusion is not normally practised in renal disease. If there is a raised blood pH, i.e., acidosis, then the doctor may prescribe sodium bicarbonate or sodium lactate to correct this metabolic acidosis.

If the serum phosphate level is raised and serum calcium low it indicates that the renal disease is causing an alteration in the bone structure. To correct this aluminium hydroxide may be prescribed orally. This medication binds phosphate to itself and prevents dietary phosphate being absorbed by the intestine.

Such modifications to the diet are a palliative measure to combat many of the distressing discomforts. **Frequent** assessment should be made to note if they are correcting features, e.g., nausea, vomiting, oedema, hypertension, anaemia, electrolyte imbalance, raised blood urea, and acidosis. If peritoneal dialysis or haemodialysis are commenced then any existing diet will also have to be reviewed.

DIALYSIS

Before the worst of the symptoms of acute and chronic renal failure develop, it is increasingly common for the doctor to commence *dialysis*. This procedure is defined as a transfer of solutes across a semipermeable membrane down a concentration gradient. The membranes which are used for dialysis are the *peritoneum* and the *aiphoran* (the artificial membrane in a haemodialysis machine).

Peritoneal Dialysis

The peritoneum is a semipermeable membranous sac partly covering or surrounding the liver, stomach, pancreas, small and large intestine, bladder, uterus, and the intra-abdominal major blood vessels. In function it supports and protects the abdominal organs: it contains a serous fluid which prevents friction as the abdominal organs move against each other, it isolates and localises any inflammatory lesion due to the many lymphatic nodes present, and it acts as a reservoir for excess body fat. The principle employed is shown diagrammatically in Fig. 3.1.

There are 2 common methods of employing peritoneal dialysis:

Intermittent peritoneal dialysis (IPD)

Continuous ambulatory peritoneal dialysis (CAPD)

Intermittent Peritoneal Dialysis

Intermittent peritoneal dialysis is used for short-term purposes. It is simple to set up, a quick means of reducing high blood urea, efficient and cost effective and does not require elaborate resources from a nursing point of view. It is often used as a temporary measure in acute renal failure until a haemodialysis machine is available. The correction of biochemical imbalance takes a little time, however, but this is to the patient's advantage as it allows for a gradual adaptation to an unusual therapy.

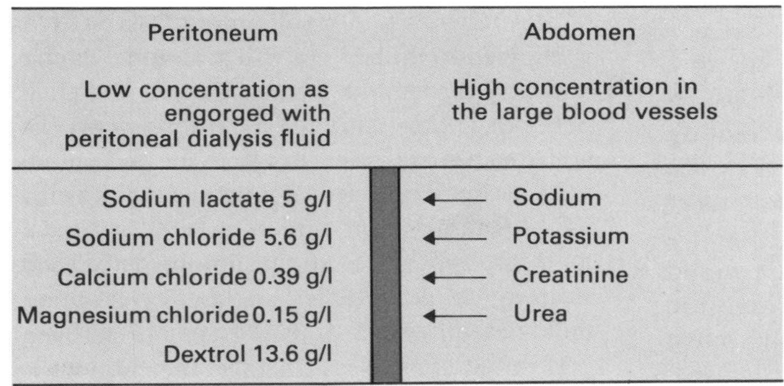

Fig. 3.1 Selective reabsorption takes place down the concentration gradient.

Continuous Ambulatory Peritoneal Dialysis

More frequently employed is continuous ambulatory peritoneal dialysis in patients with chronic renal failure until a haemodialysis machine becomes available. The patient can be taught to manage this system and so achieve a remarkable degree of independence either in hospital or at home. After a silastic catheter has been inserted into the patient's peritoneum under a local anaesthetic and the dialysis is established (Fig. 3.2), the aim will be to teach the patient the practicalities of bag exchange. The main features of such a programme would include teaching the patient:

1. How to exchange bags using an aseptic technique.
2. Observing and recording daily or more frequently blood pressure, body weight, body temperature, and reporting any abnormal readings.
3. Collecting specimens for the returned dialysate fluid.
4. Completing bag exchange at a set time interval during a 24-hour period.

When 2 bags are simultaneously infused into the peritoneum over a period of 30 minutes, they are allowed to exchange for 15–20 minutes, and then allowed to drain out for 15 minutes. The intake and output volumes are noted and compared to see if there is a positive or negative balance. This is repeated for up to 8 litre volume which would take about 4 hours. It is usual practice to leave a further 2 litres of dialysate within the peritoneum until the following day. After several supervised practices at bag exchange, the patient can achieve total control by learning how to connect the silastic catheter to the connecting tubing in an aseptic manner.

Procedure

The renal unit will have its own specific procedure and policy regarding peritoneal dialysis which the nurse will be expected to know in some detail.

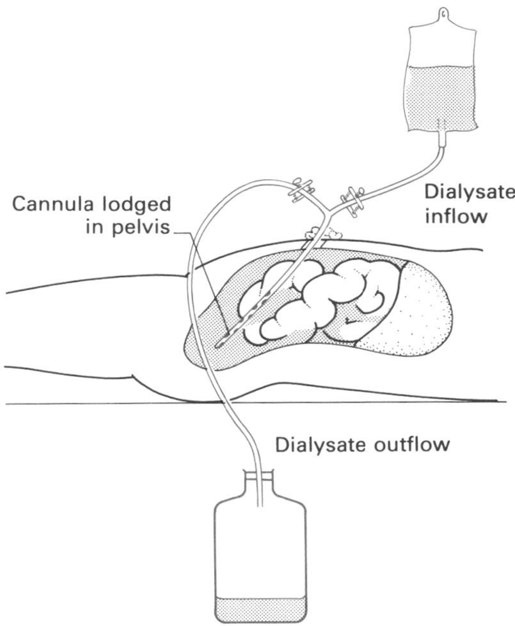

Fig. 3.2 Peritoneal dialysis.

Preparation of Patient

The purpose and duration of the therapy should be explained to the patient and if possible also to a close relative by the treating doctor. Further explanations are given by the nurse should the patient think of questions at a later time.

Prior to the procedure the abdomen would be thoroughly cleansed and shaved from the nipple line to midthigh including the pubic area. The umbilicus should also be cleansed, using a moistened cotton bud. The bladder must be emptied either voluntarily or by means of a catheter so that it is completely contracted before the procedure. The lower colon should also be empty not only of faecal content but also of gases.

A record is made of the patient's blood pressure, temperature, pulse, and weight after they have been taken accurately. A small dose of Valium may be given to calm and sedate the overanxious patient 30–60 minutes before the procedure. Some thought should be given to the clothing which the patient will have to wear during and after the procedure, since access to the abdomen will have to be available at all times. Clothing which opens at the front will be necessary.

The preferred position for the patient is either to lie dorsally or, if this proves difficult, to be only slightly semirecumbent. The doctor is better assisted if 2 nurses are available, one as the assistant to the aseptic technique, the other to remain with and reassure the patient at all times.

Commencement of Dialysis

After the abdominal wall is cleansed with antiseptic lotion and dried, the needling site is surrounded by sterile drapes and the exposed site is made pain free by an injection of local anaesthesia, e.g., lignocaine. The peritoneal catheter is then guided through the skin and muscle layers into the peritoneum approximately 5 cm below the umbilicus via the avascular linea alba.

When sited, the metal stylette of the catheter is removed and the catheter is attached to the prepared connecting tubing of the dialysis set. A small amount of the fluid is allowed to infuse into the peritoneal cavity and any discomfort for the patient noted. If necessary the catheter's position can be adjusted before being sutured to the abdominal skin. A small amount of fluid is then drained off the peritoneum and a note is made of its composition. A minor amount of blood staining is acceptable, but heavy staining indicates an organ or blood vessel has been perforated. If all is satisfactory, the catheter is further secured by a waterproof dressing. The first dialysis cycle of fluid can begin once the patient is made comfortable.

Dialysis Fluid

Dialysis fluid comes as either isotonic or hypertonic solutions. The *isotonic* solution has the same osmolarity pressure as blood and will attract all metabolic waste products into the peritoneal cavity from the intestinal blood vessels. It is therefore used to correct metabolic acidosis and uraemia. If however the patient also has oedema, a *hypertonic* solution will be used. This means that not only waste products will be attracted but also excess volumes of fluid. The main difference between the solutions is that hypertonic diaflex has more dextrose in its composition.

A normal programme consists of 2 litres of dialysis fluid per hour, the cycle of events being, 15 minutes infusion time, 15 minutes indwelling time, and 30 minutes draining time. However these times can be adjusted to meet the patient's needs.

Patient Care

During dialysis the nurse is responsible for accurate observations of the patient's 4-hourly temperature, pulse and respiration, the very strict fluid balance charting, the daily urinalysis, and checking of the daily weight of the patient.

Although difficult and cumbersome it is possible to get the patient up for short periods to sit in a comfortable armchair.

At each bag exchange the nurse should check that the temperature of the bag has

Table 3.3. Example of fluid balance during peritoneal dialysis

Date	Cycle number	Peritoneal fluid	Time in	Exchange time	Drain started	Bag weight (g) In	Out	Balance	Additives
1/12/85	1	1.36%	09.00	09.15	09.30	2200	1800	400	KCl (Potassium) 1 g
	2	3.86%	10.00	10.15	10.30	2200	2500	−100	Heparin
	3	1.36%	11.00	11.15	11.30	2200	2350	−250	Antibiotic

been warmed by dry heat to a temperature of 38° C before being infused into the peritoneum. The bag is also carefully weighed both before and after each exchange to enable accurate fluid balance charting to be achieved. A positive balance means that the output exceeds the input, while a negative balance means that the input exceeds the output. It should be noted that calculations are from the first cycle and additions or subtractions are made to each succeeding total.

Drugs may be added to the dialysis fluid and if so the bag itself should have a label attached with the name of the drug. Small amounts of heparin may be added to act as an anticoagulent since minor blood clots may obstruct the eyelet of the peritoneal catheter. Antibiotics may be either prescribed as therapeutic or prophylactic measures, and potassium chloride (KCl) may also be added if the serum electrolytes show a tendency to hypokalaemia.

At the conclusion of each cycle in the dialysis programme, the fluid may be discarded unless a specimen is requested for culture and sensitivity to detect any infection.

Complications

The problems which may arise during and following peritoneal dialysis include:

1. Perforation or rupture of abdominal organs, e.g., the bladder, bowel, and large blood vessels.
2. Excessive dialysis will restrict the movement of the diaphragm risking a chest infection from shallow breathing.
3. The dextrose content of the dialysis fluid may induce a hyperglycaemia and blood sugars may be assessed during the programme.
4. Excessive dialysis will cause intra-abdominal pressure against the musculature and may risk herniation.
5. Peritonitis is a constant hazard and requires frequent and strict observation of the patient's baseline temperature, restlessness, perspiration and abdominal pain. The drained dialysis fluid will be warmer than usual, smell sweeter and the observant nurse will notice that the exchanges need to be more frequent if peritonitis is present.

Haemodialysis

The dialysis of the blood follows a similar principle to that of peritoneal dialysis, but is usually employed as a long-term treatment until the patient is offered a renal transplant. The patient's blood is driven into the dialysis machine by the patient's own arterial pressure and it passes over a semipermeable membrane (aiphoran). On the opposite side of this membrane there is dialysate solution which attracts metabolic waste products from the blood to itself.

Although the Kiil dialyser is the most common machine used in the UK, constant improvements in design and function means that there is a wide selection and variety in size of machine available. The machine, however, is usually capable of:

Dialysis

Ultrafiltration of the blood

Monitoring the temperature of the dialysate within the machine

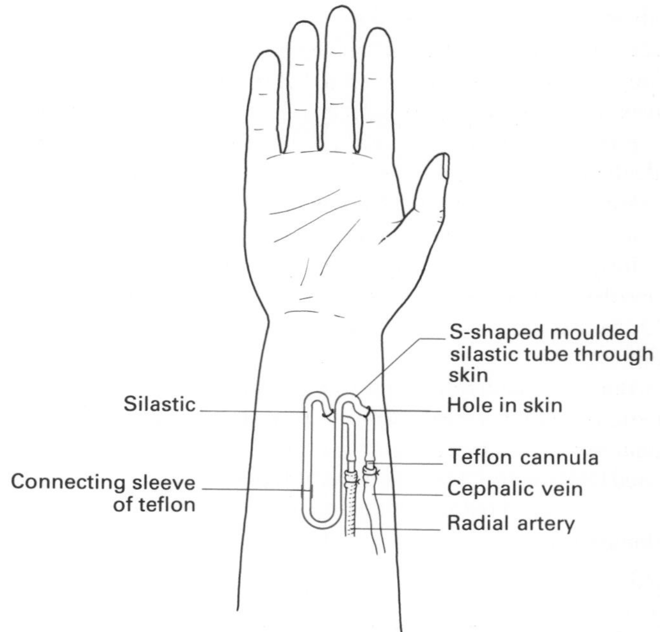

Fig. 3.3 Scribner shunt.

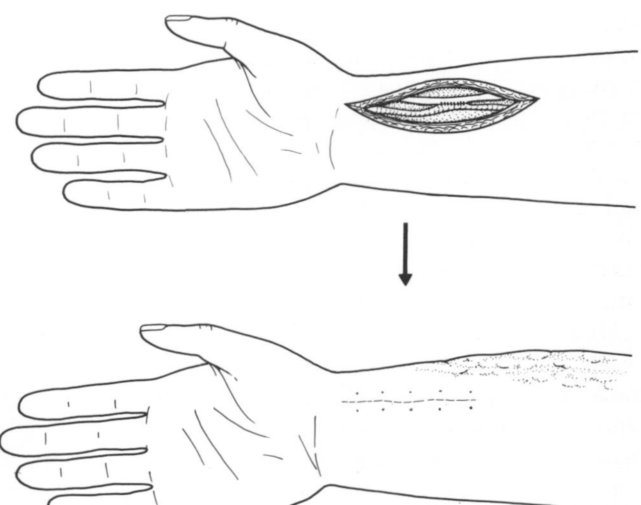

Fig. 3.4 Cimino-Breschia fistula with the radial artery anastomosed to the cephalic vein (*above*) so the 'varicose' veins in the forearm (*below*) can be used in intermittent dialysis.

Monitoring the blood-flow rate through the machine

Monitoring the blood pressure within the machine

The dialysate fluid, i.e., isotonic or hypertonic, can be adjusted to suit the patient's current biochemical status.

Preparation for Haemodialysis

Since a programme of haemodialysis may last some considerable time and in many cases it is the forerunner therapy to renal transplant, the patient requires either an arteriovenous shunt or fistula. With an *arteriovenous shunt*, narrow diameter teflon tubes are sutured into an artery and a vein. The two tubes are then connected together by a malleable silastic U loop (Scribner method). This shunt will be used as the connection between the patient's arterial outflow and venous return (Fig. 3.3). With an *arteriovenous fistula*, a vein and an artery which travel together are anastomosed side-to-side. After the anastomosis has healed it forms a tunnel through which wide-bored needles can be placed to connect the patient to the machine (Cimino–Breschia method, Fig. 3.4).

Both methods are a long-term proposal and usually once they are created they are left to heal for at least 2 weeks before they can be used for dialysis.

Home Dialysis

Following an established routine of haemodialysis the doctor will indicate if the patient should then enter into a training programme for home dialysis. The minimal teaching required is that the patient must be able to: connect and disconnect the tubing from the haemodialysis machine to the arteriovenous shunt or fistula using an aseptic technique: commence and regulate the dialysis fluid exchange; operate the basic machine controls and maintain its outer cleanliness; self assess his or her pulse and temperature, and distinguish an abnormal reading, subsequently seeking medical advice.

Should the patient meet this tremendous challenge then detailed arrangements are made to install a home dialysis machine. The team effort and its coordination requires the back-up services of a regional renal unit, and hence haemodialysis is an expensive treatment. It is also full of thorny ethical problems related to patient selection. Regardless of this it is a most successful treatment.

RENAL TRANSPLANT

All patients who are proposed for renal transplant have their names placed on a central register with details of their tissue typing. A series of immunological tests highlight the antigens which are unique to the individual, preventing or minimising the hazard to rejection. About 30 or so antigens have been identified and these lie as proteins on the surface of the cells. Specific to the individual, the antigens identify *self* and if any foreign material invades the tissues, these antigens initiate an antibody response. This comes mainly from the lymphocytes which then attack and destroy the foreign material, i.e., rejection.

Tissue Typing

Tissue typing is agreed by international standards and basically 3 tests are completed:

1. Serological defined antigens (SD test).
2. Lymphocyte detected antigens (LD test).
3. Human lymphocyte antigens (A) (HLA survey).

When a donor kidney becomes available either from a living person (usually a member of the family) or a cadaver, the same tests are carried out on the lymph fluid of the donor and the results given to the central register for tissue matching. Only 1 in 5000 are tissue type compatible. If a match can be found and the donated kidney is transplanted successfully the patient may have on average a further 2–10 years of comfortable life if not longer. The name of the matched recipient is then notified to the regional renal unit and the staff would then organise for the patient's immediate admission to hospital for transplant surgery.

The donor kidney is carefully stored in ice and packed in a flask which will maintain the temperature around the kidney at 4° C. It may be placed in a Belzer–Gambro machine which maintains perfusion of the donated kidney throughout its transit. The storage of the kidney has a limit of about 18 hours before it suffers permanent damage due to anoxia. Kidneys are not accepted from donors if they suffer from carcinoma, sepsis, hypertension, or are over 70 years of age because of atheroma.

Preoperative Care

Preoperatively the recipient patient may have had elective surgery to remove both or a single kidney: due to hypertension, if the kidney was polycystic, or because of ureterovesicular reflux. Some patients may have had a splenectomy as part of the preparation for renal transplant to overcome the problems created by immunosuppressive drugs which are given following transplant surgery.

The specific preparation of the patient for renal transplant includes completing:

1. A cross-matching of the patient's blood to obtain several units for later blood transfusion.
2. A short period of haemodialysis to correct the blood biochemistry.
3. An accurate analysis of the clotting time of blood to anticipate the risk of haemorrhage.
4. A careful assessment by the anaesthetist to consider anaesthetic risk.
5. The taking of swabs from the nose, shunt, throat, and perineum for culture and sensitivity.
6. The passing of a nasogastric tube to aspirate and maintain an empty stomach.
7. The administration of immunosuppressive therapy and antibiotics as prescribed.

A donated kidney is removed with both the renal vein and artery and a portion of the ureter. When implanted into the recipient it is secured into the iliac fossa; the iliac vein and artery are used to connect the renal artery and vein, while the portion of ureter is fashioned into the base of the bladder to prevent any urinary reflux.

Postoperative Care

Postoperatively, the patient is transferred to an isolation cubicle or area to reduce the risk of infection. This risk does not come from the operation or the possibility of rejection but because of the use of immunosuppressive drugs which suppress any tendency to rejection. Specific postoperative care, which is additional to routine care given to any patient recovering from a major operation, includes:

1. **Strict observations** of the vital signs every 15 minutes for a minimum of 12 hours. Thereafter at more prolonged intervals if they remain stable.
2. **Monitoring** of the central venous pressure. This will indicate if the cardiac pressures are within normal limits, and may accompany an intravenous infusion or blood transfusion.
3. **Frequent analysis** of blood specimens, e.g., urea, electrolytes, packed cell volume, haemoglobin, leucocyte count and creatinine. Blood samples can be collected from the shunt.
4. **Gastric aspiration** at 1-hourly intervals until bowel sounds return.
5. **Observation of the wound site** for exudate and calculation of drainage volume if a suction/vacuum bottle is secured to the site. Only when the wound exudate is minimal is the wound drain shortened, then removed, usually 48 hours later.

Risk of Rejection

The urinary catheter is left in place, continuously draining the bladder, until the threat of 'first line rejection' is over, i.e., about 10–14 days after surgery. In the meantime very careful calculation of the fluid balance is maintained. All urine passed is saved and collected for 12-hour or 24-hour analysis of the metabolic waste product levels.

The risk of haemorrhage is very high at the site of anastomosis and therefore a 'tight' anticoagulent therapy regimen is employed to try and achieve a clotting time of 20 minutes at least.

The 'portals of entry' for infection require very strict nursing management, and every technique should be considered in preventing infection gaining access via the oronasal cavity, urinary catheter, intravenous site, shunt, and the wound. Following transplant a course of immunosuppressive therapy will commence; it is usually a combined course of azathioprine (Imuran) and steroids. Of themselves these drugs cause serious side effects, the more important being to cause bone marrow depression, duodenal peptic ulceration and renal artery thrombosis.

Over a 6-week period the signs of rejection will be closely observed for and these include reporting tender painful tissue around the site of implantation, a swollen iliac fossa, increasing oliguria, and if the results of 24-hour urinalysis show poor creatinine clearance. If the patient shows any signs of rejection the patient will have to be returned to haemodialysis therapy until a second or third transplant can be offered.

The actual rejection process commences with the lymphocyte cells becoming enlarged; the immunoglobulins likewise enlarge and these deposit themselves on the intima of the blood vessels in the transplanted kidney. Over this layer of deposit the platelets accumulate to form a thrombus which leads to an occlusion of the blood supply through the organ and eventually it becomes infarcted and necrosed.

Chapter 4
Renal Calculi

In the UK it is estimated that 1 in 10 males suffer from renal stones in one form or another.

COMPOSITION OF RENAL STONES

The composition of renal stones tends to be derived from 5 different compounds.

Calcium phosphate and *calcium oxalate* are the most common and account for about 90% of those stones which are analysed. Being radioopaque they are readily diagnosed by X-ray.

Uric acid, a waste product of protein metabolism, will tend to come out of solution to form a stone if the patient cannot form alkaline urine.

Cysteine is a water soluble sulphur compound of protein.

Xanthine is a protein derivative.

Uric acid, cysteine, and xanthine form the remaining 10% and since they are all linked to protein it leads to the suggestion that the patient may have an inborn error of protein metabolism, i.e., the cause is *genetic* in nature. These 3 solutes are not opaque to X-ray and require more extensive investigations of the patient.

Predisposing Factors

Apart from studies on the composition of stones a list of predisposing factors may precipitate stone formation:

1. Idiopathic. An unknown reason or cause forms the vast majority in which it is seen that there is definite hypercalcuria but little else to indicate why.

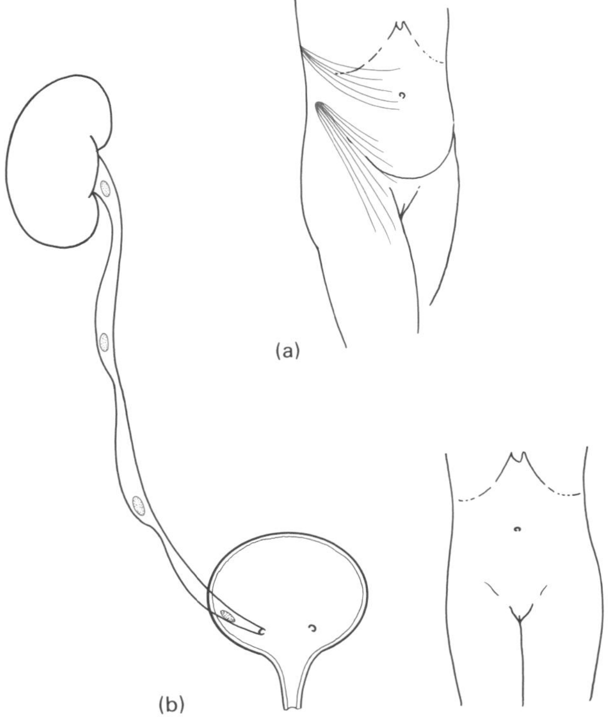

Fig. 4.1 Pain is referred from the ureter in segments, from the umbilicus (a) down to the trigone (b) as gallstones are formed.

2. Inborn errors of metabolism, especially those related to protein anabolism and catabolism.

3. Disease of the parathyroid gland. This gland controls the calcium levels and calcium metabolism in the body. If there is hyperparathyroidism, i.e., excess parathormone, or a parathyroid tumour, either will lead to hypercalcuria.

4. Acute urinary tract infections. The debris or dead tissue which occurs following the infection forms the matrix which can become the nucleus for the formation of stones. This is especially true of proteus infections and seems to occur more often in women.

5. Prolonged bedrest. Urinary stasis occurs and the calcium which would normally be excreted comes out of solution and begins to deposit along the urinary tract. Complicating the urinary stasis is a reduced renal blood flow.

6. Cancer metastasis to the kidney. This may precipitate stone formation before signs of the tumour are present.

7. Crohn's disease. If the patient has had surgery to cure this disease, the terminal ileum will have been removed. This structure in normal health would reabsorb bile salts. If they are not reabsorbed the bile salts will come out of solution and deposit in the renal tract laying the foundation for stone formation.

The primary presenting features of stone formation tends to be either *chronic* with a persistent low backache usually of or near the lumbar spine or an *acute* attack of renal colic (Fig. 4.1). Other features include haematuria, a palpable swollen kidney, dysuria, urinary frequency, and possibly pyrexia with a urinary tract infection.

ACUTE RENAL COLIC

In acute renal colic the patient clasically adopts a posture of drawing the knees towards the abdomen and rolling around in agitated restlessness and in severe pain which radiates in spasms from loin to groin. The suddenness and severity of the attack leaves the patient emotionally and physically exhausted with a marked degree of shock.

Immediate Treatment

The immediate treatment of acute renal colic is to relieve the pain using a powerful analgesic which has an effect on involuntary muscle, e.g., pethidine. Large doses are required, 75–100 mg intramuscularly. This analgesic may be combined with an anti-spasmodic drug, e.g., probanthine, which will relieve the ureteric spasm as the stone moves from the kidney towards the bladder.

In about half of all cases the stones move and, following the relief of pain, all urine passed by the patient should be sieved to search for the stone. It is surprising how something so small and gravel-like can cause so much pain. The patient is urged to drink as much as possible to dissolve the stone and encouraged to walk about in an effort to shift the stone while under the effect of an antispasmodic drug. Hot baths at frequent intervals may also prove helpful.

To Decrease Recurrence

If a stone is found it can be analysed and advice given to the patient to try and reduce any recurrence. Such **advice** may include:

1. In hot weather drink copious amounts of clear fluids and avoid any activity which encourages perspiration and the risk of dehydration.
2. If living in a geographical area where the water is known to be 'hard', take a low calcium diet, and consider purchasing a water softener for the main water tank in the house.
3. Medications may help. These include: oral neutral phosphate which combines with calcium in the food and the calcium is then excreted by the bowel. Diuretics may be prescribed if the stone is formed from uric acid. Allopurinol arrests xanthine from forming into uric acid.
4. Oral fluids of at least 3 litres per day will dissolve stones which are composed of cysteine.

After a period of this conservative approach the surgeon will see the patient again and it is routine for intravenous pyelography to be done at monthly intervals until there is no evidence of further stone formation or any residual damage to the renal tract.

CHRONIC RENAL STONES

Further Investigations

If the features are vague but suspicious the patient may then undergo a series of investigations for renal stones as an outpatient. The surgeon may tackle the diagnosis with the following in mind:

1. How frequent and severe are the symptoms?
2. Is there any present damage to the kidney?
3. What type of stone is it?
4. Is the stone unilateral or bilateral?
5. Is there any metabolic disorder?
6. Is there a dietary feature such as an excess intake of calcium oxylate-containing foods, e.g., tea, coffee, chocolate, spinach or rhubarb.

The investigations required to answer these questions include taking the level of serum calcium while in a fasting state, i.e., 2.5 mmol/l, and 24-hour urinary calcium, i.e., 250 mg in females; 300 mg in males. In parathyroid disease both these values are raised.

Type and Location of Stones

The type of stone can be measured to a limited degree by estimating the urinary calcium which is raised in idiopathic causes. If serum uric acid is raised above 6 mg/l this indicates a stone formed from uric acid. It is not possible to assess cysteine and xanthine from any known test.

The routine investigations of intravenous pyelogram, blood urea, midstream specimen of urine, erythrocyte sedimentation rate, and haemoglobin will indicate the presence and

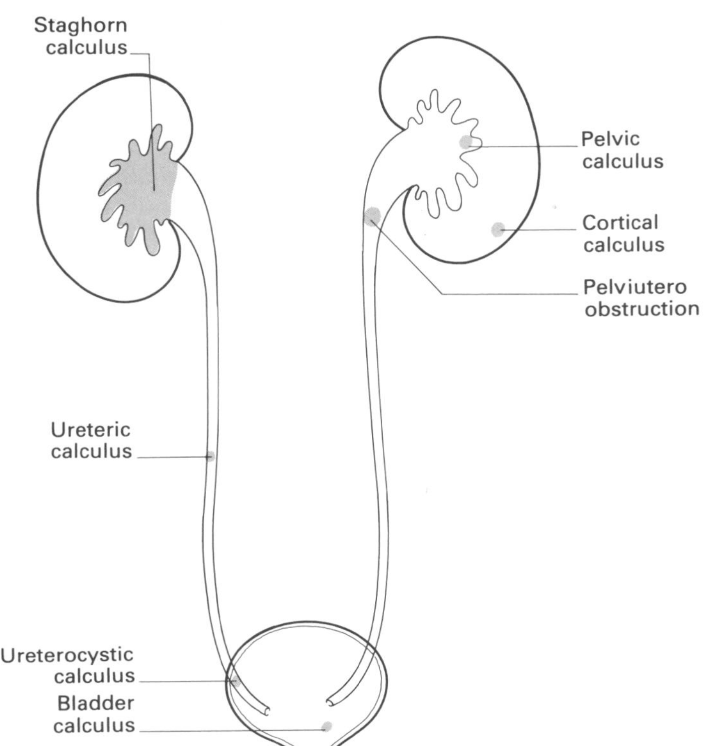

Fig. 4.2 Location of renal calculi.

location of the stone, if there is a *hydronephrosis* (dilation of pelvis of kidney), or if the stone is causing any infection, anaemia, or uraemic signs.

If there is an overt obstruction the surgeon may proceed to complete a retrograde pyelography, a renal arteriography and a panendoscopy to pinpoint the exact location of the obstruction and what effect it is having on the rest of the renal tract. If an obstruction does exist then the incidence of renal tract infection is very high.

The complications of chronic stone formation also have to be assessed and these include pyelonephritis and cystitis which may influence any decision to proceed to surgery.

Treatment

The types of operation which may be carried out depend on the site of the stone (Fig. 4.2). Surgery is usually undertaken with some speed if there is any evidence of increasing hydronephrosis as the result of a stone. More recently ultrasound therapy has been successfully used to disintegrate renal calculi enabling their removal by nonsurgical means.

Nephrectomy

Preoperative Care

As a general guideline, the specific arrangements made for a patient undergoing surgery on the kidney for the removal of a stone are:

Grouping and cross-matching of 2–4 units of blood

The patient must be free of urinary tract or pulmonary infection

The opposite kidney must be healthy and functioning

Any tendency to hypertension must be under control

The patient is capable of consuming a copious fluid intake

The patient is mentally prepared and physically ready for the postoperative period

Postoperative Care

Postoperatively the nurse should expect the patient to have a long subcostal incision of the upper abdomen, quite near the diaphragm. The wound will have a drainage tube from the renal bed which is connected to a closed drainage system. This may be either on free drainage to a disposable bag or connected to a vacuum bottle. Drainage from the bladder is via a catheter connected by a closed system to a collecting disposable bag.

Intravenous therapy or blood transfusion are usually in progress for several hours beyond the recovery period. The nursing staff have to take these points into consideration within the nursing care plan when preparing to receive the patient back from the recovery area.

Movement of the patient will at first be very limited because of the location of the incision. Respiration is painful and coughing may cause the patient to think the wound will rupture. Turning in any direction for the patient is not only painful but limited until the drains and tubes are shortened or removed. Movement therefore can only be achieved if the patient has sufficient analgesia to prevent pain.

It is desirable to commence oral fluids as soon as possible but this can only be done once peristalsis has returned and the feelings of nausea have receded. The aim should be a minimum of 2 litres per 24 hours but if possible 3 litres. The success or otherwise of this intention can only be proved if accurate fluid balance records are maintained by the nurse.

Before the wound drains are removed there may be some serous exudate or escape of urine from the wound to the skin surface which will cause maceration and excoriation of the skin surrounding the wound. A barrier cream requires to be applied until this problem has resolved. Because infection is such a high risk, antibiotics are normally prescribed, e.g., penicillin or streptomycin, but the choice of antibiotic will depend on the results of any wound swab sent for culture and sensitivity.

Chapter 5
Disorders of the Tract

DISORDERS OF THE URETER

Disorders of the ureter may originate with abnormalities of the renal pelvis.

Hydronephrosis

Hydronephrosis refers to a local dilation of the pelvis of the kidney, the most common cause being inflammation, usually ascending to the kidney via the ureter. Such inflammation deposits a ring of collagen at the pelvi-ureteric junction, which causes the renal pelvis to expand. This expansion, coupled with the inflammation, reduces the blood flow to the whole kidney and causes the organ to atrophy. As the atrophy worsens the kidney enlarges and is easily palpable. The patient notices loin pain after drinking a large volume of fluid and odd bouts of indigestion. Since the urinary flow is impeded this invariably leads to a urinary tract infection. The disease is only noted in the early stages if an excretion urogram is requested for other reasons. Causes outside the kidney include intraureteric or extraureteric neoplasms, compression of local blood vessels, e.g., in pregnancy, or vesicoureteric reflux.

Vesicoureteric Reflux

Vesicoureteric reflux, a cause of hydronephrosis, is a troublesome problem seen more commonly in children. The urine refluxes back up the ureter when the residual volume of urine in the bladder reaches a certain point.

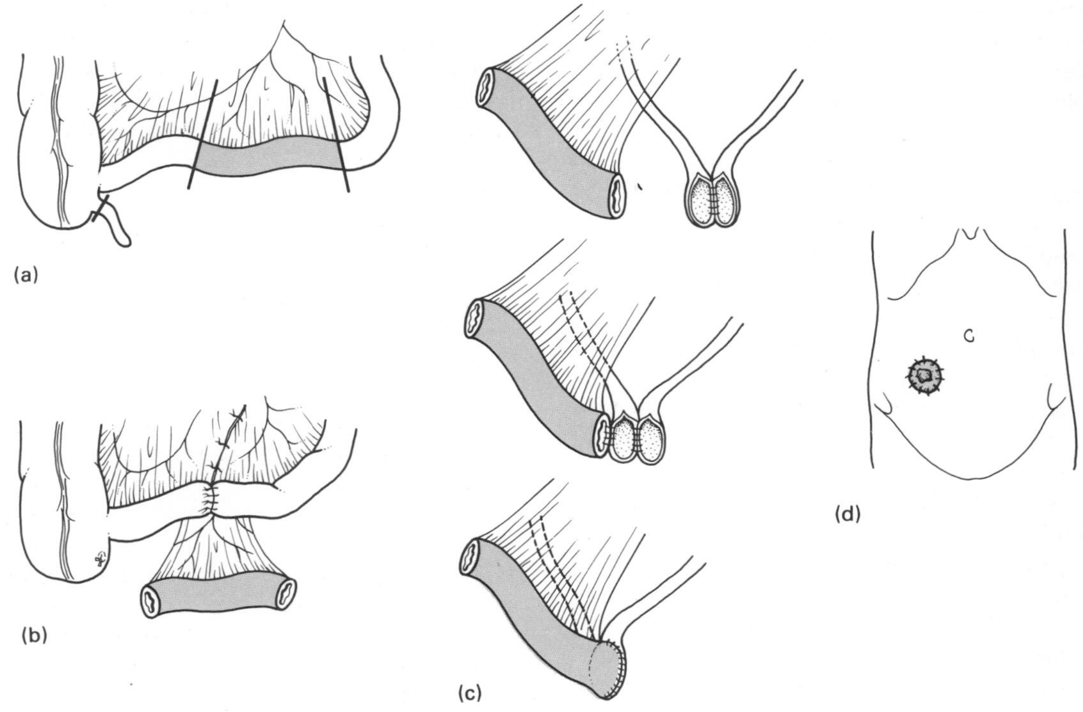

Fig. 5.1 An ileal conduit involves an appendicectomy and sectioning of the ileal loop (a) and its isolation (b) ready for anastomosis to the ureter (c). The stoma of the ileal conduit is then sited (d).

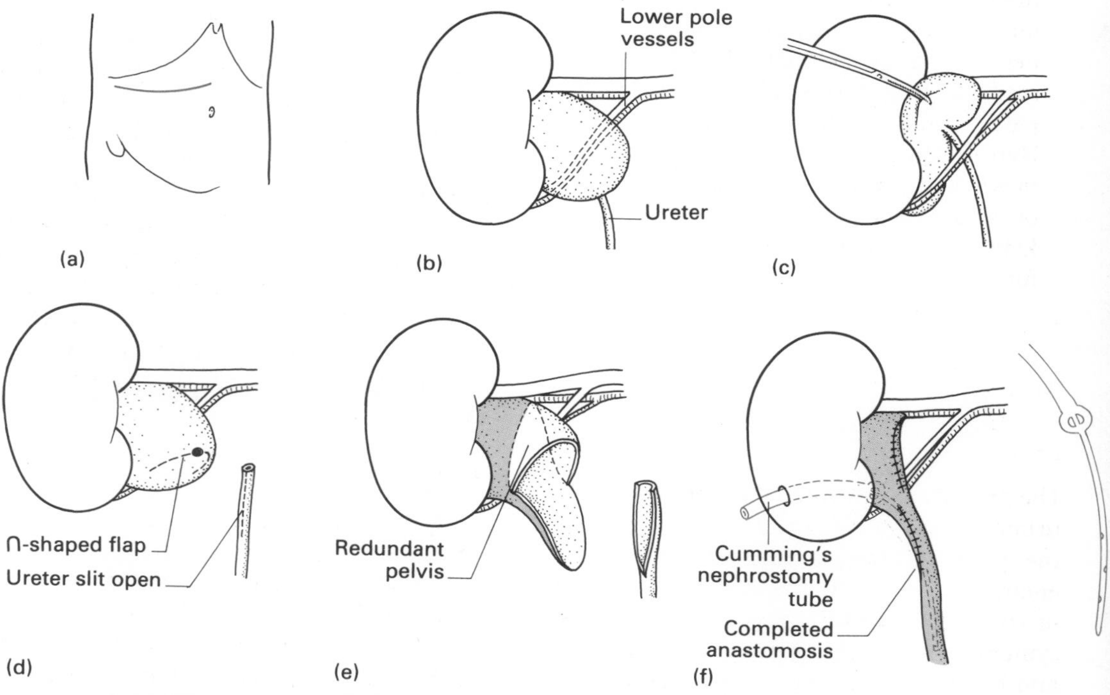

Fig. 5.2 Anderson Hynes pyeloplasty. An anterior incision (a) is made revealing the kidney (b). The enlarged pelvis is dissected away from the pole (c) and the cuts made into pelvis and ureter (d). The redundant pelvis (e) is removed and the flap is ready to be sutured into the slit ureter. A nephrostomy tube detailed (f) is put in place.

Anatomically the cystoureteric junction, i.e., the point at which the ureter enters the bladder may not be oblique enough or the folds of rugae may be inadequate to seal over the tiny ureteric portal.

Continual reflux causes the ureter to dilate, and there is usually an urinary infection and urinary frequency. A urinary reflux is diagnosed by the patient having a micturating cystogram. The dye used can be seen to reach a certain level up the ureter and may include the kidney. Depending on the level of urinary reflux, it is graded as either

Grade 1. The reflux does not extend to the renal pelvis, residual urinary infection is invariably present and antibiotics are the choice of therapy; or

Grade 2. The urinary reflux extends into the pelvis of the kidney but does not cause a distension. A prolonged course of antibiotics is prescribed and the patient considered for a ureteric reimplantation as either an ileal conduit (Fig. 5.1), or a reimplantation into the sigmoid colon; or

Grade 3. The reflux is causing a distension of the renal pelvis and reimplantation of the ureters is urgently required to prevent further hydronephrosis. If the hydronephrosis is established and affecting the medulla and cortex of the kidney the patient may require either an Anderson–Hynes operation, i.e., pyeloplasty (Fig. 5.2), in which the pelvis of the kidney is repaired or a total nephrectomy performed if the kidney is damaged beyond 50% of its function.

DISORDERS OF THE PROSTATE GLAND

Prostatism

The prostate gland, located at the base of the urinary bladder and completely surrounding the posterior urethra, can be expected to enlarge in males after the age of 40. About 1 in 10 males in the UK are expected to develop symptoms of urinary retention in one form or another as the gland tends to enlarge in every direction, including inwards thus obstructing the urinary flow along the urethra.

Early symptoms of prostatism may begin with a frequent need to void urine and a poor urinary stream, especially in the morning. The patient may notice the need to visit the toilet more frequently during the night.

Urinary Retention

The inability to void the bladder completely will lead to one of several types of urinary retention. *Chronic retention* occurs over a period of years and may or may not coexist with uraemia. *Chronic retention with overflow* is where the patient finds there is a dribble of urine between very frequent visits to the toilet. *Acute retention* occurs suddenly, in which the bladder distends upwards and outwards and is accompanied by distension pain. *Acute upon chronic retention*, where the patient has a long history of prostatism and may already be receiving investigations or palliative treatment, is when the retention becomes complete and presents as a total obstruction of urinary outflow.

The urinary retention, especially in the chronic type of prostatism, increases the residual urinary volume. This tends to stagnate within the bladder and the risk of a urinary tract infection is very high. From this the patient becomes pyrexial, tired, irritable and may also have haematuria. With this increased retention the muscular wall of the bladder can be stretched beyond its normal capacity and give rise to abnormalities. As the muscle fibres which lie obliquely across and over each other become stretched they split and create what are referred to as *trabeculations*. As these splits become worse the bladder muscle then becomes sacculated, and finally diverticuli or pouching of the wall may occur.

Anaemia

Many prostatic patients also suffer from anaemia, if there is ascending infection from the bladder to the ureters and kidney. Any infection of the kidney tends to lower the level of production of the hormone erythropoietin from the kidney. This hormone is essential to stimulate the bone marrow to release erythrocytes.

If the patient's pallor appears greyish it may suggest that the urea levels in the blood are high and this is due to dehydration. Often this dehydration comes about by the patient deliberately reducing normal fluid intake to try and combat the symptoms. It is an understandable but mistaken gesture. It may lead to difficulty in persuading the patient to drink large volumes after the retention has been resolved.

Catheterisation

For all patients with acute retention the bladder will be emptied by catheterisation. This may be by slow decompression technique in which graduated volumes of urine are released from the bladder over a specific period. Alternatively if the bladder is not overdistended the residual volume is released immediately. The degree of relief is immediate, however hospital admission is invariably required to correct dehydration, electrolyte imbalance, investigate the degree of prostatism and decide if surgical intervention can be carried out in the immediate future.

Surgical Treatment

Investigations

Whether suffering from the acute or chronic form of prostatism, surgery will ultimately be required. Preceding prostatectomy, however, a series of investigations must be completed. These usually include:

1. A catheter specimen of urine for culture and sensitivity. If infection is present then surgery is usually delayed until prescribed antibiotics or urinary antiseptic drugs are effective, e.g., the sulphonamide compounds.
2. The haemoglobin level must be known to exclude iron deficiency anaemia. If anaemia is present the iron compounds are usually prescribed in oral doses for several days preoperatively.
3. Blood urea levels are invariably raised and these are quickly restored to normal once the patient is catheterised and taking liberal amounts of clear fluids.
4. Serum acid phosphatase levels, if raised, may indicate that the enlargement of the prostate gland is due to cancer and is not merely benign, in which case the investigation will proceed to establish if it is a primary or a metastatic tumour.
5. Grouping and cross-matching of 2–4 units of blood. Transfusion will be used during and after retropubic and transvesical prostatectomy, since the amount of blood loss at the operation site tends to be large.
6. Intravenous pyelography and cystoscopy are completed in all cases to establish if the renal pathway is unobstructed and excreting urine normally and that the bladder is structurally sound.
7. A chest X-ray is a routine screening of the lungs' fields and of the heart's shape and size. This indicates in part if the patient is reasonably fit for anaesthesia or if there are any unusual shadows or features which warrant further investigation.
8. The serum levels of electrolytes are assessed to ensure that sodium and potassium are both within normal limits especially after any period of dehydration.
9. A rectal examination is carried out by the surgeon to feel the contours of the prostate gland. A rugged surface may suggest an enlargement due to cancer while smooth and rounded surfaces would suggest a benign enlargement.

In addition to establishing the clinical proof of prostatism many surgeons may request investigations to exclude prolapsed intervertebral disc, urethral stricture, diabetic peripheral neuropathy and hydronephrosis.

Preoperative Care

The objectives should be clearly stressed in the preoperative care plan for a patient about to have a prostatectomy:

1. The indwelling urinary catheter relieves the retention and is not a focus for introducing infection into the bladder.
2. The serum electrolytes have been assessed and corrected if necessary by intravenous therapy.
3. That fitness for anaesthesia implies the blood pressure is within normal limits

especially if the anaesthetist wishes to use a hypotensive agent. If during anaesthesia the blood pressure is reduced to very low levels it means that postoperatively the patient cannot sit up until his blood pressure returns to normal levels.

4. That the blood is available before the patient is taken to theatre.

5. The patient has in fact been re-educated to consume liberal amounts of clear fluids and is aware of the need to continue taking large volumes after recovering from anaesthesia.

Activities of Daily Living

Further to these specific objectives of preoperative planning, the nurse should consider the value of applying the activities of daily living to the patient's care plan.

Respiration

Suggest preoperative exercises for the patient to improve breathing techniques and encourage him to stop or reduce smoking. The nurse will need to liaise with the physiotherapist concerning postoperative physiotherapy exercises for the patient.

Nutrition

If the nutritional state of the patient is in question, then dietary measures to resolve either obesity or malnutrition should be worked out in liaison with the dietician. It is interesting to note that the size, shape, and weight of the patient may determine the type of operation to remove the prostate.

Elimination

Although the patient's main problem is that of the urinary tract, the lower colon must be empty before such a major operation so near to the bowel. This may be done by means of suppositories, aperients, enema, or more rarely by rectal washout.

Cleanliness

The fact that the patient has an indwelling urinary catheter in place does not exclude the possibility of having a shower or a bath in which a small amount of antiseptic has been added. The skin requires to be shaved from nipple to knee and includes a thorough shave of the perineum. Before and after the operation the perineum must be kept absolutely clean if the risk of urinary tract infection is to be minimised.

The patient will be unable to care for his hair following this operation and so a shampoo and possibly a haircut is to the patient's advantage.

Psychological Aspects

As with any major surgery, the patient must be told why certain things are being done, when they are likely to happen, by whom various procedures will be carried out and the likely programme of events during the postoperative period. In a word **reassurance**.

Accompanied by this need for facts, the patient also has the need for sleep and appropriate periods of rest. These must be interspersed with contact with his family and friends. If, as often happens, the patient is an elderly gentleman the nurse can act as a companion during what can be for the patient a lonely and frightening time.

Types of Prostatectomy

The nurse must know the type of operation the surgeon has decided upon to enable preparations to be made to receive the patient back from the recovery area of the theatre. There are three types of operation carried out in the UK. These are the transurethral resection, the retropubic prostatectomy and the transvesical prostatectomy.

Transurethral Resection

Transurethral resection is a relatively safe procedure especially so if the patient has cardiovascular or pulmonary disease. It is a suitable operation when the prostate gland is

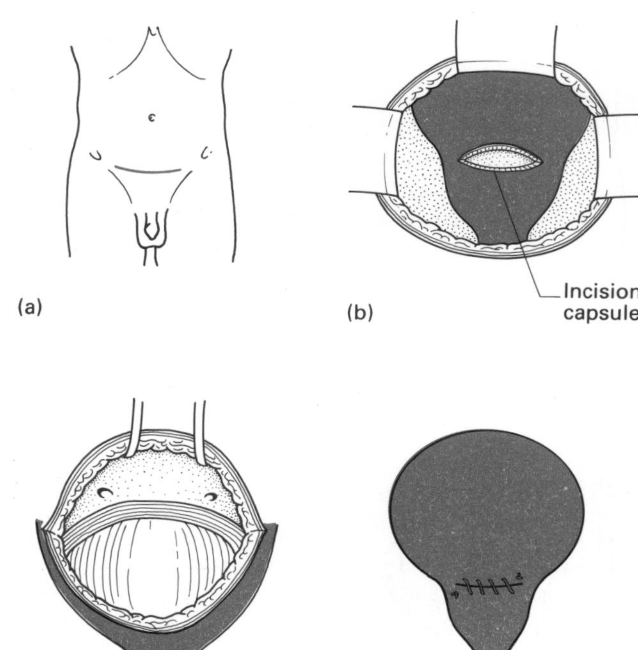

Fig. 5.3 Retropubic prostatectomy (Millin's operation): low abdominal incision (a); incision of capsule (b); gland shelled out (c); closure of surgical capsule (d).

of a small or moderate enlargement, whether it is malignant or benign. A resectoscope or cutting instrument is passed via the urethra and using a fibreoptic attachment the surgeon can see to cut away the adenomatous tissue from within the prostatic capsule. After this cutting episode the bleeding is controlled using diathermy technique and the 'prostatic chips' are evacuated from the bladder.

An indwelling urinary catheter is left in position and connected to a closed drainage system. The urine is collected into a graduated sealed plastic bag with an outlet. Since there is no wound the nursing care will concentrate on the care of the urinary drainage and, if it is required, any intravenous therapy. Normally for this type of operation the patient can expect a short hospital stay.

Retropubic Prostatectomy

A retropubic prostatectomy (Millin's operation) may be adopted for very enlarged prostate glands. The operation is preceded by a cystoscopy.

Following a low abdominal incision to expose the bladder, the bladder is tilted upwards and backwards to enable the prostate gland to be viewed. The surgical capsule is incised and the lateral lobes of the gland are shelled out and the middle lobe also removed using a diathermy needle. Disposable ligatures are used to tie off any blood vessels and the surgical capsule is also closed (Fig. 5.3).

After the muscle and skin incisions are sutured an indwelling urinary catheter is left in position. This is an extensive operation in so far as the wound can be expected to have considerable exudate, a substantial amount of postoperative haematuria and implies the patient will have a hospital stay of 10–14 days.

Transvesical Prostatectomy

While it is regarded as an easy operation, a transvesical prostatectomy (Harris or Freyer operation) is fraught with the dangers of haematuria and the prolonged use of an

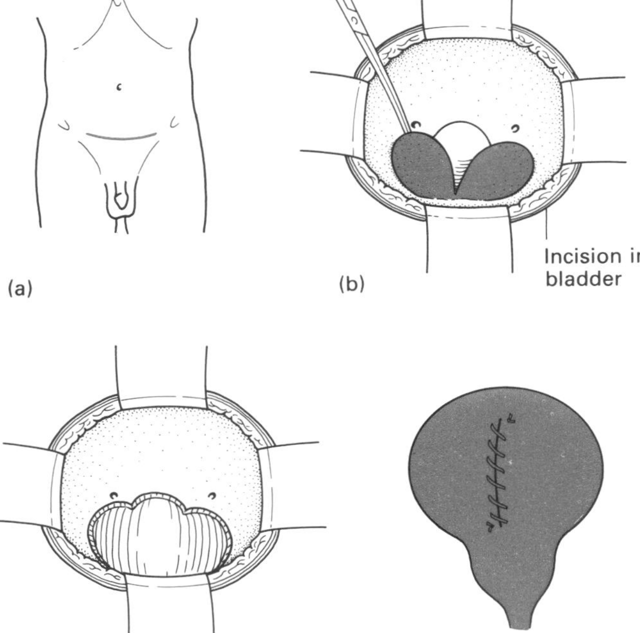

(c) (d)

Fig. 5.4 Transvesical prostatectomy (Harris or Freyer operation): suprapubic incision (a); incision in bladder (b); removal of adenomatous lobes via bladder neck (c); closure of surgical capsule and bladder neck.

indwelling urinary catheter. It is a type of prostatectomy often used for the obese patient.

Following a suprapubic incision, an incision is made into the bladder, *cystotomy*, and the adenomatous lobes of the prostate gland are removed via the bladder neck either by finger or by scissor method (Fig. 5.4). The blood vessels supplying the wall of the bladder and the prostatic bed are prolific and while the main bleeding points are either ligatured or controlled by diathermy the smaller vessels will continue to bleed until they spontaneously coagulate. Prolonged haematuria can be expected via the indwelling urinary catheter for several days following this operation.

Postoperative Care

Given that the nurse is aware of the type of operation carried out then the postoperative care plan can take into account the immediate needs of the patient on his return from theatre. Nursing features which are specific to prostatectomy include: care of the wound, maintenance of continuous bladder drainage, monitoring adequate fluid intake, provision of scrotal support, reduction of the infection risk, maintenance of urethral sphincter integrity and patient mobility.

Care of the Wound

Two drains may be present: a tissue drain which will drain tissue exudate, and a suprapubic drain leading from the operation site to the skin surface. The amount of exudate from this second drain is likely to be considerable and thus the dressing over the wound has to be changed more frequently than normal. Should the dressing become too moist then the wound covering acts as a potential source for wound infection. Gradually the wound exudate lessens allowing the tissue drain to be shortened and eventually removed after 48 hours. The suprapubic drain is usually shortened within 72 hours and removed by the fifth postoperative day.

The wound sutures should be left for at least 7 days because the underlying healing will take longer than normal because of the amount of exudate.

Continuous Bladder Drainage

To counteract the tendency to haematuria the technique of continuous irrigation of the bladder with distilled sterile water, via a 3-way urinary catheter, is often employed. This irrigation continues for as long as haematuria is an obvious fact in the collecting bag.

The nurse will need to keep a careful record of the volume of fluid used at each irrigation, usually 500 ml containers. When these volumes are totalled at the end of a 12-hour period, any excess of this volume is urine and blood. The surgeon will indicate when continuous irrigation will be discontinued and it is usually based on the improving colour of the irrigation output.

When the irrigation is discontinued, the indwelling urinary catheter will remain in position for a few more days and will need twice daily catheter toilet to reduce the risks of infection.

Fluid Intake

Intravenous therapy is the mainstay of fluid intake until the patient can commence oral fluids. The volumes used can be quite considerable because of the need to increase renal excretion. Careful assessment of urinary output is vital if overtransfusion is to be avoided, and fluid regimens should be assessed every 12–24 hours to ensure that overloading of the system is not occurring. A co-operative patient can be encouraged to try and achieve an intake of 2–3 litres of fluids orally within 72 hours of surgery, and by this time the intravenous therapy would normally be discontinued.

Scrotal Support

Since the testes are near the site of surgery, they are not only tender but may be quite swollen. The nurse should make a point of inspecting the perineum for this discomfort. While at rest and with the first attempts at being ambulated, the patient should be offered a scrotal sac to wear. This does relieve any tension within the testes and reduces a great deal of unnecessary anxiety which many patients may feel unable to voice to a nurse.

Infection Risk

It cannot be overstated that the risk of infection to the urinary tract is very high, more so when a catheter is left in position for several days. Every measure to control the risk of infection should be employed. These include using simple measures such as providing clean linen regularly, using aseptic technique in both catheter toilet and wound dressing, with thorough basic cleanliness of the patient and early mobility if and when it is feasible.

The respiratory tract is equally at risk. The patient is to a large extent kept immobile by the wound, the catheter, and intravenous therapy. The patient needs to be encouraged to do regular deep breathing exercises so long as he is confined to bed.

Urethral Sphincter Integrity

After the urinary catheter has been removed, the patient must be warned to expect difficulties in passing urine normally. Often the patient expects this function to be normal; after all what has the operation been all about? Both bladder tone and sphincter integrity have suffered, however, as a result of the indwelling catheter and therefore it may be several days before the patient regains full control of the urinary stream.

The patient should expect some frequency. To reduce this problem the bed should be sited near a toilet. A commode may be placed at the bed or a urinal left discreetly by the bedside. Each time the patient feels the need to pass urine he should be advised to exercise the sphincter by stopping the urinary flow deliberately. It takes time to regain full control and for an elderly male who has gone through a major operation the nurse must be particularly encouraging, otherwise the patient may lose heart altogether. Bladder tone may be partially regained by clamping off the catheter for defined periods of time before its removal.

Mobility

Mobility will be limited if the type of prostatectomy involves a low abdominal wound, intravenous therapy, bladder irrigation, and continuous bladder drainage. These factors will be the predominating feature of pain. With the correct use of the prescribed postoperative analgesics, pain can be prevented. In achieving this the patient will be able to co-operate with the nursing plan which has been devised to promote his recovery. Lifting and moving the patient will be easier, sitting out by the bedside although hazardous in the first few days can be achieved without too much distress. Fluids and diet will be taken more readily. Psychologically the primary anxiety of pain will be removed thus ensuring the patient can sleep fitfully and cope with the problems imposed on him by the surgery.

Complications

After a patient recovers from a prostatectomy, the nurse must be continually vigilant in observing for possible postoperative complications. These include: persistent haemorrhage; infection; clot retention; electrolyte imbalance; incontinence; urethral stricture; impotence and infertility; carcinoma; and recurrence of enlargement.

Persistent Haemorrhage

Persistent haemorrhage beyond 24–48 hours may follow either a transvesical or retropubic prostatectomy. Haemorrhage is to be expected but it should diminish as time passes. Observations of pulse and blood pressure will indicate if internal bleeding into the bladder is becoming worse, the colour and viscosity of the blood in the drainage bag or container will also help in noting if it is diminishing.

Infection

Observation of temperature every 4 hours will denote if pyrexia is developing. Other features of pyrexia should also be reported such as perspiration, restlessness, and disinterest shown by the patient in his progress.

For urinary tract infections a catheter specimen of urine can be despatched to pathology after the irrigation is concluded. Swabs can be taken from the wound at regular intervals. Inspection of the scrotal sac may indicate the beginning of an epididymo-orchitis, especially so if the patient complains of scrotal pain and swelling. Undoubtedly antibiotics are prescribed for the postoperative period but these may not always be appropriate to the organism causing the infection.

Clot Retention

Especially following a transvesical prostatectomy, the nurse should note the freedom with which the continuous drainage of urine is escaping into the collecting bag. If the fluid is draining slowly or has stopped, a gentle milking of the catheter in a downward direction away from the urethra may be sufficient to dislodge any blood clots trapped in the eye of the catheter. If this is unsuccessful it may be necessary to perform a bladder washout using 50 ml of sodium citrate as a mild anticoagulant. This may be sufficient to break down the clot which is retaining the fluid in the bladder. If the clot remains stubborn and urinary retention persists the surgeon must be informed in case a second operation is required to remove the blood clot.

Electrolyte Imbalance

Electrolyte imbalance is a particular danger following retropubic and transvesical prostatectomy. The surgeon would normally do daily assessments for as long as the intravenous infusion is required and if the bladder drainage is giving rise to concern. Unexpected infections may alter the electrolytes sufficiently to warrant their correction.

Incontinence

After the urinary catheter has been removed and several days have elapsed the patient should have regained control of the urinary stream. If, however, this is not being achieved there may be a surgical problem in that the external sphincter has been damaged. If incontinence persists the fact must be reported to the surgeon for further opinion and treatment.

Urethral Stricture

Following a transurethral prostatectomy there is a slight risk that the instrumentation used has damaged the lining membrane of the urethra. The irritation may lead to an inflammation which upon healing might cause a stricture. About 2–3% of strictures are known to follow this operation.

Impotence and Infertility

Impotence and infertility may occur if the bladder neck is involved in the surgery. This, however, is rarely viewed by the patients themselves as a problem, given their age. The urinary problem is more life-threatening than the loss of fertility.

Carcinoma

Carcinoma may arise at a later date from any residual tissue.

Recurrence of Enlargement

There may be recurrence of enlargement if there is any residual healthy tissue left within the surgical capsule.

Cancer of the Prostate Gland

If the prostate gland becomes cancerous the enlargement of the tissue is irregular. In addition to any problem related to urinary stream there are associated symptoms of perineal pain, altered bowel function, usually constipation, weight loss and anaemia. If there is spread from the prostate gland it is usually invasive to the spine in the first instance. From this the patient may complain of backache and have associated neurological disturbance depending on the level of spine affected.

Diagnosis

A firm diagnosis is made usually based on:

Rectal examination
Cystoscopy and prostatic biopsy
Serum acid phosphatase levels

Objectives

The surgeon plans therapy with 3 objectives in mind:

To relieve any urinary obstruction
To establish if the cancer is primary or secondary
To decide on the treatment

Patient Care

The nursing plan for the care of the patient revolves upon the investigations required and the treatment decided upon. The wide variety of treatments available makes it impossible to evolve a general plan of care within this textbook.

Treatments Available

The treatments which may be employed include hormone therapy, surgical removal, deep X-ray therapy, and implants. An adrenalectomy may be performed to control the pain of metastases. A hypophysectomy may be of value since the pituitary gland controls the secretion of testosterone from the testes.

There is approximately an 80% response to *hormone therapy*, and the drugs used include: stilboestrol 100 mg daily for 1 month then in decreasing doses; chlorotrianisene (Tace); and dienoestrol.

Hormone therapy is only of value if there is no disturbance to urinary flow. Should there be obstruction of the urethra then surgery may be employed.

Surgical removal involves transurethral prostatectomy combined with a course of hormone therapy. *Orchidectomy*, the removal of the testes, is beneficial since it is the production site of testosterone which seems linked as a cause of cancer of the prostate gland.

DISORDERS OF THE BLADDER

Cystitis

The acute form of cystitis is extremely common among women (see also pyelonephritis p. 21). In over half the patients seen the most common causative organism found is *Escherichia coli*, a bacterial commensal of the lower colon. To a lesser degree the organisms *Proteus* and *Pseudomonas* may be isolated in urine specimens of those patients receiving antibiotic drugs but who in fact are resistant to them. Occasionally the Chlamydia group of organism is isolated.

Chemical irritation of the bladder wall caused by immunosuppressive and cytotoxic drugs, mechanical irritation or bruising of the vagina (honeymoon cystitis) are other contributing factors to cystitis. Repeated attacks of acute cystitis necessitates the patient having a cystoscopy, and this reveals an oedematous, red epithelial bladder wall. Small areas of shallow ulcerations may also be seen. It is usual practice for the patient to undergo a complete renal screening to exclude ureteric and kidney involvement before commencing antibiotic therapy.

In the chronic form of cystitis, the oedema is accompanied by mucus aggregation, and the formation of small cysts from previous healed areas of the epithelial lining of the bladder. If these cysts become calcified they tend to bleed, hence haematuria. Apart from developing as a consequence of repeated acute attacks, tuberculosis and schistosoma (mainly in Africa and Egypt) are other causes of chronic cystitis.

To confirm the diagnosis a biopsy of the epithelial wall during a cystoscopy is essential. A therapeutic regimen similar to that outlined for chronic pyelonephritis combined with long-term antibiotic therapy is current practice after ureterocystic reflux has been eliminated as a possible complication.

Bladder Calculi

Stones forming in the bladder are more common in the elderly male who is also suffering from chronic urinary retention (see also chap. 4). The calculus invariably originates in the kidney and becomes trapped in the bladder due to prostatic enlargement. In the early stages the stone causes no symptoms but as it enlarges it irritates the bladder wall causing a cystitis. This in turn causes a urinary tract infection. If infection occurs it contributes to a further enlargement of the stone.

The main symptom is that any bladder pain is referred to the meatus when walking or moving about, but not during rest. When confirmed by X-ray, e.g., excretion urogram, it is usual to admit the patient for a lithoplaxy. In this operation a *lithotrite* is passed into the bladder via the urethra and the stones are crushed or chipped into small fragments. The fragments are then removed via a cannula attachment. Continuous bladder irrigation may follow the operation which will wash out any remaining debris.

If prostatic enlargement is also present then a cystectomy may be combined with a prostatectomy.

Neoplasm

Tumours of the bladder occur most frequently in the elderly male; there is a male to female ratio of 4:1. The principal sign is that of haematuria, hence the need for all patients with haematuria to have a cystoscopy. Frequency of, and pain on, micturition accompanied by a urinary tract infection are also present. The similarity with other bladder disorders, e.g., prostatism or cystitis, may in fact delay the correct diagnosis being made.

Types of Tumour

On cystoscopy a biopsy of the single or

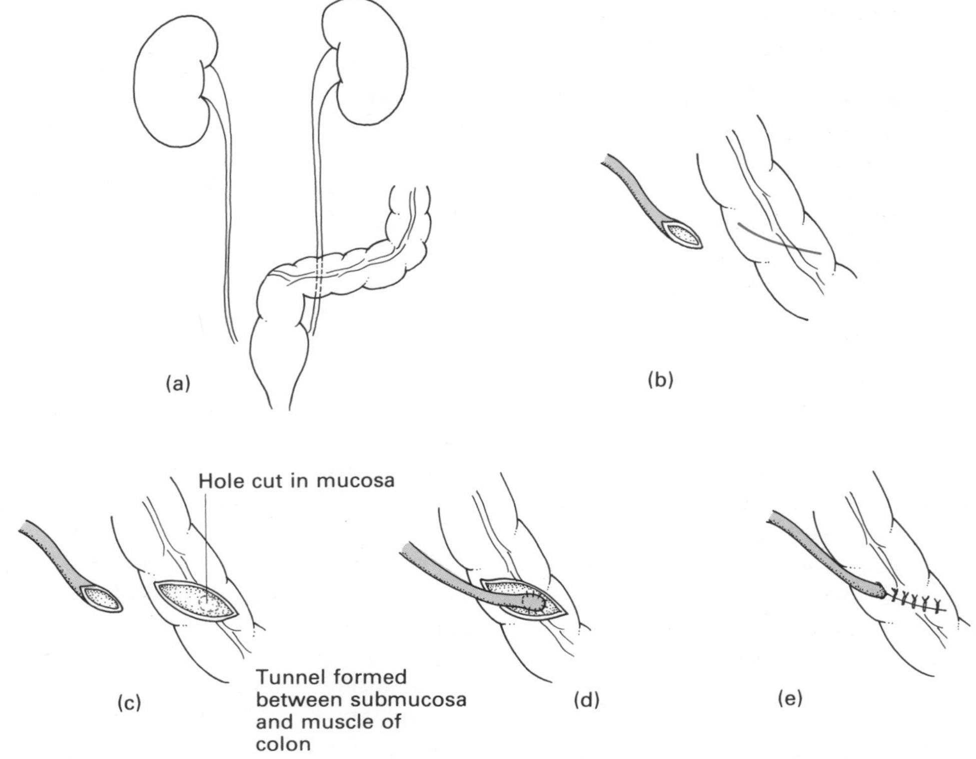

Fig. 5.5 Ureterosigmoidostomy: normal relationship (a); ureter divided (b); tunnel formed between submucosa and muscle of colon (c); ureter transplanted (d); ureter secured within colon (e).

multiple tumours is taken. Following histology studies the tumour will be classified as:

Transitional cell carcinoma. The tumour is invasive only to the depth of the epithelial wall of the bladder.

Squamous cell carcinoma. Although the tumour has invaded down to the squamous cell layer it can still be differentiated from other cells and tissues within the bladder wall.

Adenocarcinoma. This cancer is more rare and is usually located either at the dome of the bladder or the trigone area.

Stages

The stage of the cancer may be graded to indicate how far the tumour has developed:

Stage 1 is limited to the basement membrane between the epithelial and squamous cell layers.

Stage 2 means that the tumour is partly invasive to the muscle wall of the bladder.

Stage 3 implies that the whole of the muscle wall has been penetrated and the tumour has reached the lymphatic nodes.

Stage 4 means that there is metastases from the bladder to surrounding structures, e.g., the prostate gland or the vagina.

Patient Care

The nursing plan of care after the investigations have established the diagnosis will depend on the choice of therapy.

In stage 1 the outlook is very encouraging. If it is a single tumour it can be removed by either coagulation using a cystoscopic electrode, or resected with a diathermy loop. For first stage multiple tumours the antimitotic drugs thiotepa, or ethoglucid (Epodyl), may be instilled into the bladder. Alternatively if it is a large tumour the Helmstein distension technique may be used. In this, a catheter with a widely inflatable balloon is passed into the bladder. Once inflated the balloon compresses upon the tumour which gradually causes the tumour to necrose.

Stage 2 tumours may be treated by trans-urethral diathermy resection of the tumour down to the muscle layer. Alternatively a cystotomy is performed and after the tumour has been surgically removed the remnant tumour bed has radioactive gold grains implanted to irradiate any remaining cancer cells.

Stage 3 tumours invariably require a total cystectomy with re-implantation of the ureters, *ureterosigmoidostomy*, to divert the urinary outflow (Fig. 5.5) and this surgery is followed by a course of radiotherapy.

Stage 4 tumours have a poor prognosis and much of the therapy is palliative. In addition to radiotherapy and urinary diversion surgery, the widespread invasion of the tumour to surrounding structures requires specific therapeutic measures to deal with the affected structure. The pain resulting from what in many instances is inoperable cancer requires to be adequately controlled by a daily assessment of effectively prescribed powerful analgesics.

Screening

The prevention of cancer of the bladder has long been established with screening of workers in those industries which use compounds of either benzene or β-naphthylamine. Such industries include the chemical industry, dyeing, rubber moulding, rubber cable covering, pitch and gas works. Frequent analysis of urine samples from employees in these industries will reveal if the worker is excreting unacceptable levels of either benzene or β-naphthylamine.

Other causes of bladder cancer include the carcinogens from smoking and the irritation to the bladder wall from excreted waste products of analgesic drugs which are being taken indiscriminately. Hairdressers and leather workers also have a high incidence of bladder cancer but the causative carcinogen has yet to be identified.

DISORDERS OF THE URETHRA

For anatomical reasons, disorders of the urethra are more likely to occur in males. The most likely of these which the nurse will care for are: congenital lesions; inflammatory disorders; urethral stricture; and traumatic urethral injury.

Congenital Lesions

Hypospadias

With hypospadias, the external meatus is abnormally placed, so that urinary excretion is at other than the tip of the glans penis. The meatal opening may be positioned below and behind the prepuce, along the midline of the dorsal surface of the penis (*penile*) or towards the perineum (*perineal*). In addition to the abnormal siting of the meatus, the urethral length is shorter than usual and curves the penis into an abnormal shape. Occasionally, the existing meatal orifice is narrower than normal.

The standard surgical approach is to plan for a 2-stage correction. Between 8 months and 3 years old, the child is admitted to hospital to correct the shape and length of the penis, and to construct a meatal opening nearer to the glans penis. A 6-month period is allowed to elapse before the second operation, which involves a urethroplasty, is completed.

A *urethroplasty* consists of a strip of skin being folded and rolled into the existing urethra to form a complete new urethra. The child admitted for correction of hypospadias will have been prevented by this abnormality from achieving the normal phase of toilet training. In planning and giving care, the nurse must allow for this aspect and will advise the parents or guardians that toilet-training will be possible only after the operation is successfully completed.

Phimosis

When the male is about 2 years of age, the foreskin should naturally separate from the glans, allowing for retraction and subsequent cleansing of the glans. If the separation does not occur, the condition is known as *phimosis*, and it is corrected by circumcision. In parentcraft classes, parents are advised not to try to force back the foreskin of children under the age of 2.

Phimosis is also caused by ammoniacal dermatitis from napkin rash. A non-retracting foreskin will create serious hazards of infection and inflammation of the glans, such as balanitis, and, at a later point in life, painful and difficult sexual intercourse.

Circumcision

The operation of circumcision involves the foreskin being pulled forward over the glans and the excess skin being surgically removed. The remaining portion is then retracted to the prepuce and a collodion dressing is applied. The dressing should be left alone and intact until it falls off of its own accord, at which time the healing process will be complete. Because the dressing is to be left alone, the nursing plan must indicate that general bathing is not allowed for several days. In children, 'top and tailing' is practised, that is, only the hand, face and perineum are washed. In older children and adults, a warm saline bath is recommended on or after the third postoperative day. By this time the dressing readily falls from the prepuce.

Patient Care

The nurse must consider the emotional as well as physical aspects of the patient admitted for circumcision in planning and giving care. Preoperative anxiety in the patient will vary according to age and determine the reassurance needed.

Inflammatory Disorders

The majority of urethritis is due to venereal diseases, e.g., gonorrhoea, syphilis (see p. 54). *Balanitis*, or inflammation of the glans, may occur in the uncircumcised male who cannot retract the foreskin to cleanse away the underlying secretions, called *smegma*. The accumulating secretions macerate the tissues of the glans making the tissue not only inflamed but also prone to infections.

After treating the inflammation with antibiotic applications the patient should be considered for a circumcision. This operation will allow the glans to remain dry and less prone to inflammation.

Balanitis xerotica obliterans is a localised inflammation of the glans or prepuce from which a whitish discharge and weeping occurs. It is associated with a skin condition known as *lichen sclerosus et atrophicus*. One consequence of this type of inflammation is meatal stenosis. After dealing with the inflammation the patient may have both circumcision and plastic reconstructive surgery of the meatal opening. If the male patient is allergic or sensitive to any chemicals or the materials in male contraceptive devices, e.g., condoms, he may develop a contact dermatitis with inflammation of the skin covering the penile shaft.

Urethral Stricture

A narrowing of the urethra may arise from several causes:

1. Healing of the urethra following inflammation may cause scarring which narrows the urethral diameter.
2. Instrumentation may damage the meatal opening.
3. Catheterisation, especially prolonged indwelling catheters, may inflame and cause narrowing of the urethra at its midlength.
4. Gonococcal urethritis causes inflammation along the complete urethral length.
5. Ruptured urethral membrane tends to cause a stenosis at the prostatic urethra.

If left untreated the narrowing may lead to periurethral abscesses or periurethral stones from stagnating urine trapped in small amounts at the point of stricture. The degree of stricture and its location can be determined by both cystoscopy and an excretory urogram, both being completed extremely carefully to avoid causing further damage.

The treatment is by urethral *bougienage*, i.e., passing plastic or metal bougies along the urethra to dilate its diameter. If bougienage is ineffective, an internal *urethrotomy*, or slitting, of the stricture site may create an improved urethral diameter.

A third treatment and probably the one giving the best results is an *urethroplasty* where surgery is performed on the urethra to remove the stricture.

Traumatic Urethral Injury

Injury to the urethra is rarely an isolated event but rather combined with multiple injury to the perineum or pelvis. Falling from the astride position, i.e., from bicycles, mopeds, motor bicycles, horses; or impact injuries, e.g., a direct kick to the scrotum or perineum, may result in one of two possible injuries to the urethra: laceration or rupture.

Laceration

A laceration or a tear of the urethra at the bulbar portion of the urethra causes immediate bleeding into the perineum and the extravasation of urine into any haematoma which forms in the perineum. Any delay in treatment or inadequate drainage of the perineum may lead to gangrene extending from the haematoma.

Rupture

Complete rupture of the urethra is associated with fractures of the pelvis near to the symphysis pubis when the bladder and prostate gland are violently sheared upwards away from their normal positions and the violence tears the urethra apart. The bladder neck while not damaged does go into spasm which is to the patient's advantage as urine is unable to be passed. There is, however, severe urethral haemorrhage into the perineum.

The only method of assessing and planning further treatment is with the patient under the effect of general anaesthesia. A very soft catheter, no larger than 16 CH gauge, is advanced slowly and carefully along the urethra. If it reaches the bladder without difficulty and clear urine is being drained it is possible the urethra is only torn, and the catheter will be left in position to act as a splint until the urethral tear heals. A complete rupture requires the urethral torn ends to be approximated with oversplinting by means of catheterisation. In addition a suprapubic cystotomy is fashioned to allow for a urinary diversion. If there is perineal haematoma a perineal drain is sutured in position to allow for drainage of either blood or extravasating urine.

Chapter 6
Social Implications of Venereal Disease

An implied reference to venereal disease is to be found in Leviticus, the first book of Moses, presumed to be about 3000 BC. The Israelites had taken captive a group of Midianite women to their encampment. When the symptoms of disease appeared, possibily gonorrhoea, the affected Israelite males were banished from the camp for seven days, and the Midianite women were ordered by Moses to be slain. The word *gonorrhoea*, meaning *flow of seed*, is attributed to Claudius Galen a famous Greek physician of the second century AD.

EPIDEMIOLOGY

More accurate records of venereal disease begin from 1493. Spanish sailors returning from the expedition to the Americas were known to have suffered from both rashes and ulcers. After they came ashore in Barcelona, the city reported an outbreak of what was to become known as the Pox. When Charles VIII of France invaded Italy, his army consisted of some Spanish mercenaries, as also did the defending Italian army. Within a short period this military campaign of 1494 had to be abandoned because the Pox was so rife and had incapacitated both the soldiers and their camp followers.

The citizens of Germany, Holland, and Greece reported the disease in their cities during 1496. During 1497 the disease spread to England and Scotland. The town fathers of Aberdeen were alarmed at the incidence of the disease and despite severe penalties soon realised they could not control its rapid dissemination among their citizens. As a last resort they confined infected women to their homes, and banished infected males outside the town walls.

Russia and Hungary reported the disease in 1500, and in the same year, probably as the consequence of Vasco da Gama's expedition, the disease was reported from India. A similar situation followed Marco Polo's expedition in 1505 when the disease was reported from China, and in 1506 from Japan.

In 13 years the disease had spread from a small island on the American coast to sweep across Europe, India and Asia, and is the basis of the *Columbian theory* which attempts to explain the spread of the disease. A second theory called the *Unitarian theory*, states the disease has always been there and includes a proposition that the disease could equally well be caused by the increase in the slave trade bringing the disease from Africa to Europe in which case the disease would have been present in Europe from Roman times. In these middle centuries the Holy Roman Church was so concerned at the social consequences of the spread of the disease that they nominated St Denis as the patron saint of those suffering from the Pox. St Denis is also the patron saint of Paris and France, and this reflects the thinking of the period since it increasingly became known as the French Disease.

STATISTICS

The first true statistics pertaining to the incidence of venereal disease were compiled in 1850 by the armies of America, UK, Prussia and France. These first figures reveal that at that time 120 males per thousand of the male population suffered from venereal disease. Figures for both the military and civilian populations show a dramatic rise immediately after World Wars with a dramatic fall within 12 months after an end to hostilities.

During the 1960s a notable increase was observed in male immigrants into the UK from the Caribbean, India and Pakistan. Since they arrived without the disease, it is suggested that a reservoir of infectivity in the white female population of some main cities required contact tracing. During 1965, surveys made in Holland and Sweden demonstrated that 20% of all known cases in these two countries was due to casual sex between holidaymakers and prostitutes. In one London district a doctor reported that in 1966 there was a 20% incidence of gonorrhoea in practising male homosexuals.

The figures submitted by many government agencies to the World Health Organisation when analysed and totalled showed that in 1970 there were world-wide, 200 million cases of gonorrhoea and 50 million cases of syphilis. Also at this time the Vietnam War caused an all time increase in incidence in the American armed forces and in the Vietnamese female population.

The most recent figures between 1971 and 1979 for gonorrhoea and syphilis in England and Wales are shown in Fig. 6.1. During this decade the incidence of syphilis in the female population has remained static at 1000 new cases per year, while it fluctuates in the male population. The figures for gonorrhoea are showing a gradual decrease and perhaps reflect an increasing conservatism in sexual attitudes, particularly following the easy going attitudes of the 60s and 70s. This was especially so among the teenage population which suffered the greatest number of new cases.

TREATMENT

Very little reference is made to the treatment of the venereal diseases during the middle centuries. The crusaders used a salve known as Saracen's Ointment, containing mercury, to apply to the ulcers. In 1808, Wallace, a physician from Dublin, recommended the use of Potassium Iodide solution and for many years it remained the mainstay of treatment. The use of linen or fine leather condoms were originally used to prevent contacting the contagion rather than as a measure to prevent pregnancy.

In 1907, Ehrlich introduced a new treatment known as the *magic bullet*, for the treatment of syphilis. This consisted of giving an intravenous injection of an arsenic based solution known as '606' or Salversan, its

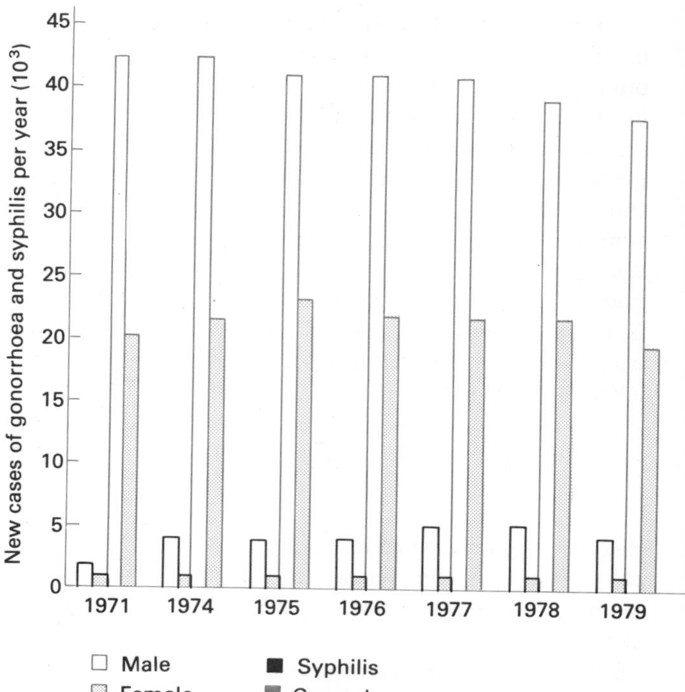

Fig. 6.1 New cases of gonorrhoea and syphilis in England and Wales (1971–79).

proprietary name being Neoarsphenamine. This contrasted with the then current practice of using mercury which in its effect was worse than the disease since it caused mercurial poisoning.

The complications of syphilis, especially those of the tertiary stage, affect in particular the nervous system which led to Wagner and Jauregg developing *Malarial therapy* to counteract the effects of neurosyphilis. By deliberately inducing malaria and causing fever, the aim was to destroy the treponema within the tissues throughout the body.

During 1921 intramuscular injections of Bismuth were combined with the neoarsphenamine (arsenic) and remained the standard treatment until the introduction of penicillin in 1943. Penicillin was considered a revolutionary treatment at the time, but it has not lived up to the then expectation that it would totally eradicate venereal disease. It is still however the first treatment of choice and should the patient be allergic or prove resistant to penicillin there is now available a wide variety of other antibiotics which ensures an almost 100% cure over an affected population.

EARLY DESCRIPTIONS

Dr Fracastor, a physician of Verona, penned a poem in 1530 which immortalised a swineherd by the name of Syphilis, and it is from this that the disease gains it name. Its title is *Syphilis sive Morbus Gallicus* (Syphilis, or, the French Disease).

> He first wore buboes [ulcers] dreadful to sight,
> Felt strange pains and sleepless passed the night,
> From him the malady received its name,
> The neighbouring shepherds catched the spreading flame.

This poem reflects one of the early attempts to describe the symptoms of the disease. Although gonorrhoea and syphilis now had separate names both diseases were considered manifestations of the same thing. This thinking continued and was reinforced when in 1766 the famous surgeon J. Hunter carried out a fatal experiment on himself. He collected infected discharge from one of his patients and infected himself deliberately. He then noted the course of the disease and concluded that both gonorrhoea and syphilis were the same thing. What he could not know was that the patient from whom he infected himself had both diseases. Due to the very high regard in which he was held the medical profession accepted Hunter's opinion and this held sway for the next 30 years.

IDENTIFICATION OF CAUSATIVE ORGANISMS

Ricord, the famous venereologist, emphatically described the symptoms and course of both diseases during 1793 and this became the cornerstone of diagnosis. In 1879 the causative organism of gonorrhoea was identified by Albert Neisser, hence the name *Neisseria gonorrhoeae*. Using dark-ground microscopy, Schaudin and Hoffman identified the causative organism of syphilis as being one of the group known as the treponemes, hence its name *Treponema pallidium*.

From this development in 1905 it was soon realised that another supposedly sexually transmitted disease, yaws, was in fact an ulceration caused by an entirely different organism, i.e., *Treponema pertenue*, and was not spread by sexual contact but rather by body contact. Further separation of other so called sexually transmitted diseases led to them being more correctly classified with the discovery of the 'virus' which explained the occurrence of genital warts, and the clarifying of the 'fungi' which explained thrush or *candida* infections of the vagina.

LEGISLATION

In the UK the first legislative measure to control the spread of venereal disease was passed in 1916. The Venereal Disease Regulations placed a responsibility on local authorities to provide:

- Special clinics for the diagnosis and treatment of venereal diseases as well as providing advice
- Contact tracing services
- Education of the public, particularly vulnerable groups
- Advertisements for the preventive aspects of the problem

These regulations made syphilis, gonorrhoea and chancroid notifiable to the medical officer of health. It also removed the legal enforcement and encouraged voluntary attendance at the clinics.

Combined with this specific legislation there were many other Public Health Acts, especially those relating to prostitution, which reflected government concern to control the spread of these highly infective diseases.

CONCLUSIONS

From this brief historical survey certain conclusions can be drawn relating to the spread of the disease:

1. There is a consistent increase in venereal diseases related to war and hostilities due to movement between countries.
2. Movement of populations, such as emigrants, to new areas also contributes to an increase in incidence but it is to be noted that the initial infectivity usually lies in the residents or natives of the area.
3. Sexual promiscuity whether between homosexuals, with prostitutes or with multiple clients, or as casual sex between consenting adults or teenagers, even when occurring in an affluent and educated society, makes a large contribution to known new cases every year.
4. Statistics at any given period of time do not qualify the actual true numbers of cases. There is no way of knowing how many cases are being treated privately, or how many individuals are ignoring their symptoms.

Chapter 7
Nursing Role in Venereology

The department specialising in the treatment of venereal diseases is referred to by one of a variety of names: special clinic, special treatment centre or department, department of genital medicine, department of genitourinary medicine, or department of venereology.

A high percentage of the patients attending the clinic are there by their own volition, seeking expert advice on a wide variety of symptoms invariably related to the genitalia, but not always as a consequence of sexual contact. Other patients are referred on the advice of their general practitioner, or by friends. Several specialist outpatient departments, notably the skin clinic, also refer patients with symptoms which may be venereal in origin. Only rarely is a patient ever admitted to the hospital from the venereal clinic. The ideal clinic functions independently within the hospital complex and is usually located near the main entrance of the hospital, so that entry and exit to the department is discreet.

TEAM SPECIALISTS

The nurse will be one of a team of specialists which usually consists of a receptionist, a venereologist who heads the team, a contact tracing officer who is either a medical social worker or a health visitor, a departmental secretary and in the larger clinics a pathology technician may be employed to collect and test blood specimens. Each team member has specific skills and knowledge which contribute to the main aims of the department which usually are:

To achieve a rapid diagnosis

To prescribe and administer effective treatment

To initiate effective contact tracing

To provide regular checks by 'case holding'

To maintain statistical information on local trends for national information

The Receptionist

Since the receptionist is the first person to meet and welcome a new patient his or her attitude is of vital importance to enable the patient to retain feelings of composure. Any hostility will only serve to increase the patient's underlying anxiety and other feelings which may be: guilt, shame, anger, disgrace or humiliation. Basic personal information is taken at this stage, and whenever possible the waiting time before examination is kept to the absolute minimum.

The Venereologist

The venereologist will normally take the history and closely question the patient before any examination takes place. To ensure confidentiality this initial interview is done in complete privacy. From experience many venereologists find that blunt and direct questions are more likely to be honestly answered than diplomatic and politely phrased questions. Apart from the history and symptoms, the venereologist begins the process of contact tracing by compiling a contact list.

Examination

The examination is divided into two phases, a close and detailed examination of the genitalia, and then a general examination, if required. For males this is best done if they are resting on a couch in the dorsal position; for females the lithotomy position is always used.

The Nurse's Role

The nurse may assist the doctor by providing the equipment necessary and helping the patient with undressing and dressing. The doctor will require equipment for vaginal and rectal examinations and such equipment is always prepared and available.

For any examination the lighting of the room must be excellent and so arranged that it casts no shadows over the patient. Since the majority of patients are young and able bodied, the general examination tends to be brief with reference being made to the condition of the skin, the mucous membranes, the conjunctiva and the throat.

Investigations

Following the examination the venereologist will decide on the investigations and tests he or she will require to confirm a provisional diagnosis.

The Nurse's Role

Since it is usually the nurse who prepares, stains, and studies the slides under the microscope it is usually she or he who collects the smears. Several skills are required including the use of the platinum loop to collect any discharge from ulcers from within the urethra or vagina.

After staining the slide it has then to be studied using a standard or adapted dark field microscope to identify a particular organism. To complement these skills the nurse requires a detailed knowledge of the anatomy and physiology of the male and female reproductive tract and the genitourinary system. With repeated use of the microscope the nurse will come to have a deeper appreciation of the various organisms which cause venereal diseases (Table 7.1). In addition to these micro-organisms the nurse may also gain experience in identifying two parasites, i.e., *Sarucoptes scabiei* (scabies), and *Phthirus pubis* (pubic louse).

Apart from taking smears the nurse may also be involved in collecting swabs which will

Table 7.1. Micro-organisms which cause venereal disease

Micro-organism	Disease
Spirochaetes	
Treponema pallidium	Syphilis
Treponema pertenue	Yaws
Treponema carateum	Pinta
Bacteria	
Neisseria gonorrhoeae	Gonorrhoea
Haemophilus ducreyi	Chancroid
Chlamydia trachomatis	Lymphogranuloma venereum
Protozoa	
Trichomonas vaginalis	Trichomoniasis
Fungi	
Candida albicans	Candidiasis (thrush)
Virus	
Papilloma virus	Condylomata acuminata
Herpes simplex virus type 2	Herpes genitalis

be cultured to grow the causative organism, and if a qualified nurse with the required training is present, the nurse learner may be allowed to collect blood specimens for specific serology tests which are done in the hospital pathology department. On some occasions the nurse will be required to assist with lymph node aspiration, lymph node biopsy, lumbar puncture, plain or invasive X-rays, and neurological assessments.

Immediate Treatment

With only a provisional diagnosis, even after examination of smears, most venereologists will prescribe immediate treatment. In giving such treatment the nurse will develop a wide range of knowledge and skills in administering drugs.

The Nurse's Role

Before *systemic antibiotics* are given the nurse must ensure that the patient does not have a known history of allergy to them. If the prescribed treatment is not effective, it is open to question if the patient may have a resistance to the antibiotic. This is now increasingly common.

Anti-inflammatory drugs may be prescribed. The complications of gonorrhoea and secondary lesions of syphilis are good examples of where steroids may be employed to control the worse effects of inflamed joints, e.g. gonococcal arthritis.

Topical applications, e.g. a wide variety of creams, lotions, and ointments, are used to control the inflammation, itching, and burning sensations of many of the venereal diseases.

In addition anti-infestation agents may be required especially those used against scabies and pubic lice.

The Contact Tracing Officer

After the rigorous interview with the venereologist and the nursing treatment, the patient is given an interview with the contact tracing officer. Such an officer is always female. It is found from experience that patients relax and give confidences more readily to a courteous and nonuniformed person especially if female.

Again the interview is strictly private to safeguard confidentiality and gain the patient's trust. The aim of the interview is to obtain more details about the sexual contacts, whether they are casual or regular. While remaining professionally objective the tracing officer may have to use plain and idiomatic language without ever appearing shocked.

The promiscuous individual may have spread a trail of havoc which severely disrupts both his or her immediate personal circle of friends, and in turn other remote acquaintances. In many instances of casual sex the names and addresses or telephone numbers may not be known, in which case the officer has to rely on a description of the contact concerned. Odd circumstances may arise when dealing with a bisexual in which the contacts present a bizarre picture. More difficult still is the contacting of wives, fiancés, or regular faithful partners.

Whatever the contact history, the officer has to decide on the best means of contacting the sexual partner(s) to encourage them to come for advice and examination to exclude venereal disease. This may be done by 'trace cards' which patients will issue to their sexual contacts which advises them to come to the clinic. If at all possible patients should be encouraged to bring their regular partner(s) to the clinic or to persuade them to attend. Direct contact can be made by the tracing officer if enough details are available. Even from a brief description it is possible for an experienced officer to trace known promiscuous people from those who attend the clinic regularly, e.g., prostitutes, homosexuals, itinerants.

The Nurse's Role

The nurse will have arranged with the departmental secretary a series of outpatient appointments, and such appointments must be kept. It is here the counselling and advisory role of the nurse must be used to reinforce not only specific advice related to any local treatment but also the need to encourage the patient to return for his or her check-up. This is best done without making any judgment on an individual's sexuality but by emphasising to the patient the need to accept responsibility for his or her own health.

To maintain records the departmental secretary will open a 'case hold' file. Since the majority of patients are seen three if not four times over the coming months their case file will contain any information required about the original prescribed treatment and its effectiveness as measured by subsequent tests, from follow-up visits. Should the patient default, i.e., not attend, then the contact tracing officer may be asked to contact the individual with a new appointment.

Statistical Analysis

Every few months the number of new patients is summarised on a statistical basis and if needed can also be plotted on a geographical chart to show if there is any specific high incidence in a part of the city. These two pieces of information are very significant and would indicate to the venereologist if any recommendations should be made to the local Medical Officer of Health. The total figures for one year of both new cases and total attendances are submitted to the Department of Health and are combined with all other figures to show the national trends of venereal diseases.

Chapter 8
Bacterial Disorders

SYPHILIS

The causative organism of syphilis is *Treponema pallidum*. This organism is one of the species of the genus Treponema, and is morphologically described as being a spirochaete, i.e., corkscrew shaped. When viewed through dark-ground microscopy with special lighting it is seen to be whitish in colour, measuring 5–20 μm in length (Fig. 8.1). It requires a warm atmosphere in which to survive and this is readily provided by human tissues. Being a fragile organism it is easily destroyed by heat, chemicals and cold and cannot survive in clean conditions. It is suggested that the rapid decline in the incidence of syphilis is due more to improved social conditions rather than advances in medical knowledge.

An important feature about *Treponema pallidum* is that it multiplies every 30 hours. Assuming that the initial infective dose is roughly 1000 organisms, the number of organisms that can be present within 18 days is considerable. Several problems arise from

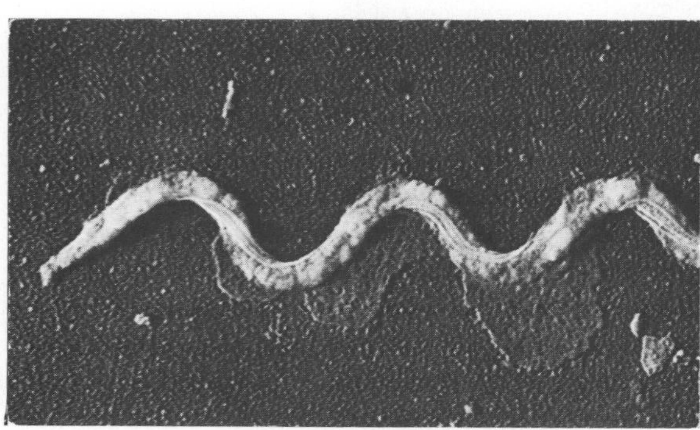

Fig. 8.1 *Treponema pallidum.*

this slow rate of division: the incubation period of the disease is quite long, confirmative diagnostic tests take longer than usual, perhaps days if not weeks, and lastly the treatment regimen must be absolute if the infection is to be controlled.

For both male and female patients the incubation period is between 9 and 90 days before the primary signs or symptoms make their first appearance.

If untreated the patient can remain an infective source for 2 years, and for this reason a detailed history of all sexual contacts within the previous 2 years are vital for both contact tracing and notification purposes. Although a notifiable disease there is no justification for any type of isolation nursing should the infected patient be admitted to a general hospital. Equally essential is that there is no immunity developed against the disease until after at least 2 years of suffering the symptoms of untreated syphilis. During the last decade approximately 1000 new cases were notified each year in the UK.

Mode of Transmission

Syphilis is an acquired contagious infection arising from direct sexual contact. The organism gains entry through the mucosa of the genitalia via a minor abrasion. Within 30 hours of becoming infected the localised invasion spreads to the blood via the lymphatic system. In male homosexuals the incidence of syphilis increases when there is a change of partner. Many of the new cases of syphilis are in fact from this group.

Increasingly rare, but still possible, is the transmission of *Treponema pallidum* across the placenta during the second half of pregnancy, i.e., the twentieth week. It is vital for all women to be screened during the first 10 weeks of pregnancy to exclude the possibility of syphilis. Since this is routinely done for all mothers it is now rare in the UK for a baby to be born with congenital syphilis. Donated blood is regularly screened for the presence of antibodies of syphilis.

Signs and Symptoms

The disease is divided into different stages according to the signs and symptoms present, summarised in Fig. 8.2. These are:

Primary
Secondary
Latent
Late or tertiary

Primary Stage

In the male the first symptom is the appearance of a raised papule on the surface membrane of any part of the penile shaft. When the covering of the papule falls off it exposes an ulcer crater, which is referred to

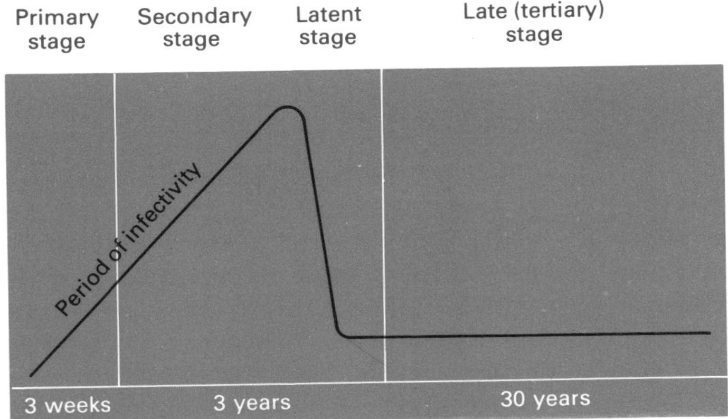

Fig. 8.2 Natural sequence of events in syphilis.

as a *chancre*. The ulcer is usually painless but is visual evidence of something seriously wrong and this will bring the patient forward for urgent advice. In the female, however, if the ulcer is within the vagina or lies between the vagina and cervix, it is hidden and being painless may go unnoticed. The ulcer heals over a period of 3–8 weeks and during this time is highly infectious. All ulcers of the genitalia should be regarded as syphilitic in nature until proved otherwise.

Secondary Stage

Between the primary and secondary stages there is usually a time lapse of 6–8 weeks, but with an overlap of signs and symptoms. The patient begins to feel unwell generally, complaining of malaise, and pyrexia. A widespread pink rash over the body, of uniform pattern, and nonirritating, but of a persistent nature, tends to last for 2 or 3 weeks. When the rash eventually flakes off and begins to heal it leaves deep pigmented areas, especially noticeable over the back and between the shoulder blades.

The lymph glands are enlarged, the inguinal, axillary, and cervical groups are enlarged and associated with this lymphadenopathy is liver enlargement. A persistent sore throat which will not resolve with any conventional treatment and occurring at the same time as sudden scalp hair loss, *alopecia*, often brings the young female patient forward for medical opinion. The appearance of flat topped warts occurring over the moist skin areas, e.g., the vagina, scrotum, buttocks, and mouth, tending to become mucus patches which leave the visual impression of 'snail-like tracks', are a symptom causing great alarm. This also prompts the patient to seek advice.

In male homosexuals these 'warts' or mucus patches may be regarded as insignificant and may be confused with haemorrhoids and thus the infected person remains an infective source for other sexual contacts.

Many patients report attempting to cure themselves of these 'ulcers' and 'warts', using a wide variety of commercially available products such as antiseptic lotions, creams, various types of sprays, and ointments. All these self-treatments are to no avail. Although they may destroy the surface organisms they do not influence the *treponemas* within the blood stream.

The secondary stage if left untreated lasts for about 3 months and during this period the patient is highly infectious to any sexual partner. The blood is teeming with *Treponema pallidum* to which the body is mounting antibodies.

Latent Stage

There are no signs or symptoms during the latent stage, but the patient remains infectious to other sexual partners. Often the diagnosis may be made accidentally when syphilis is being excluded as a possible cause of other diseases.

Late Stage

In some classifications the late stage is further subdivided into a 'tertiary' as well as a 'quartenary' stage. The first symptom of the late stage may not appear until 10 or 20 years after the original infection, and is the development of an ulcer or *gumma*. This ulcer tends to occur just beneath the skin or within bone and is extremely painful. It is prone to secondary infections and takes a considerable time to heal. The ulcer indicates that the patient although suffering from syphilis is no longer infective, and this is referred to as benign late syphilis.

Symptoms

The treponema is now parasitic to every type of tissue, especially the reticulo-endothelial and lymphatic systems which mediate the treponemal spread to every organ and system in the body. This parasitic invasiveness creates a multitude of symptoms which by their very nature 'mimic' a whole range of other classically defined disease entities. In particular the treponema affects the cardiovascular, the locomotor and the central nervous system.

Cardiovascular System

The treponema principally attacks the aorta. After the initial inflammation and subsequent healing the coats of the aorta split creating a bulge between them, i.e., an aneurysm. This in turn leads to a wide variety of systemic and cardiac symptoms which can ultimately lead to heart failure.

Locomotor System

Both the bones and the joints are invaded by the treponema. Initially there is a weakness in the matrix of the bone tissue, *osteoporosis*. This is accompanied by a loss of strength and elasticity in joint structures, e.g., the ligaments, tendons, and cartilage. The combined effect is to create postural difficulties and the development of an odd gait.

Central Nervous System

A small minority of those suffering the late stage of syphilis suffer from meningitis as the treponema becomes invasive to the coats of the brain. Another 10% suffer damage to the spinal nerve roots which increases the existing ataxia resulting from the locomotor damage.

Many behavioural changes are seen in the late stage and are usually grouped under the term 'general paralysis of the insane'. In this entity all the symptoms combine and are coupled with delusions of grandeur, depressive tendencies and psychotic behaviour. Fortunately the late stage is rarely seen today due to the effective treatment and screening carried out during the primary and secondary stages.

Examination and Investigations

Following a study of the patient's symptoms and the clinical signs, the doctor will calculate the timing factors depending on the presumed stage of the illness. From this study he or she will request from the patient details of all known sexual contacts for tracing purposes. If in the primary stage, the sexual contacts of the previous 3 months are needed; if in the secondary stage, the contacts of the previous 2 years are required.

If an ulcer is present its edges will be pressed together which causes the ulcer to weep slightly. A sample of this exudate will be collected into a sterile glass slide with a platinum loop. The collecting hand is protected by a disposable glove. The slide is prepared for microscopic examination to detect if the typical spirochaete organism is present. When a patient may have been using one agent or another to self treat the primary ulcer, they may have effectively killed off surface treponema. If this is the case the doctor may aspirate the fluid from a lymph node and this fluid will contain the organism if the diagnosis is correct.

A sample of blood will be required for specific serological testing, the results of which may not be ready for several weeks. There are a wide variety of tests available and they are summarised here with their abbreviations, since the pathology forms are usually annotated in this way to respect confidentiality.

Standard nonspecific screening tests (STS)

Venereal Disease Research Laboratory Test (VDRL) is the most popularly used of the glass slide tests and can be readily prepared and microscopically examined in the clinic.
Automated Reagin Test (ART) is based on the VDRL test but a whole batch of specimens is tested at once using automation.
Complement Fixation Tests. The Wasserman test is one of this group and requires a specimen of blood for its completion.

Specific Serological Tests

Reiter protein complement fixation test (RPCFT)
Automated RPCFT
Treponema pallidum immobilisation test (TPI)
Fluorescent treponemal antibody test (FTA)
Absorbed fluorescent treponemal antibody test (FTA—ABS)

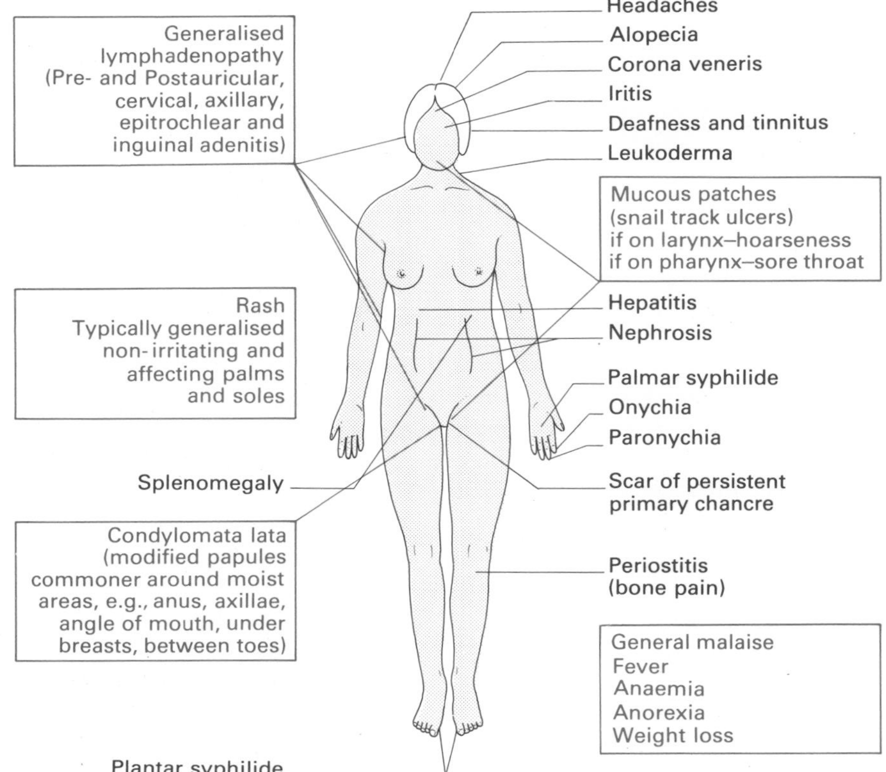

Fig. 8.3 Manifestations of secondary syphilis.

Treponema pallidum haemagglutination assay (TPHA)

All the tests require blood specimens, the results tend to take several weeks before they are available to the doctor for the patient's next visit. A further test, Price precipitation test (PPT), is repeated on each visit to the clinic and will confirm if the prescribed treatment has been effective in destroying the treponema in the blood stream.

A routine urinalysis is completed for all new patients and a visual inspection of the specimen to note any flecks or unusual deposits is carefully made in case the doctor considers it useful to perform a centrifuge test and have the deposits cultured.

In male homosexuals a rectal examination is routinely carried out, in addition to the collection of smears for culture.

For those patients who come or are referred to the clinic with latent or late stage suspected syphilis, X-rays of the skeletal system and the joints are taken to indicate the extent and degree of osteoporosis and joint destruction. A lumbar puncture may also be done to culture the cerebrospinal fluid for the presence of treponema, or their antibodies.

Treatment

Primary and Secondary Stages

In a suspected case of syphilis, treatment will be prescribed until confirmation is made from the results. Manifestations of secondary syphilis are illustrated in Fig. 8.3. The aim of treatment is to maintain a blood level of at least 0.03 μg/ml of the prescribed antibiotic for a period of 15–20 days. Penicillin is the first drug of choice and a variety of regimens have been developed to ensure that the required high blood level is maintained. Daily

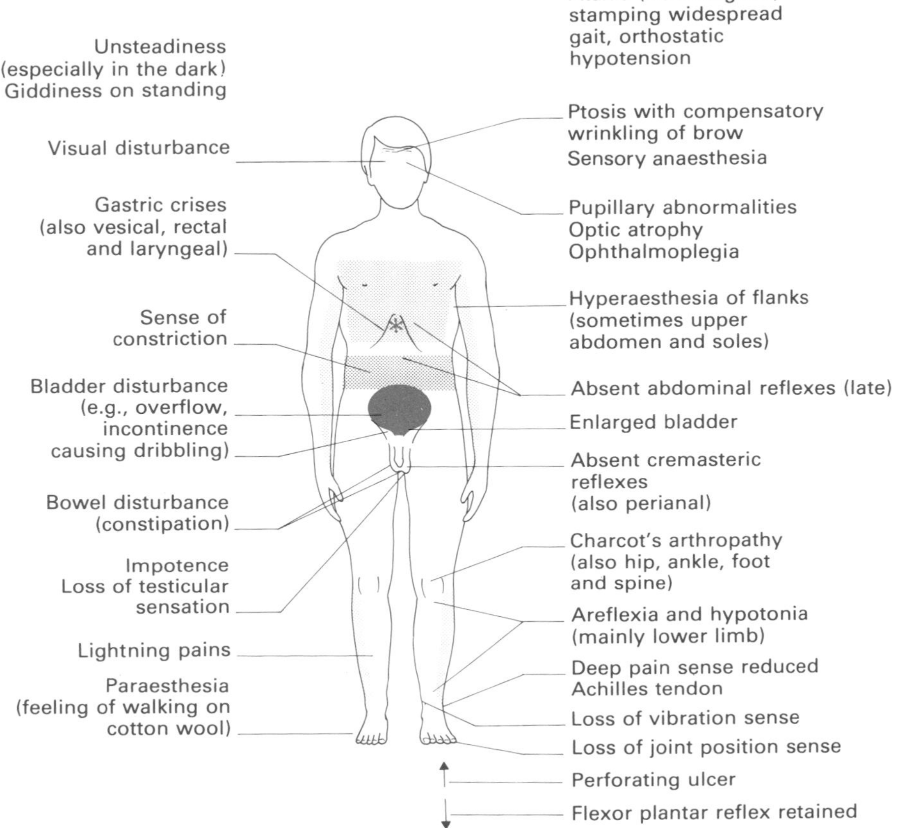

Fig. 8.4 Manifestations of *Tabes dorsalis*.

injections of penicillin may be given for 5–14 days depending on the dose prescribed. Alternatively, two massive doses of penicillin per week for 3 weeks.

Should the patient be allergic or resistant to penicillin, the second choice may be:

Erythromycin 500 mg or tetracycline 500 mg taken four times daily for 10–15 days

Cephaloridine by intramuscular injection 1 g daily for 5–14 days

Usually 24 hours after treatment a considerable number of patients develop a generalised rash accompanied by pyrexia, nausea, and severe lethargy. This is known as Jarisch-Herxheimer reaction and is taken as confirmation of the diagnosis. Due to the severity of the symptoms of this reaction all patients should be warned of the possibility of its recurrence. If the symptoms persist the penicillin may be temporarily replaced with bismuth 0.2 g once weekly for 6 weeks, after this the penicillin is recommenced.

Late Stage

In all cases of syphilis procaine penicillin is given for 21 days. The patient will be noninfective and all other treatment will be to contain the destructive process of the parasitic treponemas. The manifestations of *Tabes dorsalis* are shown in Fig. 8.4. Such measures include the administration of steroids to deal with inflammatory disorder, barbiturates to control the worst of the behavioural changes and psychiatric therapy for any psychotic disturbance.

Advising the Patient

The patients in the primary, secondary and latent stages should be reassured that if they remain loyal to their prescribed therapy and attend all outpatient appointments over 95% will be cured completely. It must be emphasised in no uncertain terms that syphilis is an extremely dangerous disease with fatal long-term consequences if treatment is abandoned. The normal pattern of outpatients' check-ups is: first check-up in 2 weeks, next in 12 weeks, then after 24 weeks and 48 weeks. The final check-up is after 2 years, and if completely cured the patient will be discharged from care.

The patient must be strongly advised to abstain from any type of sexual contact for a minimum of 1 month after the completion of antibiotic therapy. Some clinics recommend a much longer period but in practice the vulnerable groups are not in general inclined to follow advice. It is therefore more reasonable and realistic to give warnings at each visit if in fact they are still infective or otherwise.

If the patient travels a great deal throughout the country or abroad, a Surveillance Booklet (WHO) which can be taken to any clinic contains the information necessary for checks to be continued for the required 2-year period.

PINTA

The causative organism of pinta is *Treponema carateum*. Morphologically and serologically it is similar to *Treponema pallidum*, the causative organism of syphilis, but is non-venereal.

The incubation period for *Treponema pallidum* is 7–10 days.

Pinta is transmitted by skin to skin contact, but not sexual contact. It is normally passed between children while they are at play, e.g., leg to leg contact during games. It is relatively prevalent in poor and deprived areas and is confined to defined geographical areas, e.g., Mexico, South America and the Caribbean.

Signs and Symptoms

As with syphilis, the signs and symptoms of pinta appear in stages; primary, secondary and tertiary.

Primary Stage

A single papular lesion at the primary stage develops either on the legs, arm or face and eventually becomes multiform. The lesions eventually erupt and the organism is readily seen by dark-ground microscopy to be present in the serous exudate from the lesions.

Secondary Stage

During the secondary stage the papular lesions coalesce to form chronic ulcers, *pintids*, which last for several years. Not only are they ugly, but depending on their site they can be extremely crippling.

Tertiary Stage

When the ulcerated areas heal during the tertiary stage they undergo pigmentary changes, deepening in colour from a dull red to a slate blue and this change is accompanied by severe itching. Although the ulcers heal, the affected area becomes atrophic and remains visually very ugly and is the cause of much psychological suffering.

Diagnosis

In broad terms the disease remains confined to an endemic area. Serological or blood tests are positive in the second stage.

Treatment

Mass campaigns directed at improvements in cleanliness and improved living conditions have a marked impact on lowering the incidence of the disease. Those affected by the disease make an excellent response to a single injection of 120 000 units of procaine penicillin aluminium monostearate (PAM).

YAWS

The causative organism of yaws is *Treponema pertenue*, which is morphologically similar to *Treponema pallidum*.

The incubation period of yaws is 3–6 weeks.

Yaws, previously confused with syphilis, is confined to defined geographical areas which tend to be humid, e.g., Central and South America, the Caribbean, central West Africa, and South East Asia. It is transmitted by direct skin to skin contact, not necessarily sexual contact. It occurs mostly between children who are at play. It may be transmitted to other members of the family who share the same sleeping accommodation. There is some evidence that it can also be transmitted via the flies of the genus Hippelates.

As with pinta the disease is associated with conditions of extreme poverty and social deprivation. The long incubation period implies that immigrants from endemic areas can transmit the disease to a previously unaffected geographical area.

Symptoms, Investigations and Treatment

The symptoms, investigations and treatment are very similar to that for pinta disease. Both yaws and pinta confer an immunity against syphilis. Conversely the erradication of yaws and pinta by mass campaigns increases the incidence of syphilis.

GONORRHOEA

The causative organism of gonorrhoea is *Neisseria gonorrhoeae*. This organism thrives in a warm moist atmosphere. It is a kidney-shaped organism and because it is paired it is referred to as a *diplococcus*. When viewed through the microscope it is seen to lie within the pus cells (Fig. 8.5). Since it is Gram negative it is quickly diagnosed using the Gram staining technique. There are at least 5 serological types known and a further 5 morphological types each having a different virulence. The organism has a particular affinity for columnar epithelium and if and when it penetrates the tissue, it rapidly multiplies causing a submucosal inflammation.

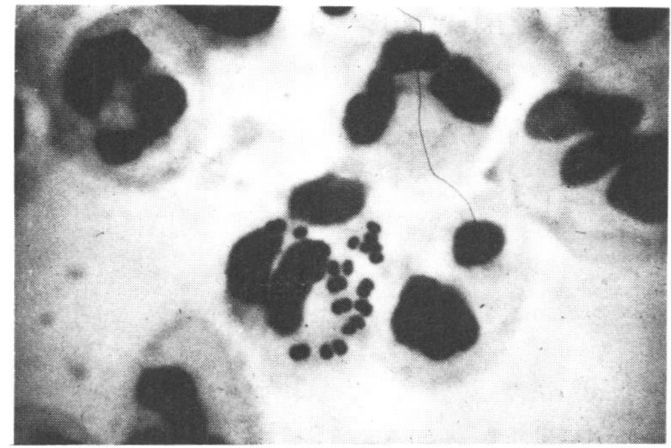

Fig. 8.5 Gonococci.

The incubation period varies between 2 and 14 days; this will depend on the virulence and dose of infectivity and the resistance of the host's body defences. In women the incubation period tends to be longer, possibly because of the shorter urethra which is more easily cleansed with micturition. In male homosexuals, or in women who have had rectal sex, the incubation period is about 14 days.

It should be noted that although gonorrhoea is an infectious disease, unlike other infectious diseases, it does not confer immunity after an attack, nor is there a vaccine or immunisation procedure against gonorrhoea.

Mode of Transmission

Sexual contact is the mode of transmission, the sexual act being taken in its widest sense:

Normal intercourse, penis to vagina
Anal intercourse, penis to rectum
Oral contact, genitalia to the mouth

Very rarely, and it should be stressed that it is very rare, gonorrhoea may be transmitted by fomites such as a towel which is being shared at the time of sexual activity.

If an individual ignores his or her symptoms, or if in fact they are asymptomatic, the disease can progress to a chronic state, in this case the individual becomes a carrier. About 25% of those suffering from gonorrhoea also suffer from and transmit non-specific urethritis. While the incidence of gonorrhoea combined with syphilis is now very rare it should also be excluded during investigation. Females with gonorrhoea at the time of giving birth

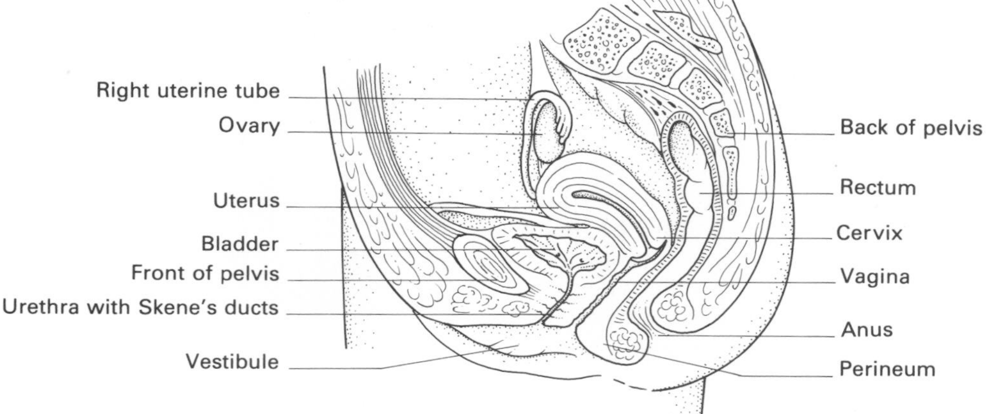

Fig. 8.6 Section through female pelvis.

may transmit the gonococcus to the eyes of the new-born infant.

Signs and Symptoms

Female Patients

The incubation period in females can be from 2–14 days. It should be remembered that 30–50% of females are asymptomatic, in which case they act as a reservoir of infectivity for further sexual partners.

Vaginal discharge is not uncommon in the healthy female, but an *altered* discharge, particularly if it is purulent and yellow, indicates a possible sexually transmitted disease. There will be a burning sensation on micturition. At a later point the patient complains of pyrexia alternating with chills, headaches and low backache.

For those females who are asymptomatic the infection spreads upwards to cause 'cervicitis'. This includes infections of the uterine cavity, oviducts, and uterine tubes (Fig. 8.6). Should these be ignored the symptoms may pass leaving the female a 'carrier' of the disease. Fortunately many patients come forward with abdominal pain or arthritic joint pain which on detailed examination may reveal the gonococcal infection.

Male Patients

The incubation period is 3–5 days and the initial symptoms are severe enough to bring the majority of male sufferers forward. These include severe discomfort of the anterior urethra, a purulent yellowish discharge, and painful burning sensations on micturition accompanied by pyrexia and headaches.

About 1 in 10 patients come forward with late symptoms, and these reflect the spread of the infection towards the upper urinary tract and reproductive organs (Fig. 8.7). The posterior urethra (upper third) is extremely painful, the prostate gland surrounding the urethra at the base of the bladder may become inflamed (*prostatitis*), inflammation of the bladder (*cystitis*) and the testes (*orchitis* and *epididymitis*) may also occur.

In male homosexuals there may be considerable rectal discharge, usually enough to stain the underclothing or bedsheets. It is of a slimy consistency. The inflammation of the anal canal may also cause the patient to need to defaecate when he already has evacuated the bowel. The sphincters are extremely irritated with persistent itching.

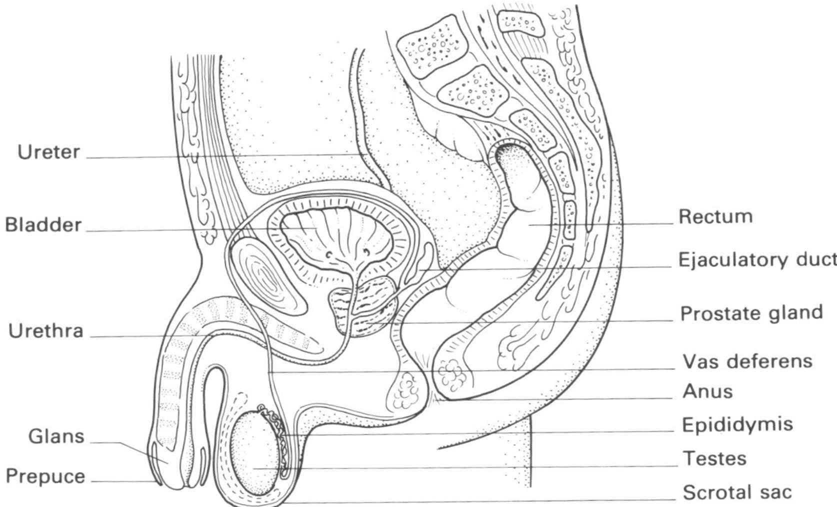

Fig. 8.7 Section through male pelvis.

Examination

Female Patients

On pelvic examination the female urethral meatus is seen to be red and swollen, the thin membrane covering the Skene's glands and the Bartholin's glands are painful and swollen. If there is abdominal pain during the examination extreme caution is required, and a rectal examination may not be done for fear of spreading the infection further. In addition to this local examination the mouth and pharynx are examined for oral and pharyngeal lesions.

Male Patients

On examination of the male genitalia, the urethral meatus is oedematous, a purulent creamy discharge is secreted on urethral massage and there is usually enlargement of the inguinal lymph nodes. A rectal examination is also done if the history indicates this is required.

Investigations and Diagnosis

The physical examination and the symptoms of which the patient complains suggest only a possible sexually transmitted disease. A smear taken of the urethral discharge (male) onto a sterile glass slide and prepared with Gram's stain will reveal the typical kidney-shaped diplococcus within the pus cells under the microscope. This is, however, only one of a series of confirmations required. It is usual though for the venereologist to proceed to treat the gonorrhoea on the basis of this first test. Three smears are normally taken from the female, i.e., from the urethra, vagina, and cervix. If the history suggests it a fourth smear may be taken from the rectum.

A second test would be to take smears for culture and sensitivity tests. The results of this test usually take 2 days, since the specimen requires to be incubated. The test will also indicate if the first antibiotic selected for treatment is the most appropriate.

A third test is to send a smear for an immunofluorescent test. If all three tests prove positive, there is a confirmation of gonorrhoea. These efforts at absolute diagnosis will prove vital if, as does happen on occasions, an innocent partner such as an unsuspecting wife sues for divorce or plans a separation.

When indicated, further tests for syphilis are usually also done at the same time.

Treatment

The immediate treatment is to give one intramuscular injection of penicillin, e.g., benzylpenicillin, ampicillin/cloxacillin (Magnapen), or procaine penicillin. Should the patient have a known allergy to penicillin then one of the other antibiotics is prescribed to be taken orally over a period of 5 days, e.g., tetracycline, kanamycin, erythromycin, Septrin, or Trobicin. Should the patient prove resistant to an antibiotic then it may be accompanied by a second drug, probenecid, which acts by raising and maintaining the antibiotic blood level sufficient to combat the blood-borne gonococcal infection.

It is the common experience of special clinics that many of their patients do not return for the follow-up appointments. Because of this, the policy of giving one injection, which is sufficient to cure the infection, has been adopted, to reduce the risks of further spread of the disease.

Advising the Patient

It is best for the patient to avoid alcohol in any form since it irritates an already inflamed urethra when the metabolised alcohol is excreted. This abstinence should continue until the next test proves negative.

Sexual contact of any type with any partner must not take place until a cure has been effected and this is proven when the smear and blood tests are negative.

Following micturition or defaecation patients much wash their hands thoroughly, be assiduous in daily washing of the perineum and genitalia, and change their undergarments daily.

Any failure to complete a course of oral antibiotics or return for further injections places patients at great risk. It is vital that the blood level of the antibiotic remains at a persistently high level which is achieved by being loyal to the treatment. Otherwise they may develop chronic gonorrhoea in which case they become carriers and are liable to suffer at a later date from gonococcal arthritis.

To enable the social welfare officer to make a complete tracing of all contacts, the patients' cooperation has to be sought in giving a complete history of their sexual contacts for the previous 3 months.

For a few days following their initial treatment, patients will continue to feel pyrexial and ill. To combat this, they are advised to rest and to consume large amounts of clear fluids to flush the renal system.

It is in the patients' interest that they attend the outpatient appointments they are given. The visits are usually once weekly for 3 weeks, and one further appointment 3 months later. On each visit patients are physically examined and have a urinalysis and several blood tests. When these are negative to tests for gonorrhoea the patient can be discharged from care.

CHANCROID

Haemophilus ducreyi is the causative organism of chancroid, or soft sores. It is a Gram-negative bacillus, and does not thrive in moderate or cold climates. The incubation period is 1–8 days.

It is a notifiable disease in the UK under the legislation of the 1916 Venereal Diseases Regulations.

Mode of Transmission

The bacterium causing chancroid is found in the hot climatic regions, notably in tropical Africa, South America, and the Far East. The organism is transferred on sexual contact or by autoinoculation and the conditions are usually those of poverty and poor hygiene. Women tend to be asymptomatic carriers. Since most patients are male, those who travel extensively through the regions mentioned may bring the disease back to their native countries.

Signs and Symptoms

Single or multiple papules which are very tender and painful appear on the glans penis. They eventually break down to reveal shallow pustular ulcers or soft sores. At the same time the inguinal glands become noticeably enlarged and they too may ulcerate if they erupt from too massive an enlargement.

Investigations

A smear is taken from the ulcer and prepared for dark-ground microscopy. Using Gram's staining technique the organism can be seen to be lying in chains. A sample of the patient's blood is taken for culture to identify the causative organism and to exclude syphilis. A small portion of the ulcer may be removed by biopsy technique for histology studies which would also diagnose the type of organism present.

Treatment

The ulcerated area is carefully cleansed with a solution of normal saline and dried thoroughly. Various antibiotics are prescribed, e.g., sulphadimidine, co-trimoxazole, streptomycin, or oxytetracycline, over a period of 14 days. Any of these drugs combined with daily cleansing should ensure a resolution of the ulcerated area.

Advising the Patient

Arrangements are made for the patient to attend the clinic each month for a total of 3 months. During these follow-up visits a series of blood tests will be completed to exclude the possibility of syphilis. Great emphasis must be placed on the strictest personal hygiene, especially with regard to daily changing of undergarments and hand-washing. If the sexual contact is abroad, which is the usual case, then the venereologist must decide whether it is worth pursuing trace contacting or informing the health authorities of the country from which the disease emanated.

NON-SPECIFIC URETHRITIS

The inflammation of the urethra has a higher incidence than that of gonorrhoea and occurs for the most part in male patients. No specific organism can be detected from smear, culture and sensitivity, or serological tests and therefore this condition is known as non-specific urethritis (NSU). Several surveys show that over 40% of male patients have a positive reaction to serological testing to the organism *Chlamydia trachomatis* (Bedsonia) but the clinical trials will not be completed for some time.

There is a definite increased incidence following a casual sexual contact, but this does not explain the cause of NSU which occurs in faithful partnerships. It is essential in the history taken from the patient that any of the following are exluded from being a possible cause:

- Urethral allergy
- Chemical or mechanical irritation of the urethra
- Recent trauma
- Presence of foreign bodies within the urethra
- Urethral scarring
- Urethral stricture
- Neoplasms
- Infections descending from the kidney, ureter or bladder
- Self-treatment with commercially purchased agents

The incubation period when there is a proven casual sexual contact, will involve the first symptoms occurring 10–30 days later. Various studies suggest that casual sex within the young promiscuous groups and other vulnerable groups accounts for over 50% of new cases seen every year, and for this reason it is regarded as a sexually transmitted disease.

Signs and Symptoms

The vast majority of sufferers are male patients. There is a variable volume of urethral discharge; it can be minimal and reasonably clear in colour, or copious and obviously purulent. The irritation of the urethral membrane causes a mild pain and urinary urgency. If there is low abdominal pain this would suggest that the bladder is also infected.

If the patient delays in reporting the

symptoms, the infection may spread to adjacent structures such as the prostate (prostatitis), epididymis (epididymitis), and the scrotum (hydrocele). The symptoms of these infections are so alarming that they usually bring the patient forward for medical advice.

A triad of symptoms known as Reiter's syndrome are a consequence of NSU. These are conjunctivitis (anterior uveitis), urethritis, and arthritis (especially of the spine and hip joints). The first two of the triad occur shortly after the infection and tend to be acute in nature, while the arthritis is more insidious, becoming chronic in nature.

Examinations and Investigations

A bead of urethral discharge, usually obtained by urethral massage, is mounted on a glass slide then prepared and stained for microscopy to exclude gonorrhoea. If the urethral discharge is minimal it can be obtained by urethral scraping. A fine platinum loop is advanced along the urethra which when removed scrapes the urethral membrane. This removes a tiny portion of the surface material which can be used for a smear test. It is not as uncomfortable as it might seem.

A swab of the urethral discharge is collected and despatched for culture and sensitivity. A variety of organisms can be expected from this test but it excludes the possibility of gonorrhoea, *Trichomonas vaginalis*, and *Candida albicans*.

Several blood specimens are collected for serology to confirm or exclude all types of Chlamydia, lymphogranuloma venereum, and syphilis.

If the patient is able to provide a specimen of urine the 2-glass urine test can be done. The first portion of urine may indicate how involved and infected the anterior urethra is, while the second portion in a second glass may show how infected is the posterior urethra. A careful visual inspection is made of each glass to detect the presence of flecks or specks within the urine. If they are of significant amounts the doctor may request the specimens to be centrifuged and the deposits to be cultured.

To indicate if the prostate gland is involved a rectal examination is usually routinely done, and a sample of prostatic fluid may be obtained by prostatic massage and be despatched for culture and sensitivity.

If Reiter's syndrome is present, conjunctival eye swabs are taken and X-rays of the spine and hip are requested to note any arthritic changes in these joints. Both tests will confirm any suspicions.

Treatment

Treatment is mainly that of broad spectrum antibiotics, the first drug of choice being tetracycline 250–500 mg every 6 hours for 3–5 days. Other antibiotics include doxycycline hydrochloride 300 mg in one dose which is taken with milk, and this drug is sometimes used in uncomplicated urethritis. Streptomycin 1 g intramuscularly for several days may also be prescribed.

Advising the Patient

The patient is advised to have no sexual contact for at least 4 weeks after the course of treatment is concluded. In every case the sex partner whether casual or permanent should also be treated. Alcohol tends to increase the patient's resistance to antibiotic therapy and on urinary excretion irritates the inflamed urethra, and should be avoided until a cure is established.

Since further attacks of NSU are quite possible the patient must attend for his follow-up appointments, these being determined by the stage and progress of the urethritis. Further appointments will include tests for serology, to note if there is any involvement of adjacent structures, and a 2-hour 2-glass urine test. For this last test the patient should come to the clinic without having passed any urine for the 2 hours previous to the appointment.

LYMPHOGRANULOMA VENEREUM

In some classification systems lymphogranuloma venereum (LGV), is also referred to as: lymphogranuloma inguinale, lymphophathia venereum and Durand–Nicolas–Favre disease. The causative organism is Serotypes LI, LII, and LIII of the *Chlamydia trachomatis*. The incubation period is 5–21 days.

Mode of Transmission

Lymphogranuloma venereum is a sexually acquired disease which is endemic in West Central Africa, Madagascar, and the West Indies. Women appear to be asymptomatic carriers for the bulk of all patients are male. It is not unusual for LGV to be concurrent with other sexually transmitted diseases.

Signs and Symptoms

The primary lesion is a small papule which contains fluid and this enlarges to become a vesicle. This vesicle eventually erupts to develop into a painless ulcer of the genitalia.

Secondary lesions are due to the lymphatic spread of the causative organism from the primary lesion. Symptoms are wide ranging from malaise, pyrexia and rigors, and weight loss, to abdominal and joint pains. Local lesions involve enlargement of the inguinal glands which can lead to enlargement of the internal iliac, sacral, femoral and aortic lymph glands. These enlarged lymph glands can erupt to cause ulcers, fistulae or abscesses of the particular glands affected and there may be infective spread to the rectum and the vagina.

Examination

A wide ranging series of tests is completed to exclude the possibility of syphilis. If it is a primary lesion it should be possible to culture the *Chlamydia trachomatis* from a smear test. The haemoglobin level and the erythrocyte sedimentation rate are also assessed due to the nature and severity of the symptoms. If there is any doubt as to the causative organism of the lymph node enlargement and infectivity then a biopsy of the lymph gland affected may be taken.

Treatment

The primary aim is the resolution of any ulcers. In addition to local dressings and ulcer toileting, antibiotics, e.g., sulphonamides 2 g twice daily for 7–14 days, or tetracycline 500 mg four times daily for 14 days, may prove effective in treating both the sexually transmitted disease and promoting the healing of ulcers. In patients who have deferred from coming for medical help the antibiotics may be prescribed for up to 4 weeks. If the abscesses have developed into fistulae in the pelvic abdomen then rectal strictures may occur and require dilation. It is also a matter of routine to exclude malignancy.

The symptoms of pyrexia, abdominal pain, and rigors require specific treatment and it is usual to recommend a prolonged period of bedrest.

Advising the Patient

Following the resolution of ulcers, if they occur, patients will be reviewed monthly for 3 months, and their sexual contacts will be traced if they are within the country where the disease was diagnosed.

Chapter 9
Fungal Disorders

TRICHOMONIASIS

The causative organism of trichomoniasis is *Trichomonas vaginalis* (TV). This organism is a species of the protozoan family of Trichomonadides. It is a pear-shaped organism about 15–30 μu long (Fig. 9.1). Since it is heavily

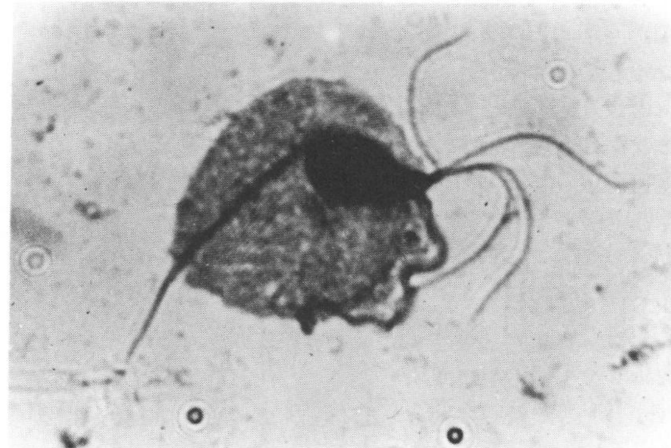

Fig. 9.1 *Trichomonas vaginalis.*

flagellated it is very motile. Its reproduction rate *in vitro* is known to be every 3.5–7 hours which would give considerable levels of infectivity following sexual contact. Since the trichomonas is found to be mixed with other organisms, and many of those who suffer TV are asymptomatic, the period between infection and symptoms arising is not clearly defined.

Mode of Transmission

For the most part trichomoniasis is a sexually transmitted disease, more so in the sexually promiscuous young age group. There is evidence that males can be carriers for short periods and with multiple sex partners such a person could infect previously uninfected women. Mothers may also transmit the disease to their daughters either at the time of birth or later when giving personal care to the infant. For surveys during the 1970s, 5–17.5% of the female population were assumed to be infected. In the male population it could account for about 15% of those presenting with NSU. It is also closely associated with the transmission of gonorrhoea.

Signs and Symptoms

Initially in females there is a slight vaginal discharge which may vary in colour, usually green or yellow. Such a discharge has a distinctive odour of *musty hay*. The walls of the vagina then become inflamed showing increasing evidence of weeping areas. This excoriation can then extend to the vulva, perineum, and inner thighs. The mucosa increasingly becomes oedematous, and the urethral meatus appears red and discharges an offensive exudate. Urinary frequency and dysuria are complained of and low abdominal pain would suggest the bladder has also become inflamed (cystitis). The combined effects of vaginitis and cystitis create difficulties with walking, sitting and moving. It is difficult to find comfortable undergarments to wear because of the intense pain caused by friction on the excoriated areas.

Males are for the most part asymptomatic, but may develop a painful urinary discharge and an obviously infected urine.

Examination and Investigations

With the female patient in the lithotomy position a bivalve speculum is inserted and local examination of the vagina may reveal a yellow green discharge. When cleared away, the inflamed areas of the vaginal wall and cervix are revealed. Bartholin's glands and Skene's glands may also be swollen and inflamed.

Smears are taken from the posterior fornix while the patient is still in the lithotomy position. Swabs are also taken to be prepared for fixed specimens so they can be stained by special techniques, i.e., Giemsa, Leishman and Papanicolaou's stains. If swabs are taken for culture and sensitivity testing they are despatched to the pathology department in a special medium. Cervical smears are also usually taken from the cervical os with an Ayre's spatula.

Since at least one third of all sexual contacts will have contracted the infection, all sexual partners will have to be traced and treated.

Treatment

A variety of antibiotics are available:

Tinidazole—2 g in a single dose

Nimorazole—1 g every 12 hours for 3 doses

Metronidazole (Flagyl)—2 g in a single dose

For vaginal and vulval oedema an application of gentian violet 1% will act as a very soothing agent to the mucosa.

Advising the Patient

Until a cure is established the patient should avoid all sexual contact. This will place a serious strain on those relationships where the partners are faithful to each other. A great deal of reassurance is sometimes required to both married partners that the disease is not always sexually transmitted.

If reinfection occurs then both the patient and the sexual consort must be treated even if one partner is asymptomatic. The female patient is usually given 3 appointments, each at a monthly interval when repeat smears are taken for culture and sensitivity to prove a cure has been established.

CANDIDIASIS

The other terms used to describe candidiasis include moniliasis and thrush. The causative organism is *Candida albicans*. This species of fungi thrives in a warm moist environment where there is a plentiful supply of carbohydrate nutrients. On staining for microscopy it appears as a flask-shaped organism radiating blue threads which are recognised as spores. It is Gram-positive and measures about 3–6 μu in length. In an innocent state this organism is part of the normal flora of the bowel.

There is no recognisable incubation period. It is calculated that about 25% of the female population in their reproductive years suffer from candidiasis, and of this number 5–30% produce symptoms. From such figures it is primarily a disease of women although it can be transmitted to a male during sexual contact.

Signs and Symptoms

Female Patients

In the female there is vaginal irritation accompanied by intense itching. Any vaginal discharge, if visible, is of a whitish colour. The inflammatory nature of the infection varies from being mild to severe and can be so intense as to cause pain and bleeding. The inflammation may spread from the vagina to include the labia, the immediate surrounding skin, the groin and across the thighs. Should the patient be obese it may involve the skin creases of the lower abdomen. The combined symptoms make it difficult to attain any comfort in sitting, walking, or wearing underclothing, and leads to both physical and psychological stress because of insomnia.

Male Patients

In the male, candidiasis is almost invariably the result of sexual contact. Initially there is urethral discomfort accompanied by a whitish urethral discharge. The inflammation of the skin can extend to the foreskin and glans penis, especially in those who are not circumcised. The localised inflammation of these two areas is referred to as balanitis, candidiasis being only one cause. The scrotum, groin and pubic region may also be involved, more so if the patient tends to obesity.

Possible Cause

In taking the history from the patient several points need to be excluded as possible causes.

1. Since the organism thrives in an environment rich in carbohydrate, diabetes must be excluded by urinalysis and blood sugar measurements.
2. The normal pH of the vagina alters in pregnancy allowing the organism to become pathogenic.
3. Currently prescribed antibiotics for another disease suppress or alter the normal flora in the vagina permitting *Candida albicans* to flourish.
4. Immunosuppressive drugs and steroids alter the normal pH of the vagina.
5. The use of the contraceptive pill if it contains oestrogen at high levels alters the normal flora of the vagina.
6. Malnutrition and debility from any cause will lower the patient's resistance and may allow micro-organisms of the gut to become pathogenic.

All of these causes have implications for those hospitalised and receiving any of the drugs mentioned. Note should be made of how quickly candidiasis can spread throughout a ward, the most likely cause of transmission between patients being the unwashed hands of the attending nurses. Fortunately in the ward situation, the disease affects mainly the oral cavity.

Treatment

After taking swabs, from the rectum and the vagina, or beneath the foreskin of the male, they will be despatched for culture and sensitivity.

One of the various fungicide creams is prescribed for topical application;

Amphotericin B 2.5%
Nystatin 2%
Clotrimazole 1%

These are applied daily to the affected areas for a period of 14 days.

Vaginal pessaries may be prescribed, e.g., Clotrimazole 100 mg, inserted high into the vagina each evening for 3 nights, or Nystatin can be used twice daily for 14 days then each night for a further 2 weeks. If the vulva is oedematous this means the patient will find it painful to sit or walk with any degree of comfort and a topical application of gentian violet 1% is soothing and comforting to the inflamed area. Its main disadvantage is that it stains purple.

Advising the Patient

In addition to the treatment the patient is advised on perineal and rectal hygiene. The undergarments should be loose fitting and made of light cotton; patients should not wear nylon next to the affected areas. Offensive body odour is a serious problem. Often the vaginal discharge smells of musty hay and a distinctive but pleasant perfume may be used to disguise the odour for the patient who is very conscious of how offensive it must be for others. Sexual partners should be traced, contacted and advised of their need for treatment especially if there are multiple partners involved.

If after the designated period of treatment the infection persists, the prescribed therapy is repeated. *Candida albicans* is a most persistent organism. If after 3 months of treatment the patient is still infected, a 28-day course of 2 povidone-iodine pessaries per day may bring about the desired cure.

GENITAL WARTS

The causative organism of genital warts (condylomata acuminata) is the papilloma virus which is morphologically similar to the virus causing skin warts. One major difference between them is that the papilloma virus prefers the moist surfaces provided by the genitalia.

The incubation period is 1–9 months but on average symptoms begin to appear after 2 months.

Between 70–90% of the incidence of genital warts is due to sexual contact. The virus gains entry into the submucosa via a minor abrasion of the mucous membrane. There is some suggestion that a second mode of transmission is by auto-innoculation, from the host's hand on his or her own or the partner's genitalia. In general terms the personal hygiene of the patient is below the accepted norm. The peak incidence for genital warts is between the ages of 18 and 24 years.

Signs and Symptoms

The first indication of the appearance of warts on or within the genitalia is a small pink or red minute swelling which grows in an upward direction. As it does so it becomes pedunculated. They can vary in size from 2 mm to 10 cm and can be either single or multiple in number. In the male, the warts appear either on the subpreputial sac, occasionally along the penile shaft, or within the urethral meatus. In the female, the warts may spread from the vulva to the perineum and perianal area. In addition they may grow on the walls of the vagina, and reach the cervix. In pregnancy there may be a rapid development of individual warts, but these are not regarded with any alarm as they usually recede within a reasonable period of time. In homosexuals the appearance of warts begins within the rectum and may spread to the perianal area.

Investigations

The clinical examination is sufficient to make the diagnosis. The venereologist may take scrapings from the warts and prepare them on a slide for dark-ground microscopy to exclude the possibility of the warts being due to syphilis, i.e., condyloma lata. A biopsy of larger warts is sometimes taken to exclude a premalignant fungating carcinoma. A careful history is essential which should evaluate the sexual contacts over the probable period of incubation, i.e., at its longest 9 months.

Treatment

Syphilis and any other condition like an accompanying sexually transmitted disease, e.g., trichomoniasis or candidiasis are eliminated or corrected before the treatment of the warts can be started. Several topical applications are available and if one fails over a defined period of time they can be tried in turn:

Trichloracetic acid
Podophyllin 20%

Both these applications are applied directly to the wart several times each week until there is evidence of the warts receding. The surrounding healthy tissue, especially the mucous membranes, is protected by firstly applying liquid paraffin to minimise the discomforts of these alcohol based substances. After 2–4 hours the application is thoroughly washed off.

Alternatively, 5-fluorouracil cream 5% is applied to the warts located within the urethra, daily, for 5–7 days and then the condition reviewed.

Cryosurgery or freezing of the wart to −70° C using a special probe with nitrous oxide, through a protective application of petroleum jelly to prevent burns, is a successful and advanced treatment. The point of the freeze probe is applied to several parts of the wart for a period of about 1 minute each. Several treatments over a period of weeks is usually organised.

Advising the Patient

Either form of treatment will take on average 2–3 weeks and during this time the strictest personal hygiene of the perineum and perianal area must be carried out daily. Obviously the patient must have no sexual contacts during the treatment period and all previous contacts must be traced and examined, and if necessary treated.

Chapter 10
Viral Disorders

HERPES GENITALIS

Herpes simplex virus type 2 is the cause of herpes genitalis. The type 2 virus is distinct from type 1 which causes the cold sores around the lips and mouth. Type 2 virus is exclusive to the genitalia and is one of 70 viruses with similar structure, e.g., chickenpox, shingles and infectious mononucleosis or the 'kissing disease'.

The virus is moderately contagious and symptoms occur 4–5 days after sexual contact.

Signs and Symptoms

Crops of minute itchy superficial blisters develop over and around the genitalia. The blisters are fluid-filled and cause intense burning and itching which leads to incessant scratching. As a result of this the blisters erode leading to minute ulcerated areas which eventually heal over, being sealed by a yellow crust. While in the ulcer stage they are painful and tender and the inguinal glands become overtly enlarged. When they erupt the blisters shed millions of viruses which are transmitted to any sexual contact. The virus remains within the body of the original infected person who therefore remains an infective host. If left untreated the ulcers tend to heal within 10 days. If a secondary infection occurs the healing is accompanied by scarring and takes about 21 days.

In males, the crops of blisters may occur over the prepuce, glans penis or along any part of the penile shaft. In females, the blisters tend to affect the labia majora, the labia minora, the clitoris and the introitus. Rarely if ever do the blisters proceed to a necrotic ulcer. There may be low back pain but this would be associated with the problems of walking, sitting, or failing to gain a comfortable position when lying down due to the persistent nature of the itching and burning sensations.

Investigations

All smear tests will prove negative, since the virus cannot be viewed through normal microscopes. Swabs or scrapings from the ruptured blisters are despatched for virology tests. It is essential to establish all sexual contacts from the previous 14 days so they also can be treated. It is a routine matter to investigate and exclude the possibility of gonorrhoea and syphilis.

Herpes genitalis tends to be of a recurring nature, the patient may be prone to as many as 6 or 12 attacks per annum. If this is the case the investigations may indicate the need to do a cervical smear for female sufferers to exclude cancer. There is a growing belief that recurring herpes genitalis is linked to cancer of the cervix.

Treatment

There is no specific treatment for herpes genitalis although there are many palliative measures which can be taken to alleviate the symptoms until they run their course. Scrupulous hygiene of the genitalia and perineum may seem obvious but it does need to be reinforced as one simple measure. Applying a mild solution of salt water to the affected area brings a great deal of relief from the itching and burning. After such douching if the area is kept clean and dry the healing is usually quicker. If the itching is unbearable an application of ethyl ether usually brings instant relief.

The blisters when ulcerating will cause severe pain especially if they are located over skin creases. Analgesia may be required to encourage the patient to rest. Topical applications of cytosine arabinoside or idoxuridine (IDU, Herpid or Kericid) applied to the affected area daily for 4 days are especially effective against gross blistering. Should inguinal adenitis be present the patient may be prescribed sulphamethoxypyridazine 0.5 mg twice daily or once a week, or a similar dose of tetracycline.

Advising the Patient

Recurrence of the blisters after a course of treatment would indicate that the virus is parasitic to the host tissues and the patient must be advised to come back immediately for further investigation and treatment.

The patient must not have any sexual contact until after the virology tests prove negative.

ACQUIRED IMMUNE DEFICIENCY SYNDROME (AIDS)

In the period between 1980 and 1985 over 7500 cases of acquired immune deficiency syndrome (AIDS) were reported in the USA. Of this number 95% were male homosexuals of which 70% subsequently died as the result of AIDS. The disease has been reported in the UK (264 cases with 20000 carriers), France, Denmark and Canada but in much smaller numbers. With a prediction factor of at least a 5% increase each year in the numbers affected it can be estimated that at least 1 million people will be affected by 1990, either suffering the full syndrome or being carriers of the causative virus.

Signs and Symptoms

The term *syndrome* implies that the patient is suffering from a variety of diseases at the same time. Classically the patient presents as a male homosexual who has been feeling progressively ill for some time. He may complain of extreme lassitude, anorexia, loss of weight and minor infections which do not respond to antibiotic therapy. His history may show that he has had a venereal disease in the past, e.g., gonorrhoea, syphilis or non-specific urethritis. Certain features will present and careful questioning usually elicits if:

The patient is sexually promiscuous and has many contacts.

Anal or oral intercourse has taken place within the last 3–36 months.

Drug abuse has been used to enhance sexual pleasure; this is a common finding. The patient usually develops certain diseases at the same time, these are: *pneumonia*, caused by pneumocystis carinii leading to fibrous scarring of lung tissue; *Kaposi's cancer*, which is a rare skin malignancy due to the Epstein-Barr virus; and *neurological disorders* of a variable nature which may present as a psychosis, seizure, flaccid paralysis, muscular weakness or dystonia, and incontinence.

Diagnosis

Present research indicates that the cause is the HTLV III (Human T cell Lymphocytic Virus). In addition in all cases of AIDS where blood has been cultured for virology, both the Epstein-Barr and cytomegalovirus have also been isolated. It is suggested that these viruses gain entry into the blood stream via the rectal mucosa or the oral cavity mucosa and that the virus is transmitted via the semen.

Once established, the virus remains latent for a long period, between 3 months and 3 years. Eventually the virus attacks the protective B lymphocytes which confer immunity upon the individual. Without such immunity the patient is prone to a multiplicity of infections from a wide source of pathogens. Pathologically a severe imbalance occurs between the B lymphocytes which are protective and the T lymphocytes which are suppressive. Their normal levels are reversed permitting the immune system to be overwhelmed.

Those at Risk

Although primarily a disease confined to male homosexuals it has affected other population groups.

Haemophiliacs are dependent on a substance called Factor VIII which promotes the clotting of blood. Since Factor VIII was mainly obtained from sources in the USA, any contaminated supplies would naturally be transmitted to innocent haemophiliac patients, some of whom have consequently contracted AIDS. The problem of Factor VIII supply and source has been overcome and the Blood Transfusion Service now routinely screen all male donors to exclude those who are homosexually active.

Haitian people are not homosexually orientated yet in the early 1980s the disease affected a significant number of their male, and a few of the female, population. The only theory that can be postulated to account for this epidemic is that bisexual males on holiday to Haiti infected the native women who in turn infected the native male population.

Prostitutes are not usually associated with AIDS but a few deaths have occurred in their number. It is possible that rectal or oral sex with a bisexual client has occurred.

Several *children* have been born to mothers who have been in sexual contact with an AIDS sufferer. The child is usually born healthy but in a few months develops all the features of the syndrome. This suggests that the virus has crossed the placental barrier and remained latent until several months following the birth.

Treatment

The final outcome of this syndrome is usually hospitalisation for intensive treatment with combination therapy of antibiotics and antiviral drugs to deal with the multiplicity of infections usually present, either: thymosin, an extract from the thymus gland known to boost immunity; phoscanite; H.P.A. 23; cyclosporin; or A.Z.T. These drugs are currently being prescribed on a trial basis and until a vaccine becomes available the prognosis remains very poor. A major consideration is that by publicising the known facts those who are prone will take sensible precautions to avoid becoming infected. It also needs to be stressed that it is a *sexually* transmitted disease and cannot be contracted by normal social interactions.

Clinical Precautions

Recommendations from the DHSS to nursing and medical staff who are dealing with patients admitted to hospital with AIDS include the following guidelines;

There is no evidence to support the assumption that the disease can be contracted by casual social contact, but clinical precautions should be taken as for any infectious disease

1. The prime risk to hospital staff is parenteral transmission by accidental self innoculation or entry of infectious material through an abrasion of the skin or mucous membranes. The utmost care must be taken to avoid self inoculation by needle injury, in dressing open wounds, when dealing with skin lesions, in the correct disposal of infected material or excreta.

2. Specimens of blood, excreta, wound swabs or saliva should be collected only by wearing disposable gloves, a plastic apron and eye goggles. Containers used should be disposable plastic, screw-capped and double-bagged with the correct coded labelling, i.e., labelled 'infected' before being despatched to the laboratory with the correctly labelled pathology forms.

3. Patients with AIDS should be nursed in isolation, preferably a single room, and the entry and exits to the room should clearly identify it as being a isolation area. This implies the wearing of gloves, plastic aprons and a strict handwashing technique before and after invasive procedures or the giving of personal care.

4. The Control of Infection Officer must be advised of the patient's admission, all other staff with direct patient contact should also be advised of the risk, without breaching confidentiality or causing embarrassment to the patient and family.

5. Personal clothing, soiled linen and bedclothing must be double-bagged, correctly sealed and labelled 'infected' before being despatched to the laundry.

6. Food waste, paper, soiled dressings must be double-bagged before being incinerated.

7. Medical and other nondisposable equipment must be thoroughly washed and dried before being employed in other ward areas.

8. Blood and excreta spills on work surfaces should be cleansed away using either Hypochlorite Solution with Chlorine, or Gluteraldehyde 2%.

9. It should be borne in mind that AIDS sufferers are prone to a wide variety of infections and additional precautions may be necessary.

10. Accidental self inoculation, i.e., needle injury must be dealt with immediately by encouraging free blood flow and liberal washing with soap and water. Such accidents must be reported to, and recorded by, the nurse manager in charge of the unit.

Chapter 11
Parasitic Disorders

SCABIES

The causative parasite of scabies is *Sarcoptes scabiei* (Fig. 11.1). This parasitic mite's preferred habitat is to burrow and thrive just below the epidermis. After the male mite fertilises the female, he dies. The female then burrows her way into the skin to lay her eggs, approximately 4 eggs every day for 8 weeks. The adult female in turn dies. Once her eggs have hatched they become known as nymphs and repeat the reproductive process.

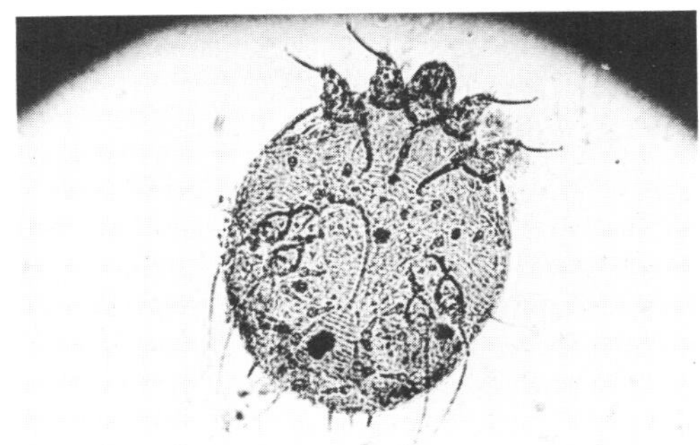

Fig. 11.1 *Sarcoptes scabiei.*

The incubation period is about 1 month before the patient shows any symptoms of the infestation. The scabies mite can only transfer from its host to another person on prolonged body contact.

Signs and Symptoms

The severe itching which the mite causes is especially noticeable at night when the body is particularly warm. The areas commonly affected by the burrowing and the resulting itching are the skin between fingers and toes, the wrists, ankles, axillae, buttocks and genitalia. These areas may appear lumpy and rather red and sore from persistent scratching. Should the skin become sensitive to the mite then the burrowed areas may erupt resulting in ulceration.

Examination

The presence of the mite cannot be viewed directly but scrapings taken from the burrowed sites and placed on a glass slide can be viewed through the microscope to reveal the mite. There will be a distinctive rash-like appearance over the areas of the body most likely to be affected. A history of recent sexual contacts or close body contacts will also be required.

Treatment

First the patient must take a very hot bath. On each succeeding night, for 3 nights, one of a number of lotions is applied over the whole body, and it is essential to emphasise the *whole body*.

Benzyl benzoate application BPC

Gamma benzene hexachloride application BPC

Sulphur ointment

On the fourth night the patient has another hot bath to remove the applied lotion and the skin should be free of the infestation.

In addition to this routine type of treatment for which hospitalisation may be necessary, gonorrhoea and syphilis are excluded by smear and serology tests.

Advising the Patient

The patient should deal with clothes and bedlinen in the same manner as with the crab louse. Since the treatment takes 4 days, he or she will have to be advised to remain out of circulation and to rest, until the treatment phase is over.

PEDICULOSIS (NITS)

The crab louse *Phthirus pubis* (Fig. 11.2) or *Pediculus pubis* (Fig. 11.3) is usually exclusive to the pubic hair. In severe cases it will also cause infestation of the perianal, thigh, chest, axillary, and eyebrow hair, but never the scalp hair. The female lays her eggs at the base of the hair, about 2 or 3 eggs per day for a week. The eggs are then cemented to the hair, and each egg is ensconced in a protective sac of a hard protein substance called chitin. It takes about one week for the eggs to hatch and then the cycle of infestation recommences.

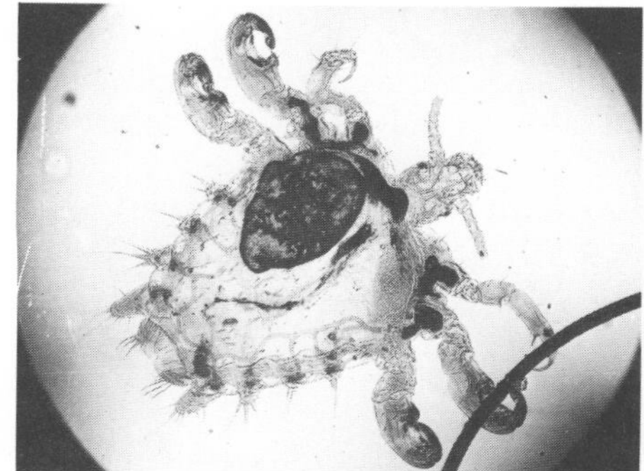

Fig. 11.2 *Phthirus pubis.*

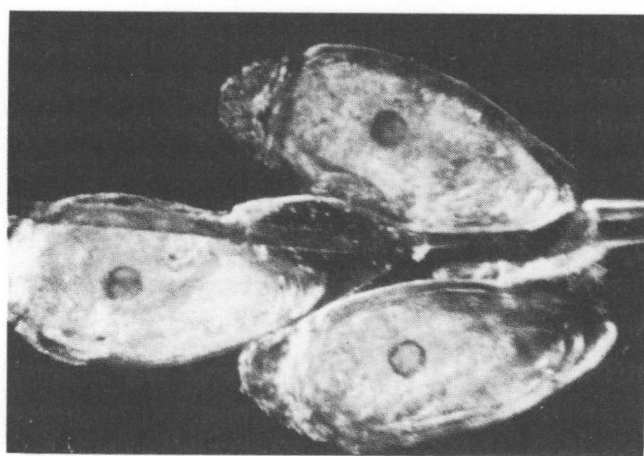

Fig. 11.3 *Pediculus pubis.*

It takes about 1 month before the initial symptoms of infestation appear.

The specificity of the region of the body which the parasite prefers indicates that it will only transfer from its host to another person who is in close proximity. For this reason, it has been grouped under the sexually transmitted diseases. It can however also be transmitted from bedclothing to those sharing a bed, towels being shared, and from toilet seats.

Signs and Symptoms

The parasite can only survive on a warm skin which also provides a blood supply on which it can feed by puncturing the skin at regular intervals. This repeated skin puncturing leads to a severe itch of the pubic region, and if the scratching is over vigorous it can lead to secondary infection of the puncture sites. On close examination of the pubic hair it is possible to see the adult louse with the naked eye. This often brings the patient forward for treatment and advice. The infestation is closely related to other sexually transmitted diseases, the symptoms of which may also bring the patient forward.

Treatment

There is a variety of skin lotions available:

Dicophane application BPC

Gamma benzene hexachloride application BPC 0.5%

Either of these are applied to the skin and hair with a small brush. The area to be covered is from the umbilicus to the knees, it includes the front and back of the body as well as the perineum. The lotion is then allowed to dry. On the second night the patient can have a bath and the lotion is reapplied and left alone for a further 2 days.

Another alternative treatment is to apply malathion lotion every day for 14 days. This treatment would ensure that the eggs are dealt with after they have hatched. The chitin sac is impervious to the malathion lotion, hence the need for treatment over 14 days.

Anyone who has been in close body contact, and this includes children of any infested adult, must also receive the same treatment. Equally, sexual contacts will require to be traced if any other sexually transmitted disease is diagnosed at the same time.

Advising the Patient

There is absolutely no need to shave the hair from the pubic area. The lotion will ensure the eventual destruction of both adult crabs and their eggs within the time scale of treatment. Some patients insist on shaving, regardless of advice.

Clothing which is worn does not require any dramatic cleansing method. It is enough to leave them hanging for 2 days undisturbed as this will ensure the adult louse will die, they require both body warmth and blood to survive.

Bedding requires the same treatment, the bedclothes should be turned back during the daytime and the bedroom well ventilated. Needless to say if there are crab lice there may be other parasites which would require stronger measures, i.e., disposing of the bedclothes by burning.

Part 2
Gynaecology and Obstetric Training

Chapter 12
Overview of the Female Reproductive Tract

The female reproductive tract is divided into two main areas: the external organs of reproduction, or genitalia, and the internal organs of reproduction. Additional to these, the nurse should include in study the accessory organs, the breasts (mammary glands), and have a working knowledge of the pelvic girdle and the muscles of the pelvic floor, to ensure a comprehensive understanding of the tract.

THE EXTERNAL ORGANS

The genitalia are collectively known as the **vulva** (Fig. 12.1) and are made up of the following structures:

Mons pubis
Labia majora
Labia minora
Clitoris
Vestibule
Vaginal orifice
Hymen
Bartholin's and Skene's secretory glands

The **mons pubis** is a raised area of fat lying over the symphysis pubis, its covering skin containing abundant hair follicles. Continuing downwards from this pad of fat are two folds of tissue, the **labia majora**, which form the lateral walls of the vulva. These tissue folds cover and protect the urethral and vaginal orifices.

Lying inside these outer folds are two thinner folds of connective tissue, the **labia minora**, which join at the back of the vagina to form the fourchette. The **fourchette** is a tissue fold which may tear during childbirth.

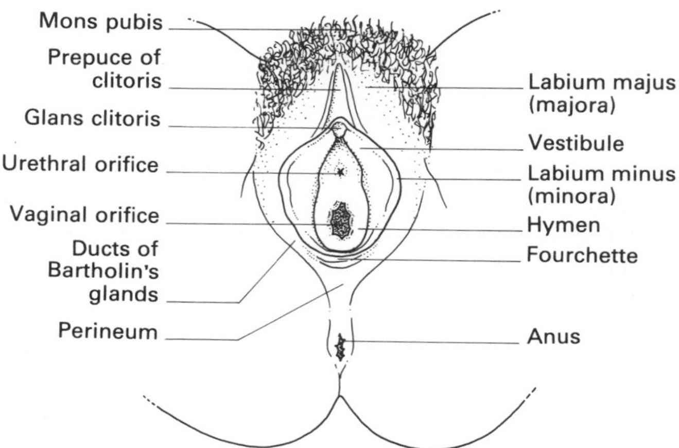

Fig. 12.1 Female external genitalia—the vulva.

The labia minora are particularly sensitive, containing erectile tissue. Anteriorly, the labia minora cover the **clitoris**, the homologue of the male penis.

When parted, the folds of the labia minora reveal the **vestibule**. This is a smooth almond-shaped area onto which the ducts of the vestibular glands, the *orifice* of the urethra and the vagina open. Partially (or sometimes wholly) occluding the vaginal orifice is a connective tissue covered by mucous membrane, the **hymen**. The hymen (maidenhead) may vary in density, though is usually thin, or may be completely absent. It will be broken following sexual intercourse and/or excessive physical activity.

At each lower end of the labia minora are the greater vestibular secretory glands, **Bartholin's glands**. Each gland is about the size of a small pea, bean-shaped, and covered with dense fibrous tissue. Both glands secrete mucus which lubricates the vaginal orifice and vulva. Bartholin's glands are not palpable in the healthy female.

The paraurethral (**Skene's**) glands are vestigial, and a homologue to the male distal prostrate glands. They are classified as the lesser vestibular glands.

The external genitalia receive their arterial blood supply from the internal and external pudendal arteries. The former rises from the internal iliac artery, while the latter arises from the femoral arteries. The vulval veins combine to form a large venous plexus which drains into the internal iliac vein. Lymphatic drainage of the external genitalia is via the superficial inguinal lymph nodes located at the groin. Minor branches of the pudendal nerve arise from the sacral level and innervate the vulva.

Extending from the fourchette to the anus is an area of skin called the **perineum**. This triangular shaped area is composed of fat, muscle and connective tissue. It is an important area of attachment for muscles from the pelvic floor. The junction created by muscles from each side of the vagina and rectum forms the perineal body. This particular area is subject to considerable stress during pregnancy and childbirth. Any weakness of this area tends to cause the contents of the pelvic floor to prolapse and press into the vagina or rectum.

THE INTERNAL ORGANS

The internal organs of the female reproductive tract (Fig. 12.2) lying within the pelvic cavity consist of:

- The vagina
- The uterus and cervix
- The right and left uterine (Fallopian) tubes
- The right and left ovaries

Related to these structures are the urinary bladder, pelvic ureters, urethra, rectum and anal canal. There is a complex lymphatic, blood and nerve supply which has deep implications for both gynaecological and obstetric problems.

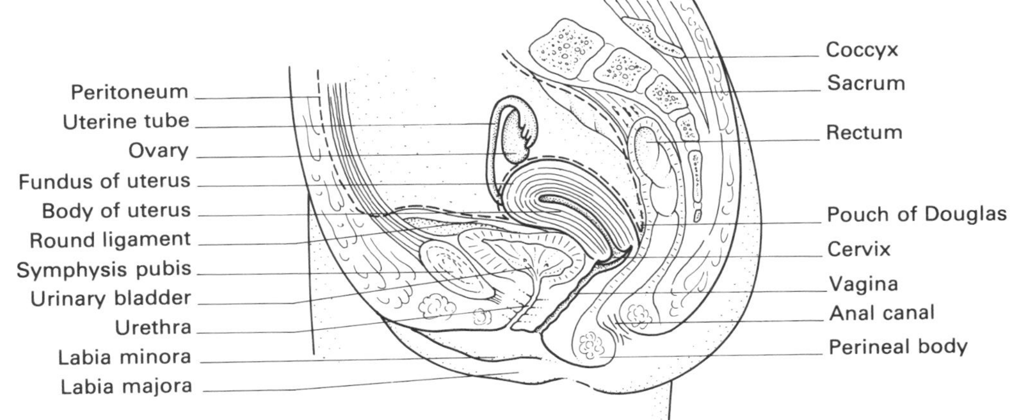

Fig. 12.2 Sacral view of internal reproductive organs.

The Vagina

Tubular in shape, the vagina extends from the vestibule to the cervix of the uterus. Its anterior wall extends for about 7.5 cm while the posterior wall is slightly longer, about 9 cm in length. It is composed of three layers of tissue which from within outwards are:

A lining of mucous membrane arranged in folds (rugae) and composed of squamous epithelium.

A middle muscular coat made of smooth plain muscle capable of great distension.

An outer layer of fibrous tissue which is continuous with the pelvic fascia.

The anatomical structures related and near to the vagina are the rectum and anal canal posteriorly, with the bladder and urethra lying anteriorly. All these structures are placed under stress during childbirth. In function the vagina receives seminal fluid during sexual intercourse, serves as the lower end of the birth canal and is an excretory route for uterine secretions and the menstrual flow.

The Uterus and Cervix

The uterus, a thick-walled hollow muscular structure (Fig. 12.3), is about 7.5 cm in length and lies in the pelvis, tilted between the urinary bladder and the rectum. Its position is anteverted, i.e., tilted forwards so that the anterior-inferior surface rests on the dome of the urinary bladder and its posterior-inferior surface is in contact with the small intestine.

The uterus is divided into 3 main anatomical areas:

The *cylindrical lower portion* which penetrates downwards and backwards into the vagina and is known as the **cervix**

The *body of the uterus*, which takes up at least two-thirds of its total size and is anatomically continuous with the cervix but at an angle to the cervix

The *upper rounded end* which is positioned beyond the line of attachment for the uterine (Fallopian) tubes and is called the **fundus.**

Although the uterus is hollow, it has 3 coats or layers which are in close approximation with each other. From within outwards these coats are:

1. An **inner endometrium** arranged in a strata of 3 special types of tissue:

The *Strata Compactum*, or compact surface composed of a layer of partially ciliated epithelium

The *Stratum Basale*, a dense layer of tissue composed of loose connective tissue

The *Stratum Basale*, a dense layer of tissue immediately connected to the middle coat and called the *myometrium*

The endometrium is of variable thickness, from 0.5 mm to 5 mm, the thickness of the coat being related to the menstrual cycle. The endometrium is where nidation takes

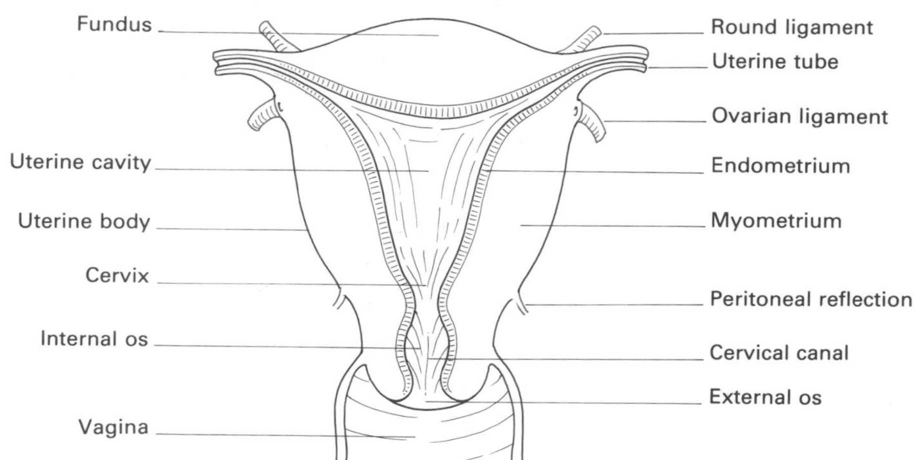

Fig. 12.3 The uterus.

place. **Nidation** (*nidus*, meaning 'nest') is the development of the epithelial lining within the uterus each month. When a fertilised ovum is received and burrows into this lining this is known as **implantation**. If no fertilised ovum is received, the lining is sloughed off in the next menstrual period.

2. The **middle layer**, or **myometrium**, is a thick muscular coat in which the smooth muscle is arranged in oblique, transverse and longitudinal layers, ensuring enlargement in every direction. The muscle arrangement also gives the uterus great strength.

3. The **outer layer** is derived from the parietal peritoneum, which is an incomplete covering for the uterus. Only part of the uterine body is covered and the cervix has no peritoneal protection, implying that surgery can be attempted on the cervix without putting the peritoneal cavity at risk.

During menstruation and following childbirth the compact and spongy layers are sloughed off and expelled either as menstrual flow or uterine excretions.

The anterior and posterior walls of the uterus are almost in contact, but in the coronal plane the body cavity is triangular, its apex pointing downwards towards the internal os which leads down into the cervical canal. At its lower end, the cervical canal constricts to form the external os which opens into the vagina. The functions of the cervix, internal and external os are to act as small sphincter muscles. During pregnancy both sphincters remain closed, being composed of mainly fibroelastic tissue. At the upper outer angles of the uterus, the uterine tubes open into the body of the uterus.

The uterus is kept in place by surrounding organs, muscles of the pelvic floor and ligaments derived from the peritoneum. Ligaments such as the broad ligaments travel from either lateral wall of the uterus to the lateral pelvic wall securing the uterus in place. Running through the layers of the broad ligament are the uterine blood and lymph vessels, and the ovary is located on the upper border of the broad ligament.

A second ligament, the round ligament, is a narrow fibrous band travelling from either lateral uterine wall through the broad ligament, down into the inguinal canal to end at the labium majorus. Between the rectum and the uterus, the peritoneum is reflected to create a small space known as the *rectouterine pouch*, or the Pouch of Douglas.

In function, the uterus receives the fertilised ovum into the endometrium (implantation), where it is retained and nourished as it develops from embryo to fetus. The myometrium, when contracted, expels the developed fetus.

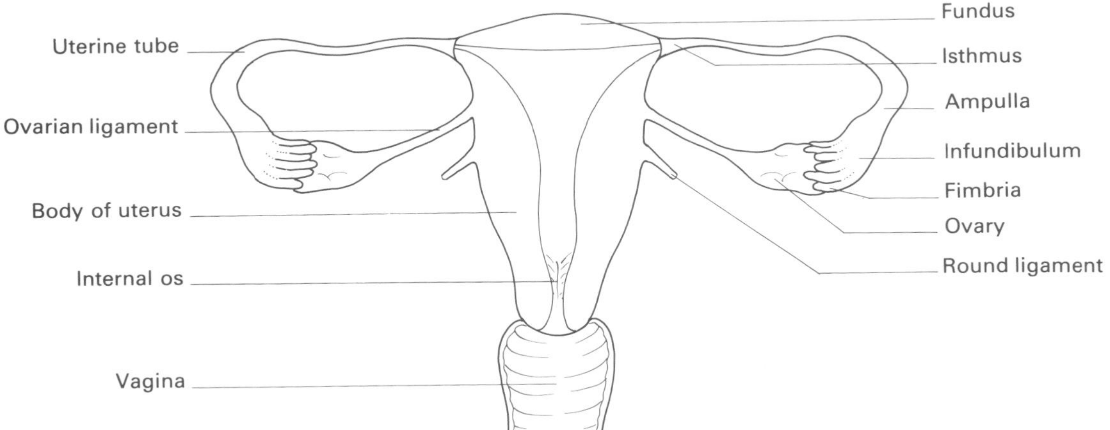

Fig. 12.4 Uterus, ovaries and uterine tubes.

The arterial blood supply to the uterus is supplied via the right and left uterine arteries which follow an extremely tortuous course, deriving from the internal iliac arteries. The uterine artery anastomoses with the ovarian artery which supplies not only the ovary but the uterine fundus. Venous drainage of the uterus is into the internal iliac veins. Lymphatic drainage is by 1 of 3 channels:

1. The fundus is drained of its lymph via the vessels travelling through the round ligament to reach the inguinal nodes.
2. The uterine body is drained by vessels travelling through the broad ligament to reach the aortic lymph nodes.
3. The cervix is drained via the external and internal, and sacral lymph nodes.

This complexity of lymph drainage needs careful thought if an understanding is to be obtained about the various operations which may be carried out on the uterus.

The Uterine Tubes

The uterine (Fallopian) tubes are about 10 cm in length. They extend from the lateral angle of the uterus to reach each ovary. Each ovary lies in the free upper margin of the broad ligament. At the ovarian end of the uterine tube there is a small orifice which opens directly into the peritoneal cavity. This orifice is surrounded by fringe-like projections called *fimbria* which have frond-like movements. The tubes are composed of 3 layers of tissue: an inner ciliated epithelium, a middle coat of smooth muscle and an outer peritoneal layer. These coats are continuous with the vagina and uterus and are relevant to an understanding of ascending infection into the tubes (*salpingitis*). Anatomically the tube is divided into 3 parts:

1. Extending from the lateral wall of the uterus, the first third of the tube is called the *isthmus*.
2. The intermediate or middle portion follows a complex course over either ovary, and is called the *ampulla*.
3. The terminal portion at the ovarian end opens directly into the peritoneum and is called the *infundibulum*

In function, the fimbria would guide a released ovum from the ovary into the mouth, or orifice, of the uterine tube. The ciliated epithelium would direct the ovum along the tube until it is discharged into the uterus. Fertilisation of the ovum by the sperm normally occurs in the uterine tubes.

The Ovaries

The ovaries are small ovoid-shaped, almond-sized endocrine glands lying either side of the uterus, each measuring about 4 cm long, 1.5 cm wide and 1 cm thick. They are held in

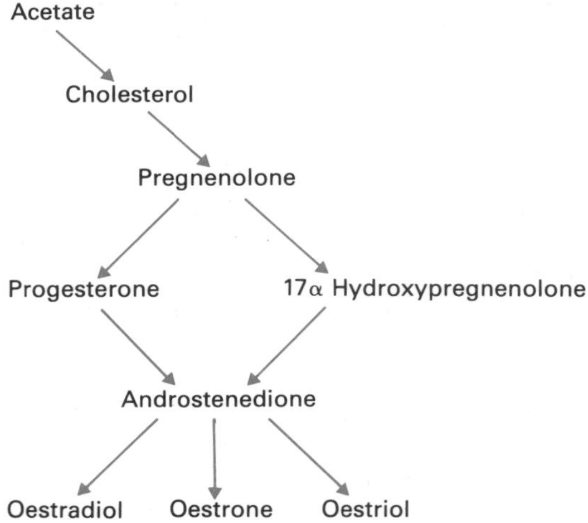

Fig. 12.5 Oestrogen biosynthetic pathways.

position by several ligaments, but are attached to the posterior surface of the broad ligament immediately below the uterine tubes.

The ovarian ligament links each ovary to the uterus, while the infundibulo-pelvic ligament connects the hilum of the ovary to the mesentery. The ovary has an external layer of germinal cells and primary underdeveloped ovarian follicles. These cells and follicles surround a central medulla of fibrous tissue or stroma, containing unstriated muscle through which run the blood vessels. At the hilum of the ovary, the ovarian artery nerves and lymphatic vessels enter, with the end branches reaching into the medulla or inner portion.

The cortex, or peripheral portion, of the gland contains the egg cells (**ova**) which will develop to different stages before being released as mature follicles, i.e., Graafian follicles. At birth the ovaries contain between 200 000 and 400 000 oocytes which will develop into various stages and then be stored until puberty and the menarche, i.e., the first period, or menstrual cycle. During the reproductive years only 400 or so eggs will actually ovulate and therefore many of the stored ova will regress.

As the ovum develops into firstly the primordial follicle and then progresses to a Graafian follicle, it releases oestrogen under the influence of the follicle stimulating hormone (FSH) secreted from the anterior lobe of the pituitary gland. After the Graafian follicle has ripened and reached the surface of the ovary, it ruptures (**ovulation**) and escapes into the peritoneal cavity. From here the released ovum is taken up by the Fallopian fimbriae and guided to the mouth of the uterine tube.

The ruptured follicle fills with a yellow pigment (**carotene**) and becomes known as the corpus luteum, or yellow body, and secretes progesterone. This secretion is influenced by the luteinising hormone (LH) which is also secreted from the pituitary gland. The whole purpose of the cycle of events of the menstrual cycle is to prepare the uterus for pregnancy. If the female becomes pregnant, the corpus luteum enlarges in diameter to about 5 cm, if not it degenerates and is shed with the menstrual flow.

Apart from the adult follicles and the corpus luteum, the oestrogens are also secreted from the placental unit and the adrenal cortex. The biosynthetic pathway for oestrogens shows that there are 3 oestrogen hormones (Fig. 12.5).

Oestrogens

In function, oestrogens are essential for:

During and after puberty, responsible for developing the female secondary sexual characteristics, i.e., broadening of the hips, fat accumulation in the breasts and buttocks, and increasing scalp and body hair.

During the reproductive years, to develop and maintain the secondary sexual structures, i.e., maintaining the excitability of uterine muscle, keeping the lining of the uterine tubes motile, rendering the cervical mucosa thinner and more alkaline for the safe transport of spermatozoa after coitus, and decreasing the circulating plasma cholesterol level.

Premenstrually, to retain sodium and water, in theory said to account for premenstrual tension.

During pregnancy, being responsible for the growth and development of the endometrium, stimulating myometrial growth, sensitising the myometrium to the stimulating effect of the hormone oxytocin, and stimulating the mammary ducts in readiness for lactation.

When the number of ova are exhausted from the ovaries and there is no further need for follicular maturation, the level of oestrogen will decline. Without this cyclical stimulation the female sexual structures will atrophy and start the beginning of the menopause.

Progesterone

Progesterone is secreted from the corpus luteum, from the placenta after the eighth to twelfth week of pregnancy and from the adrenal cortex. It should be noted that progesterone is secreted from the testes in the male.

In function, progesterone encourages secretory changes in the endometrium for pregnancy, i.e., the progestational stage. It also antagonises the effects of oestrogen on the myometrium, i.e., opposing uterine contractility in the early stages of pregnancy. Additionally, progesterone stimulates the development of the lobules and alveoli in the mammary tissue and increases the metabolic rate, body temperature and respiratory rate.

THE MENSTRUAL CYCLE

On reaching puberty, which in the Western world is approximately between 11 and 13 years of age the organs of reproduction begin to function. The ovaries are stimulated by 2 hormones released from the anterior lobe of the pituitary gland. These hormones are also known as *gonadotrophins*: the follicle stimulating hormone and the luteinizing hormone.

The menstrual cycle (*mensis* means 'a month') is a series of events occurring at regular intervals, about every 28 days and is very much a biorhythmic cyclical event during the reproductive years of a female's life (Fig. 12.6). Apart from the hormones being released from the pituitary, there are specific endometrial changes occurring in distinct phases: the proliferative, secretory and menstrual phases.

At the beginning of the proliferative

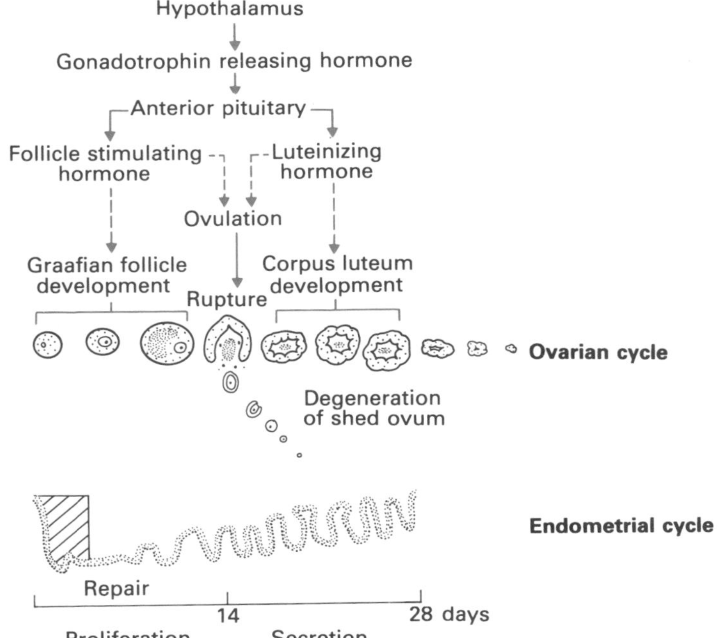

Fig. 12.6 Normal menstrual cycle.

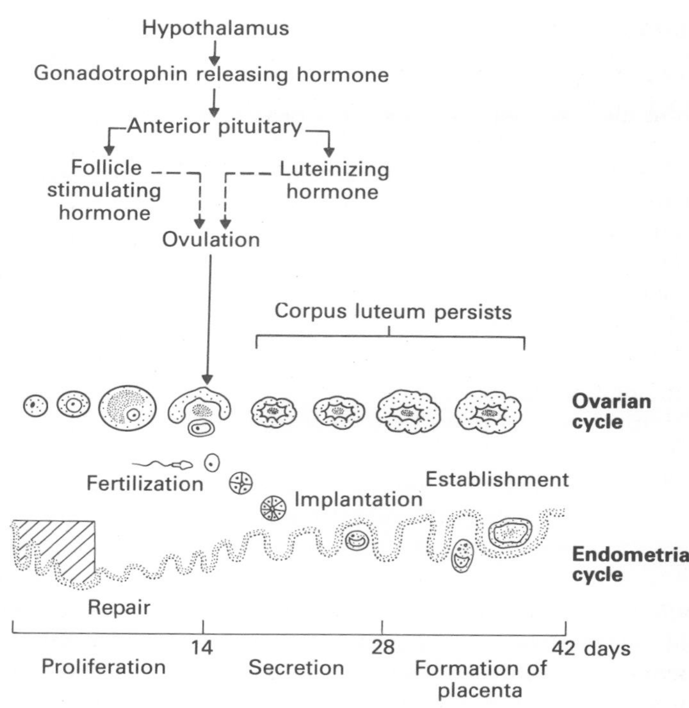

Fig. 12.7 Menstrual cycle ending in pregnancy.

(preovular) phase, which lasts for about 14 days, the follicle stimulating hormone (FSH) stimulates the primordial follicles in the ovary to grow and develop and release oestrogen. As the oestrogen is released, the FSH is diminished; an example of autoregulation.

The luteinizing hormone (LH) causes the mature follicles (Graafian) to rupture and release the ovum; this is *ovulation*. The Graafian cell wall then collapses and, in so doing, secretes oestrogen and progesterone. The progesterone now inhibits further release of the LH. Oestrogen has a direct influence on the endometrium, causing it to become thicker.

During the secretory phase, the release of more progesterone also causes further thickening of the endometrium. The endometrial glands become larger and the coat becomes more vascular. It is at this time that the endometrium is ready to receive the fertilised ovum. If this happens (Fig. 12.7), the endometrium becomes thicker and much more vascular, and is called the *decidua*. If the ovum is not fertilised, the rich endometrial coat is not required and is shed.

As the corpus luteum degenerates, the release of progesterone stops and the blood vessels supplying the endometrium go into spasm. This will result in endometrial ischaemia, causing the capillaries to rupture and ooze small amounts of blood. The cells on the surface layer begin to die, which causes more bleeding and the whole surface is sloughed off. The degenerated cells, blood, mucus and unfertilised ovum are excreted via the vagina as menstrual flow over the following 4 or 5 days.

The blood should not clot as it will have been defibrinated by the endometrial tissue. The volume lost amounts to between 50 and 100 ml of blood. Once the menstrual flow ceases, the endometrium begins to grow again to recommence the cycle.

The Menopause

Between the ages of 45 and 55 years the female reproductive years end, bringing about the menopause. Many of the physiological changes occurring at this time are summarised by the term *climacteric* or change of life. It implies that the stock of primordial follicles in the ovaries is exhausted and, without further ova, the menstrual cycle ceases. The cycle may cease abruptly, the time between menstrual periods may lengthen increasingly to eventual cessation, the menstrual flow may decrease slowly, or the cycle may become erratic or irregular before ultimately concluding.

Signs and Symptoms

Various symptoms and changes, both physical and psychological, are common. The reproductive organs and genitalia alter in size with the vulva and vagina gradually atrophying. Hot flushes resulting from vasomotor dilation produce sensations of heat, facial redness and perspiration. These may occur sporadically a few times a day or as frequently as every 10 or 15 minutes in an hour. Severe attacks often warrant treatment, either with mild sedation or small doses of oestrogen.

Psychological changes may involve irritability, lack of concentration and emotional turmoil. Some women experience severe depression, while others emerge from the menopause with a profound sense of well-being and relief.

There are certain physical changes which may take place as a result of a woman's depressed psychological state or because of oestrogen deficiency. These include: gastro-intestinal disturbances, urinary incontinence, and the growth of facial hair.

ACCESSORY ORGANS OF FEMALE REPRODUCTION

The Breast (Mammary Gland)

Each breast is a hemispherical prominence extending from the second to the sixth rib and from the sternum to the axillary midline. They lie on a layer of deep fascia which separates the breast from the thoracic muscles. The breasts are composed of three types of tissue: glandular, fibrous and fatty, or adipose (Fig. 12.8). The glandular tissue is arranged in 15 or 20 lobes, each lobe being further subdivided into lobules. In each lobule there are clusters of alveoli around a small duct.

The ducts unite to form a large excretory

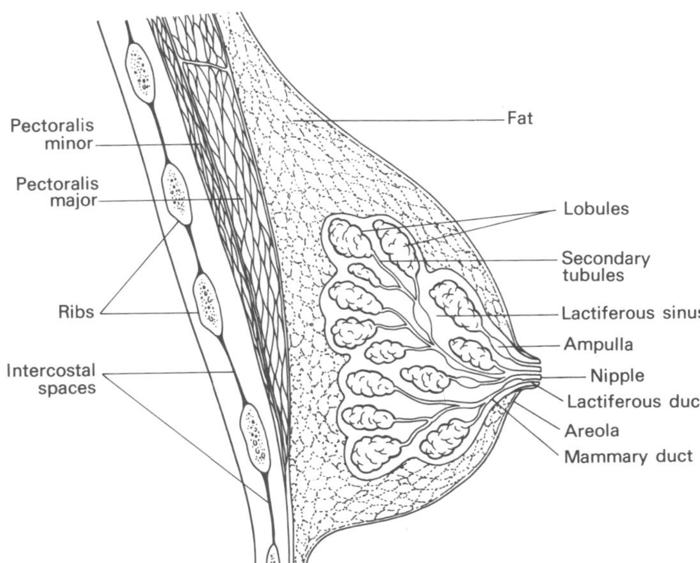

Fig. 12.8 Mammary gland (the breast).

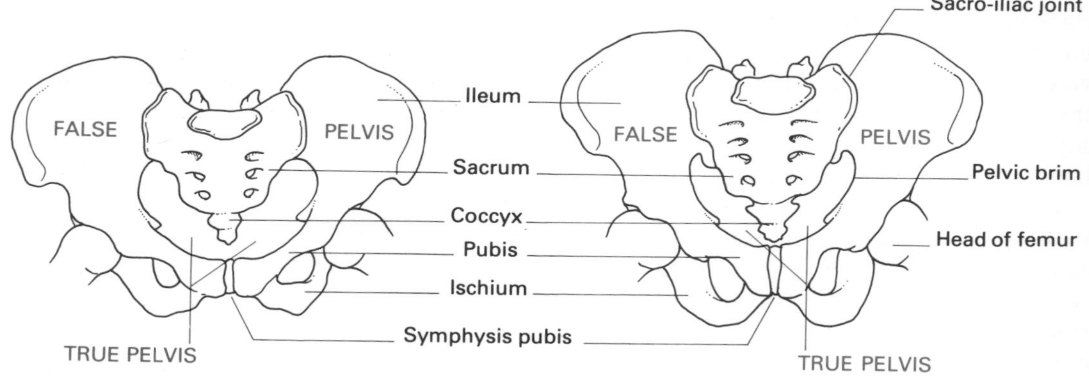

Fig. 12.9 Differences in angle between male pelvis (*right*) and female pelvis (*left*).

duct, i.e., the lactiferous ducts. These ducts converge to the centre of the breast to become dilated to form reservoirs for the milk, i.e., the *ampulla*, which become distended during lactation. Extending from these are narrow orifices which open onto the surface of the nipple. Lying between the alveoli are deposits of fatty tissue, the amount of fat determining the size of the breast. Dividing the lobules into distinct areas are bands of fibrous tissue which also help to form the suspensory supporting ligaments for each breast.

At the centre of each breast there is a conical prominence of erectile tissue which is the nipple. This is pigmented and can vary from pink, to dark brown after several pregnancies. This pigmented area is known as the *areola*, and on its surface are numerous sebaceous glands (Montgomery's tubules) which lubricate the nipple during pregnancy. The arterial blood supply is derived from the thoracic, internal mammary and intercostal arteries, while the venous drainage is via the circular venosus. This circle of veins is at the base of the nipple and drains venous blood into the axillary and mammary veins. Lymphatic drainage is quite extensive and pours into the axillary lymph nodes.

The functions of the breast are active during pregnancy and following childbirth. During pregnancy the breasts produce a substance known as *colostrum* which contains fat and protein and is present for 2 or 3 days following childbirth. The breast produces milk when stimulated by the hormone *prolactin*, secreted from the anterior lobe of the pituitary gland after childbirth. It is also stimulated by suckling, and this reflex action also produces oxytocin which stimulates milk formation.

Human milk has all the nutrients to satisfy an infant for 3 to 6 months, with the exception of iron and vitamin D. These may need to be supplemented in the infant's diet after several months of breastfeeding. Human milk contains fat, lactose, protein in the form of lactalbumen and caesinogen, calcium, phosphorus and vitamins A, B and C. It has an energy content of 70 kcal/100 ml and also confers maternal antibodies to the infant, giving immunological protection.

The Pelvis and Pelvic Floor

There are significant anatomical differences between the female and male pelvis (Fig. 12.9). These differences often account for the many discomforts and disorders seen in both gynaecological and obstetric nursing. For this reason nurses should review the structure of the female pelvis to increase their understanding of the patient's problems.

In comparison with the male pelvis, the female pelvic bones are lighter and smaller. Additionally, the pelvic cavity is shallower and more rounded, with the sacral bones being more concave. Lastly, the pubic arch has a wider angle. While the vertebral column takes the stress of body weight, such weight is transmitted through the pelvis. Excess weight and shape, as occurs in pregnancy, alters the vertebral column's centre of gravity towards the pelvis, implying the sacrum can tilt slightly backwards. It also means the pelvic bones must have great strength.

The pelvic girdle is composed of 3 bones, a right and left innominate and a fused sacral spine. Each innominate bone is a fusion of 3 smaller bones: the pubis, ileum and ischium. Anteriorly, the symphisis pubis in the female is shorter in length and points forwards and downwards to create a wider angle for the pubic arch. The sacroiliac joints are synovial in type, with supporting ligaments. During pregnancy this joint and the ligaments are made softer by hormones; this creates greater pelvic flexibility and capacity. The curve of the birth canal is formed by the concavity of the fused sacral bones and by the posterior wall of the symphisis pubis, implying that the infant must pass through the pelvis at a 90° angle.

The pelvic brim denotes the true pelvis below and the false pelvis above. In the female, the pelvic brim is heart-shaped and measures about 13 cm across and 11 cm from front to back. In the male, the pelvic brim is more triangular-shaped and much deeper. The pelvic outlet is diamond-shaped and measures about 11 cm across and 13 cm from front to back. These measurements are the reverse of each other, meaning that the infant's head must rotate as it descends through the birth canal. Viscera contained in the true pelvis must be adequately supported by the muscles of the pelvic floor.

Two sheets of muscle (the *levator ani*) arise from the lateral walls of the pelvis and join in the pelvic midline. These muscles are normally strong enough to support the pelvic viscera. Along the midline at the muscular junction, there are perforations for the openings of the rectum posteriorly, the vagina in the middle and the urethra anteriorly. Where the levator ani meet between the vagina and the rectum, they wedge together to form the perineal body. This structure is vital to the integrity of the pelvic floor. In this wedge of muscle are smaller muscles which control the anal and vaginal sphincters. This stretch of muscle covered by tissue and skin is known as the *perineum*. Weakness of the pelvic floor brought about by pregnancy may stress the levator ani and the perineal body, creating the potential for prolapse of the pelvic viscera at a later time.

Chapter 13 Examination, Investigations and Procedures

In meeting the needs of the gynaecological patient, the nurse has to be particularly sensitive to certain aspects of this specialist branch of nursing. Many patients are embarrassed in discussing problems related to their genitalia or reproductive organs. Some find it extremely distasteful to be frank and open about what may be a very personal and distressing problem. Underlying any problem of a gynaecological nature is a very real threat to an individual's own concept of her body image, i.e., her femininity. Even the most minor symptoms can be an alarming psychological threat to a person's feeling of well being.

Should the patient be from a non-Western culture, the nurse may experience the problem of religious restrictions and a language barrier. Commonly, in areas with large immigrant populations, the nurse may have to deal with the husband first and then the wife. Therefore, the nurse should be quite clear in her mind as to what degree the patient's spouse or partner is to be involved in any care or treatment that is proposed, allowing for the fact that practically all gynaecological units have an established policy of requesting the husband's written consent for many gynaecological procedures involving surgery.

If specialising in gynaecology, the nurse has to have explicit expertise and knowledge about the problems surrounding infertility, contraception, menstrual problems and the Abortion Act to advise patients with confidence. The constantly changing nature of available treatments in gynaecology requires that nursing techniques be perpetually updated and knowledge about current trends frequently reviewed. In taking a history from a patient, the nurse should obtain details about the social, personal and psychological aspects of the individual patient. Questions must specifically elicit details about the menarche, the dates of the menstrual period, problems being experienced during the menstrual cycle, if taking the contraceptive pill, or using other means of family planning, and a detailed midwifery history.

PHYSICAL EXAMINATION

For a routine physical examination, either in the outpatient department or on the ward, the nurse would need to assess and record the patient's blood pressure, pulse, and weight, and complete a routine urinalysis.

Required Equipment

In preparing to help the gynaecologist to make a full examination, the nurse would need to ensure that the necessary equipment and instruments are readily available. Endoscopy instrumentation should be clean and pretested before the actual examination.

1. An anglepoise lamp to provide an extra source of light
2. The examination couch or bed protected by clean disposable sheets
3. A lightweight blanket to keep the patient warm
4. The vaginal examination trolley equipped with:
   Sim's, Cusco's and Ferguson's specula
   Sponge-holding forceps
   Vulsellum forceps
   Sterile wool and gauze swabs
   Fetal stethoscope
   Obstetric cream or lubricating (KY) jelly
   Container for used instruments
   Disposable bag for soiled swabs
5. A proctoscope should be available
6. A tray equipped to take smears for exfoliative cytology containing:
   Ayre's spatula
   Glass slides with cover slips
   Alcohol 95% as a fixative
   Indelible pencil for marking the glass slide
   Laboratory forms.
7. A rectal tray should be available (examination of the virgin is not done via the vagina to avoid rupturing the intact hymen)

N.B. If a pregnancy is over 24–28 weeks or if the patient is aborting, a vaginal examination, if it is carried out, should always be completed as an aseptic technique. This implies that all equipment must be sterile and that sterile gloves should be provided.

Prior to Examination

Before the examination, the nurse ensures the privacy of the examining area, and advises the patient of what is involved to reassure her. Although possibly embarrassing for some, the examination is not usually painful and she will not be left unattended at any time during the examination. The patient should be free of all clothing except for a loose-fitting petticoat, nightdress or operating gown. If waiting for the examination, the patient should also be given a dressing gown to wear. As an empty bladder is essential for a gynaecological examination, the patient should be asked to pass urine, which can of course be routinely tested.

During Examination

Once the patient is resting on the examination couch and her clothing arranged to ensure modesty, the anglepoise lamp is adjusted to give added light. The examination usually proceeds in a logical pattern. The neck and thyroid are examined for obvious signs of enlargement. Both breasts and then the abdomen are palpated for obvious lumps or undue swelling. This is followed by a visual examination of the external genitalia, a digital and possibly a bimanual examination of the vagina, cervix, uterus, uterine tubes and the ovaries. A bimanual examination means that the external abdomen is palpated while the

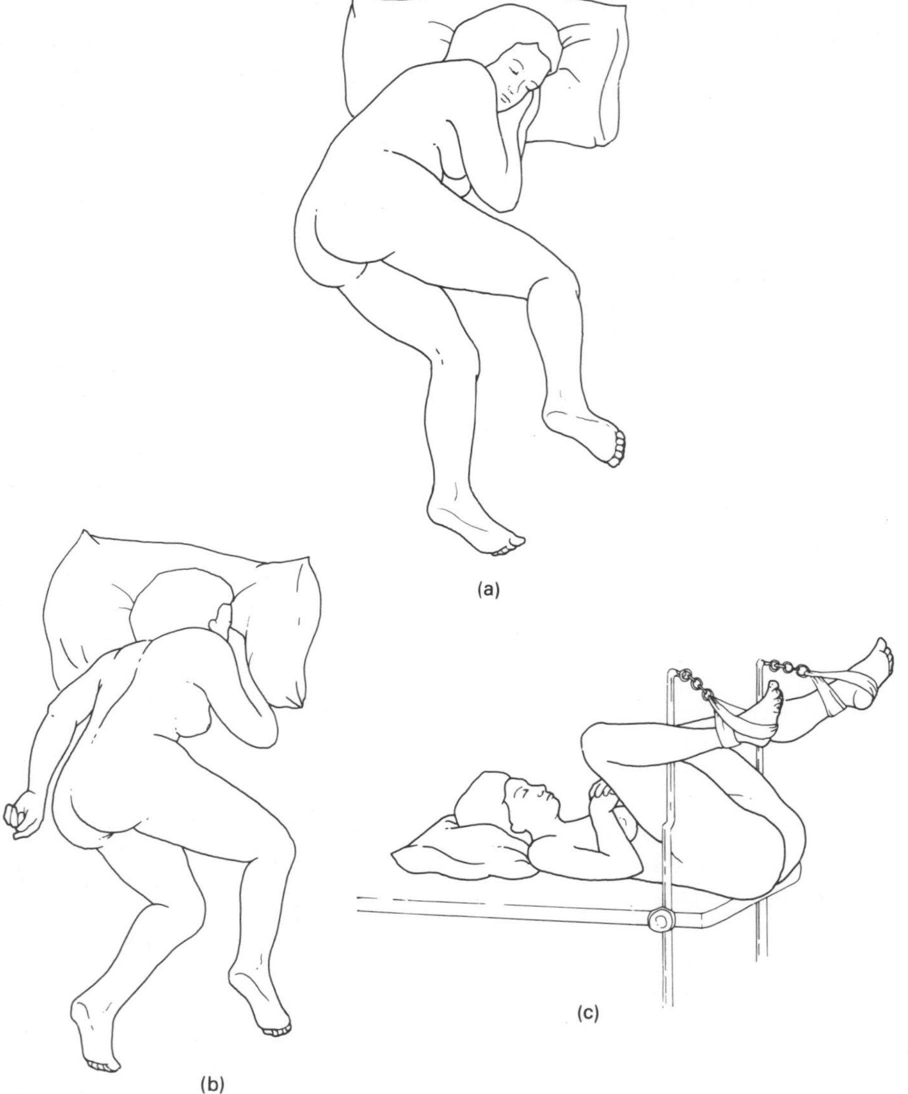

Fig. 13.1 Examination positions: left lateral (a); Sims's position (b), lithotomy position (c).

internal structures are palpated simultaneously. As the examinations proceed, the nurse has to ensure that the patient is relaxed and kept modestly covered, exposing only those areas being examined and maintaining complete privacy throughout the procedure.

During the examination, the patient may have to adopt differing positions to facilitate certain tests to be completed (Fig. 13.1). The positions commonly used during an examination include any of the following, and the gynaecologist will usually indicate the position of choice.

Dorsal Position

The patient rests on her back with both knees flexed and the thighs held apart. The arms are rested either side of the body and the head is supported with 1 or 2 pillows to prevent the abdominal muscles from becoming too tense. This is a useful position for a bimanual examination and for examination with a bivalve speculum.

Lateral Position

The patient lies on her left side, with both knees flexed and the buttocks placed parallel with the edge of the examination couch or bed. This may be used for the introduction of a Sim's speculum.

Sim's Position

With the patient remaining on her left side, the lateral position is adapted so that her left arm is brought up behind her back, the left leg is flexed to an angle of 30° at the hip and knee, while the right leg is flexed to an angle of 90°. The left leg is raised and supported while the Sim's speculum is inserted into the vagina.

Lithotomy Position

In the dorsal position, each leg is raised and supported in stirrups placed around the ankles. The buttocks are brought to the edge of a divided mattress or examination couch. This position is used during procedures requiring general anaesthesia, detailed bimanual examination, or for operations performed via the vagina.

Knee-chest, or Genupectoral, Position

The knee-chest, or genupectoral, is a kneeling position in which the head is supported on the patient's folded arms, while the buttocks are raised. Such a position permits access to the posterior fornix and allows viscera to fall away from the pelvic cavity to prevent possible injury during a colposcopy or culdoscopy. Culdoscopy is an endoscopic examination of the pelvic cavity approached via the posterior fornix and is an alternative to laparoscopy. Culdoscopy is rarely used.

Adapted Trendelenburg Position

While the patient is resting dorsally, the operating table is tilted to an angle of 45° or more. Both the head and shoulders require support with pillows and straps. A nonslip mattress surface is used. Both ankles are secured into stirrups at the end of the operating table.

After Examination

Following the physical examination, the gynaecologist may wish to take smears of the mucosa from the vagina and cervix. This is called a *Papanicolaou* smear and may detect cancer cells. Three scrapings are taken, one from the margin of the cervix, a second from the os and a third from the posterior fornix of the vaginal vault, using an Ayres' spatula.

All three scrapings are smeared onto a clean glass slide and fixed with 95% alcohol, allowed to dry, and then protected by a cover slip. The glass slide is carefully identified at its edge with the indelible pencil and, with a completed request form, despatched to pathology for exfoliative cytology. It is usual for the request form to ask for quite detailed information, which is used for cancer research purposes. Such information may include the following facts:

- The date of the patient's last menstrual period
- If she is pregnant
- Whether she is taking oral contraceptives
- The husband's occupation
- The approximate date of first coitus
- Clinical comment on the appearance of the vagina and cervix

These details are known to be useful in cancer research as they relate to the cause and incidence of cancer of the cervix. The Papanicolaou smear test is recommended as a screening test for all females over the age of 25 and those using the contraceptive pill. The test should be repeated every 2 years.

If the gynaecologist wishes, a high vaginal swab can be taken. The vulva is thoroughly cleansed and a Cusco's speculum is inserted into the vagina. A sterile wool swab is advanced through the speculum and its tip rotated on the wall of the cervix to obtain a moistened swab of the mucosa. This swab stick is then sealed in its container and despatched to pathology for culture and sensitivity tests to identify any organisms which may be causing vaginal infection.

HAEMATOLOGY

The majority of gynaecological patients are routinely screened for the following five blood tests:

Haemoglobin level to exclude or confirm iron deficiency anaemia

White blood-cell count if infection present

Erythrocyte sedimentation rate if there is inflammation present

Wasserman and VDRL to exclude or confirm venereal disease

Blood grouping, cross-matching, and Rhesus factor if the patient is either pregnant or going for surgery

Specific blood tests which may be requested are usually related to hormone levels. In summary, any of the following may be requested:

Follicle stimulating hormone
Luteinising hormone
Oestrogen levels
Progesterone levels
Tri-idiothyronine
Adrenaline and Noradrenaline
Cortisone

If requested, these blood tests usually relate to the investigations for infertility or menstrual disorder. An imbalance of any of these hormones would disturb the menstrual cycle, preventing ovulation from taking place.

URINALYSIS

A specimen of urine may be routinely collected as part of: a ward test, a midstream specimen of urine, or a catheter specimen. If a routine urinalysis is at all suspicious and suggests that there is an infection, it would then be necessary to collect a clean catchment of urine for more detailed examination.

When possible this type of specimen should be obtained from the patient in the ward bathroom. The patient should be advised to first have a thorough wash of the vulval areas, whilst having a shower or bath. Should the patient be suffering from a vaginal discharge it may be necessary for the nurse to plug the vaginal orifice with sterile cotton wool to avoid contamination of the specimen. Likewise, clothing should not be allowed to contaminate the recently cleansed vulval area or lower abdomen.

A sterile container (Boracin type) is placed over a clean bedpan without the inner rim of the specimen container being contaminated. Midway through the urinary stream, a catchment of urine is collected into the container and *immediately* sealed and correctly labelled before being despatched to pathology. If the specimens are for culture and sensitivity, they should be despatched within 30 minutes of their collection, or stored in a refrigerator.

The same procedure is followed for patients who are confined to bed, the nurse ensuring that the perineal and vulval areas are thoroughly cleansed before assisting the patient onto the bedpan. Only occasionally are specimens collected by catheter because urinary catheters, once introduced into the bladder, carry a high risk of causing urinary tract infection. However, if long-term indwelling catheters are necessary then catheter specimens are taken at frequent intervals to monitor the infection risk.

When there is a suspicion of hormonal imbalance, the gynaecologist may request a 24-hour urine collection for the assay of oestrogens, progesterone, catecholamines and 17 corticosteroids. This type of collection is commonly done in the outpatients department. There the patient is issued with special containers and given detailed instructions on when to start and conclude the specimen collection and to return the specimen to the department. If, however, the patient is unable to cope with these instructions, it may prove necessary to admit her for the 24-hour period during any weekday from Monday to Thursday.

Colposcopy

A colposcope is an operating instrument which, apart from giving a magnified view of the cervix, allows for minor cervical procedures to be completed. Although a painless procedure, it can last for a long time and does cause some discomfort so the patient requires a great deal of reassurance from the nurse during the actual procedure. Due to the anticipated discomfort, sedation may be prescribed and administered 30 minutes before the procedure begins.

Wearing only a loose-fitting operating gown, the patient is placed in the lithotomy position (see p. 105) on the operating table. The table is then tilted to an angle of 45°. Local anaesthesia may be used to dull the sensory responses of the vulva and cervix before the colposcope is introduced into the cervix. With variable magnification of up to 100 times, the instrument has several eye pieces allowing for several doctors to view at the same time. It also has a camera mount which can, if required, record the whole procedure on videotape for future reference.

The cervix is painted with a 3% solution of acetic acid or iodine to show up any abnormal areas. Tissue biopsy may be taken from any suspect areas before being treated with either *diathermy* (coagulation by heat probe) or *cryosurgery* (freezing by cold probe) for cancer in situ. Following colposcopy the patient requires a great deal of reassurance and needs to be informed of what was diagnosed and treated. The nurse should ensure that the patient has several hours' rest and that the vulva is protected by a maternity pad.

Endometrial, Vulval and Cervical Biopsies

Endometrial, vulval and cervical biopsies may be taken separately or in conjunction with a minor surgical procedure such as a dilation and curettage.

An endometrial biopsy can be obtained without general anaesthesia or dilating the os. A Novak's curette is introduced into the uterine cavity to obtain the tissue specimen. This biopsy is best taken after the fourteenth day of the menstrual cycle, in the proliferative phase, when the cells will reveal if ovulation and progesterone secretion are normal.

Vulval biopsy combined with biospy of the inguinal nodes may be pursued if there is leukoplakia of the vulva.

A cone biopsy, literally a cone-shaped piece of tissue, may be taken from the cervix in conjunction with a dilation and curettage procedure or in addition to an endometrial biopsy.

In the younger female, a cone biopsy is usually shallow. In the older female, the biopsy tends to be taken from much deeper layers of the cervix. In both cases, bleeding is a risk, and when this occurs the vagina may have to be temporarily packed with sterile gauze to encourage coagulation.

Laparoscopy

In all cases of laparoscopy, the nurse will be asked to prepare the patient for general anaesthetic. Before proceeding to the physical preparation the procedure must be explained to the patient and her spouse/partner, as to why it is being done, before the consent form is signed. It may be done for either diagnostic or therapeutic reasons. Once the patient is anaesthetised a small stab wound is made in the lower abdomen and the peritoneal cavity is insufflated with carbon dioxide gas to lift the abdominal wall free of the pelvic organs. The laparoscope, a fibre-optic endoscope, is introduced into the abdomen through the stab wound to view the internal organs of reproduction. It is possible to determine if the uterine tubes are patent, and diagnose pelvic inflammatory disease by observing the course taken by an injected dye as it travels through the uterine tubes and out into the peritoneum. The procedure may be used to:

- Ligate either one or both tubes as part of a sterilisation procedure
- Apply Filcher clips or rings as part of a sterilisation procedure
- Apply tubal diathermy

When the examination is completed the stab

wound is closed by several sutures. After the operation, the nurse should press down gently on the abdominal wall to expel any remaining carbon dioxide gas from the peritoneal cavity. If this is not done the retained gas will irritate the diaphragm and cause referred pain of the shoulder tips via the phrenic nerve. Following recovery from anaesthesia, the patient needs to be reassured and told of what was diagnosed and if the treatment required was completed. The patient should be physically fit for discharge from hospital 24 hours later. Before being sent home, the ward nurse needs to make a referral to the district nurse to call at home in 2 or 3 days' time to remove the abdominal sutures or clips.

RADIOGRAPHY

Radiography procedures may be carried out either in the outpatients department, which is the more likely, or if requiring hospitalisation, as an inpatient. In essence the majority of radiography tests are used to outline and, if possible, identify anatomical abnormalities which may account for infertility or disorders of menstruation.

Hysterosalpinography

Apart from dressing the patient in a theatre gown, it may be necessary to administer any prescribed premedication 30 minutes before the procedure begins. A radiopaque substance is directed into the uterine cavity via a cannulae placed in the cervix. The dye outlines the uterus and uterine tubes by X-ray film and will also show if the dye has escaped into the peritoneal cavity via the tubal opening, proving that the uterine tube is patent. This is quite a painful procedure for the patient and she should be informed that the dye may cause lower abdominal pain and backache for several hours, which will resolve after a period of rest.

Gynaegram

The nurse must ensure that the patient has an empty lower colon and has voided urine immediately prior to going to the X-ray department. Although the procedure is neither painful nor uncomfortable, the patient should be advised that the technique used can appear alarming. It involves air being introduced into the peritoneal cavity via a needle directed through the abdominal wall. This air will provide the contrast media for the X-rays, which will outline the abdominal organs. When the patient is placed in the Trendelenburg position, the air occupies the pelvis and should then allow the X-rays to show up any anatomical abnormality of the uterus, uterine tubes or ovaries. The patient should be reassured that the air will be reabsorbed quickly and be expelled as flatus.

Tubal Insufflation

Tubal insufflation is a simple test to determine whether the uterine tubes are blocked, and will often therapeutically clear away a minor blockage. An hour before the procedure, any prescribed sedation should be administered to the patient. Dressed in an operating gown, the patient is placed in the lithotomy position with the legs raised and supported in stirrups on the examination table.

A tight-fitting cannula is placed in the cervix to prevent the escape of air. Carbon dioxide is forced through the cannula until a pressure of 200 mmHg is recorded on the insufflator machine. As the gas enters, it distends both uterus and the uterine tubes. If the pressure remains at 200 mmHg, it implies the tubes are blocked. If a steady fall occurs, at least one tube is patent. A stethoscope placed over the iliac fossa may detect the hissing sound of the gas as it leaves the tubal opening and escapes into the peritoneum. This test may also determine if surgery is required to relieve tubal blocking.

COMMON GYNAECOLOGICAL PROCEDURES

Several of the more common procedures with which the nurse should become familiar during an allocation to a gynaecology ward include:

- Vulval toilet
  - Vulval swabbing (see Female Catheterisation)
  - Jug douche
  - Bidet douche
- Insertion of vaginal pessaries
- Catheterisation
- Vaginal packs

Vulval Toilet

The free flow of plain tap water at 32° C over the parted labia is a most comforting measure, as well as being a cleansing technique. For those patients with dry, infected or inflamed vulval mucosa from minor surgery, vaginal discharge, perineal sutures, or after removal of vaginal packs, or catheters, the vulval toilet should be routinely included in their care plan. If at all possible, the patient should be encouraged to use a bidet to allow her to determine her own needs and suitable times.

Should the patient be confined to bed and require a vulval toilet, the nurse would protect the bedsheet with an inco-pad before assisting the patient onto a bedpan. The patient is then rested back onto several pillows to help elevate the pelvis. Using a gloved hand, the nurse gently parts the labia and pours water (32° C) over the labia from a jug. It may be necessary to repeat the procedure several times to actually soothe the irritated mucosa. The vulva, groin and perineum require careful pat-drying with soft tissues before applying a maternity pad, if one is required. If the patient is unable to use a bedpan, the nurse can swab the parted labia with liberally soaked cotton wool swabs using the technique outlined in catheterisation technique.

Vaginal Pessaries

Pessaries either are in drug form or are a mechanical device that supports a prolapsing uterus. Drug pessaries are elongated soluble gelatin-based compounds which contain a specific drug such as an antibiotic or hormone. After the pessary has been advanced into the vagina with the gloved finger, it should be pressed upwards into the vault. Once it is dissolved by the local body temperature, the drug will act on the local mucosa. Two examples are: nystatin pessaries, used to treat vaginitis, and oestrogen pessaries, used to treat senile atrophic vaginitis. If the patient has a fungal (*thrush*) or trichomonal infection, the pessary should be introduced using a special applicator. The nurse should wear sterile gloves during the procedure.

Mechanical pessaries are mainly used to support and correct uterine displacement. The pessary is shaped as a compressible elliptical device, or ring, and is correctly sized so that the uterus is well supported without discomfort. To ensure a correct fitting the doctor should always insert the first pessary. Thereafter it remains in position for about 6 months and then may be changed by the nurse in the outpatients department, or by the district nurse.

On each occasion the pessary is changed, it is advisable that the patient has a thorough vaginal examination. A Hodge pessary is made of rigid plastic and should only be inserted by a gynaecologist. Such a pessary would hold the uterus in the anteverted position. When the ring is due for removal, the patient is placed in the semirecumbent position with the knees flexed. The nurse then advances a finger either side of the vaginal wall and hooks over the edge of the pessary and exerts a downwards pressure.

Female Catheterisation

Catheterisation may be requested for several reasons:

1. Very occasionally to obtain a catheter specimen of urine. It is preferable to obtain specimens by clean catchment to reduce the hazards of urinary tract infection.
2. For the relief of urinary retention. On these occasions, a small-sized catheter is used.
3. To assess the residual volume of urine left in the bladder after the patient has passed as much urine as she can in stress incontinence or bladder-neck abnormality.

4. A temporary postoperative measure following pelvic floor repair surgery.

5. For patients with caesium or radium needle implants, to reduce the nursing time spent at the bedside.

The equipment for catheterisation is usually supplied in a standard sterile pack which may contain:

2 pairs of dissecting forceps
1 pair of French bow dressing forceps
5 gauze swabs
10 wool swabs
dressing towels (disposable)
2 gallipots
1 receiver

Additional items which the nurse will need include:

Jaques and Foley catheters sizes 12 to 16 (average size required is No. 12)
Normal saline lotion (Normasol)
Chlorhexidine cetrimide solution
Sterile disposable gloves
Anaesthetic gel
Specimen container with pathology forms
Lightweight blanket for modesty and to keep the patient warm

If the light source is poor, an anglepoise lamp can be positioned to increase the illumination of the vulval area. After the equipment has been assembled, the patient is prepared, firstly, by reassuring her as to the reason for the procedure and what it will involve. The patient should be assisted to adopt the dorsal position, with the knees flexed and thighs apart, and the head supported with 2 pillows. After the lightweight blanket has been placed over the bedclothes, the top bedclothes are removed under the modesty blanket to avoid exposing the patient unnecessarily. If the anglepoise lamp is required, it is positioned and switched on.

Suggested Technique

The patient should be bathed or have a thorough perineal toilet before commencing. An assistant is required during the aseptic part of this nontouch technique, i.e., the first 5 cm of the urinary catheter **must not** be touched by either the naked or gloved hand. Thorough washing of the lower arms and hands are essential, being dried before putting on the sterile gloves.

In preparing the cleansed surface of the trolley with the equipment, the assisting nurse should be responsible for opening the sterile packs and releasing the contents onto the trolley surface. This is in addition to pouring out the lotions after they have been checked. The patient's thighs are draped with sterile towels, as is the lower abdomen, to cover the pubic area. It is useful at this point to outline the recommended swabbing technique for the vulva.

Swabbing must be done from above towards the perineum, using one swab **once only** in the following pattern:

Left labia majora
Right labia majora
Separate the labia with the index finger and thumb of the nondominant hand
Left labia minora
Right labia minora
Vestibule area over the central area of the urethra

The vestibule is then dried and the process is repeated to dry the labia minora and majora.

After swabbing, the labia are held apart to locate the urethral orifice. At this point the labia minora should **not** be touched again until after the catheter is in position. The tip of the catheter, if necessary, should be lubricated with sterile lubricant anaesthetic gel and advanced gently but firmly along the urethra into the bladder. The escaping urine is allowed to drain into a receiver placed between the thighs.

If the catheterisation is to relieve urinary retention, then the bladder is drained slowly by the use of a clamp applied to the catheter. If the catheter is to be retained for any length of time, the Foley type with an inflatable balloon is inserted and then inflated to secure the catheter within the bladder. The free end of the catheter is firstly secured to the inner and then the outer aspect of the thigh, and directed in a downward direction to the urinary collection bag. The catheter should not be positioned higher than the pelvis at any time, otherwise the risk of infection increases. The dangers associated with catheterisation include;

Trauma to the urethral mucosa

Infection of the bladder, i.e., cystitis, which may ascend to involve the ureters and kidney

Shock if there is too rapid a decompression of a very full bladder

Following the procedure, the patient is once again reassured and made comfortable. In reporting the result of the catheterisation, the nurse should note if a sterile specimen has been taken and also note if the patient should be commenced on fluid-balance recording of fluid intake and urinary output.

N.B. Care of an indwelling catheter may be found in *Nursing 1*.

Vaginal Packs

The vagina may need to be packed with sterile gauze for the following reasons:

Following an extensive cone biopsy, for 24 hours, to arrest haemorrhage

Following a vaginal hysterectomy or pelvic-floor repair if requested by the surgeon; and this is usually for 24 hours

As a preoperative measure when the pack contains Dionestrol cream to treat ulceration, procidentia, or prior to insertion of a Hodge pessary

Following abortion or haemorrage, in which instance only a doctor should pack the vagina

Equipment

The equipment required would normally include the following sterile articles:

Sim's speculum

Lubricant

A roll of sterile gauze usually 10 cm width, but 23 cm is required for haemorrhage; the gauze may be inserted either dry or be soaked with cream

A pair of large swab-holding forceps

Sterile wool swabs for cleansing

Gallipots containing antiseptic lotion

Nursing Action

Before commencing, ask the patient to void urine so that the bladder is emptied. The lower abdomen, vulva and perineum should be thoroughly washed and gently dried. When ready the patient is assisted into the left lateral position, or Sim's position, and the vulval area illuminated with an anglepoise lamp. The Sim's speculum is advanced into the vaginal vault, checking that there are no raw edges of the mucosa. Held by the forceps, the gauze is packed into the vagina from the vault downwards, ensuring that the layers of gauze reach the lateral walls. A small portion of gauze is left emerging from the vaginal orifice before a maternity pad is secured in position.

The *insertion time* should be carefully noted so that the pack is removed according to the gynaecologist's instructions and not left in for too long. While the pack is in position, the patient is requested to remain on bedrest. One problem to observe for is that the patient may suffer retention of urine as a consequence of pressure from the pack.

When it is due for removal, the nurse should use an aseptic technique with a basic dressing trolley. After protecting the bed, the nurse assists the patient to assume the dorsal position with the thighs flexed and apart, and a receiver is placed between them. Wearing sterile gloves, the nurse uses a pair of dissecting forceps on the free end of the pack and gently pulls forward. The pack is removed piece by piece in a lengthwise direction into the receiver. Following the removal of the pack the patient should be offered vulval toilet before applying a clean pad.

Chapter 14
The Menstrual Cycle and its Disorders

Disturbance and disorder of the menstrual cycle are extremely wide-ranging and affect many systems of the body, mainly the endocrine system. In the United Kingdom the average age of the menarche (first menstrual cycle) occurs between 11 and 13 years of age. A delayed menarche, however, does not usually merit serious investigation until the girl is about 17 years old, unless there is an obvious reason to do so. The prime complaint related to a disturbance of the menstrual cycle, which brings the patient forward for advice, may centre upon:

A **delayed menarche**, which in the majority of instances is idiopathic

Amenorrhoea, or the 'absence' of a period or menstrual flow (Table 14.1)

Infertility which affects about 10% of marriages in the United Kingdom

An **altered pattern** of menstrual cycle, i.e., *metropathia haemorrhagica*

Dysmenorrhoea

Premenstrual tension

The **menopause**

DELAYED MENARCHE AND AMENORRHOEA

Investigation into the delayed menarche, amenorrhoea and infertility (see later) all follow the same pattern, and will be dealt with collectively. It needs to be appreciated that any investigation will take place against a background of great emotional turmoil, and that some investigations take a long time to be completed. During this time the patient may experience feelings of severe emotional stress,

Table 14.1 Brief list of the causes of amenorrhoea*

Primary	Secondary
Delayed menarche	Pregnancy (most common cause)
Disorders of	Premature menopause
pituitary gland	Polycystic ovarian disease
ovaries	Poor luteal phase syndrome (infertility)
adrenal cortex	Postpuberty endocrine disease
Chromosomal abnormality	Emotional distress
Imperforate hymen (haematocolpos)	Debilitating disease
Endometrial disease	

* Amenorrhoea is a symptom, not a disease.

which require recognition and supportive empathy. The nursing role is not only clinical but supportive, providing a listening ear and a shoulder to lean on as the patient gets to know the nurse. Nurses can give positive encouragement to help the patient verbalise her fears and anxieties, whether real or imagined, so that she can place her feelings into a true perspective. Talking on a 'woman-to-woman' basis will help the patient assuage her possible feelings of guilt and cope with her bitterness or anger. A measure of sharing the intentions of the investigations with the patient, and if married her husband, will go far to relieve a great deal of the emotional distress.

Family History

The initial investigation is for the gynaecologist to take a complete family history to note if there is any familial, endocrine or gynaecological disorders common to the female members of the family. Detailed information is needed on the previous menstrual cycles, a complete gynaecological or obstetric history, if appropriate, and the current use of any form of contraception. In making a physical examination of the patient the following features are usually noted:

- Distribution of body hair for obvious hirsutism
- Body contour conforming to typical female shape
- Whether height compares favourably with arm span and leg length
- Compression of the breasts for milk excretion, i.e., galactorrhoea
- Abnormality of the external genitalia
- If the hymen is intact, but imperforate, to allow for escape of blood during a period

Many of these observations are a first indication of an endocrine abnormality affecting the pituitary gland and may indicate the way for further endocrine investigations.

Chromosomal Pattern

The chromosomal pattern from buccal smears may be assessed, although it is usual for chromosomal abnormalities to be obvious before the menarche, e.g., Turner's Syndrome, in which case amenorrhoea is to be expected (see Table 14.1). A progesterone plasma level above 10 nmol/litre plasma or more, 7 days before the menstrual phase, indicates the formation of the corpus luteum. Likewise, the metabolic waste products of progesterone, i.e., pregnanediol, are also raised when assayed in a 24-hour urine collection. The plasma levels of follicle stimulating hormone, luteinising hormone, prolactin, thyroxine, tri-iodothyronine and testosterone may also be completed to exclude abnormalities of the pituitary, thyroid and ovarian glands.

A 24-hour urine collection may be tested to measure the levels of 17 oxosteroids to indicate whether there is a disorder of the adrenal cortex. Any suggestion of a pituitary disorder may necessitate an X-ray of the pituitary fossa and the testing of visual fields to exclude or confirm the presence of a tumour pressing upon or arising from the anterior lobe of the pituitary gland.

Invasive Tests

An endometrial biopsy may show secretory changes which occur in the second half of the menstrual cycle and should also exclude any inflammatory condition of the endometrium. Laparoscopy is commonly used to visualise the presence or otherwise of the corpus luteum, which proves if ovulation is taking place. This investigation requires careful timing to coincide with the patient's individual cycle.

A laparotomy to examine the ovaries to see if they are polycystic may be advised and at the same time a check may be made to test the patency of the uterine tubes. Smears taken from the vagina during the second half of the menstrual cycle may reveal mucosal changes expected from the effects of oestrogen and progesterone.

The Spinbarkheit test shows the effect that oestrogen has on the mucus, which is to make it much thinner, and when placed on a glass slide will thread out to reach 7 to 8 cm long before breaking. This *mucus threading* occurs at the peak of ovulation.

A second test on cervical mucus is *ferning*. This shows that when the oestrogenised cervical mucus is allowed to dry out on a glass slide, it adopts a fern leaf pattern when viewed through a microscope. If there is suspicion of a structural abnormality of any of the pelvic organs, a gynaegram may be suggested (see p. 108).

INFERTILITY

Infertility is reported as affecting one in every ten marriages and those seeking advice are usually interviewed in the privacy offered by an infertility clinic. As mentioned, investigations into infertility usually follow the same pattern as that for the delayed menarche and amenorrhoea, but essentially the tests offered are those for amenorrhoea. Some emphasis is placed upon the daily recording of the oral temperature during the menstrual cycle. After ovulation the temperature rise, which is expected, lasts for a few days only and is inconsistent. There also tends to be a low progesterone level.

Active steps to help the patient conceive are not usually tried for about 2 years after a couple has made the initial request for help. From experience, simple techniques in the counselling of what happens following coitus and an educational approach which aids relaxation seem to work in the majority of cases.

There is also the need to screen the partner to ensure that he is fertile by asking him to complete a sperm count. The average count is in the order of 5 million sperm/2 ml of semen.

A microscopic study of the sperm may prove that they are of poor motility. The desperation which many couples feel can lead to a breakdown in the relationship unless the counselling approach is positive. Those patients going through these exhaustive tests can receive a great deal of support and specialist help from a clinic nurse. Further help can be given by interested groups such as The National Association for the Childless, Birmingham Settlement, 318 Summer Lane, Birmingham B19 3RL.

Artificial insemination by donor semen (AIDS) by either implantation or surgical technique is extremely successful, but is in general a later consideration and requires a great deal of medical and social counselling before being undertaken. External (*in vivo*) fertilisation i.e., test tube baby, is also an increasingly feasible option, but is usually offered as a last option.

DYSMENORRHOEA

Dysmenorrhoea is defined as discomfort during the menstrual phase in which pelvic pain is severe enough to interfere with normal daily activities. It may be either *primary*, i.e., there is no pelvic disease, or it may be *secondary*. If it is due to the latter, then it may be caused by:

- Menorrhagic syndrome
- Adenomyosis
- Presence of an IUCD (intrauterine contraceptive device)

Pelvic inflammatory disease
Fibroids and polyps
Endometriosis

Primary Dysmenorrhoea

Primary dysmenorrhoea is reported as having a 60% incidence in the 2 years following the menarche, and worsens between the ages of 17 and 24 years old. It gradually diminishes and is said to resolve completely after the first pregnancy, although such advice should never be given to a young girl. About one in every three sufferers requests medical help and of these about 40% respond to a prescribed mild analgesia. The pain is theoretically due to the hyperactivity of the myometrium during the menstrual flow. This hyperactivity causes a reduced blood flow to the uterus.

Secondary Dysmenorrhoea

Other causes of dysmenorrhoea are said to be stenosis of the cervix, increased vasopressin secretion, raised levels of prostaglandins, hyperactive nerve supply to the uterus and, lastly, those females who may adopt a 'sick' role, using dysmenorrhoea as a means of obtaining attention.

The investigations follow those for amenorrhoea, with particular reference paid to the type of pain, its site, nature, timing and whether the pain is related to a specific activity such as sports or heavy lifting. Three further factors, which may influence dysmenorrhoea are: the use of an IUCD, premenstrual tension, or if the dysmenorrhoea is accompanied by vaginal discharge.

A vaginal examination is not usually performed on a young girl. Advice about the patient's personal lifestyle in relationship to her sleep habits, exercise and coping with psychological stress may prove a useful avenue of therapy. From the group of drugs which inhibit prostaglandins, one may be prescribed which is to be taken immediately before and during the menstrual flow. Examples of such drugs are:

Aspirin
Indomethacin (Indocid)
Keptoprofen (Orudis)
Mefenamic acid (Ponstan)
Naproxon (Naprosyn)

Secondary dysmenorrhoea is treated according to its cause.

PREMENSTRUAL TENSION (PMT)

An increase in oestrogen levels causes a corresponding increase in the blood flow to the pelvic organs and the breasts. The patient suffers from a bloated feeling which causes a heavy sensation in the lower abdomen and a tingling sensation of the breasts. A second effect of oestrogen is to retain both fluid and sodium, accounting for a transient increase in body weight. This causes a temporary rise in the blood pressure.

Signs and Symptoms

Emotional components of the *tension* felt may include: severe depression, reduced libido, nausea, anger and lassitude. Progesterone taken in the second half of the cycle may modify the tension by counteracting the effects of oestrogen. Taking oral contraceptives with a high progesterone content between the menses is an alternative method of achieving a balance. If fluid retention is considerably marked, then small doses of a diuretic may be prescribed.

METROPATHIA HAEMORRHAGICA (CYSTIC GLANDULAR HYPERPLASIA)

A functional disturbance involving hormone imbalance when the Graafian follicle matures, but fails to rupture and secretes a high level of oestrogen is called *metropathia haemorrhagica*. The effect of this is to make the endometrium very thick, and with a diminished amount of progesterone there is no ovulation or secretion from the endometrial glands. The endometrium then becomes cystic and hyperplasic. While a minor version of this hyperplasia occurs at both puberty and the menopause, it mainly affects women in the middle years of their reproductive life who have never had children, i.e., they are *nulliparous*.

The periods are heavy, grossly prolonged and painless, with a loss of the cyclical pattern. These symptoms are due to the endometrial hyperplasia. The initial treatment is usually curettage, but this can be replaced by the gynaecologist's prescription of high doses of progesterone within a contraceptive pill to help regulate the cycle. Apart from these two approaches, it is usual to exclude cancer of the uterus before proceeding to a hysterectomy, if all other treatment fails.

It has to be appreciated that there is much emotional conflict during this time, but whether this is due to hormonal imbalance or social factors is very difficult to determine. Nevertheless the nursing approach should continue to be one of sympathy and support, regardless of the treatment prescribed.

MENOPAUSE

The cessation of menstruation usually occurs between 45 and 55 years old. It may occur suddenly, be preceded by increasingly irregular periods or by odd irregular periods. There are usually many systemic changes immediately before and after, and the term *menopause* should take these other changes into account.

Organic changes include the atrophy of the labia, uterus and vaginal epithelium, all being due to lower plasma levels of oestradiol. At the same time, increased hormonal secretions from the anterior lobe of the pituitary gland cause vasomotor flushing, perspiration, obesity, hirsutism and emotional turmoil. The bones tend to become osteoporotic after the menopause and the plasma cholesterol levels tend to rise with the increasing risk of atheroma. It is also at this time that uterine prolapse and vaginal infections increase in frequency.

Fortunately, many women in fact do not suffer any undue discomfort, but for some it is a time of intense emotional havoc. For these patients oestrogen therapy by tablet, injection or pellet implant may be considered necessary. Those patients with premature menopause due to irradiation therapy or surgery require replacement oestrogen therapy until at least the average age of the menopause, if not longer.

Chapter 15
Ovarian Disorders

Arising from within and around the ovaries are a vast array of differing types of cyst or tumour, large and small, benign or malignant, many of them existing without causing any symptoms. Of passing interest to the nurse is the classification of the tumours as outlined in Table 15.1. Only the more common of these are discussed in the text.

CYSTS AND TUMOURS

Of the 15 different types of possible tumour suggested in Table 15.1, the more common are:

Follicular cysts
Serous and mucinous cystadenomas
Dermoid cysts
Fibromas
Carcinoma of the ovaries

Follicular Cysts

Follicular, or benign water-filled, cysts of the Graafian follicle, which have failed to rupture, are extremely common and may be caused by:

1. A response to natural or therapeutic gonadotrophin in the treatment of infertility.
2. As a response to oophoritis, i.e., inflammation of the ovary. In this the tunica albuginea becomes thickened and prevents the rupture of the mature Graafian follicle.
3. In association with the Stein Levanthal Syndrome, which means there is a failure of the ovarian enzyme systems. The ovaries

Table 15.1 Classification of ovarian tumours

Tumour	Cell origin	Type	Incidence (%)
Benign			
Cysts	Graafian follicle and corpus luteum	Cystic	60
Serous cystadenoma	Coelomic epithelium	Cystic	10
Mucinous cystadenoma	Coelomic epithelium	Cystic	12–15
Teratoma (dermoid cyst)	Oogonia	Cystic	15–20
Endometriomata	Ectopic endometrium	Cystic	
Fibroma (and Brenner)	Mesenchyme	Solid	5
Malignant			
Serous cystadenoma	Secondary changes of above Cystic or semisolid		common
Mucinous cystoadenoma	Secondary changes of above Cystic or semisolid		common
Granulosa/theca	Oestrogen producing tumour (feminising)	Solid	rare
Androblastoma (Arrhenoblastoma)	Androgen producing tumour (masculising)	Solid	rare
Disgerminoma	Germ cells	Solid	rare
Teratoma	Embryonic tissues	Solid	rare
Secondary carcinoma			
Krukenburg tumour	From the stomach	Solid	rare
Adenocarcinoma	From the uterus	Solid	rare

N.B. International staging of ovarian cancer:

1. The cancer is limited to one or both ovaries.
2. The cancer involves both ovaries, but is limited to the pelvis.
3. The cancer is widespread intraperitoneally.
4. The cancer has widespread metastases.

become enlarged, cystic and develop a thickened fibrous outer surface, and there is failure to ovulate.

Rarely does the cyst cause symptoms unless there is an occasionàl menorrhagia, or dysmenorrhoea. If there is lower abdominal pain, it may mimic appendicitis, cystitis, pyelitis, or ectopic pregnancy. On examination the lateral fornix may be tender and the ovary may be palpable. In many patients the conservative approach of 'wait and see' is followed, in the hope that the cyst will resolve spontaneously. If the cyst is still present after 3 months the patient would then have a detailed examination while anaesthetised and, if necessary, a laparotomy is performed to remove the cyst.

Corpus Luteum Cyst

The corpus luteum cyst is a single cyst that forms in the corpus luteum after ovulation has occurred. It may bleed, which gives rise to abdominal pain, often mimicking an ectopic pregnancy. Such a cyst may present in the early weeks of pregnancy, but should regress by the twelfth week. If the cyst is still present after 3 months and exceeds 5 cm diameter, it is removed via a laparotomy incision. It is at this time that there is no threat to the uterus. If the corpus luteum fails to involute, the secretion of progesterone continues causing disturbed menstrual cycle, e.g., amenorrhoea, dysmenorrhoea or menorrhagia.

A cyst of a significant size can cause abdominal pain in either the right or left iliac fossa. These cysts may form as a consequence of treatment with gonadotrophin or clomiphene, which are used to induce ovulation in those suffering from infertility.

Serous Cystadenoma

Serous cystadenoma is a benign cyst and is rare before the age of 35. It is bilateral in about one third of affected patients, and the risk of developing malignancy is very high. Unless the cyst gives rise to complications such as haemorrhage, torsion or ruptures, it tends to remain asymptomatic. On a bimanual examination, a lump may be felt. If the patient is young, she may wish to have a family and in this case hopefully only the tumour may be removed. An older patient may have an oophorectomy, after which the patient should be followed up for 10 years in case of malignancy.

Mucinous Cystadenoma

Mucinous cystadenoma is described as a 'multilocular cyst', meaning it is compartmented, with each compartment filled with a mucus-like gel. It has the potential to grow into considerable dimensions out of the pelvic cavity up into the abdomen. It occurs more frequently in females between 30 and 40 years of age, and in about 50% of cases can become malignant. It is asymptomatic until a lump can be felt in the lower abdomen. Occasionally it may give rise to haemorrhage, torsion, or rupture. In the younger female, the treatment of choice is an oophorectomy. In the older female, i.e., over 40, a total abdominal hysterectomy and bilateral salpingo-oophorectomy may be completed.

Dermoid Cyst (Teratoma) (Benign Cystic Teratoma)

A dermoid cyst arises from the primordial germ cells and may contain the most bizarre elements of any type of tissue. Teeth, hair, skin, nails, muscle, cartilage, bone, or glandular tissue may be found within the thick unilocular wall. Such a tumour may grow to 10 or 12 cm in diameter, but rarely becomes malignant. An abdominal X-ray showing something as odd as a tooth is usually diagnostic of a dermoid cyst. Because they are asymptomatic, these cysts are not discovered until a routine pelvic examination is being undertaken, such as in early pregnancy, or a routine abdominal X-ray is taken. For the younger female, an ovarian cystectomy is usually attempted. For the older female, an oophorectomy is the treatment of choice.

Fibroma

A fibroma is a solid tumour arising from the ovarian mesenchyme; it is benign and tends to occur in the postmenopausal female. The tumour can grow up to 10 or 12 cm in diameter, pushing upwards into the abdominal cavity and may cause an ascites, i.e., abdominal effusion. If the tumour is large enough, it may also cause a right-sided pleural effusion which is sometimes referred to as Meigs' Syndrome. A fibroma is readily diagnosed and requires an oophorectomy.

Carcinoma of the Ovaries

As can be noted from the classifications in Table 15.1, a malignant tumour may be either primary or secondary, and cancer of the ovaries is very common (Fig. 15.1). Each year there are about 4000 deaths attributed to this type of cancer. An ovarian tumour in the prepuberty age, while rare, is very likely to be malignant. The older the female the more likely an ovarian tumour is to be malignant, and this seems to occur between the ages of 45 and 55.

Should the tumour be primary, it remains silent or asymptomatic until contiguous spread occurs. Neighbouring structures which may be invaded by seedling cancer cells are the peritoneum, endometrium, bowel, uterine tubes and the urinary bladder. Lymphatic spread of the cancer cells tracks to the para-aortic nodes and from there to distant sites. Initially there may be a palpable lump, but it is more usual for the patient to present with the classical triad of weight loss, anaemia and ascites, i.e., a *cachexic* patient. Diagnostic measures, which are completed as rapidly as possible, include cytology of the aspirated ascitic fluid, laparoscopy, and rarely a culposcopy or a laparotomy.

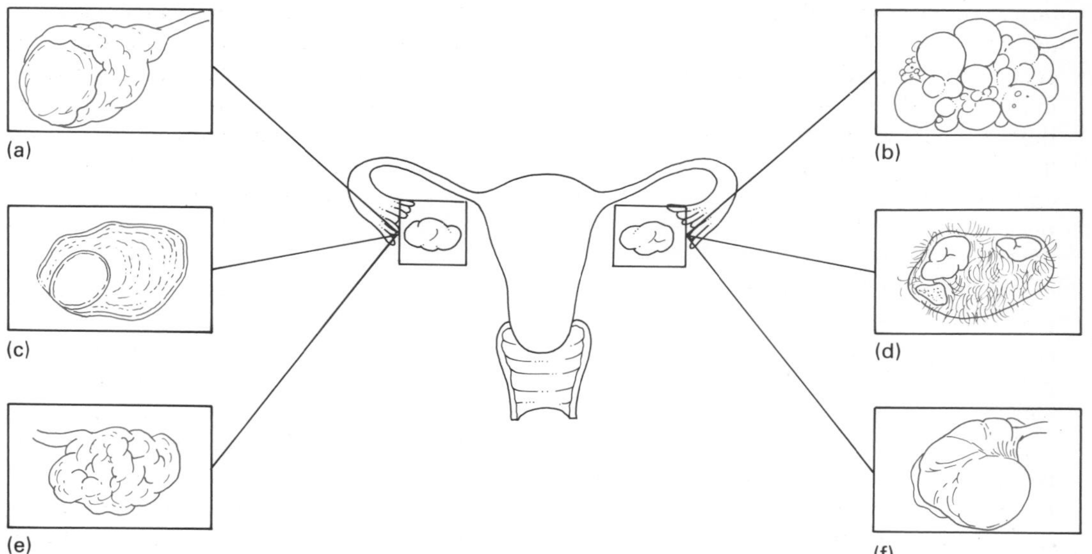

Fig. 15.1 Ovarian tumours: follicular (a); serous ovarian cyst (b); carcinoma (c); papilliferous (d); dermoid (e); torsion (f).

Nursing Action

The treatment plan on which the nursing care centres may be a total hysterectomy with bilateral salpingo-oophorectomy, pelvic radiotherapy or systemic chemotherapy (see Oncology). In those patients with advanced cancer, the nursing care would centre upon caring for the terminally ill patient. The essential features applicable to ovarian cancer include:

Controlling and containing the abdominal pain

Relieving the abdominal distension, due to the ascites, by frequent tapping of the fluid, i.e., paracentesis abdominis

If possible preventing intestinal obstruction

Preventing vomiting by the use of antiemetic drugs

Maintaining the patient's fluid balance

The outlook for these unfortunate patients remains bleak. Heroic efforts to save life must take into account that there is an 85% mortality rate within 5 years of the initial diagnosis being made.

Assessment

The assessment for ovarian tumours would incorporate the following features, which should be included in the nursing plan of care:

Pain	Nutritional aspects
Abdominal girth	Bimanual examination
Pressure symptoms	Ultrasonic screening
Menstrual disturbances	Pregnancy test
	Psychology

Pain is unusual, unless the tumour complicates. If there is lower abdominal pain without gross enlargement of the abdomen, then there is a possibility of endometriomatosis or malignancy. A large tumour will obviously cause distension pain, but is not usually malignant and would have been diagnosed as malignant long before it reached a significant size.

Abdominal Girth. The patient may have noticed small changes, such as clothing becoming restrictive, a pelvic swelling, and amenorrhoea which may make the patient believe she is pregnant. Girth measurements should be taken routinely if ascites is present, or is being treated by tapping.

Pressure Symptoms. If the tumour mass is confined to the pelvis, it may cause displacement of related pelvic organs. If the urethra is distorted, retention of urine may occur and pressure on the urinary bladder may cause frequency of micturition. If there is pressure upwards into the abdomen, it may cause gastric upset, heartburn and embarrass respiration causing dyspnoea in severe cases.

Menstrual Disturbances. The three main disturbances to the menstrual cycle are amenorrhoea, menorrhagia and dysmenorrhoea. A careful note should be made of the patient's observations about her menstrual cycle and reported to the gynaecologist.

Nutritional Aspects. Obesity undoubtedly confuses abdominal palpation and bimanual examination. It is also a surgical risk, having many postoperative dangers for the patient. An early loss of weight, vomiting, nausea and disinterest in food combined with ascites suggests malignancy and the nurse should note if the patient is becoming increasingly cachexic.

Bimanual Examination. If requested to assist with such an examination, the nurse should ensure that the patient has first emptied the bladder. The examination will help the gynaecologist determine the size of the tumour, if it is free moving or fixed, has a pedicle, if the uterus is displaced, if there are adhesions or inflammation of the pelvic organs. A test is carried out to examine for the Hegar's sign, in which the body of the uterus feels as though it has separated from the cervix.

Radiography is usually only contemplated in the nonpregnant patient and is usually confined to plain abdominal X-ray films to determine pelvic organ outlines.

Ultrasonic Screening is a more popular investigation, which is noninvasive and will determine the position and size of any tumour mass.

Pregnancy Test can be done on the ward using the Pregnosticone Planotest. The substance is mixed with a few drops of an early morning urine specimen. If it remains milky, it is a positive indication. If it curdles, it is a negative reaction to pregnancy. There are two essential points here. A tumour can coexist with a pregnancy, so a positive test does not preclude the existence of a tumour. Equally, the patient may think she has a cyst but is in fact pregnant. The ward test is only an indication and urine specimens should be despatched to the laboratory for more exact pregnancy tests.

Psychology. A most important part of medical and nursing assessment is to ascertain the patient's own attitudes to future family planning. The wish for children at a later time will have a great influence on the therapeutic approach. This is especially true for the younger female. The older female, although still in the reproductive years, may have already come to a definite decision about not having any more children. There is an undercurrent of fear in the patient's own mind about the word *tumour* or *cyst* and knowing the truth as soon as is feasible may be more harmful than denying the patient knowledge.

Whenever possible, the husband or partner should be included in the discussions about intended nursing care. Certainly, the nurse should refer the husband to the gynaecologist for exact information about the diagnosis and treatment. In good practice, the husband is routinely seen by the examining physician and the senior nurse at the outset of treatment. Both partners will then have the same information on which to base their future plans for having a family. The patient should be given the opportunity to voice any fears she may have about losing her femininity or alteration to her body image. Vocalising fears allows the patient to get her anxieties into perspective.

Complications of Ovarian Tumours

An ovarian tumour may complicate to torsion, rupture, infection, haemorrhage, impaction or incarceration.

Torsion

If a cyst has a pedicle which has freedom to move, the pedicle may wrap itself around the uterine tube. It can unwrap itself, in which case the torsion it exerts is spontaneously resolved. If, however, the torsion is increased, its effect is to compress the tubal veins initially and later the arteries. The patient experiences sudden low abdominal pain, pronounced shock and suffers from repeated vomiting. Another feature of the torsion effect is to increase the size of the ovarian tumour, causing further abdominal tenderness. Left untreated, the compression of the local blood vessels will inevitably lead to tubal gangrene.

Rupture

Spontaneous rupture of an ovarian tumour is rare, but may occur as the direct result of a bimanual examination. The consequences of a rupture depend on the type of tumour. Small cysts release a watery content without undue damage, or there may be bleeding similar in type to an ectopic pregnancy. If it is a malignant tumour, widespread dissemination of seedling cancer cells may occur. An immediate laparotomy is usually advised if the type of tumour is already known and diagnosed.

Infection

The results of an ovarian infection resemble inflammation of the uterine tube, i.e., salpingitis. Abdominal pain is intermittent, pyrexia occurs and, on examination, the vaginal mucosa is extremely tender. A laparotomy to remove the infected ovary, plus a course of antibiotics, is usually the treatment of choice.

Haemorrhage

Bleeding may occur from or into the ovarian tumour. As with any internal bleeding, the blood lost can only be roughly calculated from the degree of shock from which the patient is suffering. Associated with an obvious pallor, tachycardia, hypotension and possibly air hunger are low abdominal pain and abdominal swelling arising from the pelvis. An emergency laparotomy is arranged and immediate grouping and cross-matching of blood is completed before the patient is transferred to theatre for ligation of the ruptured blood vessel and removal of the tumour, if not also the ovary.

Impaction

Impaction is a rare complication and implies that the ovarian tumour has impacted itself into the pelvic girdle. More usually the tumour will grow out of the pelvis, up into the abdomen. A tumour impacting the pelvis will impede delivery of the newborn through the birth canal and may necessitate a caesarean section if the tumour is not diagnosed until after the twenty-eighth week of pregnancy.

Incarceration

The tumour mass may become fixed in one part of the pelvis, such as the Pouch of Douglas. The tumour mass would then exert pressure on the related structures such as the bladder, ureter, and their blood vessels. Such incarceration would initially cause urinary retention, hydronephrosis, venous stasis of the lower limbs and obvious ankle swelling. After diagnosis and because of the risk of gangrene around the fixed mass, the nurse may be asked to prepare the patient for an emergency laparotomy to excise the tumour.

Treatment of Ovarian Tumours

There are many surgical procedures tor the treatment of ovarian tumours. Essentially, the nurse is planning to prepare the patient for lower abdominal surgery and would ensure that the routine preoperative management has been completed. However, the nurse can never be certain of the postoperative needs of the patient until after surgery is completed.

Exploratory Operation of Laparotomy

The patient may return to the ward with an ovarian cystectomy, an ovariotomy or oophorotomy, or an ovarian tapping.

Ovarian cystectomy is the enucleation of the tumour from its capsule and excision from the healthy ovarian tissue. The operation is completed with the patient in the Trendelenburg position. A long abdominal incision is made so that a detailed examination of the uterus and both ovaries can be made. The cyst is tapped or drained of its fluid content before being enucleated by dissection. If there is a pedicle, it is unclamped and divided. If a torsion is present, it is dealt with in the same manner.

Ovariotomy or oophorotomy is an incision into the ovary to facilitate the excision of a tumour.

Ovarian tapping is a palliative measure to drain the tumour of its fluid content if the patient is unfit for more radical surgery, or has respiratory embarrassment due to the size of the tumour.

If the tumour removed is suspected of being malignant, it is possible the surgeon may also do a hysterectomy in the older female for prophylactic reasons. For a proven malignancy, it is usual for the patient to have a total hysterectomy with bilateral salpingo-oophorectomy.

Chapter 16
Tubal Disorders

Inflammation (salpingitis) and ectopic pregnancy are the two principal tubal disorders to which student nurses should address their studies.

SALPINGITIS

Inflammation of the uterine tubes is mainly due to infection, the causative organisms gaining access to the tubes by direct transmission from such structures as the appendix, colon and uterus. An indirect spread may occur from the lymphatic system, or be blood borne. The causative organisms which are mainly found include the following species:

Streptococci and *Staphylococci* are the most common and are found particularly following either abortion or normal delivery.

Eschericia coli and *Streptococcus faecalis* may gain access to the tubes from the intestinal tract.

Clostridium welchii is only rarely found, but should be suspected in intractable infections.

Gonococcus (*Neisseria gonorrhoeae*) is now extremely common, gaining access to the tubes after sexual intercourse. Because it is asymptomatic in the early phases, it may not be suspected by the patient until the inflammation becomes chronic.

Tubercle bacillus (tuberculosis), if present, invades the tubes by the bloodstream and causes chronic salpingitis.

There is, however, a major problem from a diagnostic point of view in that many of the swabs taken from the vagina and cervix do not reveal the causative organism, which often delays treatment of a specific nature. This is especially so for chronic salpingitis. Inflammation due to infection follows the normal pathological pattern as for any type of tissue, and may proceed to involve the ovary so that the patient develops salpingo-oophoritis. As a consequence of the inflammation, both ends of the uterine tube close due to oedema and allow pus to collect within the tube. This is referred to as *pyosalpinx*. Since the inflammation also damages the inner epithelial wall, and this is combined with tubal closure, the tube tends to retain fluid and become rather distended. This is referred to as *hydrosalpinx*.

Acute Salpingitis

Acute salpingitis has a sudden onset of lower abdominal pain, an elevated temperature, usually about 39° to 40° C, and a toxaemia may prevail. A foul, purulent vaginal discharge, if present, may accompany urinary frequency and dysuria. A swab of the discharge should be taken and a urine specimen (MSU) collected and sent for culture and sensitivity tests.

Assessment

On examination there is a marked tenderness over both iliac fossae. On vaginal examination, localised tenderness may be so acute that a pelvic examination has to be abandoned. If the causative organism is gram negative, then the patient may be in extreme shock due to toxaemia and at risk from peritonitis. The diagnosis is sometimes confused with appendicitis, pyelonephritis, torsion or haemorrhage of an ovarian cyst and ectopic pregnancy. For this reason an exploratory operation (laparotomy) may be done. A suspected acute appendicitis cannot be ignored or left to conservative measures.

Nursing Care Plan

When a diagnosis is relatively straightforward, the nursing plan of care would dovetail with the typical prescribed regimen of bedrest until the pyrexia resolves and the vaginal discharge becomes minimal. This would involve the nurse in offering cooling measures to keep the patient comfortable and giving frequent vulval toilet.

Observation of the temperature and pulse should be taken at least every 4 hours until the pyrexia has resolved for at least 48 hours. While on bedrest the patient should be encouraged to adopt a recumbent posture, well supported by pillows.

If the patient uses an intrauterine contraceptive device, this should be removed at the earliest opportunity before vulval and perineal toilet is commenced.

Applying heat, i.e., a warm towel or a poultice, to the lower abdomen is a very comforting measure and if applied above the symphisis pubis, will take away a great deal of the pain.

Although anorexic and with little appetite for normal foods, the patient **must** be encouraged to maintain a fluid intake of up to 2 litres in every 24 hours because of perspiration and pyrexia. If the patient is toxaemic this fluid intake may have to be increased.

Prescribed sedation will assist the patient to rest, an essential part of the healing process. Another advantage is that anxiety will be reduced. However, it implies that the nurse arranges the care plan to allow for suitable periods of rest.

While awaiting the results of bacteriology tests, the gynaecologist would normally prescribe broad spectrum antibiotics, e.g., amoxycillin or Cotrimoxazole. If, however, the causative organisms are gram negative, it may prove necessary to commence intravenous therapy. Therefore more powerful antibiotics, such as gentamycin, carbenicillin or cephaloridine, are usually prescribed. If these measures prove inadequate the nurse may then be asked to prepare the patient for laparotomy or drainage of a pelvic abscess. If the acute inflammation does not respond to therapy the risk of chronic salpingitis and infertility is very high.

Chronic Salpingitis

Chronic salpingitis is a possible sequel to the acute form, or may be the result of gonorrhoea, tuberculosis or puerperal sepsis. There is usually a prolonged history of general ill health without a specific cause. The features include headaches, weight loss, lassitude, anorexia and disturbed sleep, none of which point to any single cause of feeling unwell.

More positive indications which the patient may experience include an intermittent dragging pain in the lower abdomen, and backache. A foul-smelling vaginal discharge is one feature which would bring most patients forward for medical advice. The menstrual flow is usually heavy, with dysmenorrhoea. Sexual intercourse can be painful and difficult due to pelvic tenderness, i.e., *deep dyspareunia*. Due to the damaged ciliated epithelium lining of the uterine tube, there is infertility. Chronic inflammation may cause abscesses to form within the peritoneal cavity, or in the ovary, and adhesions of the uterine tubes to related structures.

Observations and Treatment

On examination the iliac fossa are tender over the affected side and a palpable mass may be felt to be rising out of the pelvis. In doubtful cases, blood tests may show a neutrophilia and a leucocytosis with a raised erythrocyte sedimentation rate. A conservative approach may be for the patient to have a prolonged course of antibiotic therapy for 3 to 6 months. A short course of shortwave pelvic diathermy may help to improve the condition. The alternative regimen is for the patient to be prepared for surgery, usually a salpingectomy with or without an oophorectomy, or an hysterectomy if the patient is postmenopausal.

Tuberculosis of the uterine tubes requires that an endometrial biopsy is taken and that other investigations are made to find the primary source of the disease, e.g., the lungs. However, patients usually respond well on a 2-year course of antituberculosis drugs. Following recovery the patient may be offered a salpingotomy to re-establish patency of the uterine tubes for future pregnancies.

Patients with gonorrhoea, apart from being treated with antibiotic therapy, should also be referred to the venereologist as there may be a need to follow up the patient's sexual contacts in the previous 12 months to 2 years, bearing in mind that the inflammation is chronic and may have been asymptomatic for some time.

ECTOPIC PREGNANCY

Ectopic pregnancy is defined as an extrauterine pregnancy, occurring when the fertilised ovum implants itself at a site other than the uterine endometrium. The ovum is usually fertilised at the outer end of the uterine tube and anything which impedes its propulsion towards the uterus risks the implant being at another site. About 1 in every 300 pregnancies are ectopic. The majority of ectopic pregnancies (99%) occur in the uterine tubes, a few in the ovaries and even fewer in the abdominal or pelvic cavity. By far the greatest area of ectopic implant is into the uterine ampulla (55%), the uterine isthmus has a 25% incidence, and the fimbria only 17%. Least of all, a 2% incidence is found in the interstitial portion of the tube (Fig. 16.1).

The trophoblast, or outer cells of the morula, burrows into the inner epithelial wall of the tube in search of a blood vessel from which it can obtain its nourishment. However, lacking the uterine decidua, the developing trophoblast or embryo will either terminate as a tubal abortion or rupture into the peritoneal cavity. Secondary abdominal pregnancies are very rare.

Causes

The principal cause of ectopic pregnancies is salpingitis, which distorts the normal shape of the uterine tube. Other causes may be:

1. Delay in the propelling of the fertilised ovum through the tube towards the uterus.
2. Fertilisation being delayed after ovulation.

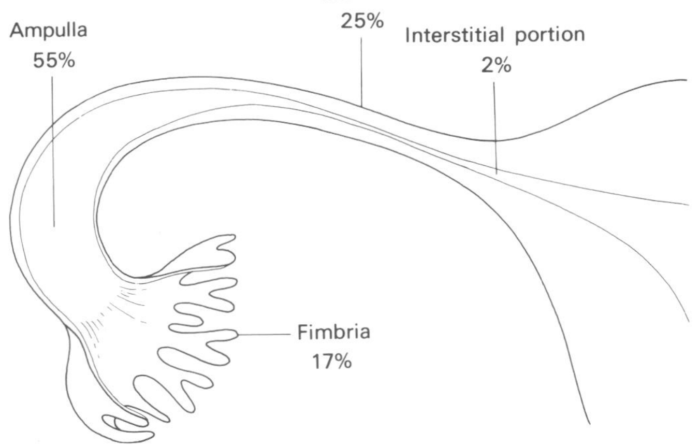

Fig. 16.1 Ectopic pregnancy.

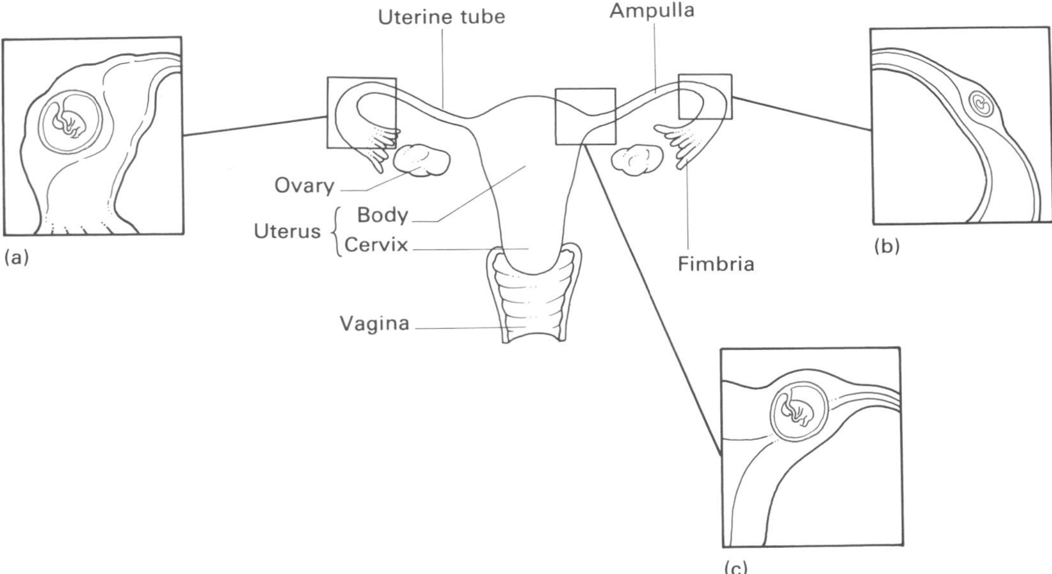

Fig. 16.2 Abnormal implantation: ampillary (a); interstitial (b); tubal abortion (c).

3. Congenital abnormality of the uterine tube, e.g., hyperplasia or diverticuli.
4. The use of an intrauterine contraceptive device, which has a high incidence.
5. Taking a progesterone only contraceptive pill.

Tubal Abortion

The conceptus may be absorbed completely or may pass into the peritoneal cavity from the fimbria and be absorbed. If the conceptus remains in the tube, it becomes surrounded by a blood clot, i.e., a *tubal mole*. Less obviously the tubal abortion may cause a gradual bleed, into either the Pouch of Douglas or the broad ligament. This slow bleeding may accumulate to form a pelvic haematocele and can, at first, be confused with the symptoms of acute appendicitis.

Ruptured Ectopic Pregnancy

The tubal wall becomes eroded to cause a sudden severe intraperitoneal haemorrhage of up to 2 litres or more of blood. This bleeding may occur before the patient is even aware that she is pregnant. Since it is about the only cause of intraperitoneal haemorrhage in the young female, the condition is usually rapidly diagnosed.

Signs and Symptoms

Should the patient suffer a massive haemorrhage, all the signs and symptoms of severe shock and sudden collapse will occur. A typical history may reveal that a patient has amenorrhoea, perhaps missing a period in the previous 4 to 6 weeks. Immediately prior to her sudden collapse there may have been a low abdominal, colicky type of pain. If there is vaginal bleeding, it will be scant but brown in colour due to oestrogen withdrawal.

Intraperitoneal haemorrhage always follows the abdominal pain. On examination the gynaecologist may find a vague palpable abdominal mass. However, palpatation may precipitate a catastrophic haemorrhage and severe abdominal pain. Palpation should **never** be undertaken, except in controlled conditions such as a hospital. The abdominal pain may at first resemble appendicitis, radiating to the epigastrium from the right iliac fossa, and then be referred to the shoulder tips as the phrenic nerve is irritated by blood.

Nursing Action

The diagnosis of ruptured ectopic pregnancy is obvious when associated with the degree of shock, collapse and abdominal signs. In subacute cases, however, the signs may be somewhat vague, with a low haemoglobin level, a normal white blood cell count, a slight pyrexia and a positive pregnancy test. A palpable mass and tender fornices would suggest an ectopic pregnancy and a laparoscopy would confirm a suspicious diagnosis. In doubtful cases, the gynaecologist may request the nurse to prepare the patient for a pelvic examination under anaesthesia. Such an examination is however fraught with danger and the operating theatre should also be prepared for an immediate laparotomy in case of haemorrhage.

In extremis, a ruptured ectopic pregnancy is an emergency. On arrival at the hospital the patient may already have received morphine or pethidine from the general practitioner in an attempt to control the haemorrhage and reduce the hazards implicit in moving a severely collapsed patient. It is strongly recommended that the patient is **not** moved from the emergency trolley but kept resting and still while being treated for shock. Until transferred to an emergency theatre, the patient's pulse and blood pressure are monitored at very frequent intervals, with the doctor advised **immediately** of any further hypotension or worsening tachycardia.

Prior to being sent to the operating theatre an intravenous infusion of either plasma, rheomacrodex, or blood group O Rhesus negative may have to be transfused. To overcome the problem of Rhesus incompatibility, it may be possible to tap the patient's own blood from the abdomen and reinfuse it after it has been filtered. Grouping and cross-matching of blood is urgently completed so that blood is available for the patient when in theatre and for use in the postoperative phase.

Postoperative Care

In theatre, the patient has an emergency laparotomy, drainage, suction and irrigation of the peritoneum combined with a salpingectomy of the affected tube to prevent a recurrence. Following surgery the nurse would implement a standard care plan for a patient with lower abdominal surgery. Keeping in mind that the operation is of an emergency nature, there may be considerable postoperative shock.

Physical recovery takes between 7 to 9 days. The emotional content of the 'shock' may contrast with the physical improvement, as the patient mentally realises the implications for her own future. The threat of not being able to have a family may be a prominent feature of the patient's anxiety. It is always best if both the patient and her partner are counselled together by the surgeon, who is the best person to guide them on the findings of the operation and what had to be done. The surgeon will also have a more accurate idea of hope for future pregnancies. Encouragement to verbalise fears or hopes for the future will help the patient gain a perspective on how to cope with the future.

Chapter 17
Uterine Disorders and Hysterectomy

The uterus may be affected by congenital defects, displacement, endometriosis, benign tumours, cancer of the cervix, trophoblastic diseases and infections. Because most of these disorders may be resolved by hysterectomy, it is included within this chapter.

CONGENITAL DEFECTS

While uncommon, congenital defects may not be found until after puberty. Symptoms such as a delayed menarche, amenorrhoea, infertility, abortion and malpresentation during delivery may be the basis for initial investigations. In the developing female fetus, the two Müllerian ducts have to fuse between the sixth and twentieth week to ensure a normal anatomical uterus. Failure of these ducts to fuse may lead to one of the following defects:

Uterus didelphys. The individual has 2 uteri, 2 cervices and 2 vaginae.

Uterus bicornis bicollis. While the uterus and cervix are normal the vagina is fused.

Uterus unicornis. One of the Müllerian ducts fails to develop and a rudimentary horn remains on one side of the partially developed uterus.

Uterus septus. The uterus is divided by a septum at the fundus.

Arcuate uterus. The fundus is both wide and distended.

Uterus aplasia. If there is complete failure of the Müllerian duct system during fetal life, there is a complete absence of uterus, cervix, tubes and upper vagina.

Radiography, such as a salpinography, would show the majority of these defects, many of which are amenable to surgical repair. For example, a vaginal fusion can be divided, or the rudimentary horn can be excised to allow normal pregnancy to take place. Endocrine investigations would clarify if the menstrual cycle requires replacement therapy. Normal pregnancy is not necessarily precluded, providing the need for a caesarean section is kept in mind.

UTERINE DISPLACEMENT

The adult uterus adopts the anteversion position, i.e., at a 90° angle to the plane of the vagina, inclined forwards and over the posterior wall of the bladder.

Retroversion

In about 15% of women the uterus is retroverted, i.e., on the same plane as the vagina and inclined backwards towards the sacrum. Retroversion may be either **congenital** or **acquired**.

Congenital retroversion is rare and does not usually affect a pregnancy.

Acquired retroversion may be due to childbirth, endometriosis, pelvic infection or tumours.

Signs and Symptoms

A typical history shows the patient to have suffered from dysmenorrhoea, persistent backache, incomplete defaecation and deep dyspareunia. The last symptom is due to the ovaries falling behind the retroverted uterus into the Pouch of Douglas. When bimanually examined, the uterus is found to be enlarged and fixed in the retroverted position.

Interventions

One conservative technique employed to return the uterus to the anteverted position is for the gynaecologist to insert a Hodge pessary. This is a firm elliptical-shaped device which is placed between the posterior fornix and behind the symphisis pubis. The pessary is retained in this position for up to 12 weeks. If dyspareunia is relieved, the patient may then be offered surgery.

Several surgical procedures can be considered. The Crossen-Gilliam operation is a technique of ventrosuspension, and involves the round ligament being pulled through the internal abdominal ring and sutured to the back of the rectus sheath. Alternatively, the round ligament is shortened by pleating and suturing. If the patient is postmenopausal, a hysterectomy may be considered.

Prolapse

A uterine prolapse implies that the uterus is displaced in a downward direction into the vagina. The cause of such a displacement may be that the supporting uterine ligaments or the levator ani muscles of the pelvic floor are weak. Invariably, the patient has had one or more children. The prolapse may appear soon after childbirth, which is rare these days, or not until after the menopause which is the more likely.

Contributing factors to a weakness of either the uterine ligaments or the pelvic floor muscles include:

Obesity

Straining on defaecation (constipation)

Chronic coughing, e.g., in chronic bronchitis

Increased uterine weight due to a tumour

Preceding or accompanying a prolapsed uterus may be any of the following:

Urethrocele, a protrusion of the urethra onto the anterior vaginal wall

Cystocele, a prolapse of the bladder onto the anterior vaginal wall

Rectocele, a prolapse of the rectum onto the anterior vaginal wall

Enterocele, or prolapse of the Pouch of Douglas high onto the posterior vaginal wall

Stages

The uterus may prolapse to a variable degree and this is staged according to the level of collapse:

1. The cervix is below the level of the ischial spine.

2. The cervix is at the level of the vaginal entrance (*introitus*).

3. The fundus is at the level of the vaginal entrance, with vaginal eversion. This last stage is known as *procidentia*.

The patient's awareness of prolapse may be at first a feeling of a lump in the vagina and a sensation of bearing down. Urinary frequency may occur on its own or be related to signs of an infection with low backache. Stress incontinence and incomplete defaecation may add to the patient's problems. If the procidentia rubs against underclothing, it may cause ulceration of the cervix, localised bleeding and an infection.

Interventions

A temporary prolapse, i.e., stage I, may respond to *pelvic floor exercises* and these are especially useful in the young female who has just given birth. A stage 2 prolapse is significantly helped by the insertion of pessaries if she is not fit for surgery.

Pessaries which may be inserted include the Water Spring type, rubber ring, Gelhorn and the plastic ring, which is held in place by suction. While the pessary is in place for perhaps up to 12 weeks, the patient is supervised by the district nurse. The pessary is usually replaced after 12 weeks. If during this time bleeding occurs outside the normal menstrual cycle, the pessary must be removed and further investigations carried out.

Surgery may prove essential for stages 2 and 3 where the following operations may be considered:

Anterior colporrhaphy; a repair of the anterior vaginal wall to restore the urethra and bladder to their normal position, i.e., for urethrocele and cystocele.

Posterior colporrhaphy; a repair of the posterior vaginal wall to restore the rectum to its normal position for a rectocele.

Vaginal hysterectomy; a radical operation to remove the uterus and shorten the ligaments and strengthen the pelvic floor, i.e., the levator ani muscles. This operation may be done if the patient feels she wants no more children.

Fothergill's operation (*Manchester Repair*); the cervix is amputated and the ligaments shortened to repair the weakness of the pelvic floor. It is usually done, again, if the patient feels she wants no more children.

ENDOMETRIOSIS

Endometriotic tissue is found in abnormal sites and behaves in a similar way to the normal uterine endometrium during the menstrual cycle. Endometriosis rarely occurs before the age of 30 years and is more likely in childless women. Although the cause is unknown, there are several theories which attempt to account for abnormally sited endometrial tissue:

Retrograde menstruation: the endometrial cells are carried backwards through the uterine tubes embedding themselves in the ovaries and the Pouch of Douglas.

Lymphatic and vascular transport of the endometrial cells to more distant sites.

Metaplasia, i.e., embryonic endometrial cells are already deposited in abnormal sites and activated by circulating hormones.

The abnormal sites may be confined to the myometrium, i.e., *adenomyosis*. Other ectopic sites include the ovary (*chocolate cysts*), Pouch of Douglas, broad ligament, sigmoid colon and rectum. Less commonly, endometrial tissue may be found in the cervix, bladder, round ligament, appendix, umbilicus and the uterosacral ligaments.

Ectopic endometrium undergoes the typical changes during the menstrual cycle, i.e., oestrogen and progesterone secretion and stimulus, and bleeding during the menstrual flow. In ectopic sites the blood cannot escape and is partly absorbed, leaving behind a cystic, thick, tarry residue, hence the name 'chocolate cysts'. The cysts can be of any size, and if they rupture they will cause an inflammatory reaction. A consequence of endometriosis may be the formation of dense adhesions which bind the uterus into retroversion. Adhesions may also affect the intestine, omentum and the Pouch of Douglas.

Pain

Endometriosis is often diagnosed incidentally, as 25% of patients are asymptomatic. A patient being investigated for infertility may have asymptomatic endometriosis. For those with symptoms, pain is the most significant factor and should be closely questioned, for it has the following features:

Congestive dysmenorrhoea.

Pain before the period, becoming worse during the period because of oedema of the ectopic endometrial tissue.

Constant pain, if the endometrial cyst is large.

Deep dyspareunia, i.e., pain on sexual intercourse, usually due to adhesions, retroverted uterus, oedema of endometrial deposits, or the ovaries being adherent to the Pouch of Douglas.

Painful defaecation, which may suggest adhesions of the gut or the omentum. The diagnosis is usually made after a bimanual examination which demonstrates that any cysts present are tender, with tenderness of the posterior vaginal wall, Pouch of Douglas or the ovaries.

Interventions

There are three avenues of treatment. The first is the prescription of mild analgesia which the patient may take when the symptoms cause undue discomfort. Should the patient be prepared for surgery, the operation usually will involve the excision and removal of any cysts, the division of any adhesions and the correction of a retroverted uterus. If surgery is proposed for the younger female, as much reproductive tissue and organs as possible will be preserved to ensure future pregnancies, while in the older female a hysterectomy may be performed.

A third treatment is for the gynaecologist to prescribe hormone therapy with the intention of inducing a pseudopregnancy, the principle being that the condition does improve following a pregnancy. Therefore by inducing a pseudo state, the endometriosis will resolve. A drug such as norethisterone acetate (Primidos) is prescribed in daily doses of 2.5 mg which are increased each fortnight over a 9-month period until the maximal dosage of 15 mg daily is achieved. Basically, this progesterone-based drug will alter the endometrium into a pseudodecidua, during which the patient can expect to become amenorrhoeic but the pain will disappear and she should regain her general feeling of well-being. Other drugs are available from the progesterone group which in normal physiology is concerned with the continuation of pregnancy.

BENIGN TUMOURS

The incidence of benign tumours (*fibromyoma fibroids*) is unknown, since the majority of patients suffer no symptoms. However, a calculated guess is that about 30% of the adult female population will suffer from a benign tumour.

In the main, the tumour takes the form of an innocent swelling in the smooth muscle of the uterus, i.e., the myometrium. The cause of these innocent tumours is unknown, but seems to be linked in some way with a high secretion level of oestrogen. This type of tumour is seen more often in childless women, or those who have not conceived for several years. Most tumours remain small, i.e., about 2.5 cm, but some can grow to a weight of 11 kg. The majority are sited in the myometrium (70%), some grow inwards towards the uterine cavity (10%), while the remaining 20% grow towards the peritoneal surface.

Pathology

According to where the tumour is sited it may be classified as being intramural, subserous or submucosal, this siting being relevant to the eventual outcome of the tumour. Some tumours become pedunculated, i.e., they develop a narrow irregular shaped part which may act as a support for the tumour. Examination by microscope shows the tumour to be arranged as spindle-shaped cells lying in a network of fibrous tissue (hence the term *fibroids*), which is encapsulated in a layer of connective tissue separating the tumour from the myometrium. This capsule does permit easy enucleation or shelling out of the tumour during surgery. Typical of benign tumours, they grow slowly and have a poor blood supply, and may atrophy at the menopause, reducing the need for treatment.

Apart from atrophy, other pathological changes which occur include the hyaline content of the tumour degenerating, altering the solid tumour to that of a cyst. In pregnancy, this tumour may suddenly degenerate giving rise to the typical *acute abdomen*. At operation, this degeneration may cause the tumour to take on the appearance of raw beef due to the blood cells releasing haemoglobin. If pedunculated, the narrowed extension of the tumour may cause either a *torsion* or a *volvulus*, both being surgical emergencies. Another pathological change is that the tumour may become calcified, and lastly but rarely the tumour may become malignant, i.e., a *sarcoma*.

Signs and Symptoms

As already stated the patient may have no symptoms, the tumour being diagnosed incidentally or in association with other investigations, e.g., infertility, when the tumour distorts the shape of the uterus preventing implantation into the endometrium. Intramural and subserous tumours may cause menstrual cycle disturbances, such as menorrhagia, hypermenorrhoea with blood clots and dysmenorrhoea. If the patient has a continuous discharge of blood, usually she will be obviously anaemic. A subserous tumour causes bleeding as the tumour may rupture causing abdominal swelling with a risk of intestinal adhesions which in turn initiate digestive upsets. If large enough, the tumour will cause pressure symptoms of both the bladder and the bowel.

Fibroid Polyps

A fibroid polyp may not cause any problems but it may follow one of two other possible pathological changes. Should the fibroid become necrotic and infected, there will be a bloodstained, offensive vaginal discharge. Alternatively, if the patient is pregnant, the fibroid polyp may endanger the pregnancy with abortion, premature labour, malposition, malpresentation, obstruction of the birth canal or postpartum haemorrhage.

Interventions

On bimanual examination the uterus may be felt to be unevenly enlarged by one or several rounded masses which move with the uterus. Tests to exclude pregnancy and malignancy are completed before treatment is prescribed. It is common practice to adopt one of two approaches. First, the gynaecologist may recommend that the patient be kept under observation until the menopause. Second, regular outpatient appointments are arranged and, on each visit, the patient is carefully examined to note if there are any significant changes.

At the menopause the benign tumour will usually atrophy, in which event no further treatment is required. Alternatively, if surgery is proposed this may either be a *myomyectomy*, to shell out the benign tumours from their capsule after cutting into the myometrium. This operation is usually done via the vagina and may lead to many lower abdominal discomforts in the postoperative phase. Myomyectomy is preferred in the younger female patient who has not completed her family. A second operation for the older female who has decided on having no more children is a *total hysterectomy*, when the fibroid-bearing uterus and cervix are removed.

CARCINOMA OF CERVIX (SEE ALSO ONCOLOGY NURSING)

The visible part of the cervix which projects into the vagina is covered with stratified squamous epithelium, as is the vagina. At or near the external os this changes to columnar epithelium. Where these two tissues meet there is a red area which is surrounded by a white colouration of the junction. This area is known as the *ectropion* or *eversion* and is of considerable interest since early malignant changes can be detected at this junction. If changes do occur, and these can be detected by regular checking with the Papanicolaou smear test, it would suggest that more detailed investigations and increased observations should be made for the early detection of cervical cancer.

The incidence of cervical cancer occurs in about 2% of the adult female population, and at least 50% of this total progress to renal failure, fatal infections, or metastasis because diagnosis was made too late. However, only 3% of those detected by regular 2 yearly screening with the Papanicolaou smear test progress to invasive carcinoma. This last point should be stressed to females who are between 25 and 35 years of age. After 40 years of age, the existing cancer tends to be invasive before it is diagnosed. The majority (95%) are squamous cell cancers, 4% are adenocarcinomas and the remaining 1% is a sarcoma, lymphoma or melanoma.

Causes

Causes of cervical cancer attract great attention as they seem to suggest that social behaviours can and do have an impact on the health of an individual. The causes are said to be:

1. It is common in the sexually active female who from adolescence has had multiple partners. Whether this is a result of the effects of smegma from the uncircumcised male on the female cervix has yet to be proven.
2. It has a low incidence in orthodox Jews who follow the Law of Niddah, which states that sexual intercourse is forbidden during the menstrual flow, for 7 days after, during pregnancy, or for several months following the postpartum.
3. Theoretically, it is suggested that the DNA of herpes virus II and from spermatozoa may be donated to the cervical tissues during a period of hormonal imbalance at adolescence and the donated DNA invokes a new line of cells which become malignant many years later.
4. Premalignant conditions which predispose to cervical cancer include *metaplasia*, i.e., a change in tissue type at the ectropion, *dysplasia* similar to metaplasia but the premalignant changes occur at the basal cell layer carrying a very high risk of malignancy, and *carcinoma* in situ. This latter premalignant change refers to a full thickness epithelial cancer which remains localised for up to 10 years before breaking through the subepithelial layer to become invasive to the cervix. A cone biopsy via a colposcope is usually necessary to prove the existence of carcinoma in situ.

Stages

Cervical cancer is staged according to its invasiveness:

0. Intraepithelial cancer only
1. Invasive, but still confined to the cervix
2. Invasive to, but not beyond, the pelvic wall or lower third of the vagina
3. Invasive to the pelvic wall and lower third of the vagina
4. Invasive to the bladder and rectum

Early detection at Stages 0 and 1 offers a good prognosis, with early treatment by single or combined techniques of ionisation, irradiation or cauterisation. If a Stage 2 cancer is diagnosed, current statistics show that the patient has a survival rate of between 50 and 70% beyond 5 years following radical surgery.

In Stages 3 and 4 the prognosis remains poor because of the metastasis. Combined therapy with radical surgery, irradiation to limit the metastasis, and cytotoxic drugs may control the worst of the symptoms of pain and cachexia, but there is at the moment an inevitably early death due to its invasive nature (for nursing care, see Oncology).

Malignant changes in the endometrium seem to occur in the postmenopausal female between 55 and 65 years of age. Usually the patient is unmarried without any children. There is a causal relationship between the malignant changes and obesity, hypertension, diabetes or an oestrogen secreting ovarian tumour.

Signs and Symptoms

The first unusual sign the patient notices is vaginal bleeding, although she is postmenopausal. The bleeding may only be slight but be either a thin watery or brown coloured discharge with an offensive odour. On bimanual examination the cervical os may be obstructed by a blood cyst or could be infected, in which case the patient will have signs of toxaemia.

When palpated, the uterus is felt to be enlarged and quite tender. The actual diagnosis of endometrial cancer is made at operation, i.e., at curettage. The curettage may reveal the cancer, in which case serial smears are taken from the cervix, body and uterine fundus. Microscopic examination of the smears determines the actual type of cancer. It is usually an adenocarcinoma of the upper posterior wall of the uterus with slow endometrial growth. If the cancer has been established for some time it may also involve the myometrium.

Apart from differentiating if the malignant cells are well-distinguished from normal cells, the cancer can be staged for its invasiveness:

1. Dysplasia of the endometrium, i.e., the basal cell layer only
2. Confined to the corpus
3. Invasive to the cervix
4. Extended beyond the uterus, but within the true pelvis
5. Metastasis to the bladder and rectum

In Stages 1 and 2, a simple hysterectomy may eradicate the cancer entirely. A radical hysterectomy is usually undertaken for Stage 3. For Stages 4 and 5, radical surgery combined with deep X-ray therapy or radium/radon implant usually produce the best results. Hormone therapy may be a combined part of the total therapeutic approach.

TROPHOBLASTIC DISEASE

Trophoblastic disease is a rare condition that refers to either a benign or malignant tumour developing in the uterus during a pregnancy. It is estimated that 1 in 6000 European births are affected by this disorder.

In benign tumours there is abnormal development of the placenta, which has multiple cysts with the appearance of very distended villi, a so-called *hydatidiform mole*. About 10% of these hydatidiform moles become malignant, and the trophoblastic tissue invades the myometrium causing extensive destruction and rapid spread of malignant cells to the lung, liver and brain.

A malignant tumour of this nature is referred to as a *choriocarcinoma*. During the pregnancy, the patient may experience vaginal bleeding. If this occurs after the fourteenth to eighteenth week, it is not usually due to abortion. Along with the bleeding, the patient may have hypertension and peripheral and systemic oedema. On examination the uterus is much bigger than it should be for the date of pregnancy, no fetal parts can be felt, and there is no fetal movement or heart sounds. A 24-hour urinary specimen is usually collected to test for chorionic gonadotrophin level, which remains elevated.

Interventions

The patient after admission to hospital is prepared for a therapeutic abortion with the full involvement of the patient's husband or partner. If a hydatidiform mole has been diagnosed, it is digitally removed from the uterus. A few days later the patient has a second operation of dilation and curettage.

A great deal of emotional supportive therapy has to be given at this time. The treatment for a choriocarcinoma is extremely urgent due to the destructive nature of the malignant cells. Initially, the patient is started on a course of methotrexate, a cytotoxic drug. Following this, the patient may have a hysterectomy and then a further course of methotrexate.

Several problems can be immediately identified. These are the natural disappointment of a lost pregnancy, the cytotoxic effects of methotrexate, and the surgical hazards associated with a hysterectomy. Even overcoming these problems the patient still has an uncertain future. In the following 6 months, she has to be seen each month to detect for any further malignant changes. If in the following 2 years she is free of malignant changes, the patient may then if she wishes start a family.

INFECTIONS OF THE UTERUS

Uterine infections may be acute or chronic, and commonly involve the endometrium (*endometritis*) or the cervix (*cervicitis*).

Endometritis

Acute or chronic inflammation of the endometrium, in the main, is due to the invasion of pathogenic bacteria:

Gonococcus neisseria
Streptococcus
Staphylococcus
Tubercle bacillus

Many females are prone to endometrial infection and inflammation immediately following menstruation, abortion and childbirth. In the acute infections, there is likely to be a rapid response to therapy because the endometrium will shed naturally within a defined time period.

In the chronic type, however, the deeper layers of the endometrium are affected and the inflammation will tend to remain persistent. The patient experiences the symptoms of inflammation: menorrhagia, dysmenorrhoea, a purulent offensive vaginal discharge, pelvic pain, backache, urinary frequency, bouts of pyrexia and an extreme lethargy.

On examination, the uterus is felt to be enlarged and is tender to the touch, when moved with palpation. Swabs are taken and despatched for culture and sensitivity. Until the results are known, the patient is usually prescribed a broad spectrum antibiotic. Once the swab results are known, specific antibiotics can be given.

Intervention

If there is any sign of toxaemia or pyrexia, the patient is cared for with bedrest. Frequent vulval toilet is introduced into the nursing care plan. Should the cause of the infection be attributed to an abortion, she may have a dilation and curettage at a later time. If gonorrhoea is confirmed, the patient should be referred immediately to the venereologist so that all sexual partners can be traced and contacted for treatment.

Tuberculosis of the endometrium is treated conservatively with a triple regimen of 3 of the following antitubercle drugs:

Streptomycin	Isoniazid
Paramino-salicylic acid	Rifampicin
	Ethambutol

The drugs are continued for a 2-year period, and usually give a good response towards a cure.

Cervicitis

Like endometritis, cervicitis may occur in acute or chronic form, and may be the result of invasion by:

Candida albicans
Trichomonas vaginalis
Haemophilus vaginalis

Similarly, it follows childbirth, with the cervix, or neck of the uterus, noticeably red and oedematous. Generally, it is accompanied by a malodorous vaginal discharge, pain and bleeding may occur on touch. The last aspect usually precludes sexual intercourse temporarily for the patient and her partner.

After a smear has been taken for culture and sensitivity, the patient with acute cervicitis is usually prescribed an antimicrobial regimen. Whereas, the woman with chronic cervicitis may be prescribed a topical treatment, although cauterisation, hot or cold, may be the most effective method of relief.

HYSTERECTOMY

Surgery to remove all or part of the uterus may be recommended after investigations confirm a preliminary diagnosis of the following conditions:

Cancer of the body of the uterus. Of all those diagnosed 67% are of squamous cell carcinoma and 37% are adenocarcinoma

Cancer of the cervix which seems to be more common in women under 40 years of age

Endometriosis
Menorrhagia
Procidentia (prolapse)
Uterine polyps
Endometritis

It is most unusual for this operation to be done as an emergency. Therefore, it is usual and preferred to admit the patient 24 hours in advance of the scheduled surgery. Patients for Wertheim's operation would normally have to be admitted for a much longer preoperative preparation period because the surgery is radical, with as much of the vagina as possible being excised, and a detailed assessment is needed on the patient's physical, psychological and nutritional state. This preparation time allows the patient to orientate to her surroundings, to meet the nursing and medical staff and to be physcially prepared without undue haste. In devising a nursing care plan to meet the patient's specific needs, the nurse needs to know the surgeon's intentions, the type of hysterectomy and the surgical approach.

The uterus may be removed either via an abdominal incision or via the vagina. An abdominal approach is usually employed when the ovaries and uterine (Fallopian) tubes are also to be excised. A vaginal hysterectomy (Mayo's operation) is usually reserved for surgery confined to the uterus.

Types of Hysterectomy

The extent of surgery (Fig. 17.1) is categorised as:

Subtotal hysterectomy, removal of the body of the uterus, leaving the cervix intact, is usually done for benign conditions confined to the uterus

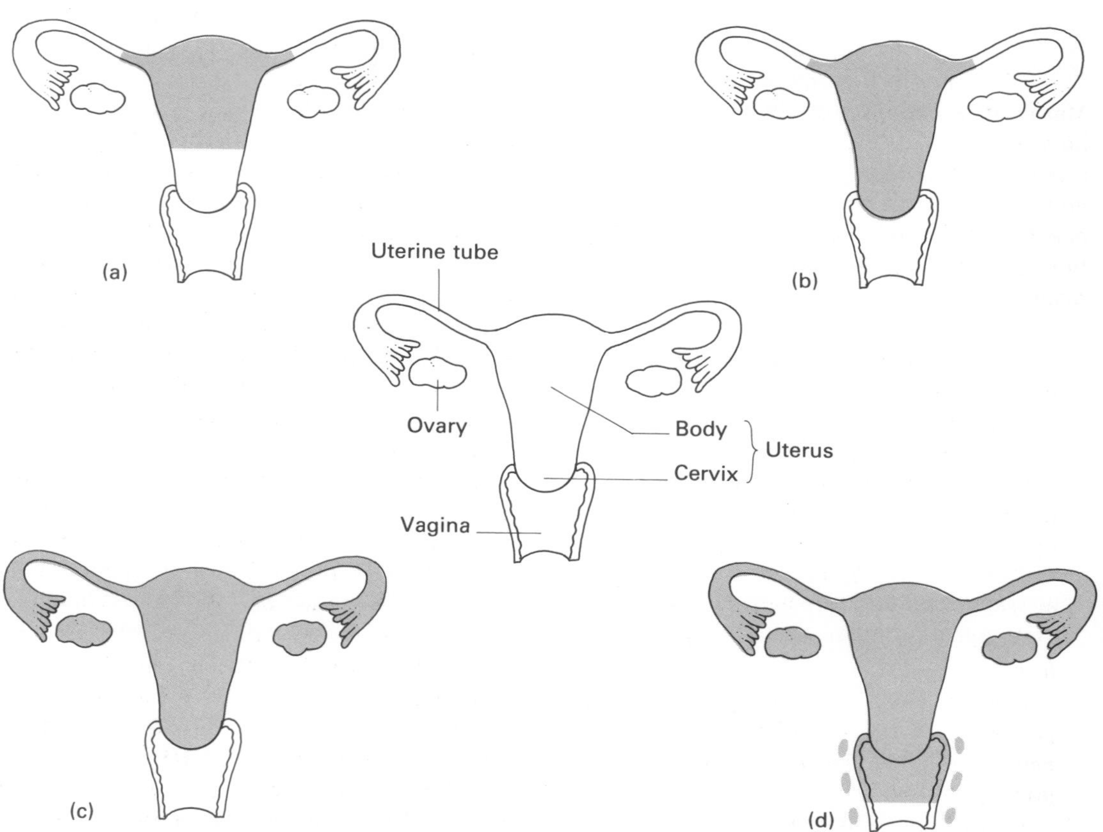

Fig. 17.1 Hysterectomy: subtotal (a); total (b); bilateral salpingo-oophorectomy (c); Wertheim's (d).

Total hysterectomy, removal of the whole uterus and the upper portion of the cervix

Total hysterectomy, combined with removal of the ovaries and uterine tubes, i.e., a bilateral salpingo-oophorectomy

Wertheim's operation, in addition to excising the uterus, the uterine tubes and the ovaries, there is extensive excision of the connective tissue surrounding the uterus (*parametrium*) and lymphatic tissue from the pelvic cavity and the upper third of the vagina. This removal of all the reproductive organs is to clear cancerous tissue and as much risk of metastases as possible. The patient usually has a history of either receiving radiotherapy or chemotherapy. Their physical, psychological and nutritional state all require detailed assessment, hence the need for a longer preparation time.

Investigations

Many of the preoperative investigations will have been completed while the patient was attending the outpatient departments. The ward nurse, however, has a responsibility to check that the following standard investigations have been completed and the results are available:

Chest X-ray

Electrocardiographs, if the patient is postmenopausal

Full blood count

Electrolyte levels

Haemoglobin level to exclude anaemia; usually repeated immediately before the operation

Two or more units of blood, grouped, cross-matched and available for theatre

Serum level of urea to determine renal function

Intravenous pyelography for those patients with cancer of the uterus, who usually also have recently had a dilation and curettage

Wasserman and Kahn tests to exclude venereal disease

Preoperative Preparation

After a social history has been taken and evaluated, the general preoperative physical preparation can begin. Both the surgeon and the anaesthetist will wish to examine the patient to determine her fitness for surgery and the type of anaesthesia to be employed. Vaginal and rectal examinations are usually part of this assessment. The consent to surgery is signed by the patient, witnessed by the doctor and, when applicable, is usually also countersigned by the husband, depending on local policy. This is especially so for premenopausal women.

Physical

The specific preparation of the patient for hysterectomy includes:

A midstream specimen of urine is despatched for culture and sensitivity. The risk of an ascending urinary tract infection is a real hazard and often prophylactic antibiotics are prescribed to counter this risk.

Ward urinalysis of a specimen of urine is done to exclude glycosuria or proteinuria.

A suprapubic shave is completed without causing abrasion or cuts to the soft tissues of the labia or abdomen. This is best done by using warm soapy water and afterwards asking the patient to have a shower or bath to remove any vestiges of hair. Apart from an obvious infection risk, pubic hair is removed because the patient invariably has a self-retaining urinary catheter in place postoperatively.

The lower colon must be emptied and cleansed, mainly to avoid undue straining of the lower abdominal muscles in the first few postoperative days. Glycerine suppositories, or a small enemata, are usually sufficient for this purpose. A note should be made of the patient's personal habits to anticipate any postoperative problems with constipation.

Vaginal discharge of any type or volume should be reported. Menstrual bleeding does not imply that the operation has to be cancelled. The surgeon may prescribe vaginal and perineal douching after a high vaginal swab has been collected. For Wertheim's operation, some surgeons may, for antibacterial purposes, request that an antibiotic vaginal pack (penicillin) be inserted in the vaginal canal for several hours in the immediate preoperative period. This pack is removed immediately prior to the actual operation.

The physiotherapist introduces the patient to the advantages of deep breathing exercises, specific abdominal muscle movements and leg exercises. Pamphlets are available which demonstrate these exercises and the nurse must encourage the patient to do them so they are able to cope during the postoperative period. If the patient smokes, every effort should be made to persuade her to abandon the habit while she is in hospital.

Insomnia due to natural anxiety about the operation is detrimental to the outcome of surgery and sedation is routinely prescribed to ensure a deep and restorative sleep.

A check should be made that the patient has a good supply of lightweight cotton panties. These will secure vaginal or maternity pads in position; larger than usual pads are used. As part of the preparation for the patient to cope in the postoperative period, it is always a wise precaution to make sure that the patient can use a bedpan.

Psychological Preparation

A great deal of work has been done to highlight the many problems faced by patients following a hysterectomy. These basically centre upon the emotional distress consequent upon alteration of the hormones and the loss of the menstrual cycle. Many surgeons do in fact delay hysterectomy, if they can, until the postmenopausal age. For patients with fibroids, these sometimes recede of their own volition thus avoiding an unnecessary operation.

All patients should have the operation explained to them in terms they understand. This often comes better from a female nurse. Details of what to expect in the first few postoperative days will reduce anxiety levels with less demand for analgesia. For the younger female, this operation is a threat to her body image and her femininity. In practical terms, this means a direct threat to her marriage or personal relationships even if she appreciates that the surgery will be of therapeutic benefit. For this reason the husband or partner should be involved in the preoperative discussions as any insight gained by the husband or partner will prepare him for her needs during convalescence, which may be a very trying time for the patient.

Encouragement for the patient to verbalise her fears may be better done by introducing the patient to someone who is making steady progress after a hysterectomy. This woman-to-woman chat can put many minor worries into a better perspective and also allow her to phrase questions which will elicit the answers being sought. This is an important psychological point, without information we carry on worrying unnecessarily and it has a physiologically detrimental effect in the postoperative period.

Postoperative Care

Immediate

Following recovery from anaesthesia, the ward nurse should check with the theatre nurse exactly what observations and instructions have been written by the surgeon and anaesthetist.

Pain is prevented by powerful analgesics, e.g., pethidine. It is standard procedure to administer prescribed analgesia every 6 hours for at least 30 hours.

Intravenous therapy is continued for 12 to 24 hours to maintain hydration and to counter the tendency to shock.

Urinary bladder drainage is continuous. The catheter should be correctly fixed to the inner thigh so that drainage is always downwards to counter the risk of infection.

If there is a **vaginal pack** in position, any blood loss will have to be checked for and reported on at frequent intervals. The surgeon should indicate when he or she wishes this pack to be removed, usually at 24 hours.

If there is an **abdominal wound**, the

covering dressing is checked to ensure that it is intact and whether it is bloodstained.

Pulse and blood pressure are frequently recorded and evaluated to detect if shock is being contained or becoming worse.

Antiemetics, e.g., metoclopramide (Maxolon), are a standard prescription following hysterectomy and may be administered twice in the first 24 hours of postoperative care.

On return to the ward it is best to nurse the patient in the lateral position, with the head supported by one pillow. A prolonged period of rest and sleep is allowed before sitting the patient upright and making her physically comfortable by changing her personal bedwear, washing her hands and face, giving a refreshing mouthwash and checking to see if her level of pain warrants administration of analgesic.

Subsequent Care Plan

A nursing care plan for a patient with hysterectomy usually follows a predictable pattern over a 10- to 14-day period. Observations of pulse, temperature and blood pressure are taken 4-hourly to evaluate if shock or infection are present. These baseline observations should be continued until the patient has been free of either risk for at least 48 hours.

Dependency

The plethora of wound drains, intravenous infusion tubing, packs and bladder drainage increase the dependence of the patient during the first 48 hours of postoperative care. Additional to the problem of recent surgery is that hysterectomy patients tend to tire easily after any prolonged procedure. This requires the nurse to plan for adequate periods of rest during the first 7 days of care. Until the drains and tubes can be removed, the patient is obviously limited in how much she can do for herself. Very basic attention to skin cleanliness, oral hygiene, good bedmaking, and frequent changes of position are welcomed by the patient as they increase her comfort.

Mobility

The patient's mobility is obviously limited because of the drains and tubes. If possible, the patient is given a few minutes armchair rest on the first postoperative day. Thereafter, graduated mobility is planned over the next 7 days. After the vaginal pack and urinary catheter have been removed, usually by the third day, the patient is encouraged to attempt a walk to the ward bathroom. A shower, bidet, or kneeling bath is much appreciated at this time, being refreshing and comforting to the perineum.

The value of physiotherapy taught in the preoperative stages is now realised as the patient practises deep breathing, regularly flexes the ankles and feet and uses the extension pole to lift herself up and down from the bed. Correctly done, these exercises contribute to the prevention of chest infection and deep vein thrombosis. Since the patient tires so easily, visitors should be advised to limit the time of their stay to enable the patient to have adequate periods of rest, especially in the afternoon.

Wounds

The vaginal pack serves the purpose of keeping the anterior and posterior vaginal walls apart until healing can begin. It would normally be removed 24 hours after surgery, and 30 minutes after the administration of analgesic. Some bleeding is expected, so the pack may be stained with capillary blood. After its removal the nurse should be alert to the risk of increased blood loss from the vagina.

Vaginal swabbing is carried out to cleanse and comfort the labia and perineum, and a large maternity pad is applied to absorb any further vaginal discharge. Occasionally an infection high in the vaginal wall occurs on the suture line and a swab should be routinely taken and despatched for culture and sensitivity.

If there is an abdominal wound, the incision line may be secured by clips or by sutures. In either case, the wound should be left alone for

5 days. When it is dressed, the incision line is checked for any signs of inflammation or infection. If present, a wound swab is routinely taken and the surgeon informed. If the wound is healthy the clips are removed on the fifth day and sutures between the seventh and tenth day.

Nutrition

Hysterectomy usually leaves the patient with a poor appetite for many days after the operation, the implication being that the patient will prefer a light diet after the intravenous therapy has been discontinued, i.e., when bowel sounds return. Once *peristalsis*, i.e., intestinal movement, begins the patient commences on gradually increasing amounts of clear oral fluids and progresses to a light diet usually within 48 hours. Haemoglobin levels are assessed at regular intervals and, if necessary, iron compounds given to supplement the light diet.

Elimination

The urinary catheter remains on free drainage until the patient has commenced free fluids and the bladder outflow is satisfactory. While the catheter remains in position, it requires to be cleansed twice daily and a strict fluid balance chart should be maintained. When the catheter is removed, it is useful to collect a specimen of urine for culture and sensitivity as a precautionary measure to identify any infection.

Two problems may arise as a consequence. The patient may suffer a degree of urinary incontinence, which should resolve once mobility is increased. Alternatively, the patient may go into urinary retention. This is judged by oliguria for 12 hours and increasing distension of the suprapubic abdomen, in which case the patient should be recatheterised for immediate relief.

The bowel is kept quiescent for at least 3 days to avoid undue abdominal straining. After this time it is advisable to administer 2 glycerine suppositories to help the patient void a soft motion from the rectal colon. If abdominal distension occurs due to trapped intestinal gases, a flatus tube is the quickest and most effective method of relieving this complication.

Convalescence

Convalescence is a prerequisite following this type of surgery. Some surgeons indicate at least 3 months is required before the patient regains physical and psychological well being. This has major implications if the patient has domestic or work responsibilities, and any supportive rearrangements should be dealt with in detail before the patient is sent either to a recovery nursing home or directly to her own home.

Counselling Prior to Discharge

During the 3-month convalescence, the patient must avoid heavy lifting. In fact, she will not even feel like doing physical work of any kind for some time. However, some patients feel they must make some effort to meet their family and domestic responsibilities, but they must be strongly warned against doing so. Actions such as carrying heavy shopping bags or hanging out washing will leave her totally exhausted and at risk from a hernia.

Sexual Intercourse

Sexual intercourse should be avoided until after the first outpatient appointment. The abdominal and vaginal examination carried out at this time will indicate if intercourse can recommence. The younger patient may require reminding that she will be amenstrual and may experience sudden menopausal symptoms such as emotional irritability, flushing, weight gain and some atrophy of the labia. Depression is quite common and should be dealt with by the patient's general practitioner.

Complications

Many of the complications already mentioned, e.g., chest infection, deep-vein thrombosis, paralytic ileus, flatus, constipation, retention of urine, sudden menopausal symptoms, depression and secondary haemorrhage, can be prevented or anticipated by good nursing care. For patients with a Wertheim's operation, the nurse should observe for the possibility of a ureteric-vaginal fistula. This tracking wound between the ureter and vagina usually occurs because of the extensive clearance of connective tissue from around the ureters. In the process, the delicate ureters may have been traumatised. Such a wound takes a long time to heal and it may necessitate the patient returning to theatre at a later time for irrigation and packing of the wound to promote healing.

Chapter 18
Vaginal Disorders

The causes of sudden, dramatic, vaginal haemorrhage include the following:

Abortion. All women with vaginal bleeding are considered pregnant until proved otherwise

Advanced carcinoma of the cervix

Leiomyoma uteri, or benign fibroid tumours of the uterus

Disturbance of hormonal secretions during the menstrual cycle associated with:

- Contraceptive pills
- Intrauterine devices
- Ovarian disease
- Systematic disease, e.g., blood coagulation defects
- Leukaemia, which accounts for about 10% of all cases of vaginal bleeding

Postpartum haemorrhage

Dysfunctional uterine bleeding, when no other organic cause can be found

Secondary haemorrhage following gynaecological surgery

ASSESSMENT

No matter what the cause of the vaginal bleeding the nurse will be dealing with a patient who will be in *shock*, both haemorrhagic and neurogenic. Such shock is more pronounced by a rapid visual assessment of the patient's pale, anxious expression, dilated pupils, cyanosis of the periphery and lips and, in severe cases, sighing respiration which denotes air hunger.

The haemorrhage may be associated with pain, and this has to be questioned as it is relevant to the diagnosis. Posture and gait can also indicate how severe the bleeding is. The patient **must** be placed at rest in a semirecumbent position and vaginal pads secured in position to absorb the blood. A rapid assessment should be made of the pulse, blood pressure and temperature. If the patient is pregnant, the fetal heart sounds should be monitored. When changing the vaginal pads, the nurse should check for the presence of any blood clots and also for odour. All pads **must** be retained for the physician, as an estimate of actual blood loss has to be made as part of the physical examination. When undressing the patient, the nurse should be careful to note if there is abdominal rigidity, distension, or rebound tenderness. After being undressed, the patient **must** be kept warm, but **nothing** should be given by mouth until after the physical examination.

The medical and nursing assessment of the patient's initial examination should be able to determine the following aspects before treatment is prescribed: the volume, character and duration of bleeding and a comparison between this and the normal period, and the number of vaginal pads used since the bleeding began.

Menstrual History

An accurate menstrual history should include the date of the last period, whether the periods are regular or irregular, and if the bleeding has been lighter or heavier than usual, as well as answers to the following questions:

Does the patient use any form of contraception? If so, in what form, i.e., the contraceptive pill, an intrauterine device, etc.?

If the patient thinks she is pregnant, are there any confirming signs such as breast tenderness, lassitude, early morning sickness or urinary frequency?

If there is pain, can the patient describe its nature, duration, location and onset?

Has there been any history of lower abdominal or perineal trauma?

Is there a history of previous pregnancies, infections of the reproductive system, previous episodes of vaginal bleeding, other than menstruation, and a history of any miscarriages? (The term *abortion* should be avoided at such a crucial time in case it evokes feelings of guilt or remorse.)

Preparing the Patient

After the assessment, the nurse should prepare to assist the doctor in stabilising the patient's condition. If bleeding is profuse, the following steps are taken immediately:

An **intravenous infusion** is established to enable a blood transfusion to be given.

Oxygen therapy via nasal catheters should be given if the respiration is laboured.

Blood samples are taken to do an emergency estimation of the haemoglobin, erythrocyte sedimentation rate, blood urea and electrolytes. The blood is also grouped and cross-matched for both the ABO system and the Rhesus factor. Until this blood is available, blood group O Rh negative may be used.

During this intensive care, the patient should be reassured with an explanation of the procedures and by the continuing presence of the nurse. The patient should **not** be left alone at any time. Vaginal examination is usually delayed until the patient's physical condition is more stable, but the nurse would continue to dress the perineum and vagina each time the vaginal pad is changed.

After emergency treatment a possible outcome of a specific diagnosis may be that:

1. If the bleeding is due to hormonal imbalance, the use of an intrauterine device, dysfunctional uterine bleeding or ovarian cysts, the patient may be referred back to her general practitioner for further care and follow-up.
2. If the bleeding is due to ectopic pregnancy, uterine cysts or abortion, the patient is usually admitted into hospital. Initially they may be prescribed bedrest, sedation to aid sleep and tranquillity and a vaginal pad count.
3. The nursing care plan would then concentrate on promoting physical comfort until the gynaecologist decides if surgery is required. Only if a firm diagnosis has been made can the nurse offer any firm guidance

or counselling on the likely events, except to say that at this point of care the very real and natural anxieties require skilled placation.

ABORTION

Abortion is a major cause of vaginal bleeding during the reproductive years. It is defined as the natural termination of a pregnancy at any time before the fetus has attained viability. Fetal viability is stated as being 28 weeks in the Infant Life Preservation Act 1928, but this point of law is contended by pressure groups who regard viability of fetal life as occuring much earlier. About 15% of all pregnancies terminate with natural abortion.

Physiology

The physiology of abortion is that a haemorrhage occurs in the decidua leading to a local necrosis and inflammation. The ovum then becomes partially or totally detached and behaves as a foreign body. This detachment causes uterine contractions and a dilation of the cervix. If occurring before 12 weeks the abortion is most likely to be *complete*, whereas if it occurs between the twelfth and twenty-fourth week the fetus is likely to be expelled but the placenta retained, i.e., an *incomplete* abortion.

Types

The types of abortion which the nurse working on a gynaecology ward would need to know are: threatened; inevitable; missed; septic; habitual; and therapeutic.

Threatened Abortion

Technically, there is bleeding from the placenta before the 28th week, but not severe enough for a natural abortion to occur. The pregnancy has a very good chance of proceeding to full term if the bleeding remains slight and the cervix remains closed. The bleeding is not retroplacental and may be due to cervicitis, cervical polyp and, very rarely, carcinoma.

Interventions

The usual treatment plan is to keep the patient on bedrest for at least 48 hours. This will improve the uterine blood flow and reduce mechanical pressures on the uterus. A pregnancy test should be completed to confirm that the fetus is still viable. A mild sedative drug may be prescribed to help the patient achieve rest and peace of mind.

After 48 hours, the gynaecologist will examine the cervix to ensure that it is still closed. If uterine contractions are strong, then pethidine or morphine may be prescribed. Should the pads show blood, it is possible for a prognosis to be made if it is clear what colour it is. If the blood is *bright red*, the pregnancy has a 10% chance. If there is a *brown* but persistent discharge the pregnancy has a 55% chance of continuing. If coloured both brown and red the pregnancy has a 45% chance.

A vulval toilet should be carried out at frequent intervals to enhance the patient's comfort. Once it is clear that the fetus is safe, the mother is reassured as to the possible cause of the bleeding and advised on suitable rest periods. Before being sent home, she is given a letter of explanation to hand to her obstetrician in the antenatal clinic, which would be helpful for further care and guidance during the pregnancy.

Inevitable Abortion

Although the vaginal bleeding may only be slight, it is retroplacental and the ovum is already dead. The uterus will begin to contract, the os open and the cervix begin to dilate. If occurring before the twelfth week, the fetus will be expelled completely, i.e., a *complete* abortion. If, however, there is bleeding between the twelfth and twenty-fourth week, only the fetus is expelled and the placenta is retained. This is an *incomplete* abortion. It should be noted that bleeding will continue and, after suffering from uterine contractions, the patient reports having 'passed something' via the vagina.

Incomplete Abortion

For those patients with an incomplete abortion, surgery is planned so that the remaining products of conception can be removed. Prior to this, however, the patient may be prescribed either morphine or pethidine for the abdominal pain, and intramuscular or intravenous ergotamine 0.5 to 0.25 mg to help control the bleeding.

A careful aseptic examination of the vagina is completed by the gynaecologist to remove any obvious conceptive products from the cervix or vagina. Blood grouping and cross-matching must be completed, as blood will have to be available to the theatre staff in case of further haemorrhage during surgery. The standard preparations for any operation are carried out by the nursing staff. Once the patient has been anaesthetised one of several procedures may be done:

Digital curettage. External palmer pressure is exerted onto the fundus of the uterus and its contents simultaneously removed by internal digital clearance, removing blood clots and other debris remaining from the products of conception.

Forceps removal of the placenta. The patient is given 5 units of oxytocin to induce uterine contraction and a thickening of the uterine wall. The open blades of a placental tissue forceps are rotated in the uterus until they grasp and then withdraw the retained products of conception.

Curettage. The concave side of a blunt or sharp curette is pressed against the wall of the uterus and pulled downwards and outwards. This process is repeated several times to different parts of the uterine wall.

Temporary uterine pack. If haemorrhage remains a risk, and oxytocin proves ineffective, the uterus is packed with dry sterile gauze and left for 12 hours to encourage haemostasis.

Following surgery the patient requires frequent vulval toilet and observations of any vaginal discharge reported on. At this time, ascending infection is a very real **hazard** so the nurse must be extra vigilant with cleanliness of the patient's own bedwear and bedlinen. In some instances, the patient may require to remain in hospital for a second curettage if the discharge remains a problem. Before being sent home, the patient does require advice from the gynaecologist on future pregnancies and will require help to suppress lactation.

Missed Abortion

The ovum dies without any external symptoms and is retained for several weeks. There may be some vaginal bleeding, but this will usually have been treated as for threatened abortion. As the days pass, the normal signs of pregnancy regress, the breast tissue returns to its normal size, and the uterus remains small for the known dates. A pregnancy test will prove negative.

It is possible for a complete abortion to occur up to 12 weeks, but be missed by the patient. If the ovum is retained until gestation, it may conclude either as a carneous mole or a macerated fetus. In many instances, however, a missed abortion is expelled spontaneously, but carries with it a high risk of bleeding due to a coagulation defect. A large retained aborted fetus requires the administration of prostaglandin E2 via an extra-amniotic route to aid contractions and expulsion of the dead ovum.

Septic Abortion

Any abortion which becomes infected carries with it a high risk of systemic septicaemia, i.e., a blood-borne infection which can lead to a very serious and alarming toxic shock. Infection can occur within an intact uterus if there is delay in removing the products of conception, or if surgical evacuation has been inadequate, or if there has been a criminal attempt to abort the fetus. In any event, ascending pathogens from the perineum and vagina gain entry via the cervix. If the cervix is traumatised, for instance by a small tear or perforation, it may delay natural healing and can lead to a more generalised infection such as *peritonitis*. The causative organisms tend to be commensal to either the vagina or perineum, and are commonly found to be the

Streptococcus or *Escherichia coli*. Less commonly, *Clostridium welchii* and *Bacteriodes necrosis* are the cause and these two can lead to septicaemia.

Investigations and Interventions

Slight vaginal bleeding, which has an offensive odour associated with a pyrexia, tachycardia and exceptional anxiety are usually noted on the initial assessment. A suspected septic abortion requires rapid diagnostic measures which include bacterial smears taken from the cervix and vaginal vault.

Blood cultures should also be despatched. Whilst a white blood count may reveal a serious leucocytosis, a urinalysis may show a high specific gravity with heavy cast deposits, the blood urea may be elevated and the electrolytes imbalanced. While the test results are awaited, powerful broad spectrum antibiotics are prescribed, e.g., cephaloridine.

Since the uterus must be cleared of infective material, a curettage is carried out as soon as possible. If necessary, the uterus is drained via a perforating wound and occasionally a hysterectomy may have to be done. Where possible the degree of infection is graded to give some idea of its severity. If only the decidua is infected then the infection is mild. If it has affected the myometrium and uterine tubes the infection is moderately severe. Beyond this, the infection is extremely serious with a probable peritonitis.

If the bacterial swabs reveal the pathogen to be *Clostridium welchii*, the patient would require antigangrene serum. The nursing care plan will have to revolve around the care required for a pyrexial, exhausted patient. If extremely toxic, intravenous therapy is utilised to ensure adequate hydration and maintain a normal electrolyte balance. Recovery from both the infection and its toxic effects is very slow and indicates the need for a prolonged period of convalescence.

Habitual Abortion

If a woman has had 3 abortions successively and spontaneously, she is said to be *habitually* aborting. The actual cause of this is unknown, although investigations may be completed to exclude congenital defects related to recessive genes or inborn errors of metabolism. Congenital defects of the uterine tract may prevent development of a successfully implanted embryo. Equally, uterine fibroids or uterine retroflexion may be the root cause.

A common finding is an incompetent cervix, i.e., the cervix is either weak or torn. If this is the case the cervix can be repaired either by reconstructive surgery, or by the insertion of a Shirodkar suture.

Treatment

The Shirodkar suture technique involves the use of nonabsorbable suture material such as nylon, which is threaded into the layers of the cervix as high as possible and then pulled together and tied tightly. This suture would remain in place for the full 36 weeks, or until the risk of a habitual abortion is over, when it is then removed.

A second form of treatment is the administration of progesterone in the form of Primolut Depot or Gestamin. This may be done if vaginal cytology, the ferning test, or a 24-hour urinary pregnandiol excretion test shows a progesterone deficiency.

Therapeutic Abortion

The Abortion Act 1967 allows for a pregnancy to be terminated as a therapeutic measure providing that two registered doctors are of the opinion, formed in good faith, that a continued pregnancy would involve a great risk to the mother's life, involves risk or injury to the physical and mental health of the mother, places at risk the physical and mental health of existing children, or that if the pregnancy were allowed to continue the child, when born, has a substantial risk of mental or physical handicap.

Responsibility of the Nurse

From a legal point of view, the registered doctors must sign a form, which is retained for

3 years. A second form must be sent to the chief medical officer of the Department of Health and Social Security within 7 days of the operation and terminations of pregnancies must be carried out in approved hospitals or nursing homes.

The Act carries a conscientious clause for those nurses and other health workers who object to aiding with therapeutic abortions on moral or ethical grounds. In respecting this legal clause, nurses can be exempt from witnessing or actually helping with such abortions but this does not exempt the nurse from aiding the patient in her recovery or in giving all other nursing care that she may require.

Sociological Aspects

Several social dimensions have evolved since the introduction of this Act. The first is the change in social attitudes towards sexual taboos, which has reduced criminal abortion to negligible figures. Additionally, the national birth rate has fallen and, along with it, the number of illegitimate births. On the other side of the coin, the degree of sexual freedom may have contributed to the alarming rise in the figures for venereal disease. Ultimately, sexual freedom will also be seen to carry with it a greater degree of personal responsibility and discretion.

Techniques

The techniques used to induce a therapeutic abortion include:

Vacuum aspiration, which involves applying suction to the uterine wall followed by curettage. This technique is used up to the tenth week of pregnancy.

Vacuum aspiration with a metal suction catheter and followed by curettage. This use of metal suction catheter is employed between the tenth and thirteenth week of a pregnancy.

Abdominal hysterotomy via a small abdominal incision. The uterus is brought to the surface and the fetus removed. This technique is done when the fetus is over thirteen weeks.

Intra-amniotic instillation, using either hypertonic saline or prostaglandins which are instilled into the uterus between the fourteenth and twenty eighth week of the pregnancy. From the twenty eighth week onwards, the fetus is legally viable and would not usually then be aborted.

Regardless of the method used, many surveys show that the patient goes through a grief reaction which may last for many months. There is also a related problem of hormonal imbalance, which may not resolve itself for the full 9 months. This hormonal imbalance may be countered by the gynaecologist prescribing either oestrogen or progesterone, which may also help to suppress lactation in some females.

After a therapeutic abortion, it may be necessary to offer counselling with regard to future pregnancies. Such advice would be given by the gynaecologist and further reinforced by the nursing staff. It is always useful to consider whether the patient would benefit from a discussion on family planning and the various techniques used to prevent either fertilisation or implantation.

COMMON VULVOVAGINAL DISORDERS

Apart from a copious watery vaginal discharge at birth, the female child does not usually suffer any further vaginal discharge until the menarche. Vaginal discharge in the prepuberty years should always be investigated as the discharge may be due to an infected foreign body. At school, the girl reaching the age of puberty should have several educational sessions regarding vaginal hygiene, the use of tampons or pads and the menstrual cycle in preparation for the menarche. This should be in addition to advice and support from her mother.

At the menarche, cervical secretions moisten the vaginal walls. In addition, the influence of oestrogen lays down a glycogen content which encourages the growth of *lactobacillus*. This organism, the *Doderlein's bacillus*, converts glucose to lactic acid, ensuring an acid environment within the vagina. Such an environment acts as a natural defence barrier against the normal commensal organisms to be found in the perineum and vagina. Anything which reduces the acid pH of about 4 to 5 to a higher alkali pH predisposes the vagina to the risk of infection. It should be noted that the vaginal pH is about 8 in the premenarche and postmenopausal female.

During the reproductive years, commensal organisms are of little consequence. However, the use of the oral contraceptive pill with its oestrogen content may increase the glucose content of the vagina, with the risk of thrush. Vaginal discharge other than the menses is quite common and consists of cervical secretions and natural desquamation of the cells from the vaginal walls.

Excess discharge is **not** necessarily due to infection, and is referred to as *leucorrhoea*. Although this is an innocent discharge, it does cause the patient some distress and she should be reassured that she does not require treatment. However, persistent vaginal discharge other than the menses should always be investigated. In cases where the cervix or uterus are involved, cancer should never be ruled out as a possible cause.

The common factors affecting the vagina are the pathogenic organisms of gonorrhoea, staphylococcus, thrush and trichomonas, foreign bodies, and senile atrophy of the vaginal mucosa in the postmenopausal years.

Candidiasis (Vaginal Thrush)

The causative organism *Candida albicans* (formerly referred to as *Monilia albicans*) is a yeast and thrives in an environment which is warm, moist, has an acid medium and a glycogen content. These environmental factors are enhanced in pregnancy due to the increased oestrogen, in diabetes mellitus due to excess glycogen, after a recent course of antibiotics, after a moderate pyrexia, or when the patient is taking oestrogen oral contraceptive pills.

There is a very understandable degree of distress and social embarrassment as the patient copes with a thick creamy white vaginal discharge. An irritation and an itching of the vulva (*pruritis vulvae*) causes restless behaviour and insomnia, which of itself may cause the patient to withdraw from social interactions. Sexual intercourse is both painful and unpleasant due to the vulva being inflamed, red and sore (*vulvovaginitis*).

On examination there are grey/white patches in and around the vagina which, if removed will cause mucosal bleeding. A smear of the discharge is swabbed onto a glass slide and, when tested with stain, is gram negative. When viewed through the microscope, the typical threadlike hyphae of the yeast organism are clearly seen.

Treatment

Several tests should be completed before any treatment is prescribed. Pregnancy and diabetes mellitus should both be excluded by routine urinalysis tests. Invariably, the patient is prescribed:

Nystatin pessaries (Natamycin) are inserted into the vagina, one each evening for the following 2 weeks.

Oral nystatin. If the patient has a history of repeated monilial infections, oral drugs are preferred since the source of the infection may actually be the bowel.

Nystatin cream is prescribed for young females and is more appropriate for children. It is inserted into the vaginal vault via a small bore catheter, the treatment being repeated each evening for 10 nights.

Vaginal painting. A solution of 1% gentian violet in water is not only comforting, but is most useful when the organism is proving resistant to drug therapy.

Counselling

Since it is most probable that the patient's partner is also affected, he too should be examined and treated. Some patients will need to be advised about their vulval toilet as undoubtedly the infection may be due to unhygienic habits. Nylon underclothing does not absorb perspiration, if anything it tends to raise the local skin temperature. Therefore the patient should be advised to wear cotton pants with a wide gusset. In her daily toilet she should avoid the use of cosmetic creams, lotions, sprays, soaps or powders until the infection has completely cleared up.

Trichomonal Vaginitis

The causative organism is a protozoa, the *Trichomonas vaginalis*. It flourishes on red blood cells and is therefore more likely to occur during the menstrual flow than at any other time in the menstrual cycle. This infection is rare before the menarche and after the menopause, but quite common during the reproductive years. It is transmitted via the male urethra, in which the organism may be lurking in the seminal vesicles or prepuce.

Signs and Symptoms

The main differences in the symptoms are that the discharge tends to be greenish in colour, is rather frothy, irritant and has an offensive odour. The infection may cause a dysuria in addition to dyspareunia, vulvovaginitis and pruritis vulvae. After a vaginal examination, the mucosa may bleed. A smear of the vaginal discharge is swabbed onto a wet slide and diluted with normal saline. On microscopic examination, the protozoa can be seen to be swimming freely. A protozoon is about the size of a white blood cell and has the typical four flagellae.

Treatment

In addition to the advice outlined for moniliasis, the patient is usually prescribed a course of metronidazole (Flagyl) oral tablets, 200 mg three times daily after meals for 7 days. Other treatments which may be offered include a local application of di-iodohydroxyquinolone (Fluoraquine) in a pessary form, which is inserted into the vagina each morning and evening for 7 days. Miconazole cream may also be prescribed for application each evening for 2 weeks. As with monilial infections, the partner or husband should be simultaneously treated for trichomonas infections.

Non Specific Vaginitis (Bacterial Vaginitis)

Pathogenic bacteria become invasive to the vagina usually as the consequence of trauma. Such trauma may take the form of a 'lost' tampon or other foreign body. Allergy to cosmetic substances used for perineal/vulval toilet may alter the chemical protection of the vagina, allowing bacteria from the perineum to gain entry. A malignant tumour will usually always be associated with vaginal infections, as will diabetes mellitus and senile atrophy of the vaginal tissues.

Signs and Symptoms

The symptoms are in fact very similar to those of monilial and trichomonal infections and include pruritis vulvae, offensive vaginal discharge without a classical appearance, dysuria, dyspareunia and local inflammation. The diagnosis is somewhat more perplexing, as it requires a vaginal examination to search for either a lost tampon or, if suspected, a foreign body such as a ring pessary. The gynaecologist will also want to rule out the possibility of tuberculosis, cancer, cervical ulceration and diabetes mellitus.

Treatment

Swabs taken from the vaginal vault are sent for culture and sensitivity. While the cause of the bacterial infection is being established with these investigations, a broad spectrum antibiotic is prescribed. Local applications of an antiseptic such as Povidone iodine 10% may reduce a great deal of the discomfort, as well as cleanse the infected mucosa.

After the menopause, senile atrophy of the vaginal mucosa does make the patient far more prone to infection. This problem, coupled with the ageing process, does require the nurse to be very sympathetic as the infection is one more problem in addition to the many others imposed by age. Initially, the investigations of the cause of the infection should always exclude cancer. Once this has been done, the therapy is very localised to teaching the patient how to douche the vagina each day with a weak acid-based solution; in the home, this can be diluted vinegar.

Applications of local antiseptic creams will soothe the vulval irritation and inflammation. Alternatively, oestrogen creams may restore some of the lost tone of the labia. Alternatively, replacement hormone therapy (RHT) with oestradiol 0.01 mg twice-daily may be tried if the patient is suffering from repeated vaginal infections.

Leukoplakia of the Vulva (Hypertrophic Dystrophy)

Leukoplakia is the appearance of white patches over the epithelium of either the perineum or vulva. The white patches, or marks if present, are noted to be on the inner aspects of the labia majora, labia minora and clitoris. The cause of these patches is unknown, but the epithelial thickening (*keratinisation*) causes intense itching and irritation. Trauma from scratching may superimpose minor injury over the patches. After several years the underlying basal layer breaks through the keratinised basement membrane and may establish a squamous cell carcinoma. Essentially, leukoplakia in the postmenopausal female is a premalignant condition. It requires vigilant follow-up to detect for early changes of a possible malignancy.

Interventions

In the early stages of the condition, the patient should be taught how to apply hydrocortisone cream to the vulval patch areas, and should be supervised on the method she uses to keep the vulval area clean and dry. Later, it may be necessary to admit the patient to hospital to have biopsies taken from several of the patchy white areas to rule out or confirm malignant changes.

Surgical intervention may then be proposed. If cancer is found in a very early stage, a simple vulvectomy may be all that is required. If a more radical vulvectomy is proposed, the patient requires a great deal of psychological support and understanding to face such a major operation. This is a mutilating operation necessitating a prolonged stay in hospital; both points are a major threat not only to the patient but to the family.

Pruritis Vulvae

Irritation and itching of the vulva is symptomatic of an underlying disease. It is a common feature of vaginal infections, diabetus mellitus, vulval disease, systemic illness such as jaundice or Hodgkin's disease, and may be an extension of pruritis ani if the patient has intestinal parasites, i.e., worms.

The intensity of the itching causes the patient to scratch and further insult the irritated area with scratch injuries. Scratching persistently through the day and during sleep leads the patient into a vicious circle of restless behaviour and irritability because of insomnia. Many patients adopt a home remedy to counter the severe itching, and it is a useful precaution to know what they have been doing to relieve the situation. Often patients have to be advised against using various cosmetic sprays, lotions, soaps and powders until the actual cause of the pruritis is diagnosed.

A routine urinalysis should be made to exclude diabetes mellitus. Bacterial swabs should be routinely taken from the vulval areas to detect if there is any infection. A detailed history may actually pinpoint an underlying cause, and this can often be confirmed by a thorough physical examination. Occasionally, pruritis vulvae is of a psychogenic nature, the pruritis being the outward sign of an inner conflict regarding sexuality, body image or a deep-rooted guilt complex.

It is most important to allow the patient adequate rest and sleep. Therefore night sedation and tranquillisers may be prescribed to ensure uninterrupted restful sleep for several nights. Simple cleansing of the vulva, followed by the application of a hydrocortisone cream (e.g., Betnovate), should reduce the irritation in the majority of cases and allow time for detailed investigations to determine the actual cause.

During the healing phase, it is better for the patient to have showers or bidet douching rather than warm baths, to wear very loose cotton undergarments with a wide gusset and to avoid using cosmetic toiletries. In a child, a pruritis ani may be the original source of a pruritis vulvae, and she should be examined carefully in case of parasites, e.g. threadworms.

Vaginal Fistulae

A fistula is an abnormal channel or tube formed by fibrous tissue which connects one body cavity with another. It is a possible consequence of either a disease or local wound. The vagina may connect via a fistula with the rectum, anus and colon posteriorly, or the bladder, urethra and ureter anteriorly. Such fistulae may occur as a consequence of trauma, surgical wounds, irradiation therapy, venereal disease, or as a complication of a malignant tumour.

The diagnosis, while obvious, is rather distressing to the patient, i.e., the passing of urine or faeces via the vagina. Nursing such a patient through what is a degrading insult to her body requires a great amount of tact and gentleness. In confirming the diagnosis with a retrograde pyelogram, the exact site of the fistula is determined and a basis is formed for determining the best type of surgery. A second test is to pass a dye into the rectum and then note the dye stain on a vaginal tampon.

Interventions

To reduce the hazards of urinary and faecal infections ascending into the reproductive tract, a self-retaining urinary catheter is passed into the bladder and continuously drained. Bowel washout may or may not be advised, but is usually not done in the case of a rectovaginal fistula.

The patient is then routinely prepared for one of several possible operations depending on the actual site of the fistulae:

Vesicovaginal Fistulae or fistula. An operation is carried out between the vagina and bladder. Continuous bladder drainage is maintained. The existing wound is cleansed frequently with antiseptic solution until it shows signs of healing. A temporary suprapubic cystotomy may be done to aid this healing. When the wound is sufficiently healed, it is closed by suture. Several days later the cystotomy is also closed.

Uterovaginal Fistulae. Urgent surgery may have to be implemented if damage to the kidney on the affected ureter is to be avoided. The affected ureter can be divided and the fistulae excised and the remaining portion of the ureter anastomosed. Alternatively, the affected ureter can be reimplanted into a lower part of the urinary bladder. A third possibility is for the surgeon to do a nephrectomy if renal investigations show a severely damaged kidney.

Anovaginal Fistulae. Initially a broad spectrum antibiotic is prescribed to reduce the intestinal bacterial flora. The patient is routinely prepared for a general anaesthetic and the fistula is closed on both sides, i.e., on the anal wall and on the vaginal wall.

Rectovaginal Fistulae. A very similar plan is followed as for anovaginal fistulae, but the patient is given a temporary colostomy until the fistula heals naturally, or is sufficiently healthy to allow closure by suture.

Vaginocele is a type of fistulae that is very rare, i.e., a channel between the vagina and colon. Extensive investigations have to be completed to rule out a local or metastatic cancer, after which the patient is given a temporary colostomy until the fistula heals.

Chapter 19
Overview of Obstetric Training

Throughout a six- or eight-week allocation to the maternity unit to complete training in maternal care and care of the newborn, the learner nurse can expect to work in several specialist areas. These include the labour ward, delivery suite, postnatal wards, nursery, neonatal unit, outpatient clinics, parentcraft classes and perhaps working for several days with a district midwife in the community. During this experience the nurse may become aware of many cross-currents of opinion from midwives, obstetricians and from mothers. To understand the various points of view it is useful to take a brief look at the history and development of obstetric nursing.

HISTORY AND DEVELOPMENT OF OBSTETRIC NURSING

Until about 1850, the midwife was the dominant force in the labour room, being thoroughly expert in the problems of pregnancy and delivery. The dominance of males in obstetrics started when King Louis XIV of France insisted on being present and witnessing the birth of his mistresses' children. This introduced the male attendant, and also for the first time the dorsal position during delivery to better the view of the birth of a child.

Parallel to this, other surgeons were insisting upon and introducing new techniques such as asepsis, anaesthesia and new surgical techniques such as Caesarean section. Male dominance in obstetric practice was further extended with male attendants being present at almost all of the births of Queen Victoria's children. For some time this male ascendancy relegated respected female practitioners to their expertise being confined to helping the poorer income groups and the working classes. Within a few years the acknowledged experts were men, with the female midwife being regarded as a rather poor substitute, who was probably rather ignorant and ill-educated. Back-street abortions would seem to stem from this decline in female influence in pregnancy and obstetric practice.

Midwives Acts

Realising the very impoverished state of midwifery, a group of semiprofessional women banded together to form the Midwives Institute in 1881. As a consequence of their work, Parliament passed the first Midwives Act in 1902. This permitted midwives to formulate a statutory training programme with formal examinations, enabling midwives once again to resume their rightful place in the nursing services.

The Act conferred on qualified midwives some unique clinical privileges. They were allowed to give controlled drugs and administer anaesthetic gases without referral to a doctor, and of course be responsible for a mother throughout her pregnancy and delivery. It should be noted that this was against a social backdrop in which the majority of confinements were in the home, *not* within a hospital. Professional development continued with the establishment of the College of Midwives in 1941, being prefixed with the 'Royal' in 1947.

The Midwives Act was amended in 1951 and again in 1979 to incorporate it into the Nurses, Midwives and Health Visitors Act 1979, an Act which enables all branches of nursing to be brought under the aegis of the Central Council of Nursing for the United Kingdom. This professional development is paralleled with steady and gradual improvement in social living conditions for the majority of the population. There is no doubt that social deprivation and squalor is directly proportional to infant mortality, implying that the 'social' work of a midwife can be seen as a quite separate issue to her clinical role.

Centralisation

With the advance of technological innovation, mainly in diagnostic techniques, the need arose to centralise obstetric practice so that the greatest advantage could be made of new and life-saving technology. Maternity units developed at a rapid pace at the expense of the district midwifery service. For example, at the present time, 98% of all births take place in hospital in England and Wales. Midwives then found themselves once again feeling subservient to obstetric aims and goals.

Home versus Hospital Confinement

The argument for home versus hospital confinement is not a clear-cut issue. The following recommendations are usually followed if a mother insists on a choice:

Hospital confinement. Specialist services are available on a 24-hour basis for those who may experience a prolonged or difficult labour. The mother has a temporary freedom from the dual responsibility of caring for a home and family, and delivering a baby. If social circumstances indicate poverty or overcrowding it is in her own interest to be hospitalised. Expert supervision can be offered to the mother with a firstborn child to boost her confidence. Hospitalisation is always recommended for the first, fourth and subsequent pregnancies where difficulties are always expected.

Home confinement is possible if the mother has enjoyed a trouble-free pregnancy, if the pregnancy is the second or third and problems are minimal, if she is between 17 and 35 years old and if a district midwife is available.

The Odent Method

The debate over 'home versus hospital' confinement has been going on for a long time, and recently has taken on a new dimension with the wide publicity given to the Odent method for childbirth. Dr Michael Odent working in France bases his obstetric practice on the philosophy of natural childbirth without the use of drugs. The word *natural* in this context means that the mother adopts her own position of choice for each stage of labour and during the delivery of her baby. This opposes the concept of the *traditional* method where the mother usually has to lie in the dorsal position for both labour and delivery. Providing the midwife has access to the vagina to aid the baby during its emergence, there is no particular reason why the mother cannot adopt whichever position she wishes or indeed follow her natural instincts.

In this natural philosophy, the idea of a labour ward and delivery suite is replaced by the *birthing room*. Within such a room there is usually subdued lighting, quiet music playing and the attendant midwives although present throughout the whole labour and delivery are never intrusive. The mother and father support each other during this time, with the father actively encouraged to help the mother at each stage of labour and during and after delivery, sometimes being allowed actually to cut the cord at the discretion of the midwives. Drugs are **NOT** allowed at any time and therefore for the natural method the mother must have a normal pregnancy; a fact overlooked by many advocates.

Implications of the Odent Philosophy

The Odent philosophy, however, has many implications and does challenge many aspects of traditional practice. As a result, many maternity units have taken a hard look at the midwifery service they offer. Some units have made considerable progress in this direction, while others lag behind in supplying the necessary birthing chairs and specialist beds required for the natural method.

Equally, the environment within the unit itself has to be altered and such changes take time and money along with managerial commitment. Pressure for change is also coming from outside the profession as many women are increasingly aware of their right of choice and are vigorous in their right to practice choice. A direct benefit for many midwives has been a reaffirmation of their clinical, supportive and educative role for those who allow the natural method of childbirth. They have also overcome their uneasy feelings of being the subservient nurse in an age of overwhelming technological gadgetry.

Research in America and in Europe does indicate that traditional obstetric methods leave many mothers feeling unsatisfied after their pregnancy and childbirth. These feelings of failure may arise if the mother is unable to breastfeed, has had a Caesarean section (an increasing practice), has been induced for no good reason or when she is deliberately restrained from expressing her natural instincts.

Some mothers report on how odd it feels to be treated as a 'patient' when in fact their pregnancy is a perfectly normal and healthy thing. This may be a reflection of the fact that hospital-based nurses do tend to see the mothers as patients and not as 'client consumers'. The incidence of postnatal depression is higher in the traditional method, whereas it is rarely if ever reported following a natural childbirth.

The strongest argument for hospital confinement however is a most compelling one in that the majority of mothers can be reassured of a safe birth and a healthy baby.

Chapter 20
Maternal Physiology

FERTILISATION

Fertilisation of the ovum by one of many millions of spermatozoa can occur 48 to 72 hours after ovulation. A fertilised ovum (a *zygote*) carries 22 pairs of somatic chromosomes (*autosomes*) and 1 pair of sex chromosomes. Twenty-three chromosomes are donated from each parent. The sex chromosomes are identified as either XY for a male child or as XX for a female child. While the father determines the sex of the child, all other genetic features are conferred by both parents.

Development following Fertilisation

As the zygote moves along the uterine tube, assisted by ciliated epithelium and muscular contraction, it divides and further subdivides (Fig. 20.1). Within 3 or 4 days, the fertilised ovum has the appearance and shape of a small mulberry about $\frac{1}{2}$ mm in diameter. Between the sixth and eighth day following fertilisation, the zygote, now called a *morula*, enters the uterus, and it is from this tiny cyst that the fetus will develop.

The cystic cavity within the morula is known as a *blastocyst*, while the outer layer is called the *trophoblast*. It is the trophoblast which will find and take nourishment from the uterus and develop into the placenta. The cells of the trophoblast secrete a proteolytic enzyme which digests away the superficial endometrial layer until a trench is formed. It is into this trenched area that the blastocyst will embed itself and will continue to do so

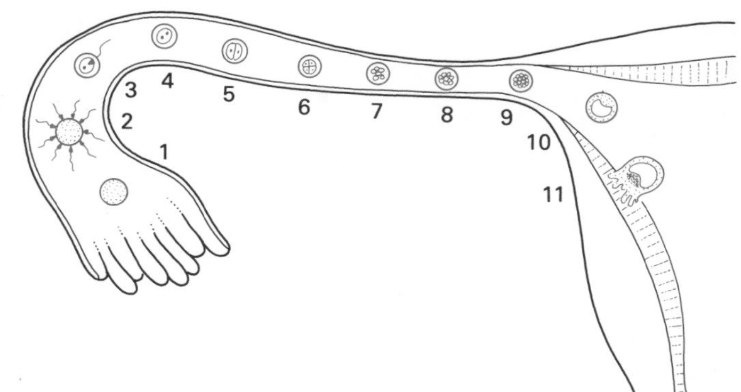

Fig. 20.1 Stages from fertilisation of ova by sperm to implantation of trophoblast.

until the blastocyst is completely entrenched into the endometrial layer of the uterus, which takes about 10 days.

Another function of the trophoblast is to produce a hormone which will inhibit the next menstrual cycle and simultaneously cause the endometrium to become thicker. This much thickened endometrium is called the *decidua*. It is very vascular and will provide the necessary nourishment for the blastocyst.

Small fringe-like projections (villi) develop from the trophoblast and their function is to obtain nourishment from the maternal blood vessels. These vessels, the *chorionic villi*, grow and develop into a many branched tree-like structure. Some of the villi anchor themselves into the decidua, while others float within the maternal blood spaces. From this arrangement, fetal blood vessels grow from the villi and provide the necessary nutrients and oxygen to pass from the maternal blood into the fetus. At about the twelfth week of pregnancy, the chorionic villi begin to proliferate to become the placenta, and other nutritive villi degenerate to develop into the chorion.

Simultaneous growth is occurring within the blastocyst from which the fetus will develop. The inner cells differentiate into 3 layers: the endoderm, mesoderm and ectoderm. As these layers develop, 2 defined cavities also begin to form. The amniotic cavity and the yolk sac, between which lie a layer of mesodermal cells.

Amniotic Cavity

The amniotic cavity is lined with the ectodermal cells which form the amnion and amniotic fluid. The amnion is an inner smooth transparent tough protective membrane. Amniotic fluid, or *Liquor amnii*, is strawberry coloured and is 99% water containing protein, glucose, minerals, urea, desquamated fetal cells, lanugo, which is hair, and the vernix. The ectodermal cells within this cavity will develop into the nervous system, skin, hair, nails, lens of the eyes and the tooth enamel. Amniotic fluid surrounds the yolk sac and body stalk.

Yolk Sac

The yolk sac, or cavity, is lined with the endodermal cells which will develop into the alimentary tract, liver, pancreas, lungs and thyroid gland. The yolk sac itself will be ultimately incorporated into the alimentary tract. The body stalk eventually develops into the umbilical cord which carries the maternal arteries and veins. This cord extends from the placenta to the fetal umbilicus. It is about 50 cm in length and 2 cm in diameter, being composed of connective tissue covering a substance known as *Wharton's jelly*. The cord contains an umbilical vein which conveys oxygenated blood and 2 arteries conveying deoxygenated blood.

Mesodermal Cells

Between the two cavities lies a layer of mesodermal cells which will eventually form the heart, blood vessels, blood, lymphatic system, bones, muscles, kidneys, and the reproductive organs. Organ formation, e.g., the heart, brain, eyes, etc., is completely differentiated by the twelfth week of pregnancy. The remaining period of the pregnancy is devoted to complete growth and maturity of the established fetus.

The Placenta

The placenta which has developed from the trophoblast and chorionic villi grows into a round flat organ and weighs about one sixth the weight of the fetus at full term. On average it will weigh between 500 and 600 g, be 20 cm in diameter and 2.5 cm thick. It has two surfaces:

The fetal surface is very smooth, a shiny bluish mauve colour and covered in amnion. The umbilical cord is attached to the centre of this surface with its blood vessels radiating in all directions.

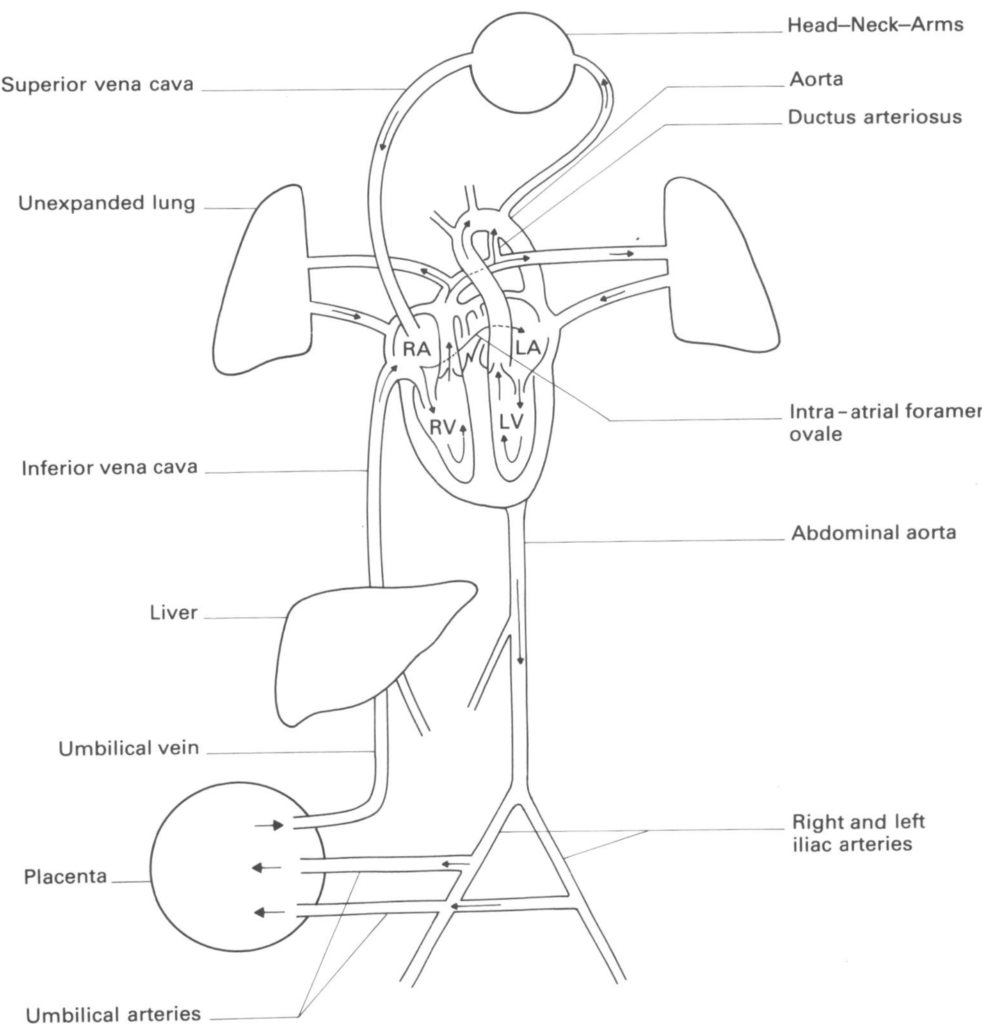

Fig. 20.2 Fetal circulation.

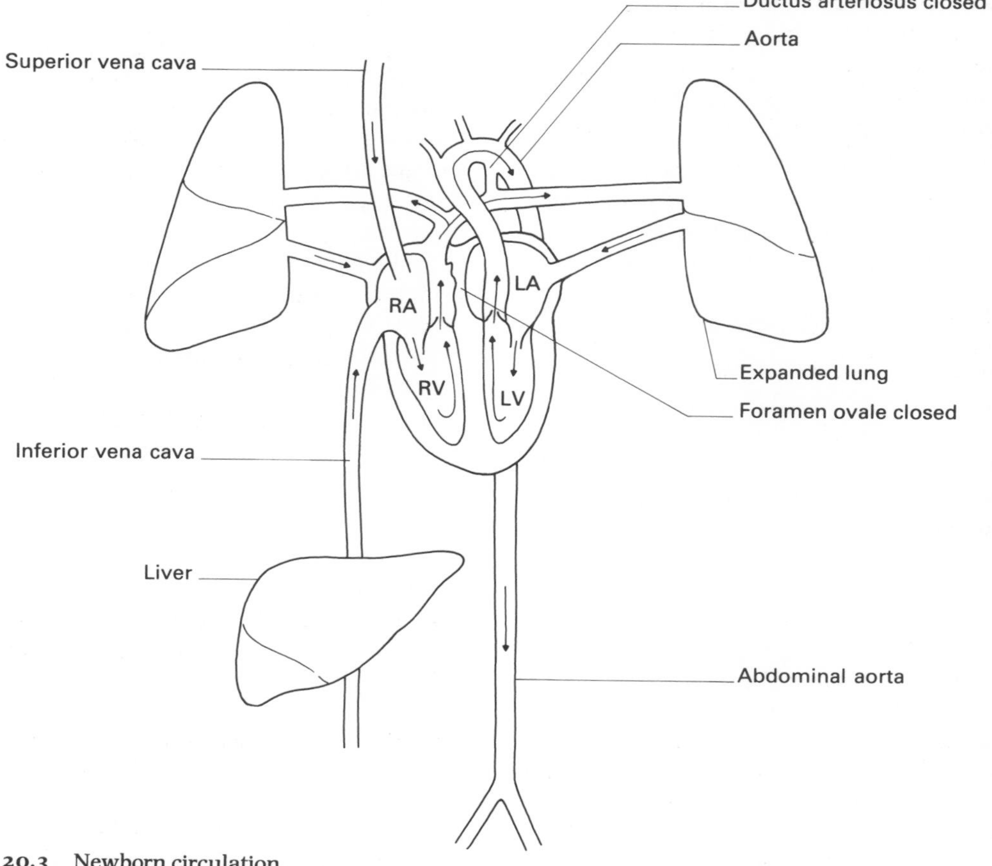

Fig. 20.3 Newborn circulation.

The maternal surface is attached to the decidua, is rough in texture, reddish in colour and consists of masses of chorionic villi which are arranged in distinct lobes. These lobes, or *cotyledons*, number between 15 and 20.

Functions

The functions of the placenta are vital to the health and development of the fetus, and they include:

1. To act as the kidney, lungs, liver and intestines for the fetus.

2. To produce hormones: Human chorionic gonadotrophin (HCG) which is secreted into the maternal urine and forms the basis of the pregnancy test; oestrogen and progesterone from the twelfth week of pregnancy; human placental lactogen (HPL), which is secreted into the maternal blood and can be measured to assess placental function.

3. To permit oxygen and carbon dioxide exchange between the fetal and maternal circulation (Fig. 20.2). Figure 20.3 shows how newborn circulation differs.

4. To ensure an increased blood supply to the uterus, i.e., 20 times greater than normal; the fetal haemoglobin level can exceed the maternal haemoglobin.

5. To allow substances of a molecular weight below 1 000 to cross between the fetal and maternal circulation. Thus water, mineral salts, amino acids, glucose, fatty acids and vitamins can be delivered to the fetus, and urea can be removed. Antibodies exceeding 1 000 molecular weight can also cross, but how this happens remains a

mystery. Excretion of waste products is via the amniotic circulation and then into the maternal circulation. Additional to these nutritional functions, the placenta also stores glycogen which can be converted to glucose in times of stress.

SYSTEMIC MATERNAL CHANGES

Pregnancy will naturally produce many changes throughout all the systems of the body. Such changes are usually monitored continuously, particularly at each trimester. The mother herself can be advised of these expected physical changes and encouraged to monitor her own progress throughout the pregnancy.

Urinary System

At about the sixth week of pregnancy, there is an increased blood flow to each kidney. Paradoxically, this leads to lesser volumes of urine being produced as absorption by the renal tubules is increased, but at the same time the mother complains of increasing urinary frequency. The ureters and bladder at this time tend to lose their muscular tone due to the level of circulating progesterone. Uterine enlargement begins to exert mechanical pressure on the dome of the bladder. Both factors will cause urinary frequency.

With the loss of some muscle tone, urine will tend to stagnate in the bladder which in turn leads to the risk of urinary tract infection, e.g., pyelonephritis. Urinary tract infections are quite common in pregnancy. At each clinic visit a urine specimen should be tested for glycosuria. With the increased renal blood flow, there is likely to be 'spill over' of glucose from the blood into the urine. If present, a glycosuria must be recorded and reported so that further investigations can be completed to discount diabetes mellitus. If the odour of urine has a fish-like smell, it is suggestive of an infection. A fresh specimen of urine should be collected and despatched for culture and sensitivity tests to determine the appropriate antibiotic required.

Respiratory System

During pregnancy, the uptake of the oxygen is increased by 20% to meet increased metabolic activity. The depth of respiration can be noted by the increased movement of the diaphragm and the greater expansion of the rib cage. *Tidal volume*, i.e., inspiration of air while at rest, increases from an average 250–500 ml to 450–700 ml of air. Correspondingly, the minute volume rises from an average of 7–10 litres of oxygen. Apart from meeting metabolic requirement, the increased respirations ensure a high arterial oxygen pressure ensuring adequate fetal oxygenation and the rapid removal of carbon dioxide.

Cardiovascular System

The cardiac output increases from an average 5 litres to over 8 litres of blood per minute, to meet increased metabolic activity. The double effect of increased metabolic activity and oxygen uptake combine to create more heat and the mother has a pleasant feeling of warmth and well being. The rise in body temperature which one would expect is compensated for by vasodilation of the peripheral vessels which contributes to the 'glow' so often noted in early pregnancy.

Blood volume as measured by the haematocrit and other blood tests shows an increase of up to 40%. The heart rate increases from an average 70 beats up to 90 beats per minute. The blood pressure, however, remains constantly normal due to the vasodilation of the peripheral blood vessels, and reduced viscosity of blood. Generally speaking, the cells increase in number; erythrocytes by about 18% to allow for extra haemoglobin to carry the extra oxygen required. The leucocytes, platelets and plasma proteins also increase in volume with the exception of plasma albumen, which decreases, thus reducing plasma viscosity.

Local changes in the blood vessels of the lower limbs can be very striking. Such changes are in part due to the poor venous return caused by uterine pressure on the pelvic veins. Venous return to the heart and kidneys can be impeded, mainly by a

Table 20.1 Nutritional needs in the second and third trimester (per day)*

Kilocalories	2400 (10 MJ)	
Protein	44–60	grams
Calcium	1.200	mg
Iron	15	mg
Vitamins A	1.2000	μg
C	60	mg
D	10	mg
Nicotinic acid equivalent	18	mg
Riboflavin	1.6	mg
Thiamine	1	mg

* HMSO recommendations: Manual of Nutrition.

prolonged standing posture. Inadequate rest periods can lead to ankle oedema and varicose veins.

Alimentary System

The average dietary intake in the nonpregnant state is about 2000 kcal per day. By full term this should have increased to roughly 2400 kcal to ensure fetal development, placental growth, and breast enlargement in readiness for lactation. An average weight gain of between 10 and 12.5 kg is to be expected (Table 20.1).

Glucose

Glucose derived from carbohydrate foods is the immediate energy source for fetal growth. The maternal blood glucose level tends to remain raised for longer than usual to permit glucose to cross into the fetus via the placenta. It is suggested that such a high blood glucose level can only remain high for a prolonged period if insulin is being opposed by an antagonist such as a corticosteroid. One effect of this persistent high blood glucose level is that some glucose will spill over into the urine once the renal threshold for glucose has been breached.

Metabolism

Simultaneously, the body's metabolic pathway is adjusted to convert carbohydrate into reservoirs of body fat in preparation for lactation. Dietary fat is the principal form of stored energy. The mother should have reserves totalling 4 kg deposited in the abdominal wall, back, thighs, buttocks and retroperitoneum. The blood cholesterol levels increase from about 180 mg to 280 mg per 100 ml of blood. It should be noted that while the maternal glucose levels are high there is no glucose reserve in the liver and therefore ketoacidosis is more likely during labour.

Protein

By the twenty eighth week of pregnancy the mother should be in positive protein balance with reserves amounting to over 500 g held in the liver. The fetus and placenta will utilise about 50% of all protein intake, while the remainder will contribute to the growth of the uterus, breast enlargement and maternal blood volume increase. Protein is essential for overall growth and replacement of cells and tissue. During pregnancy, the mother should have a protein intake of between 44 and 60 g per day.

Iron and Calcium

Iron and calcium are two essential minerals which should be continuously monitored in the diet. The iron contributing to the development of the red blood cells and essential for haemoglobin will automatically be increasingly utilised by both the fetus and mother. Stored iron reaching levels of 375 mg for the fetus and 750 mg for the mother can only be assured if the mother is taking at least 15 mg of iron per day. This is often prescribed in the form of ferrous sulphate 200 mg three times a day to ensure a good reserve. Both the erythrocyte count and haemoglobin levels are routinely measured on each clinic visit. As the pregnancy proceeds the haemoglobin tends to fall, but only because the dietary and prescribed iron is being increasingly utilised.

At the first trimester the haemoglobin level should be 13 g/dl, at the second trimester 12 g/dl and at the third trimester 11 g/dl of blood. Folate deficiency, if it occurs, may lead to a macrocytic anaemia and can be prevented by taking folic acid 15 to 20 mg per day.

The developing fetus requires calcium for growth of the skeletal, muscular and nervous systems. Additional to this, extra calcium is required by the mother in readiness for lactation. Vitamins A, C and D are also required and usually are to be found in generous quantities in a typical Western diet. If the mother is a strict vegetarian, or belongs to a specific cultural group with dietary restrictions, it is often necessary to supplement the diet by oral medications.

Endocrine System

With the increased metabolic activity there is a corresponding increase in the secretion of the appropriate hormones regulating many of the body's activities. The thyroid, pituitary, parathyroid and adrenal glands increase slightly in size and in their secretion.

Chapter 21
Initial Assessment and Guidelines in Pregnancy

On her first visit to the doctor, the expectant mother has almost self-diagnosed her pregnancy if there has been amenorrhoea for 4 weeks after the last period was due. Confirmation of the pregnancy is rapidly completed by a urine test which proves the presence of human chorionic gonadotrophin (HCG) in the fresh specimen of urine.

HISTORY-TAKING

Sociological

A detailed personal history is taken with the aim of establishing what factors, if any, would affect the health of the developing fetus. The social circumstances are significantly important. It has long been recognised that infants born to mothers in Social Classes 4 and 5 are at greater risk than those who are born to parents in the professional, skilled or semi-skilled social groups. Regular attendance at antenatal clinics and classes for monitoring, while emphasised for all pregnant women, is poorly supported by those in the lower income groups. Apart from social circumstances, it may also be their poverty of education which accounts for those at greatest risk who tend to avoid regular attendance at antenatal clinics.

Medical

The past medical, surgical and obstetric history is of equal importance in planning for the individual needs of a mother-to-be. Previous or current medications, allergies or medical conditions should be clearly indicated in the obstetric notes, e.g., diabetes, asthma or cardiac conditions. The current immunisation status should be checked, especially for vaccination against Rubella. The causative virus of this infectious disease – if crossing the placenta – may induce either a visual or hearing handicap in the developing fetus.

Previous pelvic or abdominal surgery carries a risk of adhesions or hernia, either of which would hinder the growth of the enlarging uterus. Women with a history of previous abortions will require strict supervision throughout the whole of their pregnancy; usually there has been or is an underlying gynaecological condition which persistently causes spontaneous abortions.

Psychological

It is always useful to know if the pregnancy was planned, is accidental, or if the baby is in fact unwanted. In any of these circumstances the obstetrician, midwife and nurse will have a better understanding of the client's psychological approach to her pregnancy. If the baby is unwanted, it is a well-established fact that such a child after birth may be subject to child battering by the parents. Appropriate consultation with the primary health care team may help towards establishing the well being and safety of the child.

PHYSICAL EXAMINATION

The initial physical examination follows a set pattern and would normally include the following points:

Height and weight are recorded and compared against standard desired weight charts. Obvious obesity will require the mother to be given advice on dietary changes which are commensurate with her pregnancy.

Blood pressure changes in pregnancy, if they occur, tend to be towards hypertension and on each examination the blood pressure should be taken and recorded.

Heart and lungs are both auscultated to detect any abnormality.

The breasts are examined to determine their enlargement, and the nipples inspected to see if they are everted, which is important if the mother expresses the wish to breastfeed.

A specimen of blood is taken for a variety of tests. The haemoglobin level is assessed at regular intervals throughout the pregnancy. The client's blood group, both the ABO and Rhesus, must be known in case of the need for a blood transfusion at a later time or in case of Rhesus incompatability between the mother and the fetus.

Wasserman and Kahn blood tests are completed as a matter of routine to exclude syphilis and gonorrhoea.

A specimen of fresh urine is routinely tested for glucose. *Glycosuria* can occur during a pregnancy. It may be only of a transient nature due to altered metabolism; nevertheless it should always be reported so that diabetes can be excluded by completing blood tests for glucose.

Abdominal palpation, with the client in the dorsal position, determines the size and location of the uterus.

Internal examination of the vagina and cervix is usually only done twice, at the initial physical examination and then at the thirty sixth week of pregnancy. Apart from the health of these structures, the examination will determine if the os is closed by a mucous plug.

Pelvic measurements may be taken if the mother has an obviously small and shallow pelvic girdle, which means she has a very narrow birth canal. Conversely, a large pelvis may have a weak muscular pelvic floor which may not adequately support an enlarging heavy uterus.

The lower limbs are examined for varicose veins and ankle oedema. Pregnancy will further embarrass either of these conditions and the appropriate advice and treatment should be offered.

Following this first examination the doctor will try to calculate the estimated delivery date (EDD). This is predicted by determining the first day of the last menstrual period and then adding 9 months and 1 week. It should be noted this is only an estimation and not an accurate prediction, but it does give the obstetrician a firm basis on which to plan care over the following months of pregnancy. Subsequent antenatal care is planned at this first assessment and the mother given details of the clinics she should attend, usually at monthly intervals. She would also be normally 'booked in' at the local maternity hospital and allocated to a specific obstetrician for all further care.

GUIDELINES FOR THE EXPECTANT MOTHER

On the first and subsequent visits to the antenatal clinic, the expectant mother should have several counselling sessions with her midwife. Aspects of maternal health and the commonly expected changes during a pregnancy make a good basis for communication. The attentive nurse may also be alerted to associated problems during routine checks and informal conversation. An experienced nurse should be able to counsel on all aspects of pregnancy.

Counselling

Cleanliness

During a pregnancy there is an increased vulvovaginal mucoid secretion and increased perspiration. Although quite normal, it can be uncomfortable and lead to offensive body odour. Daily perineal toilet and regular changing of undergarments are advised, especially if the domestic circumstances suggest there is no bathroom in the house. If neglected, the skin creases of the perineum become excoriated and the **risk** of infections such as *Candida* (Thrush) or *Trichomoniasis* are increased.

Exercise

Additional to the normal exercise obtained from caring for the home and family, the expectant mother will also receive classes on those exercises which will help her both relax and tone up her musculature. While sporting activity may be continued, the mother should reconsider those activities where there is a **risk** of falling, such as horseriding.

Coitus

Only if there is a risk or history of habitual abortion should sexual intercourse be avoided for the first 12 weeks of pregnancy. During the last 4 weeks of pregnancy, sexual intercourse should be avoided, mainly due to the **risk** of infection from the male partner.

Clothing

Girdles, suspenders and other forms of constrictive clothing should be avoided. As the breasts enlarge, a firm supportive bra may prove necessary. Since the body's centre of gravity will shift away from the spine, it is a useful precaution to wear shoes with a heel height not exceeding 4 cm ($1\frac{1}{2}$ inches). A fashionable sensible shoe will avoid postural imbalance. Loose-fitting attractive maternity clothes are readily available from commercial stores or can be made from patterns.

Smoking

The nicotine in cigarettes causes vasoconstriction of both the maternal and fetal blood vessels. The effect of such vasoconstriction is to deprive the developing fetus of oxygen, essential for its growth and development. When born, the infant is likely to be very small. The expectant mother should be encouraged to give up smoking.

Alcohol

There is a statistical correlation between the abuse of alcohol and congenital defect or underweight infants at birth. For this reason the expectant mother should be advised not to have any alcohol. If she insists, the rule is only one drink per day of a **low** alcohol beverage.

Dental Care

Free dental treatment is available to expectant mothers during pregnancy and for a further year after the baby is born. The use of local anaesthetics or gases for dental treatment does not usually affect the fetus in a healthy pregnancy. The demand on the maternal sources for minerals such as calcium can quickly lead to dental caries. Foods containing rich sources of calcium should be included in the diet.

Bowel Habit

Constipation is to be expected as a consequence of increased intra-abdominal pressure. Increased secretions of the hormone progesterone may also contribute to constipation. A diet containing high fibre foods such as fruit, salads and vegetables can help to avoid this tendency to constipation. If required, laxatives may be prescribed but they should be very mild and sufficient to ensure a bowel motion at least once every 2 days.

Haemorrhoids may also be a consequence of increased uterine weight and, because they are so painful, may lead to constipation. An anaesthetic gel applied to the anal sphincter and then a suppository inserted into the rectal canal may be sufficient to aid evacuation of the rectal content without distress.

Urinary Frequency

Urinary frequency can be expected for the same reasons as constipation, i.e., increased intra-abdominal pressure. As the pregnancy advances in time, the pressure down into the pelvic cavity increases and exerts pressure onto the dome of the urinary bladder. Apart from its nuisance value of frequent visits to the toilet, the expectant mother also finds she has to plan in detail any long journeys to ensure the availability of toilet facilities as the need arises.

Increased Weight

At the very outset of pregnancy the mother should establish if she is obese, overweight, or underweight and correct these problems in the first month. In the following 2 months, the mother may in fact lose weight due to morning sickness. During the last 6 months of pregnancy, the fetus will increase its weight by two-thirds. A maternal weight gain of about 1.5 kg per month is desirable. If by the estimated date of delivery the mother has gained between 10 and 12.5 kg, it is regarded as ideal.

Conversely, if the mother is gaining less than 0.80 kg per month there is a need to investigate her dietetic intake. To achieve the desired weight gain an expectant mother should have increased her dietary protein intake by 100 g of protein per day. The ultimate weight gain is usually derived from 6 factors:

Breast enlargement	1.0–1.5 kg
Uterine enlargement	0.5–1.0
Maternal subcutaneous fat; Liver protein reserve	4.0–4.5
Growing fetus and placenta	5.0 (on average)
Increased water retention	1.0–1.5 litres
Total weight gain	11.5–13.5 kg

Breasts

Coupled with breast enlargement, which is in readiness for breastfeeding, by the sixteenth week of pregnancy, there is the secretion of a substance known as *colostrum*. The colostrum must be washed away carefully with hot soapy water or it will form crusts which can lead to localised infections. The nipple itself becomes increasingly pigmented and the accessory lactiferous ducts (*Montgomery's ducts*) begin to make their appearance.

During the last 2 months of pregnancy, the mother should be taught how to massage her breasts to help express milk. This will help to prevent the lactiferous ducts from becoming blocked. Should either nipple be **inverted**, the wearing of a suction shield (*Waller's*) will help the nipple to become everted. The suction shield is worn beneath the bra cup throughout the pregnancy. Once everted the nipple will be ready for breastfeeding. Wearing a firm supportive bra throughout the latter half of the pregnancy is essential to avoid ache of the local musculature due to the breast enlargement.

Work

Should the expectant mother wish to continue working, either full or part time, she should be advised to request her maternity leave from the twenty-seventh week, i.e., 11 weeks before the estimated date of delivery. She should then be entitled to both Maternity Grant and Maternity Benefit plus the fact that her job is protected for her until she returns to work after her confinement. It is always a good idea to suggest to the expectant mother that her claim forms to the DHSS be scrutinised by a social worker or midwife as she may be entitled to other benefits depending on her circumstances, e.g., the single mother.

If the mother wishes to work beyond the twenty-seventh week, she should do so **only** if it does not involve prolonged standing. Combined with pregnancy, prolonged standing after the twenty-seventh week can lead to varicose veins of the lower limbs. In any event, a working mother-to-be should be advised that she must have a defined 1 hour's rest period each afternoon and at least 8 hours rest or sleep at night.

Relaxation Classes

Techniques of relaxation are taught on a regular basis at parentcraft classes in the antenatal clinic. Specific exercises are taught with the dual purpose of achieving:

Muscular relaxation
Improved muscle tone

as aids during the initial and second stages of labour when the contractions begin on a regular basis.

Simple exercises are done to strengthen the back, abdominal and thigh muscles. These include spinal stretching and flexion, alternate leg raising from the dorsal postion and knee flexion and straightening in the standing position. A variety of relaxation positions are demonstrated and then tried by the mother, one of which should be suitable for her. These are done either in the dorsal position with the head supported by one pillow or on the right or left lateral positions. Both the exercises and relaxation techniques should be practised each day until they become part of the daily routine.

The midwife will also teach and discuss with the mother the process of labour and how relaxation techniques can positively aid her at this time, in addition to coping with the pains of her contractions through breath control. Advice should also be given on the drugs used to relieve unbearable pain, e.g., inhaled anaesthetic gases, or an epidural injection to produce regional anaesthesia.

Parentcraft Classes

The main aim is to dispel ignorance and fear, usually best achieved on a sharing basis with small groups. The expectant mother will be told about the physiological changes which are occurring in her body and so help her understanding. Films are usually shown on the birth of a baby, again to reassure the expectant mother of what happens and who is there to help. A great deal of emphasis is given to first-time mothers and fathers about the 'physical' care a newborn baby requires, i.e., feeding, bathing, nappy changing and cuddling.

Travel

Long journeys are not recommended during the last 2 months of pregnancy, in case of premature labour. If travelling is absolutely necessary, then the mother must be accompanied and precautions taken to advise the appropriate authorities, e.g., family doctor, travel firm, or airline.

Minor Expected Complaints

Each expectant mother is unique; some go through their pregnancy without the least problem while others have a variable response to the expected discomforts. In some instances, they can be quite severe. It is a wise nurse who believes the mother-to-be's complaints and does not assume generalisations from reading or any short experience of maternity nursing. It is usual for the obstetrician to assess what are loosely phrased as 'minor complaints' at each clinic visit, but in many instances, it is reassurance that is usually required.

Some common minor complaints are heartburn, postural aches, morning sickness and insomnia.

Heartburn

Heartburn is most likely caused by lower oesophageal reflux of the acid gastric contents due to an increased intra-abdominal pressure. There can be a risk of hiatus hernia. The mother can be advised to adopt an upright seated posture for sleeping, well-supported by pillows. This will prevent the acid from the stomach entering the oesophagus. If heartburn is persistent both day and night then antacids may be prescribed.

Postural Aches

Backache, leg cramps and sciatica are only a few examples of what can happen once the body's centre of gravity is shifted away from the spine. A maternal change is the softening of ligaments within and around the pelvic cavity, which is in preparation of the birth canal but contributes to backache. To help deal with this problem, the expectant mother should be advised about her shoes, i.e., a sensible low-heeled court shoe, and have defined rest periods each day on a firm surface, e.g., fracture boards underneath the mattress.

Morning Sickness

No clear explanation is available for this all too common phenomenon. It invariably occurs in the morning and is most likely due to a combination of circumstances. Gastric motility is reduced, as is liver function, but the circulating oestrogen level is raised and this would lead to vomiting. In many instances a very light breakfast of easily digested food, combined with a short rest period after eating, is enough to contain the problem. Persistent vomiting throughout the whole day or prolonged over several months does require help with a prescribed antihistamine, which helps by reducing gastric spasms.

Insomnia

Insomnia is often coupled with a dietary fetish. The expectant mother has inexplicable cravings in the middle of the night for the most outlandish food combination. Again why this occurs is not readily explained, but most husbands or partners easily acquiesce to meeting these cravings. It is usually unwise to recommend tranquillisers to an expectant mother to help deal with insomnia.

N.B. On no account should an expectant mother self-prescribe or purchase commercially available drugs to deal with her minor complaints. In every instance, the expectant mother should be strongly advised to consult her doctor before taking any drugs, and equally to report if she is feeling unwell.

Chapter 22
Screening Tests for Fetal Development

Those tests which may be offered to a client are in the main to investigate fetal viability, growth and development. Of equal importance is their predictive value in determining if a fetus is abnormal and if an abortion should be offered. During the first and second stages of pregnancy, screening tests can be done to measure the degree of stress being endured by mother and child. Any single test must be seen in the context of the mother's gynaecological, obstetric and family history and must be relevant to any risk factor in the mother's history. Surrounding these tests are a plethora of gadgetry and technology, but if the equipment being used is simply explained most patients will cooperate when their natural curiosity or anxiety has abated.

AUSCULTATION AND PALPATION OF THE FETUS

Auscultation and palpation remains the mainstay of obstetric and midwifery examination of the abdomen. Listening to the fetal heart with a fetal stethoscope (Pinard's) from the twenty-fourth week onwards for both fetal cardiac rate and volume will tell the expert examiner about the progress of the fetus.

Palpation of the uterine fundus can tell of the height achieved by the uterus during a pregnancy and so also indicate if the fetal growth is normal (Tables 22.1 and 22.2).

At the same time the uterine weight should gain by 0.25 kg per week in the last 8 weeks of pregnancy. This type of examination is very rule of thumb and can only give average

Table 22.1 Fetal growth

Weeks	Length in cm	Anatomical characteristics
4	1.0	Head, tail fold and limb buds
*		
8	2.5	Nose, external ears, fingers, toes The head is flexed into the chest wall
12	8.5	Eyelid fusion, neck formed External genitalia established but undifferentiated Organ formation established
16	18.0	Skin red but transparent External genitalia differentiated
20	25.0	Hair and lanugo
24	30.0	Eyelids separated, eyelashes and eyebrows present Skin is wrinkled
28	35.0 (weight 125 g)	Fetus legally viable outside uterus Skin covered with lanugo Testes descend Subcutaneous fat deposited
32	40.0 (weight 400 g)	Fingernails formed Increased subcutaneous fat deposited Skin covered by sebaceous material, i.e., vernix caseous
36	45.0 (weight 2500 g)	Skin pink and covered with lanugo Further increase of subcutaneous fat
40	50.0	Skull bones hard Testes descend into scrotum Decreased amount of lanugo

* From the 6th week the embryo becomes a fetus and various anatomical developments can be clearly identified

Table 22.2 Uterine enlargement

Week	Hegar's sign present, i.e., isthmic region is softening
12–14	Uterus palpable in the abdominal cavity
18	Fundus between the upper edge of the symphisis and umbilicus Fetal movement felt by mother
20–24	Fundus level with umbilicus
30	Fundus midway between umbilicus and xiphisternum
36	Fundus level with xiphisternum
40	Fundus lower than xiphisternum by 7.5 cm

predictive values of fetal growth and development.

DAILY FETAL MOVEMENT COUNT (DFMC)

After the thirty-second week of pregnancy fetal activity falls from an average of 90 movements in 12 hours to 50 movements at full term. If the movements become less than 10 per 12 hours, it is suggestive of fetal hypoxia and requires immediate investigation of the fetal heart rate. Providing the expectant mother has common sense and is fairly objective about her pregnancy, there is no reason why she cannot monitor her own baby's fetal movements each day and record them on a provided chart. The fetal count is usually taken between 9 A.M. and 9 P.M. each day. If over a period of 48 hours she observes a noticeable decline in the fetal movements she is advised to seek obstetric advice immediately.

ULTRASONOGRAPHY (ULTRASONIC CEPHALOMETRY)

Two measurements are taken and displayed on a cathode ray screen. The first is the fetal skull diameter (biparietal diameter), and its increase confirms that fetal growth is occurring. The skull size is also used to determine fetal weight and maturity. The second measurement involves cross-scanning the maternal abdomen to provide information about the position of the fetus and placenta. Measurements of the fetal thorax and abdomen can also be made.

Apart from the clear picture it provides, which often delights the parents-to-be, ultrasound scanning has many other uses. It confirms a pregnancy by the sixth week, diagnoses abortion or multiple pregnancy, diagnoses fetal abnormality, identifies the placenta before amniocentesis, and can identify malpresentation. Smaller portable sound scanners are available for ward use and provide the same information as static larger scanners, but the picture provided is not so clear.

FETAL HEART MONITORING (FHM) (FHR)

The static scanner can detect fetal heart movement as early as the eighth week. For those expectant mothers with hypertension, known retarded fetal growth, and other risks, it is useful to obtain a 30-minute recording each week after the thirty-fourth week. The normal fetal heart rate is between 120 and 160 beats per minute. A sudden or unexpected deceleration of this value suggests fetal hypoxia, requiring possible obstetric intervention.

Fetal heart monitoring can be done continuously during uterine contractions and is normal practice in difficult deliveries. Additionally, a fetal electrocardiograph can also be obtained by attaching an electrode to the fetal scalp but this can only be done if the membranes are ruptured and the scalp, or cap, presenting.

FETAL BLOOD SAMPLING

The fetal blood pH may need to be compared with the maternal blood pH during a normal labour. Sometimes the mother develops a metabolic acidosis, but even then her pH should remain between 7.38 and 7.42 while the fetal pH is more acid, between 7.30 and 7.35. The blood sample is obtained via a special tube with a guarded blade which is inserted into the cervix to reach the fetal scalp from which a small sample of blood is obtained. This method is quite troublesome and a difficult procedure during a labour. It should be done only if there is retarded intrauterine growth or placental insufficiency, and a proven metabolic acidosis which requires correction.

AMNIOCENTESIS

Procedure

Amniocentesis cannot usually be done until the fifteenth or sixteenth week of pregnancy, when the fetal cells are most numerous. It involves obtaining a 20-ml sample of amniotic fluid via a sterile needle inserted through the anterior abdominal wall (Fig. 22.1). The needling technique, if done by an expert, requires the minimal amount of local anaesthetic and leaves the patient without any discomfort. Prior to the procedure the maternal blood would have been tested for the level of alpha-fetoprotein. If its level is twice that of the expected normal, i.e., 30 to 40 mg/l between the fourteenth and sixteenth week, it suggests that the fetus is abnormal, and confirmation is required by direct examination of the amniotic fluid. As a precaution, an ultrasound scan is taken to identify the exact location of the placenta to avoid any damage from needling. If the obtained sample is bloodstained, it is likely to give false readings.

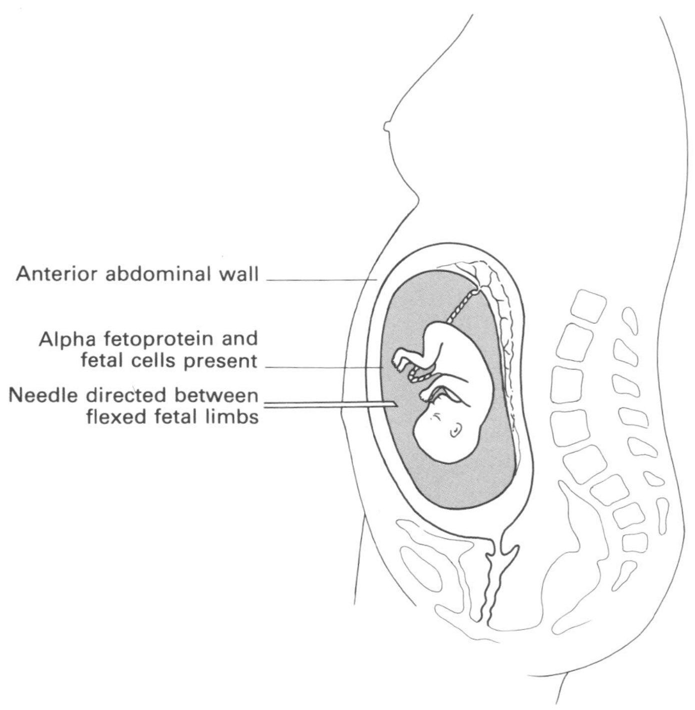

Fig. 22.1 Amniocentesis.

Outcomes

Several tests are done on the amniotic fluid. It contains fetal cells, chromosomes, fetal urine and alpha-fetoprotein. Examination of the fetal cells may indicate a sex-linked disease such as haemophilia. The chromosome pattern may reveal whether the fetus has Down's Syndrome, i.e., mongolism. Fetal urine can be tested to determine if there are any inborn errors of metabolism, and the alpha-fetoprotein will confirm if there is a neural tube defect (NTD) such as spina bifida or anencephaly.

If the results of any of these tests are positive, then the obstetrician may feel obliged to offer the mother an abortion. There are many legal and moralistic questions regarding this topic of abortion and it needs very sympathetic but careful handling to ensure that the expectant mother has all the necessary information before she makes a choice. If an abortion is carried out then the fetus should be examined to confirm the antenatal diagnosis.

Amniocentesis is not without some **risk**, about 2% of expectant mothers may naturally abort as a consequence of needling. There can be placental injury, uterine infection, haemorrhage or sensitising of a Rh negative baby if the mother is Rh positive.

FETOSCOPY

The fetal respiration movement in the third trimester varies between 30 and 90 per minute. It is mainly a diaphragmatic movement, but there is no gaseous exchange. These movements can be seen on ultrasound scanning. To observe these movements more closely, a fibreoptic endoscopic instrument of exceptionally narrow diameter (1.77 mm) can be passed into the amniotic sac under ultrasonic control. At the same time, a skin biopsy and placental blood sample can be taken for neural tube defect tests. With the fetoscopy technique, a contrast medium can be injected into the amniotic sac to give more accurate information, i.e., an amniography.

URINARY OESTRIOLS

From the many oestrogens there are mainly 3 of great interest during a pregnancy: oestrone, oestradiol and oestriol. Oestrone and oestradiol are synthesised in the placenta, and their level should be rather low as the pregnancy progresses. Oestriol, however, requires fetal precursors for its manufacture and is produced in considerable amounts between the eighth and fortieth week of pregnancy. Since these hormones are excreted via the maternal urine they can be measured quite accurately in a 24-hour urine collection. Low levels of oestriol may indicate the need for further tests as it suggests retarded fetal growth or placental insufficiency, especially in the last week of pregnancy.

HUMAN PLACENTAL LACTOGEN (HUMAN CHORIONIC SOMATOMAMMOTROPHIN)

Lactogen is a substance produced by the placenta and can be measured from a sample of maternal blood, by radio-immunoassay. Low levels in late pregnancy, i.e., below 4 μg/ml, may indicate fetal hypoxia.

ANTENATAL CARDIOGRAPHY

Each time the fetus moves, the fetal heart rate should increase by about 20 beats per minute. This measurement can be taken by attaching electrodes over the maternal abdomen. Each time the fetus moves, there is a painless uterine contraction with a corresponding increase in fetal heart rate. A quiescent fetus may be in danger of fetal hypoxia if the fetal heart rate does not rise following a fetal movement.

CHORION BIOPSY

Chorion biopsy is a recently developed technique which permits a small fragment of the chorion to be removed and studied microscopically as early as the eighth week of pregnancy. It gives an early predictive warning of fetal abnormality, much as the amniocentesis does. Because it can be done at a much earlier time in the pregnancy, it is likely it will overtake amniocentesis.

A major advantage is that abortion, if it is offered and accepted, can be done much earlier and with greater safety. This is not possible with an amniocentesis because if an abortion is offered following amniocentesis it may have to wait until the twentieth week of pregnancy. The later the abortion the more physical and emotional trauma is suffered, and if left too late it may not be possible to carry out the abortion because of the current legislation.

Chapter 23
Normal Labour

When pregnancy has reached full term (280 days or 40 weeks) the uterus will begin to contract or go into 'labour'. During the last 4 weeks of pregnancy, there are irregular painless contractions (*Braxton Hicks contractions*). These serve to 'thin out' the lower part or segment of the uterus. The precise trigger for the actual onset of true labour is unknown, but is thought to be due to a fall in the levels of the hormone *progesterone*. Normally, this hormone would prevent uterine contractions. The physiological activity of labour is divided into 3 stages (Fig. 23.1):

Stage 1. Lasts from the commencement of regular contractions until the cervix is fully dilated, on average by 10 cm.

Stage 2. Commences when the cervix has reached full dilation until the baby is delivered. During this phase the uterus and vagina become an elongated tube, the pelvic floor muscles and the perineum stretch backwards, the bowel is compressed and the bladder forced upwards towards the abdomen, and the urethra is fully stretched.

Stage 3. Follows childbirth immediately and continues until the placenta and membranes have been expelled.

TYPICAL EVENTS DURING LABOUR

Stage 1

For some unknown reason, many expectant mothers have a sudden burst of energy prior to the commencement of true labour. They compulsively busy themselves with many household chores until they experience their

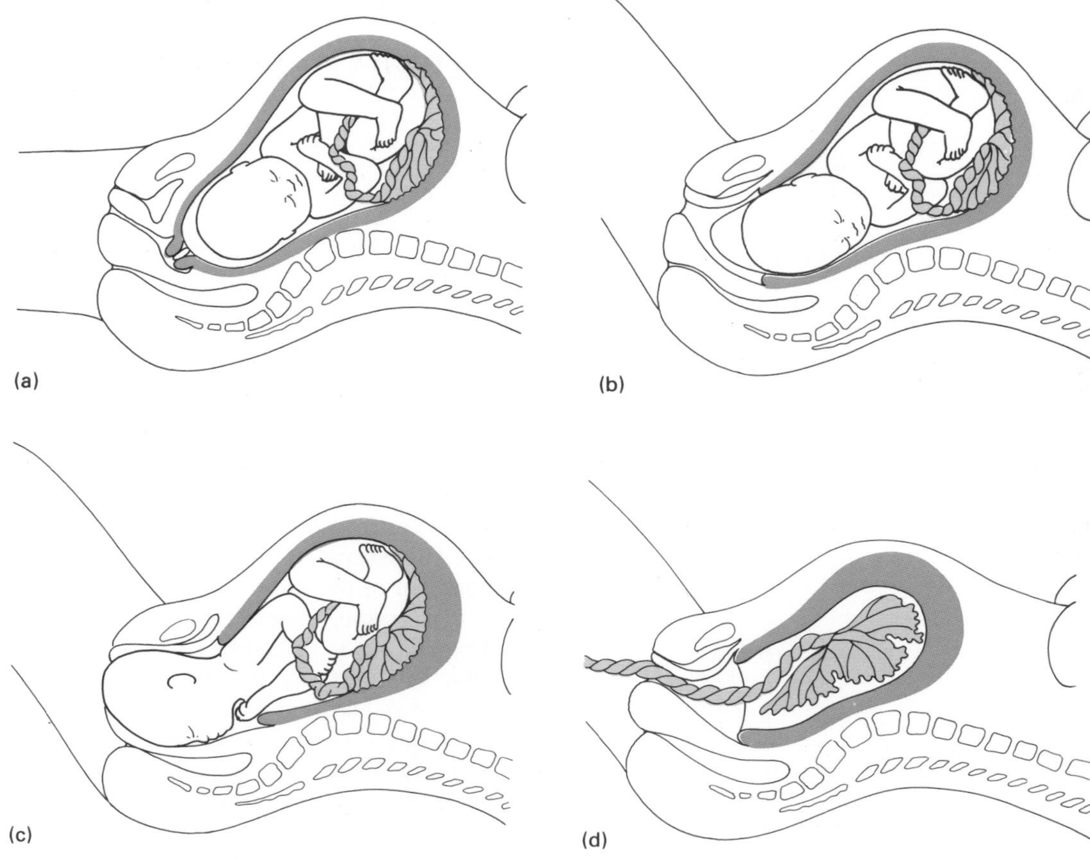

Fig. 23.1 Normal stages of labour: the womb at full term (a); first stage of labour (b); second stage of labour (c); third stage of labour (d).

first true contraction. A sign of a positive diagnosis of labour is the *show*. The show, or showing, refers to a mucous plug streaked with blood which escapes from the cervix and is passed via the vagina. There may be an escape of some amniotic fluid (*rupture of the membranes*). If this occurs in large amounts, it may unduly alarm the expectant mother unless she has been informed of its potential likelihood and assured that it has minimal effect on the delivery.

Contractions

The first contraction is felt in the lower abdomen and back. It is in effect a continuation of the Braxton Hicks contractions from late pregnancy. These pains are intermittent and should occur between every 15 to 20 minutes. The contractions become more pronounced and prolonged until they occur every 7 minutes. What the contractions do is to dilate the cervical canal until the fetal head can pass into the vagina (Fig. 23.2).

Each involuntary contraction begins from the very muscular fundus and spreads downwards over the uterus to reach the lower segment of the uterus. The ring of fibrous muscular tissue at the cervix is 'thinned out' to create a clear passage for the baby. Each contraction increases the intrauterine pressure which causes the pain felt in the lower abdomen. The interval between each contraction should be pain-free.

If it is the first baby (*primigravida*), Stage 1 of labour may last for 12 to 18 hours.

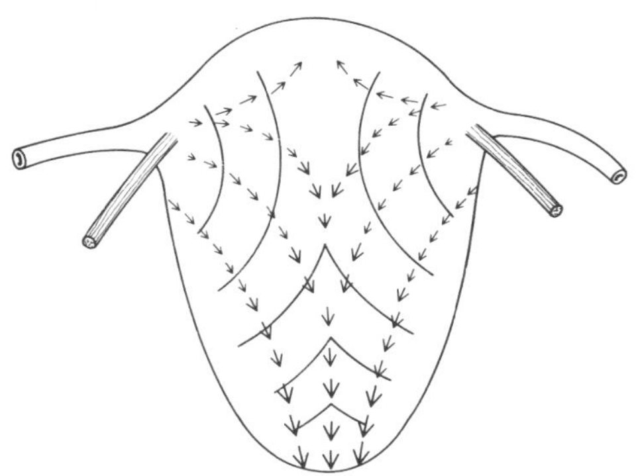

Fig. 23.2 Patterns of propagation of uterine contraction impulse.

Normally, the expectant mother would be advised to stay at home until her contractions are occurring every 7 minutes. False alarms do occur, and it may be something of an inconvenience or embarrassment to be sent home to wait for true labour to commence. Nevertheless, the mother should be encouraged to follow her own instincts and seek help.

Admission and Care

On admission to the maternity unit, the antenatal care given is reviewed and a brief history of the labour is taken.

A standard care plan followed by many maternity units, with some variations, could be summarised as:

1. A small *enema* or suppositories may be given, if necessary or requested by the mother, to cleanse the rectum. It also stimulates uterine activity. However, strong aperients or purgatives are **never** used in place of an enema.

Table 23.1 Standard equipment in a delivery suite

Tiltable delivery bed, well protected by absorbent sterile sheeting
Sterile leg and abdominal drapes; towels and sheets
Ample supply of swabs and gamgee pads
Anaesthetic gases
For episiotomy
Local anaesthetic agents
Syringes, 2, 5, and 10 ml, with needles
Episiotomy scissors
Suture material and needles
For umbilical cord
Pressure forceps
Plastic clamps
Cord ligatures (for tying off)
Scissors
For infant care
Sterile towel to wrap the baby in
Mucus extractor or suction catheter
Oxygen cylinder
Laryngoscope
Prepared cot or incubator
Drugs for emergency use
naloxone (Narcan)
levallorphan (Lorfan)
In case of haemorrhage
Oxytocic drugs
Syringes, 2, 5 and 10 ml, with needles
Pressure forceps to apply to vessels of the perineum
Measuring jug to assess blood loss of third stage
For midwife and attendants
Sterile gowns, masks, caps and gloves (the delivery, if conventional, is an aseptic procedure)

2. The pubic area and the perineum are either *shaved* or cropped of excessive hair.

3. A *shower* is preferred to a bath, this not only refreshes the mother, but will reduce the risk of introducing infection into the vagina.

4. Every *specimen of urine* that is passed is tested for albumen, sugar and ketones. If there is ketonuria it indicates starvation or dehydration or both. In this event, the obstetrician may want to establish intravenous therapy of normal saline and dextrose. Should intravenous therapy be started it would confine the mother to bed. It is important that the bladder be empty before the second stage of labour and if necessary a urinary catheter be passed to empty the bladder.

5. During Stage 1 of labour, the midwife will observe constantly:

Maternal blood pressure, pulse and temperature

Fetal heart rate

Duration, frequency and strength of the uterine contractions

Fetal descent by abdominal examination

Vaginal examination to determine cervical dilation

If the cervix is only half dilated after 4 hours of labour, an analgesic such as pethidine or promethazine may be required for the pain. If the labour is making very slow progress then regional anaesthesia by either epidural or paracervical anaesthesia may be done to ease the pain

6. During a normal labour, the expectant mother should remain up and about if she wishes and encouraged to walk about. This can be alternated with armchair rest and doing the breathing exercises learned in the antenatal relaxation classes; she should if possible have her husband or partner with her at all stages of labour. As the contractions shorten in duration, the midwife will have prepared the delivery room/suite in readiness for Stage 2 of labour. It is preferred that any food or drink are kept to the absolute minimum during Stage 1 because drugs and anaesthetic agents may have to be used.

Stage 2

The membranes must have ruptured before the fetal head can be delivered. In this second stage, which may last for 1 hour and should never exceed 2 hours, the mother has a distinct need to *bear down* and naturally assist the involuntary uterine contractions to expel the baby. All the maternal musculature is used to this end and to aid in this process, the mother can adopt a variety of positions to help expel the baby.

Positions for Birth

Two conventional positions are either to lie prone on an absorbent surface with the legs flexed and elevated or to lie in the left lateral position. The increasing use of *birth chairs* which can be adjusted for height allow the mother to adopt a seated posture. The principle which is most important is that the adopted position **must** allow the midwife to gain immediate access to the head of the baby as it crowns the perineum.

The need to push, or bear, down is of some importance as in general the more pushing the mother is capable of the lesser the pain. It should be possible for the mother to push 2 or 3 times in unison with each contraction. As it descends through the birth canal the baby's head has to rotate through 90°, since the birth canal is curved through the same angle.

When the forehead, face and chin appear, the baby's head will rotate back to its normal position. If the umbilical cord is trapped around the neck, it is released by gentle manipulation. The midwife will then support the head with both hands and guide it backwards to allow the anterior shoulder to emerge. The head is then brought forwards to permit the posterior shoulder to escape. Once both shoulders are free the remaining body should emerge without any further difficulty or delay.

Episiotomy

During this stage, careful observation is made of the pressure exerted on the perineum.

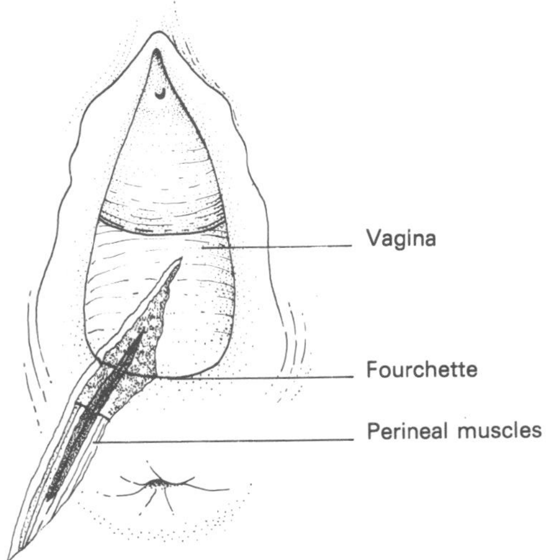

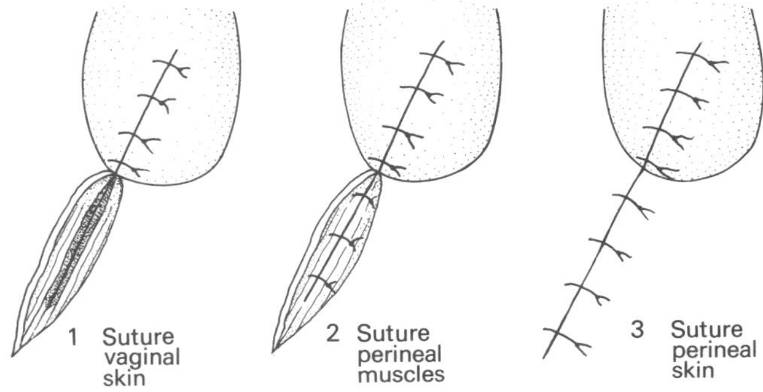

Fig. 23.3 Repair of an episiotomy.

Should it bulge unduly it means that there is some **risk** of the surrounding soft tissues tearing. Inhalation anaesthesia, if required, may be self-administered, e.g., nitrous oxide 50% and oxygen 50% or trilene with air (trichlorethylene 0.35% to 0.65%). If used, these gases should be inhaled at the beginning of each contraction.

Once the head descends into the perineum, a local anaesthetic may be injected into the superficial tissues of the vagina and fourchette. If the perineum becomes so stretched by *crowning* that it is in danger of tearing, an episiotomy is performed. Correctly timed, this scissor cut under local anaesthesia into the perineal tissues will assist in the delivery of the head without further damage to the perineum (Fig. 23.2).

After the head has been delivered an intramuscular injection of syntometrine 0.5 mg (oxytocic drug) is given to the mother to aid in delivery of the placenta and membranes during the third stage. On delivery of the baby, its nose and mouth are cleared of mucus by either mucus extractor or catheter, and breathing should commence within 30 seconds.

The Umbilical Cord

The baby is placed on its mother's abdomen while the umbilical cord is left to pulsate for several minutes. The cord can be milked towards the baby as it contains useful blood. It is then clamped, one plastic clamp towards the fetal end and the other towards the maternal end of the cord. After this the cord is divided or cut with scissors. If the cord is very thick then it may be tied off with nylon suture. It is strongly advocated that the baby is put to the mother's breast to suckle as soon as possible. This suckling is said to aid in the expulsion of the placenta, and be helpful in establishing maternal baby bonding. During this stage, the father can be of great value in supporting the mother in her various positions during the delivery.

Stage 3

The mother will have several minutes of well-deserved rest before the syntometrine injection begins to take effect. This drug will cause a sustained contraction of the uterus. While waiting for this drug to take effect, the maternal end of the umbilical cord is placed in a receiver positioned between the mother's legs.

The Placenta

The midwife palpates the abdomen until she detects a hardened uterus and presses downwards. This will prevent the now empty flattened uterus from filling up with blood. When the uterus is felt to contract and feels very hard the midwife exerts gentle traction on the umbilical cord. As she pulls, the placenta should shear away from its bed on the uterine wall.

The membranes should also follow as they too peel away from the lining of the uterus. Both placenta and membranes are closely inspected to make sure they are complete. At the same time, there is an expected blood loss of about 100–200 ml. If an episiotomy was necessary, it is now repaired with either catgut or Dexon soluble sutures, using a local anaesthetic.

Care of Mother and Baby

The baby should by now have been wrapped in a warm towel and placed in either a cot or incubator. Initially, it is best to tilt the cot slightly so that the baby's feet are higher than its head to allow free drainage from the nose and mouth. The mother is given a gentle bath, dressed in her own clothing, and given a maternity pad to apply over the vagina and perineum. A drink is most welcome before being allowed to rest or sleep in the postnatal ward.

INDUCTION OF LABOUR

Between 25% and 35% of all pregnancies are induced by external controlled means. The reasons for aiding or accelerating a labour are manifold (Table 23.2). The methods used to induce labour may be combined or used singly, and 95% of those pregnancies which are induced deliver within 12 hours. The commonly used methods include:

Drugs, e.g., oxytocin (Syntocinon) and prostaglandins

Surgical techniques such as cervical stimulation, amniotomy or intra-amniotic injections

Table 23.2 Induction of labour

Maternal conditions	Fetal conditions
Diabetes mellitus	Rhesus sensitisation
Pre-eclampsia (hypertension)	Unstable lie or breech
Primipara over 35 years old	Fetal abnormality
Previous difficult obstetric history	Fetal death
Prolonged pregnancy, i.e., over 42 weeks	Placental malperfusion
	Post-maturity, i.e., over 42 weeks.

Drugs

Oxytocin (Pitocin, Syntocinon, 0.5–1 ml of 5–10 units)

Oxytocin may be administered as a tablet to suck, since the essential active ingredient is absorbed through the mucous membranes of the mouth; if swallowed, it is inactivated by the stomach. Alternatively, it can be given intravenously in a solution of dextrose saline. An infusion pump such as the Cardiff or Palmer type should be used to regulate the flow rate. The dose is usually set 1 ml per minute and doubled every 10 minutes until uterine contractions are established.

The drugs are synthetic preparations of the hormone oxytocin, which is naturally stored in the posterior pituitary and secreted from the hypothalamus. Once the drug has been given the nurse must not leave the patient alone at any time. Careful observations are taken of the uterine contractions, preferably by tocography. The fetal heart rate is assessed by the fetal monitor. If the contractions are too vigorous, or the fetal heart rate too rapid, the obstetrician must be informed and the infusion flow rate reduced. Before the contractions begin for Stage 2 of labour the membranes should have ruptured. This drug may also be used to control postpartum haemorrhage, but it is not as effective as ergometrine for this purpose.

Prostaglandins (Prostin E_2 and $F_{2\alpha}$)

These substances, i.e., prostaglandins, are formed by most cells in the body, being released by a variety of stimuli, and generally have a very localised effect. In particular, the derivatives Prostin E2 and F2 alpha have oxytocic properties causing the uterine muscle to contract. The drugs may be given either to induce labour or to abort an early pregnancy.

Prostin E_2 is given orally at a dose of 500 μg hourly while Prostin $F_{2\alpha}$ is given via an intravenous infusion at a dose of 2.5 μg per minute for at least 30 minutes. More uncommonly, these drugs may also be administered intravaginally as pessaries, extra-amniotically via a fine catheter, or intra-amniotically by direct injection. As with oxytocin, the fetal heart rate and strength and frequency of contractions are monitored every 15 minutes and the obstetrician informed of any untoward changes.

Surgical Techniques

Cervical Stimulation

Near term, the cervix may be stretched by passing a gloved finger through the cervix in the hope of stimulating uterine contractions.

Amniotomy, or Artificial Rupture of Membranes (ARM)

Before the amniotomy is started it is advisable to administer a mild sedative to the mother. The *forewaters* or the *hindwaters* or both are deliberately brought on with a Kocher's forceps (Fig. 23.4). Alternatively, a disposable plastic hook is used for the forewaters and a metal catheter for the hindwaters.

A forewater amniotomy is usually used because it is generally regarded as the safer of the two. The procedure is an aseptic technique. The amount of liquor released, although not critical, is examined for both colour and bloodstaining. With this method of inducing labour it is imperative that the baby be delivered within 24 hours, if necessary by proceeding to Caesarean section.

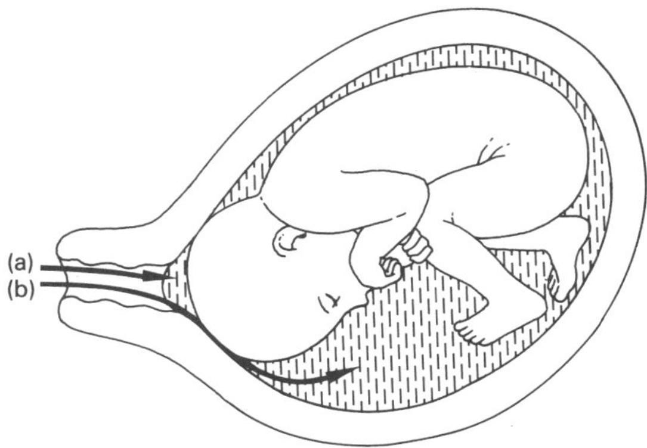

Fig. 23.4 Artificial rupture of membranes: low rupture involves the forewaters (a); high rupture involves the hindwaters (b).

Intra-amniotic Injections

If an intra-amniotic injection is to be used, the technique is once again aseptic. A local anaesthetic is required to numb the superficial tissues of the abdomen before a needle is directed through the abdominal wall into the amniotic sac. About 50 ml of the amniotic fluid are removed and a second prepared syringe containing 50 ml of either a hypertonic solution or a hormone solution is introduced into the cavity. This technique is repeated until 200 or 300 ml have been exchanged.

At the same time, an oxytocin intravenous infusion is commenced to reinforce the uterine contractions. Delivery can be expected within at least 12 hours, at most 18 to 24 hours later. The **risk** of introducing infection is high and a prophylactic antibiotic is usually added to the exchanged injected fluids.

Chapter 24
Anomalies from Normal Labour

EMERGENCY CHILDBIRTH

Occasionally, the childbirth is so quick that there is no time to summon a midwife or doctor and it would be dangerous to travel to a hospital. Nevertheless, an ambulance should always be summoned as the ambulance crew will have basic training and the required equipment. If advised that it is an emergency childbirth, the ambulance station normally gives it top priority.

The mother requires the verbal reassurance that although it is a quick labour, this is normal and there is no threat to the baby, and each different stage is naturally accelerated. Initially, the mother must be persuaded to empty her bladder, preferably into a receptacle (for specimen investigation) and not the toilet pan. Restrictive clothing around the waist, ribcage and neck are released and the lower garments removed.

During Delivery

The first-aider must be conscientious about cleanliness and if possible wash his/her hands thoroughly before assisting with the birth.

Time permitting and if at home, several items are gathered together, the most helpful being bowls or jugs of hot water, warm towels, cotton wool, soap and nail brush, scissors and thread or thin string which should have been immersed in boiling water. Absorbent sheeting should be placed beneath the mother. If at home, the infant's cot can be made ready.

Contractions

The contractions of the first stage of labour can be timed and in an emergency childbirth they will soon reach 3-minute then 1-minute intervals. During this phase, the mother is encouraged to practise the breathing and relaxation exercises learned in antenatal classes. Regular inspection of the perineum and vagina will reveal when the *show* has occurred. This is a piece of bloodstained mucus expelled via the vagina and is the first warning of the membranes about to rupture and allow the escape of some amniotic fluid.

When the mother feels she wants to bear down, she is encouraged to push down in unison with each contraction. The first-aider should advise and support the mother to flex her knees and press her heels into the mattress or surface upon which she is lying to give her more leverage while pushing downwards. If during these contractions and bearing down there is a bowel motion, any faeces are cleansed away using cotton wool and wiping from the vagina towards the perineum to reduce **risk** of infection of the birth canal.

Birth

As the baby's head emerges it will stretch the vulva and perineum. This stretching needs to be controlled by cupping the head with both hands and asking the mother to take panting breaths which will in effect temporarily stop her from bearing down.

When the baby's head is free, a check is made that the umbilical cord is not trapped around the neck. If it is, it **must** be looped forward and brought over the baby's head; otherwise, as the baby advances the cord will tighten around the baby's neck.

The head is still supported until the shoulders are free. Once this stage is reached the first-aider can support the baby under the axilla and gently pull forwards and upwards and then outwards. The baby should be held upside down for a few moments, to help drain the mouth and nose of any mucus, and wiped clean.

Respiration

The baby should cry within 30 seconds, if it remains silent for 2 minutes then artificial respiration may be necessary. If so, air is gently blown into the nostrils or mouth to help the baby start breathing. When the baby's breathing is assured, a warm towel is wrapped around the baby, and he/she is gently rested beside the mother. It is best to lie the baby with the feet slightly higher than the head to allow free drainage from the nose and mouth.

After Delivery

The last stage of labour involves expelling the placenta and the membranes (*afterbirth*), which takes place 5 or 10 minutes after the actual childbirth. The placenta, when delivered, should be collected into a receptacle and retained for the doctor's or midwife's inspection. If there is significant bleeding, the first aider is advised to apply palmer pressure onto the abdominal wall at the level of the mother's umbilicus and firmly massage the area where the now collapsed uterus or womb is positioned. This should help to arrest the bleeding.

The Umbilical Cord

When possible, the umbilical cord should be left for the doctor or midwife to deal with. If, however, 10 minutes after the placenta has been delivered help is still unavailable, the cord **must** be tied off in two places.

Using a strong thread or thin string the first-aider places the first tie about 15 cm and the second tie at 20 cm from the baby. The cord is cut between the two ties. The end of the baby's umbilical cord should be checked for any bleeding. If it is bleeding then another tie should be applied, making an even tighter knot. A piece of clean tissue or cotton wool is placed over the cord to keep it clean.

Care of the Mother

The mother will now need some help to tidy herself; a wash and change of bedlinen and

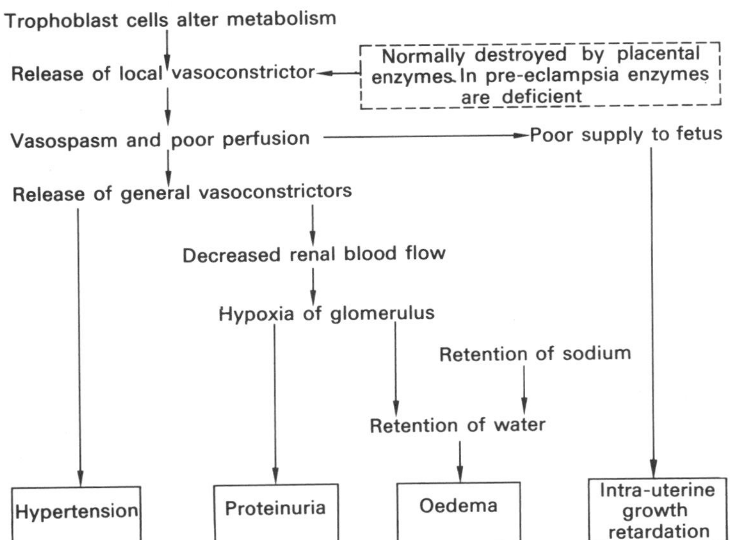

Fig. 24.1 The most likely theory of the aetiology of pre-eclampsia.

clothes are obviously necessary. A sanitary towel should be placed over the vagina and perineum. While waiting for medical attention a hot drink should be given and the mother and baby allowed to rest. The first-aider should, however, remain with the mother until either the doctor or midwife arrive.

TOXAEMIA OF PREGNANCY (PRE-ECLAMPSIA)

The word *eclampsia* means 'convulsion' and if prefixed by *pre* means that a toxic condition is present before the event of a convulsion. The *toxaemia* takes the form of a hypertension-related pregnancy, and if uncontrolled can lead to a classical eclampsia. Roughly 10% of pregnancies are hypertensive related and toxaemia of pregnancy remains one of the most common causes of maternal and perinatal mortality.

Signs and Possible Causes

The 3 classical signs of toxaemia of pregnancy are:

Hypertension, the blood pressure reading being consistently at or above 140/90 mmHg, even after 15 minutes rest from doing active work

Proteinuria, especially if albuminuria is consistently found on repeated urinalysis

Oedema of the fingers, hands, face and feet (*peripheral oedema*)

In isolation, any one of these signs may not be of great significance. Oedema, for instance, is quite common during pregnancy. However, when they coexist, it implies the need to increase the screening tests, especially for the fetus, to twice each week.

On further investigation, the mother may have a sudden weight increase, a raised plasma urea and creatinine level and uric acid retention. Blood coagulation tests may show an increased coagulation time. There may also be evidence of oliguria.

The true cause of pre-eclampsia is unknown, although there are many theories. The most likely cause is shown in Figure 24.1, which suggests that placental ischaemia releases a vasoconstrictor which causes a persistent arteriole constriction. It seems to occur most frequently in women who: are primaparous, have a twin pregnancy, have diabetes mellitus, are older women, or have an existing hypertension, renal failure or a hydatidiform mole. Its onset is usually detected from normal screening tests between the thirtieth and thirty-fourth week of pregnancy. Whenever possible, the pregnancy will be allowed to continue, but with some restrictions placed on the mother.

Treatment

Treatment and the restrictions placed on the expectant mother depend on the degree of the pre-eclampsia, which may be mild, chronic, acute or sudden. In the milder case the mother is advised to take plenty of rest and is prescribed sedation to ensure plenty of bedrest. For the more serious cases (acute, chronic or sudden) hospital admission is invariably recommended to supervise the mother and ensure that she remains on bedrest, which is the mainstay of treatment.

Treatment is mainly symptomatic, sodium amytal 100 mg three times a day, and in increasing doses for the chronic or sudden hypertensive states. Blood pressure recordings are taken 4-hourly each day until the thirty-eighth to fortieth week. The underlying threat to the fetus requires twice-weekly fetal assessment, and from these tests the obstetrician will decide if labour should be induced, or whether to carry out a Caesarean section.

ECLAMPSIA

Eclampsia is now a very rare occurrence since the risk can be so easily detected in screening at the thirty-fourth week of pregnancy, hence the need to emphasise accuracy in all routine tests. Both toxaemia and eclampsia occur in unison. Preceding the epileptic type convulsion, the mother may complain of headaches, vomiting and oliguria, associated discomforts which closely resemble those of an imminent cerebrovascular accident.

Patient Care

The mother requires to be nursed in a quiet, darkened room as noise and bright light may precipitate another convulsion. Immediately after the convulsion, the airway must be cleared and oxygen therapy given. The position of choice is to nurse the mother in the lateral position with the chin tilted forwards and downwards.

Observations of pulse, blood pressure, respiratory rate and level of consciousness are frequently taken and recorded to indicate recovery or a potential second convulsion. The mother tends to remain drowsy after the convulsion and any brain damage such as cerebrovascular haemorrhage may be difficult to diagnose.

Drugs which may be administered to contain the hypertension and toxaemia include:

Hypotensives, such as hyallazine combined with diazepam (Valium)

One of the **anticonvulsant** drugs

Diuretics such as frusemide (Lasix)

Once adequate control over the toxaemia and hypertension is established, the baby is induced surgically followed by an infusion of Syntocinon, or a Caesarean section is undertaken.

Complications

The possible complications from eclampsia, if it remains uncontrolled, are cerebral haemorrhage, cardiac failure and intrauterine death from placental separation.

CAESAREAN SECTION

Caesarean section is a surgical procedure whereby the baby is removed from the uterus via an abdominal incision. Over the years, this technique has become extremely safe with advanced techniques in both surgery and anaesthesia. There are many reasons why this operation may prove essential, but the more common circumstances are:

1. The baby is too large to pass through the bony pelvic birth canal
2. A previous difficult obstetric history
3. Fetal stress being endured during the first stage of labour
4. Ovarian cysts or large fibroids
5. Severe pre-eclampsia
6. Severe antenatal haemorrhage
7. Malpresentation of fetus
8. Twin or triplet pregnancy

During the antenatal screening, there may be advanced warning of the need for this procedure which allows plenty of time for planning this elective surgery. In those cases where it is an emergency, the mother can be positively reassured that it is a very safe procedure in the majority of cases without any danger to either the baby or the mother. Because the baby will not pass through the bony birth canal, the fetal scalp is not moulded and therefore Caesarean section babies tend to have round heads.

Surgical Techniques

There are two surgical techniques: the classical method and the lower segmental section, the latter being the acknowledged safer method. Prior to surgery, the mother is prepared as for any abdominal operation and in addition has her blood grouped, cross-matched and several units saved for post-operative transfusion.

Classical Section

The classical section involves approaching the uterus via a midline abdominal incision. The abdominal organs are retracted to expose the uterus and an incision is made into the upper segment of the uterus, the placenta is cut and ignored, the baby's feet are located and the baby is then pulled out of the uterus feet first.

The baby is handed over to the attendant midwife who will give immediate postnatal care, ensuring that the oronasal cavities are sucked out to guarantee the airway. After this, the infant is placed into a prepared cot or incubator and removed from the theatre.

In the meantime, the mother is given a solution of ergometrine to assist separating the placenta and membranes from the uterine wall. Once this is completed, the wound is closed in 3 layers and a suction drain secured into the wound by a suture.

Lower Segmental Section

The preferred method, or lower segmental section can be regarded as a pelvic operation and as such carries fewer postoperative risks. The lower segment of the uterus is approached via a transverse suprapubic or vertical subumbilical incision. The pelvic organs are retracted, the peritoneum is cut, a transverse incision is made into the uterus, and widened digitally so that the head can be engaged and the baby delivered head first.

Postoperative Care

With either technique, the nurse can expect to plan the care of the patient involving an intravenous infusion or blood transfusion, nasogastric aspiration, and an abdominal wound with a suction drain.

Essential in the planning is to mount those observations which can detect the potential complications of paralytic ileus, abdominal distension, peritonitis and pulmonary embolism, especially if the classical technique has been used by the obstetrician. The lower segmental section, being a pelvic operation, may embarrass urinary continence and sometimes requires a self-retaining Foley catheter and the requisite care. In either operation it is most likely that the patient would have to have a 5- or 7-day course of antibiotics to counter the **risk** of pelvic or abdominal infection.

On recovery from the operation, the mother and baby should be brought together as soon as possible for obvious psychological reasons. There is the need to advise the mother that future pregnancies are neither necessarily threatened by Caesarean section nor is there any limit on the number of children born by this method to a mother, providing only a lower segmental section is used.

MULTIPLE BIRTHS

The theoretical incidence of having a multiple birth is based on Hellin's rule, which when quoted, shows that the chances are

Twins, a 1 in 80 incidence

Triplets, a 1 in 6 400 incidence, or 80 × 80

Quadruplets, a 1 in 512 000 incidence, or 6 500 × 6 400

Quintuplets, a 1 in 4 096 000 incidence, or 512 000 × 512 000

These figures, however, are based on a *naturally* occurring multiple birth. The increased prescription of the oestrogen-based fertility drugs for infertile women alters the figures quite dramatically. Naturally occurring multiple births are more common amongst the Negroid races, particularly in Africa.

Identical twins

Other terms to describe twins who are identical include: *monovular*, *monozygotic* and *monochorionic*. For identical twins to occur, the single ovum is fertilised by a single sperm, and at the blastomere stage the developing embryo divides into two identical halves, each twin being of the same sex. Identical twins are usually born to a mother aged between 20 and 35 years old.

Nonidentical twins

Other terms to describe nonidentical twins include: *binovular*, *dizygotic* and *dichorionic*. In this instance, two ova have been fertilised by two separate spermatozoa at the same time. The twins are not necessarily of the same sex. The incidence of nonidentical twins is 3 or 4 times more common in mothers over the age of 35.

Diagnosis of Multiple Births

Diagnosis is relatively straightforward, but about 5% of multiple births are missed in the antenatal clinics, much to everyone's embarrassment at the time of delivery. The maternal family history may indicate the likelihood of twins occurring in previous generations, which would suggest that clinical tests should look for a twin birth.

Signs

The uterus enlarges much faster than normal for the gestational age, particularly from the twenty-fourth week. There tends to be excessive vomiting during the early phase of pregnancy. The mother notices and feels excessive movement in the abdomen.

On palpation, a multiplicity of limbs may be felt as can be two heads. When the twin heartbeats are counted simultaneously by two observers, there should be a difference of 10 in the count. At the tenth week an ultrasound scan may confirm the diagnosis, and later in the twenty-fourth week, a plain abdominal x-ray may be advised if the diagnosis is still uncertain.

Management During Pregnancy

Management during a multiple birth pregnancy should emphasise the need for the mother to take extra iron and folic acid in a high protein nourishing diet. There is a need to check with the mother that she is taking her extra medication and to double-check her haemoglobin and folic acid levels from blood tests.

To reduce the **risk** of pre-eclampsia or premature labour, the mother must have several hours more rest each day, this is particularly true where the expectant mother has an over reliant family group. If necessary, the mother should be admitted to hospital to ensure she has adequate rest.

Possible Risks During Pregnancy and Labour

A multiple birth carries with it multiple risks (Table 24.1) and for this reason the delivery should always be in hospital where specialist personnel and equipment are centralised and immediately available to the mother. Apart from the nursing team, it is usual for the obstetrician to be assisted by an anaesthetist and for a paediatrician to be available.

During Delivery

The stages of labour are as for a single birth but the second twin is born 15 to 30 minutes after the first. The obstetrician will have taken great care to ensure that the firstborn has a longitudinal presentation (Fig. 24.2), if necessary using version to correct its position. If for any reason the firstborn's position cannot be corrected, then Caesarean section may be performed. After the membranes have rup-

Table 24.1 Possible risks in multiple pregnancy

In pregnancy	During labour
Abortion Premature labour (pre-38th week) Pre-eclampsia risk increased threefold Iron deficiency anaemia Folic acid deficiency Hydramnios Antepartum haemorrhage abruptio placenta placenta praevia	Prolapse of the umbilical cord Second twin has higher mortality rate Postpartum haemorrhage

tured there is an immediate check to ensure that the cord has not collapsed.

During delivery there is a constant check made on the fetal heart. After the first twin is born the cord is clamped and the baby given directly over to the midwife for the immediate care of the newborn. After an interval of 10 to 30 minutes the second twin should be born. Ergometrine is not administered until after the second twin is safely delivered.

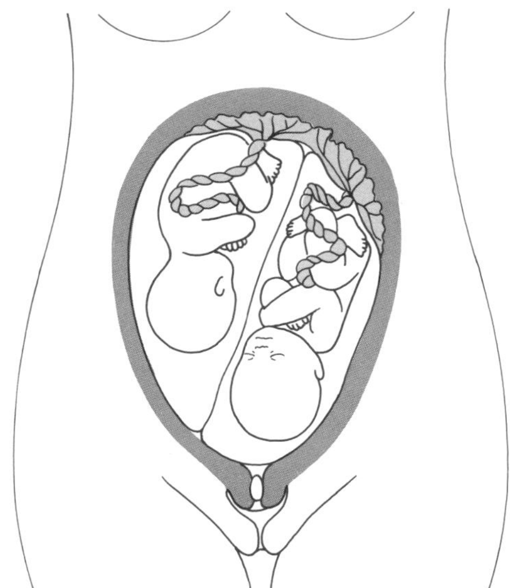

Fig. 24.2 Position of fetuses in womb (multiple birth).

THE PRETERM BABY (PREMATURITY)

Prematurity is defined as a delivery before the thirty-seventh week (259 days) and occurs in 7–10% of all births in the United Kingdom. The two possible indications of a premature birth are a premature rupture of the membranes and/or premature contraction of the uterine muscle. The predisposing causes of a premature labour are regarded as being:

Pre-eclampsia and **maternal hypertension**
Abruptio placenta
Placenta praevia
Multiple pregnancy
Congenital abnormality
Rhesus isoimmunisation

Body Weights

A premature infant is likely to weigh less than 2.5 kg (5 lbs) and below this weight, even if born at full term, is regarded by WHO (World Health Organisation) as being premature. This definition, however, is only a guideline, as premature infants can in fact be born in quite a mature condition while full-term babies may be born extremely small and be *light for dates* (Table 24.2). In general, a baby below a birthweight of 2.5 kg requires intensive nursing until the recognised risks of prematurity are overcome (Fig. 24.3).

Risks

There are risks in a premature birth to both the mother and the child. The maternal

Table 24.2 Comparison between the preterm and light-for-dates baby

	Preterm	Light for dates
Skin	Red with vernix	Dry without vernix
Subcutaneous fat	Insufficient	Insufficient
Umbilical cord	Wharton's jelly	Hardly any jelly
Muscle tone	Hypotonic	Active
Facial expression	Fetal	Alert
Possible risks	Hypothermia Respiratory distress syndrome Jaundice Infection Cerebral haemorrhage	Hypothermia Hypoglycaemia

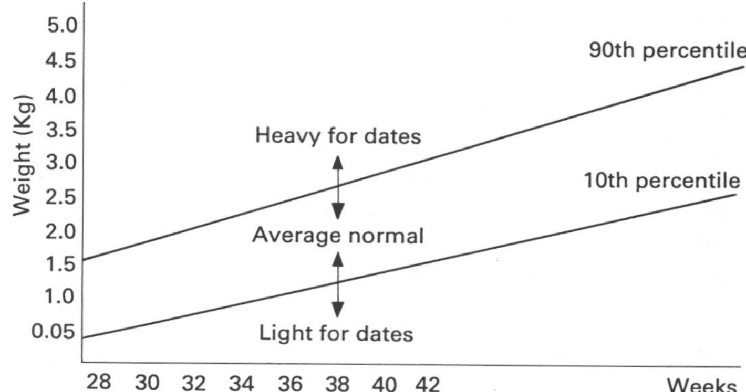

Fig. 24.3 Gestational estimation for body weight.

difficulties are that the birth canal has not yet physiologically stretched to accommodate the baby, and an episiotomy has to be done for a vaginal delivery. A second major hazard is that the uterus is prone to infection, against which antibiotics are not effective. For these two reasons there is an increasing tendency to deliver the baby by Caesarean section.

The premature infant has several distinct problems which threaten its survival:

1. The respiratory tract is anatomically and physiologically immature, with a high risk of respiratory distress syndrome.

2. The temperature control mechanism is underdeveloped, and body heat loss from perspiration is a marked risk, i.e., *hypothermia*.

3. The immune system is underdeveloped and the infant is more than usually prone to serious infection risk.

4. There may be a neurological reflex deficit, i.e., the absence of a suckling reflex preventing the infant from taking feeds.

Management and Delivery

If the fetus threatens to deliver before the thirty-fifth week, the obstetric management is usually aimed at preventing the birth until at least the thirty-seventh week. This is achieved by treating the mother while on bedrest. If the cervix is not dilated beyond 4 cm, a cervical suture, e.g., Shirodkar, may be employed to close the uterine opening. However, if the contractions continue this would have to be cut.

The uterine contractions may be arrested by infusing one of the beta adrenergic drugs via an intravenous infusion, usually by electronic pump method. Examples of the drugs used include:

Alcohol 9.5% solution 15 ml per kg

body weight, assessed every 2 hours until the contractions have stopped

Isoxuprine 250 µg every minute as an initial dose then increasing the amount if required until the contractions stop

Salbutamol 2 to 20 µg per minute until the contractions stop and then continued orally

Ritodrine 50 µg every minute in the initial stages and then after 12 hours continued with oral Ritodrine

Whichever drug is prescribed, the nurse is responsible for monitoring the pulse and blood pressure at 15–30 minute intervals for adverse effects from the drugs.

If, however, the labour commences at the thirty-fifth week or over and the membranes rupture, the labour is accelerated by giving intravenous oxytocin. The reason for accelerating the delivery is because of the high risk of intrauterine infection. Since the infant's respiratory centre is so immature, pethidine is not used during any of the stages of labour.

After Delivery

On being safely delivered, the premature infant is immediately placed in a controlled environment (an *incubator*). This apparatus allows the infant to be nursed in an environment which has a high temperature, 28°–30° C which is humidifed with a rich supply of moistened oxygen.

Feeds

If there is no suckling reflex, a narrow bore paediatric nasogastric tube is passed into the stomach and feeds are commenced every 2 hours. The baby should have about 10 feeds within every 24 hours and this is maintained until weight gain is obvious. Oral feeding is attempted when the paediatrician indicates that the baby may be lifted from the incubator for short periods each day.

Isolation

The enforced separation from the mother may be ameliorated by taking photographs of the baby. Apart from this, the mother should have frequent verbal reports on how her baby is progressing. From necessity, there has to be very strict control to prevent cross-infection, which in effect will limit access to the baby by the parents and other relatives. In handling the baby and giving direct care via the portholes of the incubator, the nurse has a special responsibility to follow the current rules in force in the intensive care to limit the spread of infection.

LIGHT FOR DATES BABY (FULL TERM)

A baby reaching full term may also present with the same problems as the preterm baby if its weight is below 2.5 kg. In this instance, the baby is below the tenth percentile for its gestational age. Diagnostic monitoring will usually indicate if the baby is light for dates. Since the baby is at grave **risk** from intrauterine hypoxia, delivery **must** take place without delay. If the baby survives the management techniques employed for the premature infant for 72 hours, the prognosis is very good.

POSTPARTUM HAEMORRHAGE (PPH)

If there is blood loss from the birth canal exceeding 560 ml within 24 hours of childbirth, it is classified as a *reactionary* postpartum haemorrhage. If occurring after 24 hours, it is a *secondary* haemorrhage. In the 10 to 12 days following childbirth, the uterus should regress to its prepregnant shape and size by a process known as *involution*. This process, however, begins after the placenta has sheared itself free from the uterine wall in the third stage of labour.

Causes of Postpartum Haemorrhage

Causes of postpartum haemorrhage include:

Failure of the uterus to contract and control bleeding from the placental site (the most common and dangerous form of postpartum haemorrhage)

Failure of the placenta to separate completely, thus preventing the uterus from contracting

Retention of placental fragments (retained *secundinae*), again preventing the uterus from contracting and sealing off the endometrial blood vessels

Vaginal or cervical tears, including episiotomy

Formation and detachment of thrombi from the uterine wall due to poor involution from the sixth to fifteenth day after childbirth

The potential to suffer from a postpartum haemorrhage should always be considered in mothers who

have **excessive uterine distension** e.g., twins)

are suffering from **malnutrition**

are **multiparous**

have required a **surgical delivery** (i.e., a Caesarean section)

are suffering **placenta praevia**

Any severe bleeding from the vagina will quickly lead to a marked hypotension, extreme shock, and a very frightened patient facing the possibility of death. In a moderate bleed, apart from the expected severe shock, the patient will suffer from anaemia and have a very real fear of future pregnancies.

Care and Treatment

Care and treatment is of any emergency nature with the treatment of shock of paramount importance. The patient requires to be nursed in a bed with the end of the bed elevated, using an additional blanket for extra warmth, if needed.

Continuous monitoring of the pulse and blood pressure will give a guideline as to the severity of the shock and the urgency with which the haemorrhage should be dealt with. The volume of blood loss is assessed by calculating only what can be collected in a receiver placed between the thighs. An intravenous infusion should be established as urgently as possible and plasma infused to restore the circulating volume and increase the blood pressure. Added to the infusion is the drug Syntometrine, which has oxytocic properties, i.e., a combination of oxytocin and ergometrine. The drug has an immediate effect on the uterus, causing it to contract. These contractions will seal off the blood vessels which are oozing the blood. The patient must remain on bedrest for some time, certainly until the anaemia has been treated and both pulse and blood pressure are within normal average levels.

Other methods of treatment include applying digital pressure and massage to the fundus of the uterus. It may be necessary, if Syntometrine and massage do not work, to prepare the patient for theatre so that a saline pack can be inserted into the uterus as an emergency measure to control the bleeding.

Once the bleeding has been controlled and the patient is ready for discharge to home, an appointment is arranged for the patient to have a dilation and curettage at a later time, to remove the retained products of conception.

INTRAUTERINE DEATH

Intrauterine death is an increasingly rare situation due to the tremendous advances made in obstetric diagnostic techniques. The causes are:

Abruptio placenta (accidental haemorrhage after the twenty-fourth week of pregnancy)

Coagulation defect of the blood, usually due to a deficiency of fibrin or a rhesus defect

Diabetes mellitus which has not been diagnosed

The detection of intrauterine death is suspected when the fetal heart beat cannot be heard, if there is a reduced fetal movement, if on palpation the uterus feels wooden and hard and if plain abdominal X-rays show a solid mass.

Once confirmed, the treatment is to induce labour with the aim of saving the baby if at all possible. If the diagnosis is made after the twenty-fourth week, a Caesarean section is usually attempted with the aim of saving the baby.

STILLBIRTH

As the term suggests this is the birth of a dead fetus. In descending order of incidence the following shows the main causes of a fetus becoming inviable:

Premature labour

Intrauterine hypoxia (reduced blood supply to the fetus)

Congenital abnormality (e.g., anencephaly, spina bifida)

Birth injury (forceps delivery)

Eclampsia

Potential **diabetes mellitus**

The nurse has an extremely important role to pursue in helping a mother come to terms with the loss of her baby. Some mothers wish to hold or see their baby, despite any advice to the contrary, and this should be allowed. The emotional responses may vary, but in general they are those of grief. Anger against nursing staff or feelings of intense guilt can be experienced and good counselling can help the mother to put both of these reactions in perspective.

Counselling is required for the need to register a stillbirth as well as receiving from the obstetrician a certificate of stillbirth. By law, both these are required before the infant can be given a funeral. It is advisable to keep the grieving mother in hospital for at least a few days to permit arrangements to be made at home so that she is not left alone for long periods.

A great deal of emphasis is placed on the statistics related to perinatal death, i.e., stillbirths and neonatal deaths. These figures show a dramatic reduction as obstetric and midwifery skills and social standards have improved. For stillbirths, the mortality rate has fallen from 40 per 1 000 births in 1930 to 10 per 1 000 births in 1980. Neonatal deaths, i.e., death during the first week of life, have fallen from 22 per 1 000 in 1930 to less than 10 per 1 000 in 1980.

Chapter 25
Examination and Assessment of the Newborn Child

INITIAL CARE OF THE NEWBORN

Immediately on delivering the baby, the midwife lightly wipes away any mucoid material from the baby's eyes, nostrils and lips. The universally accepted method of assessing the risk of asphyxia in the newborn is to assess the Apgar score at 1 minute, 4 minutes and at 10 minutes after birth (Table 25.1).

Establishing Patent Airway

The use of a mucus extractor may be sufficient to extract a small mucus plug from the nostrils or mouth by applying gentle suction to remove the mucus into a small plastic container. Supporting the baby in the upside down position will also aid the removal of mucus by natural drainage of these cavities. For more tenacious stubborn mucus a suction catheter may need to be inserted into the nostrils or oropharynx and positive vacuum pressure used to release the mucus.

Respiration

Within 30 seconds to 1 minute of birth the baby should reflexly cry with the first exhalation. If the respirations are slow and shallow, it may be necessary to administer oxygen via a mask or nasal catheters to supplement the baby's own efforts. *Delayed respiration* is a medical emergency and would require the paediatrician to pass a paediatric laryngoscope to inspect the vocal cord rima and insert an endotracheal tube and supply oxygen under pressure. Any intubation is

Table 25.1 Apgar scale (score)

Sign	Score		
	0	1	2
Colour	Pale	Blue	Pink
Heart rate	Absent	Below 100	Above 100
Respiration	Absent	Gasping	Loud cry
Muscle tone	Limp	Limb flexion	Strong movement
Reflex response	None	Facial grimace	Loud cry

Score interpretation
8 to 10: good physical condition
7 to 4: may develop asphyxia
4 to 0: is shocked and has asphyxia

usually of short duration, being removed as soon as the baby can breathe independently.

The infant's respiration may be affected by *drugs*, such as morphine or pethidine, if used in the delivery period. The antidote to these two drugs is nalorphine and should be available in the delivery room. The causes of asphyxia in the newborn are intra-uterine asphyxia, drug induced, intracranial damage during delivery and mucus plug obstruction.

Circulation

Having established a clear airway for the newborn baby, the midwife will then concentrate on the physical comfort of both baby and mother. Shortly after being born, the baby's colour should alter from a greyish blue to a warm pink, indicating that the circulation of blood is well-established. Should the baby remain bluish it may imply that there is a congenital heart defect.

TESTS AND OBSERVATIONS

Within the next few hours the midwife will make a series of tests and observations to assess the baby's health status. These assessments are a mix of objective and subjective measurements, but the attending midwife would report immediately if any of the following tests showed a marked variation from expected normal average values:

Occipito-heel length	Respiratory rate and depth
Conjunctival-lacrimal inspection	Rectal temperature
Birth weight	Obvious congenital deformity
Pulse rate and volume	Inborn errors of metabolism
Skull circumference	Feeding difficulties
Neurological defect	

Skull Circumference

The average diameter of the skull is between 33 and 35 cm. Any bulging or collapse of the tissues over the anterior or posterior fontanelles should be reported as it may indicate interference with the flow of the cerebrospinal fluid (*hydrocephalus*).

Occipito-heel Length

The average length between the occiput and the heels is between 45 and 50 cm. The child may be small for dates or, alternatively, large if born to a diabetic mother. In normal physiology, the baby should double its length during the first 12 months. This original measurement is helpful in postnatal assessment.

During this measurement note should be made of the roundness and movement of the limbs and a finger run along the length of the vertebral column to detect for unexpected depressions or swellings (e.g. *meningocele*).

Conjunctival-lacrimal Inspection

The conjunctiva are inspected for any obvious mucoid secretion. If present, it could be suggestive of gonorrhoea, i.e., *neonatorum gonococcus* infection, which requires an eye swab to be taken and prescribed antibiotic ointment or drops immediately instilled. The lacrimal apparatus is still incomplete and, therefore, the newborn child is unable to shed tears. Both conjunctiva should be slightly moist, and do not require cleansing. The colour of the iris in the newborn is always blue, the true eye colour develops after 6 weeks.

Birth Weight

It is quite normal for the baby to lose between 200 and 300 g in body weight in the first few days of life. This loss is normally regained by the fifth day when the feeding regime is firmly established. Any failure to gain weight is regarded as a failure to thrive and there is usually an underlying cause, e.g., *metabolic* or *anatomical*, which requires deeper investigations.

Pulse Rate and Volume

The pulse rate is usually taken by auscultation at the apex of the heart and on average measures between 120 and 140 beats per minute. It is not routinely recorded unless there is prematurity or a congenital heart defect, when a cardiac monitor would be used for accuracy.

Respiratory Rate and Depth

Once the threat of asphyxia has been removed, the respiratory depth is usually shallow and the baby breathes at about 30 respirations per minute. Crying does deepen the inhalation and expand the lungs. The lung tissue at birth is exceptionally delicate and for premature infants a controlled environment such as an incubator is necessary until the tissue is relatively safe and mature.

Rectal Temperature

The temperature should record between 36.7° and 37° C on a rectal thermometer. In all newborns, the heat regulating centre located in the hypothalamus is immature. This implies that none of the normal mechanisms for keeping warm or cool is utilised in infancy. The tendency is for an infant to lose heat by radiation rather rapidly, hence the need to keep the baby warm and nurse the baby in a warm environment. In premature infants, a controlled temperature is vital; they must be nursed in incubators where the required temperature can be constantly maintained.

Obvious Congenital Deformity

Physical testing, handling and visual assessment are normally done to detect the more obvious congenital defects. These are:

Undescended testes have no immediate treatment as the testes may descend spontaneously in the early postnatal period. However, **note** should be made of this defect so that it can be a reminder in the health screening after discharge from hospital.

Imperforate anus can be noted at the time of recording the rectal temperature. The baby would have to be referred for further surgical opinion for possible reconstructive surgery at a later date. Faecal incontinence into a fistula is a major hazard requiring careful nursing techniques to keep the perineum especially clean following each bowel motion.

Talipes, or clubfoot, is rather obvious from the shape and unnatural alignment of the ankle, and requires referral to the orthopaedic surgeons for their opinion as to when surgery or conservative treatment should be started.

Cleft palate, or harelip, may not be very obvious until feeding begins. A small defect in the anatomy of the upper or lower mandible where the right and left halves of the jaw meet means that there is a direct connection between the mouth and the nasal floor space. (See *Nursing 1* for further detailed coverage.)

Meningocele, Spina Bifida, and Hydrocephalus may all be detected by running the finger over the fontanelles and along the spine to feel for any unusual depressions or swellings which require to be reported at once.

Incomplete genitalia, such as hypospadia, incomplete or absence of a urethra require very close visual inspection for detection and should be referred to the surgeon to determine when reconstructive surgery should be offered.

Congenital Dislocation of Hip (CDH) is assessed by employing Ortolani's Test. Either leg is capable of a 90° abduction when it is flexed, with the baby lying in a supine position. Any clicking noise or resistance to this flexion sugests that the head of the femur is not rotating in the acetabulum of the pelvis. There are a variety of early treatments during childhood and these are discussed in *Nursing 1*.

Mental Handicap, such as Down's Syndrome, may or may not be visually obvious at birth, the shape of the head often being used as a sign to detect its presence. Neurological testing is often completed if there is a suspicion of its presence.

Inborn Errors of Metabolism

The more obvious of the inborn errors of metabolism, *phenylketonuria* (PKU), is proven by the Guthrie Test after a milk-feeding regimen has been established. A specimen of urine is obtained either from a nappy or a paediatric urine sampling bag and tested with a reagent strip (Phenistix). Other inborn errors of metabolism may not be so readily assessed until the baby shows evidence of failure to thrive, such as in cystic fibrosis.

Feeding Difficulties

Reflex behaviours of rooting and suckling are usually present from the outset and encouraged by placing the baby to breast within 4 hours of birth. The lip-areolar contact is sufficient to initiate the suckling reflex. Anatomical defects of the mouth, throat or oesophagus may, however, impede the swallowing reflex, causing the baby to vomit or regurgitate any feeds offered.

If the mother is not breastfeeding, the first feed is usually composed of warm sterile water with sugar added. When this is taken without difficulty, the baby is commenced on a 4-hourly feeding regimen. The timing of feeds is more variable with breastfeeding. If required, the mother can have her milk expressed and saved for the baby. If the baby has not had a feed in the first 18 hours of life, for whatever reason, it strongly suggests a paediatric assessment is required to establish the deeper cause of such a feeding difficulty.

Neurological Tests

Prior to the infant and mother being sent home, the paediatrician may wish to test several of the many reflexes to assess if normal development can be predicted with any certainty. The suckling and swallowing reflexes, along with blink and pupil reflexes, will already be established.

To assess **motor development**, the reflexes controlling muscle tone and coordination can be tested. The Moro reflex is used to test whether the baby will abduct and extend the arms in a crucifix fashion when the head is released from a supported position. This reflex is also present in the premature infant, but should disappear between the third and fourth month of life. Its absence before then indicates a muscular condition of *hypotonia*.

The **startle** reflex tests the baby's ability to hear sounds, which should be present from birth. After a loud noise (clapping) is made the baby's head should flex and the eyes turn towards the source of the noise. A hearing handicap is often difficult to determine in its severity at birth, but a negative startle reflex suggests a vigilant follow up in the postnatal period.

A **grasp** reflex of the fingers flexing around an object placed in the baby's palm and then gently pulled away is also suggestive of good coordination. When the baby is supported on its feet there should be an indication of both the stepping and walking reflex. On stroking the sole of the foot, the toes should turn upwards away from the ground, i.e., the opposite of the plantar reflex in the adult.

The value of all these tests is not immediate, but the results if carefully recorded in the baby's notes will be scrutinised in the postnatal examinations held at the mother's health clinic. The mother herself should also be guided as to the value of the tests as they form the basis of specific counselling the paediatrician may offer the mother on the future care of her child.

SPECIFIC NURSING CARE OF THE BABY

The specific nursing care of the baby is the prerogative of the mother, but in the hospital environment the nurse can offer a great deal of support and education. The baby's cot is usually placed at the mother's bedside and the temperature of the environment should be between 18° and 21° C. The baby will sleep most of the time, only being interrupted by the discomforts of hunger and incontinence.

Feeding

A regular feeding pattern is desirable within 18 hours of birth and if the baby is being bottlefed would usually take on a 4-hourly pattern. The nurse can offer to feed the baby at this early stage to allow the mother to rest during the first 24 hours. If the mother is breastfeeding, there are many physiological advantages which outweigh bottlefeeding, but the nurse may have to advise on care of the nipples and breasts and a suitable bra.

The Umbilicus

The clamps attached to the umbilical cord are left alone as the umbilical stump will dry and atrophy, receding into the umbilicus of the abdomen within a few days. In the meantime, the umbilical stump is kept clean and dry, with sometimes a Sterivac powder being lightly dusted over the stump.

Elimination

The baby's first bowel motion is usually a green-coloured meconium, after this the stools are a yellow colour. Obviously, the infant has no control over bowel motions, with perhaps a bowel evacuation 3 or 4 times in 24 hours. Frequent perineal hygiene is given. After cleansing it is usual to apply a nonallergic cream to the skin to protect it against the excoriating effects of urine and faeces.

Infection Control

The infection risk in neonatal wards is very high and the nurse, apart from having a high personal standard of cleanliness, must follow the strict policies regarding the handling and disposal of soiled nappies and cot linen. Feeds which are delivered from the milk kitchen where they have been prepared with sterility and extreme care, require strict cleanliness. The bottles may be of the disposable type. If not they should be soaked in Milton 1 in 80 strength, as should the teats before being returned to the milk kitchen. If the baby becomes ill it is usual practice to insist on parents wearing protective clothing to prevent the spread of infection.

Identity Bracelets

The identity of the baby is most important, even where individual rooms are provided, or if there is a multiple birth. Bracelets are attached to the ankle giving the baby's surname and if decided the forename along with the number on the parents' notes. Should the baby be born prematurely, or require specialised care in neonatal intensive care, the parents should be asked if they would like the baby to be baptised, or in the case of non-Christian infants the parents should seek counsel from their spiritual adviser in respect of their religious customs.

Chapter 26
The Puerperium

In the earlier part of the twentieth century, the puerperium was regarded as an extremely dangerous period because of the high incidence of infection. Since the advent of antibiotics, safe aseptic techniques, good antenatal and postnatal care, the incidence of such hazards as puerperal fever and sepsis have been eradicated.

The puerperium is defined as 'the time between delivery of the child and the return of the uterus to its normal position and size', usually 6 weeks. During this interval, the caring team have a fourfold plan of care:

To restore the mother to normal physiological and psychological well being

To **maintain** the infant's health and welfare

To **establish** and monitor the infant's feeding regime

To educate both parents on their own and their child's future health

MANAGEMENT DURING NORMAL PUERPERIUM

The immediate management during a normal puerperium is divided into eight areas to help achieve the aims of the plan of care. These areas of assessment and evaluation are:

1. Clinical observation
2. Dealing with after pain
3. Promoting a normal sleep pattern
4. Encouraging postnatal exercises
5. Establishing infant feeding
6. Giving psychological support
7. Arranging discharge from hospital to home

8. Advising on future health care arrangements

Clinical Observation

The **axillary temperature** should be recorded every 4 hours for at least 24 hours to detect for any pyrexia; this would imply an early infection. A persistent **tachycardia** without any obvious cause should be noted and verbally reported. Any signs of **calf pain** or **oedematous ankles** may indicate a deep-vein thrombosis and require to be reported immediately. The **blood pressure** should be monitored every 4 hours for 48 hours if the mother suffered from pre-eclampsia in the antenatal stage, or labour was deliberately induced.

Vaginal discharge (**the lochia**) should be observed. It will alter from fresh blood to a yellowish white discharge over a period of 10 days. Offensive odours and extremely soiled maternity pads may indicate a uterine infection requiring further investigation.

A **diuresis** is to be expected within 48 hours of childbirth and may last for 3 days as the body readjusts its renal function. If the **haemoglobin level** is below 11% dL, or the mother is obviously anaemic, then supplements of oral iron may be prescribed in addition to a nutritious diet. After 48 hours, it is usual pratice to offer the mother a mild aperient to aid **defaecation** as the pelvic floor muscles are still stretched, implying the mother is prone to constipation for several weeks.

After Pains

Uterine contractions may continue for sometime after the baby is born and are extremely uncomfortable, requiring potent analgesia if the pain persists. The perineum itself may also be very painful and uncomfortable, more so if an episiotomy proved necessary.

The vagina, cervix, vulva, urethra and bladder have all been considerably stretched, which adds to the overall pelvic discomfort. Sitting upright can be most uncomfortable and nursing measures to relieve perineal pressure include the use of analgesia, applying ice packs to the area and, of course, the use of an air ring or cushion. At the 24-hour and then 48-hour interval, the perineum should be checked for healing if an episiotomy has been performed.

Sleep

After delivery the mother is naturally exhausted, but may also be excited and sometimes overwhelmed. The conflicting emotions may mitigate against rest and sleep, making the mother quite restless. If necessary, mild sedation may prove useful if in the nurse's opinion the restlessness or lack of sleep hinders the mother's ability to care for her baby.

Exercises

Following a normal birth, the mother is usually assisted with her physical needs for the first 24 hours and thereafter gently guided towards self-care, such as with personal toiletting and hygiene. The muscle tone of the stretched areas is particularly weak; these areas involve the pelvic and abdominal recti or rectus muscles.

Consciously contracting and relaxing by the mother of these muscle groups for 15 minutes twice daily will help to increase their tone. The advantages of these exercises are that they improve bladder and bowel function, improve venous blood flow from the lower limbs and flatten the stretched abdominal muscles. If deep-breathing exercises are also done, then the mother's overall feeling of well being is further enhanced.

Infant Feeding

About 40% of mothers opt to breastfeed their baby. In those who prefer or have to bottlefeed, it may be necessary to suppress lactation. This suppression is usually achieved by the administration of a prescribed drug such as quinestrol (Estrovis) 4 mg for 48 hours, in addition the oral fluid intake is reduced and the breasts are not expressed.

Breastfeeding

Breastfeeding has many advantages over artificial methods as the supply of human milk contains the correct proportions required by the infant: 2% protein, 4% fat, 6% carbohydrate and 0.2% mineral salts. Apart from human milk being sterile, it also contains antibodies which will confer immunity on the baby for some months. The mother–baby contact is directly reinforced and the loving bond is established very early.

During the antenatal period the nipples should be everted and massaged with a soothing cream and any colostrum expressed. A healthy baby will suckle at birth and, if put to the breast immediately after delivery, not only will reassure the mother but also helps with uterine contractions in the last stage of labour. It is about 3 days before milk is secreted in quantity and a routine is soon established, most babies requiring to be fed at 4-hourly intervals.

Before and after each feed the mother should wash her hands and nipples and during the feed should relax either in a sitting posture or lying on her side supporting the baby towards the breast in her flexed arm. In the first five minutes of suckling, most of the milk is secreted, but the remainder of the time the physical contact give both baby and mother a great deal of pleasure. If the breast is very engorged, the baby will be unable to grasp the nipple between the lip and hard palate. In this instance, it is necessary to rest the breast, otherwise the nipple will become painful and cracked. In this circumstance, the milk may be expressed by hand, by a hand pump or with an electric breast pump (Humilactor). Before breastfeeding, the baby's napkin should be changed as babies sleep following a breastfeed, and change then would disturb them.

Psychological Support

On or about the fifth day, the mother may confess to a feeling of depression. She should be reassured that this is quite a common experience following childbirth. There is often a combination of factors contributing to this feeling of the 'blues' (postpartum depression). The mother may feel inadequate and unable to cope with a new baby. Additionally, there are many physical discomforts to contend with and the breasts may be painfully engorged. A great deal of support can be given by just allowing the mother to express her fears and by doing so place them in perspective.

Leading questions may be asked by the nurse to pinpoint the exact areas of the mother's concern. Often it defines those aspects of baby's care or welfare within the home and with the family. If the mother is depressed, there may be some advantage in allowing the baby's father to visit more often, and to extend the same opportunity to other members of the family. There is a wide selection of pamphlets and literature available from many sources which may help answer specific anxieties, particularly where a mother is faced with trying to anticipate the needs of a handicapped baby.

As a last resort, the use of sedation or antidepressants may be prescribed but this choice does not really get to the root of the mother's problems. Particular signs which should be reported are *insomnia*, *restless behaviour*, *ignoring* or *rejecting* the newborn baby, or *behaving* 'out of character'. These may be early signs of puerperal depression (**psychosis**), a serious form of depression requiring psychiatric opinion and treatment.

Discharge from Hospital to Home

As stated earlier, following a normal delivery the mother would be assisted with her physical needs for the first 24 hours and then guided gently towards self-care. In the majority of cases, the mother and baby can be discharged from hospital to home after 48 hours. This, however, is only possible if it is a *planned early discharge*. This would mean that the mother has had excellent antenatal care and has arranged in detail for the care of the baby at home. Prior to discharge there must be a firm appointment for the district midwife's first visit to the home within 1 week.

Problems

Particular problems require different solutions. There may be poor housing conditions, a single-parent family, medical problems, multiple birth or adoption procedures. In these examples, the discharge from hospital would be delayed until the referral agencies had made their decision and arrangements.

Community

A letter is forwarded to the general practitioner about the birth, appointments are made for a first postnatal examination, with the infant welfare clinic and with the family planning clinic. If the registrar of births does not visit the maternity hospital on a daily basis then, by law, the birth must be registered by the parents within 14 days. In some districts the baby's name is placed on a computer for later immunisation schedules.

FUTURE HEALTH CARE

On the first postnatal examination either at the hospital or with the mother's general practitioner, the following plan of care is usually pursued:

1. Maternal health is checked
2. The infant's health is assessed
3. Contraception techniques are discussed

Maternal Health

A physical examination usually determines if the vulva, urethra and vagina have regained their shape and tone. The urethra, having been stretched, may have caused problems of urinary dribbling but by this first visit they should have resolved. If not, the bladder tone and pelvic muscle tone may be inadequate with a consequent **risk** of urinary tract infection.

Palpation of the uterus will show if it has returned to its normal pelvic position. This it usually does by the tenth to twelfth day following childbirth. The process of uterine involution involves atrophy caused by a reduced level of oestrogens, the uterine blood vessels thrombose, there is shrinkage of the myometrium and the endometrium regenerates between week 2 and week 5–6. The cervical stretching causes a permanent alteration of shape, as with the external os.

Following examination, a cervical smear is taken for cytology screening. Healing of an episiotomy scar should be well-advanced, with no sign of either infection or inflammation. The blood pressure and body weight should have returned to prepregnancy levels. If the mother is breastfeeding, the breasts are checked for mastitis and cracked nipples.

Infant Health

It is recommended that the infant has weekly weight checks at the infant welfare centre and that any feeding problems are discussed with the health visitor. The atrophied umbilical cord stump should have fallen away without leaving any scarring or infection and the mother reassured that any slight protrusion of the umbilicus is quite normal.

The genitalia are again checked for any possible congenital defect. If the posture of the baby indicates any hypotonia, the baby may undergo a neurological assessment either at the clinic or at the hospital. The health visitor will have an opportunity to discuss with the mother any problems she is experiencing in her care of the baby and many anxieties can be resolved regarding the infant's welfare.

Contraceptive Techniques

Of the many clinics to which the mother is referred, the family planning is the most important (see also chapter 27). Previously used contraceptive techniques are reappraised and their future suitability assessed. This is particularly so for the pill and requires expert advice and guidance for medical reasons. Whichever technique is advised and adopted has to be commenced from the sixth week following pregnancy. Sexual intercourse during the puerperium is not advised since there is a **risk** of infection in this period.

Chapter 27
Family Planning

As the nurse gains experience she/he will repeatedly observe situations where elementary advice on family planning could have prevented illness or unnecessary distress. In obstetrics and gynaecological practice there is an obvious need for the nurse to possess a command of family planning techniques in order to counsel effectively. However knowledge of family planning is also of value in paediatrics, psychiatry, community nursing and in venereology. Although there are many agencies who specialise in advising on family planning, it is often the nurse who has primary contact and is the first to appreciate the patient's need for such counselling.

In Western cultures there are obvious advantages if parents plan when to have their children and the interval between each child. These advantages are:

1. Nationally, there is a need for the population to match the natural and manufactured resources it can provide. Population trends projected over the next 20 years in the United Kingdom show an increase in the population by 15 million. This upward trend has been compensated by already calculating that the average married couple have 2.4 children. Additionally, the figure takes into account the expected longevity of the existing population. What is not calculated is that if family planning was more positively pursued, it would in fact reduce the consequences of a population explosion.

2. The specific health of the female population and their children shows a marked improvement when the family size has been deliberately planned and thought about

deeply. Children who are wanted create harmony, strengthen family bonds and are assured of caring happy parents. This leads to a better health outlook for all members within the family unit. The continual struggle against poverty, overcrowding, ill health and ignorance is more obviously contained if married couples are encouraged to seek out information and help with family planning.

3. Family planning is a positive health measure in those women with a history of: unnecessary abortions, difficult pregnancies, or complicated deliveries.

4. Those couples experiencing the subsequent problems associated with subfertility are indirectly helped by family planning counselling and can be directed to the correct sources for further advice and treatment.

5. For the single person entering into a sexual relationship, a knowledge of contraceptive techniques is vital if either partner wishes to avoid an unwanted pregnancy. Even if living in an enlightened and compassionate society, the single mother remains a disadvantaged citizen from every point of view. The social, economic and lifelong commitment of being a mother can and does cause physical and psychological distress, leading to illness. Apart from the single mother, the father also has stresses to contend with, usually of a psychological nature. The extended family may feel quite bitter about an unplanned child, the end result being that the child is disadvantaged from the very outset of its conception.

6. Although there are wide and varying beliefs and moralities of different cultures and religions, one or several of the established contraceptive techniques are usually acceptable. There is no single perfect contraceptive technique; therefore, the nurse needs to consider all the techniques currently available.

AVAILABLE CONTRACEPTIVE TECHNIQUES

The majority of couples usually discuss the size of the family they would like and the spacing of intervals between each child. It is to be encouraged that the couple not only discuss their future family, but seek out professional advice if they are not familiar with contraceptive techniques.

In all marriages (or relationships) there has to be a period of adjustment until a suitable contraceptive technique is adopted which also allows for sexual gratification to both partners. Quite a number of marriages do not have this 'communication' because of embarrassment or ignorance, and it is at this point that counselling from an expert can help save, if not improve, the marriage or relationship. Many mothers freely admit that their pregnancy was a mistake, and the nurse should gently enquire if the mother has ever consulted a family planning clinic, Brook Advisory Centre, her own doctor, or has read any of the many helpful pamphlets available from health education departments. This type of question may permit the nurse to help the mother consider a more positive approach to family planning.

Many youngsters today have a sketchy background knowledge of the 'pill' or the 'sheath', even though most schools have sex education as part of their curriculum and some emphasis is given about available contraceptive techniques. Assuming this background of social awareness, many nurses are constantly surprised at the ignorance about family planning and the use of contraceptives. Ignorance on this topic, or an indifferent attitude, is most noted in those from social groups 4 and 5, and it is within this population group that the most work has to be done.

All techniques used in family planning follow either one of two principles: the technique either prevents the fertilisation of the ovum by the sperm or prevents the fertilised ovum from embedding into the wall of the uterus. The most common methods or techniques are:

Drugs	The contraceptive pill
Mechanical devices	Intrauterine contraceptive device (IUCD) or (IUD)
	Sheath (condom) and spermicides

	Diaphragm or cap method with spermicides
Surgical techniques	Sterilisation: tubal ligation (female)
	Vasectomy (male)
	Clinical abortion
Natural methods	Safe period
	Withdrawal method
	Abstinence

Drugs

The Contraceptive Pill

The contraceptive pill contains low doses of both oestrogen and progesterone which, while similar, are not exactly the same as their counterpart physiological hormones. These two hormones in combination prevent ovulation from taking place by:

Hindering the transport of the ova to the uterus from the ovary

Increasing mucus secretion in the cervix which traps the sperm

Impairing endometrial development after menstrual bleeding

Ovulation usually occurs 14 days before menstruation begins and will be inhibited if the pill is taken daily for 10 days before and 10 days after the calculated ovulation dates. This technique is often referred to as *21 days on/7 off* or *22 days on/6 off*.

When taking the pill for the first time, the female is advised to count the first day of her period as 1 and from day 5 to commence taking her prescribed pill. In the initial stages, it is best if the female keeps a diary, not only to remind herself to take the pill each day but to note down any untoward side effects. This information is very useful to the prescriber when considering any side effects of the drug and such information is especially useful during the first 2 months of using this contraceptive technique.

Side Effects

Expected side effects of the pill are well-documented from the research accumulated since the pill was first used in Peru in 1956. Since then, over 20 million women have been prescribed the pill and relatively few problems have arisen, considering the numbers involved. It is a point of great reassurance that many of the earlier side effects have been eliminated by careful readjustment of the oestrogen and progesterone doses carried in each pill.

Some women will suffer from nausea, headache, enlarged breasts, irregular vaginal bleeding, a single event amenorrhoea and weight increase. Fortunately, many of these side effects recede after 2 months, hence the need to keep a diary. If the problems remain persistent the woman should be strongly advised to seek advice from her doctor.

Contraindications

The following circumstances are contraindications for prescribing the pill:

Diabetes mellitus. Both the oestrogen and progesterone would further embarrass the existing disorder of carbohydrate metabolism.

Thrombophlebetic tendency. In the female population the risk of thrombosis, phlebitis and embolism is 9 times greater in those taking the pill as compared to females who do not. Those women who are to have surgery should discontinue the pill for at least 4 weeks before the operation is carried out to reduce the **risk** of deep-vein thrombosis. Those women with lower limb varicosities can take the pill providing their varicose veins are correctly treated. In sudden emergencies and admissions to hospitals, women of childbearing age should be routinely questioned if they take the contraceptive pill.

Jaundice or gallstones. A previous history of either jaundice or gallstones implies the liver may be incapacitated. Both oestrogen and progesterone are known to raise the level of circulating cholesterol. Since cholesterol is eventually metabolised in the liver, it may be unable to carry out this function if it has been previously damaged.

Breastfeeding. Following a pregnancy, a mother expressing the wish to breastfeed should be advised not to recommence taking the pill until her child has been weaned off the breast. Oestrogen and progesterone inhibit milk production.

Menopause. The pill may prolong menstrual bleeding at the menopause. This often confuses the woman who has reached the menopausal years and is wary of discontinuing the pill in case she falls pregnant. If unwilling to use any other form of contraceptive at this crucial time, she would require the expert advice of a gynaecologist as to the best time to stop taking the pill.

Cancer of breast or genitalia. Although sexual contact is not likely when such a diagnosis has been made, the pill must be discontinued. Not only will the hormones in the pill increase the likelihood of metastases, it will confuse the prescribed treatment for these types of cancer.

Following Instructions

Apart from the aforementioned circumstances, the pill is 100% effective **providing** the instructions are followed. The packaging and labelling of these pills are such as to guide practically anyone. It is always wise to check with those who have become pregnant by 'accident' if the patient can remember omitting a dose, has borrowed from a friend while waiting for a new prescription, or had a spell of vomiting in the past few months. The pregnancy may be due not to the pill but to a fault somewhere in the patient's handling of her prescription.

Mechanical Devices

Intrauterine Contraceptive Device

An IUCD is a flexible loop or coil of radiopaque plastic material. It is introduced and inserted into the uterus by a gynaecologist and left in place indefinitely. Once in place, the coil springs open and will prevent the fertilised ovum from becoming embedded into the endometrium or inner coat of the uterus. There is a wide variety of designs, the more popular being Lippes Loop, Saf-T-Coil, Dalkon's Shield and Copper 7.

Two threads extend from the coil down towards the vagina and can be readily identified on vaginal examination. These threads permit the coil to be removed when the female wishes to become pregnant.

The IUD's principal *disadvantage* is that it may cause a heavier and more prolonged menstrual period. It has a *limited use* in the following circumstances:

1. For several months following a Caesarean section
2. For 6 months following a successfully treated salpingitis
3. Congenital abnormality of the uterus
4. In those women with established dysmenorrhoea

Common Problems

The common problems associated with the coil are those of extrusion from the uterus down into the vagina. Very rarely, it may cause a perforation of the uterine walls and occasionally is the cause of a localised infection. These problems tend to arise if the coil is badly selected and inexpertly fitted. It is very useful for those women who are generally indifferent to all other forms of contraceptives and would prove unreliable if they were given a choice.

The technique, however, is 97% successful in preventing unwanted pregnancies.

Sheath (Condom) and Spermicides

The *sheath*, or condom, is composed of thin latex rubber and is commercially available in a wide variety of styles and sizes. When used correctly, the male should roll the sheath down and over the erect penis **before** penetrating the vagina. In love foreplay, the male may feel it is safe to penetrate the vagina unprotected, **but** sperm can be ejaculated without any sensation.

Although a very popular and reliable method, its efficacy is enhanced if the female also uses a spermicide. *Spermicides* are pharmaceutical substances commercially available as pessaries, foams, jellies or suppositories and contain a chemical harmful to sperm.

Spermicides should be inserted into the vagina 10 or 20 minutes before intercourse. On their own spermicides are **not** a contraceptive technique. When used correctly and if combined with spermicides, the sheath is almost a 100% contraceptive technique. An advantage is that the sheath does reduce the **risk** of contracting venereal disease via the genitalia.

Common Problems

Common problems related to the use of the sheath are:

1. The male fails to apply the sheath correctly or waits until it is too late.
2. The sheath is too large for the penile length, and sperm escape from a loose-fitting sheath or the sheath slips off while in the vagina.
3. Re-using the sheath when it is meant for single use. Only those which are washable can be safely re-used. Even then, any breach in the integrity of its structure, however minor, may allow 1 sperm from the 200 million ejaculated to reach the uterus and fertilise the ovum.
4. Some males find it interferes with sexual gratification and are reluctant to use this technique.
5. A few men are allergic to latex rubber.

Cap method (Diaphragm and Dutch Cap) and Spermicides

For many centuries females have used a wide variety of substances and articles to act as a barrier to the entry of sperm into the uterus. Sponges, cotton wool, linen patches and rancid butter are a few examples, but these have come to be replaced by the diaphragm or the cap. The cap or diaphragm is a thin cone shaped disc of latex rubber encircled by a rim of spring recoil metal. The diaphragm has to be a very precise fit, hence they vary in diameter from 50 mm to 100 mm and the initial fit should always be done by a gynaecologist or nurse trained in the technique.

The recoil rim is pressed together in an 8 shape and the cap advanced into the vagina covering the cervix at the back and wedging against the pubic bone in the front. It is then allowed to spring open into place. After this initial fitting, the female must be supervised while she inserts and removes it several times to ensure that she can correctly fit the device.

When it is used it must be smeared with a spermicidal cream, including especially around the edges, to prevent any sperm from escaping between the rim and the cervix wall into the uterus. It should be inserted 30 minutes before intercourse and left for a further 6 to 8 hours after intercourse before it is removed. If the cervix is unsuitable for a fitting, it is possible for a cap which fits directly over the cervix to be adapted to act as a barrier at a lower point in the vaginal vault.

This is a very reliable method (96%) providing the following rules are carefully followed:

1. The timing given above is absolutely crucial to prevent any sperm entering the uterus.
2. Spermicides **must** be used.
3. After insertion, the cervix must be felt to be covered by the diaphragm (similar to 'feeling the tip of the nose' covered by latex rubber).
4. The cap must be thoroughly cleansed after its removal, carefully inspected for tears or damage and stored in its provided container to keep it dry and clean.
5. If either partner is aware of the cap during intercourse, it is fitted incorrectly, and pregnancy is a real risk.

Surgical Techniques

Sterilisation: Tubal Ligation

Tubal ligation is a surgical procedure that involves tying off the uterine (Fallopian) tubes so that the sperm is prevented from reaching the ovum. *Hysterectomy* and *oophorectomy* are procedures which would also render the patient sterile, but such major surgery would only be considered if the uterus or ovary were diseased.

The patient should be counselled very

clearly, preferably with her husband, that the operation is **irreversible** and the joint written consent of both husband and wife is required before proceeding. It is a technique with a 100% contraceptive success. The use of a laparoscope introduced through a small abdominal incision allows the uterine tubes to be visualised and then cauterised. Although a general anaesthetic is used, it is a relatively minor procedure. There are associated but minor discomforts such as abdominal distension and localised pain around the incision site. In the majority of cases the hospital stay is not longer than 48 hours.

Tubal ligation is usually offered to women in the following circumstances:

1. An existing medical condition which would make pregnancy difficult, dangerous or fatal.
2. If the female conceived a child with a possible fatal hereditary disorder.
3. Difficult and multiple pregnancies.
4. An excessive number of children in a short period of time.
5. When no alternative contraceptive technique is acceptable to either partner.
6. In those females who are mentally handicapped, sexually precocious, and would not use an alternative contraceptive method with reliability.

Vasectomy

Vasectomy is the most reliable contraceptive method yet devised. It should not be confused with castration and has **no** effect on sexual urge or performance. An essential preliminary before this procedure is carried out is to obtain the joint consent of both husband and wife, ensuring that the husband is not being pressurised into the operation by his wife but has rather come to the decision by himself. It should be made quite clear to the patient that the operation is **irreversible**, despite the many claims of surgeons to the contrary. The patient should also be asked if he has projected his thoughts to the possible situation where he may remarry at a later time in his life and his new wife may wish to have his children.

The operation itself is a relatively minor procedure which is completed in 10 minutes by an expert, and can be done in an outpatients or private clinic during any working day. The patient does not usually require any sick leave or time off.

A local anaesthetic is used to dull any pain sensations of the scrotal sac, two small incisions are made into the scrotal sac and the vas deferens identified. These two tubes, which convey the sperm from the testes to the urethra are then tied off and cut, a small section of the tube being removed. One or two sutures are inserted to seal the incisions and the resulting wound heals in the next 48 hours. Very occasionally there may be problems of scrotal oedema, minor bleeding, or infection, but these are easily dealt with and leave no residual problems.

Following the procedure the patient should continue to regard himself as fertile until 2 specimens of semen show a negative sperm count, with a month's interval between each specimen. The reason for this is that stores of sperm are held by the epididymis for some time after the operation. It is necessary then for the patient to continue using another contraceptive technique until his specimens prove negative. This may take as long as 3 to 4 months until the sperm reservoir is exhausted.

Vasectomy is usually considered suitable for those males who have a:

1. Transmissible hereditary disease
2. If his wife must avoid pregnancy for medical reasons
3. If he voluntarily accepts full responsibility for birth control of his children

It should not be readily offered to healthy batchelors, for those who show the least hesitancy about the operation, if the marriage is unstable, and for those who are proven to be psychiatrically ill.

Clinical Abortion (see chapter 18)

Safe Period (Rhythm Method) (Mucothermic Method)

The safe period method refers to avoiding sexual intercourse during the fertile phase of the menstrual cycle. The period of fertility is calculated from the first day when bleeding stops.

From day 1 and on each succeeding day the female notes, by daily observation, when her vaginal discharge becomes thin and mucoid. Secondly, she should take her body temperature and record the results on a chart and note those days when her temperature is 0.5° to 1° C above her normal pattern. This temperature rise should occur 2 to 3 days after the vaginal discharge becomes thin and mucoid, and indicates the period of ovulation fertility has begun.

Intercourse should be **avoided** from the time when the vaginal discharge becomes thin and mucoid and then for a further 3 days after the body temperature rise occurs. This cyclical pattern of events is *most unreliable* since it varies from period to period. Equally, interpretation of the temperature recordings can often lead to mistakes. It carries a very **high risk** of pregnancy.

Withdrawal method (Coitus Interruptus) (Interrupted Intercourse)

The male partner withdraws the erect penis from the vagina immediately before ejaculation and sheds the sperm outside the female body. This is a **most unreliable** method as the male can ejaculate sperm in the early phase of coitus without any sensation, and secondly neither partner are sexually gratified which may lead to marital conflict.

FUTURE CONTRACEPTIVE METHODS

In conclusion of this brief look at family planning techniques, it is possible that in a few years time further techniques will be available. Undergoing clinical trials are the following suggestions:

Subcutaneous Injection of Depo Provera which prevents implantation for up to 3 months. The technique is suggested for those who live in remote communities and have limited access to clinics or medical facilities. It does, however, carry some serious and unpleasant *side effects* such as: severe dysmenorrhoea, nausea, headaches and depression. These side effects are unacceptable to most women and the technique has lost favour, even in its earlier trials.

The **morning after pill** has a high dose of progesterone, but as an alternative to ordinary contraceptive pills it is of doubtful value except to say it may be of some use in those victims of rape. The effect of the pill is to produce a 'mini abortion', and the most recent recommendation is that it is used in an emergency only.

The **once a month contraceptive pill** contains a high dose of prostaglandin and would be taken 'once a month'. Similar to the morning after pill, it produces a mini abortion. Because of the evocative word *abortion*, many women feel that the pill is being used for immoral purposes and that it would be unethical to take part in clinical trials.

MORALS AND ETHICS VS PROFESSIONALISM

The nurse who becomes involved in giving family planning advice or counselling may also have to consider the moral question of whether family planning is ethically acceptable in the first place. It is against the dogma of the Roman Catholic church and a staunch Catholic may take great offence at being offered family planning even if very ill from habitual abortion. While this has little to do with the nurse, it is important to realise that the nurse may be the one person to whom a teenage girl will turn for advice before seeking out medical help. Nurses, therefore, must have their attitudes and thoughts correctly asserted in their own mind before proceeding to advise others.

Part 3
Cardiovascular and Thoracic Nursing

Chapter 28
Blood Vessels

Each type of blood vessel is structured to perform a specific function. The arteries branch and divide to form arterioles, these terminate as capillaries, which in their regrouping form venules and these come together to form the veins (Fig. 28.1).

STRUCTURE

In structure the larger arteries possess 3 coats or layers:

An **outer layer** mainly composed of fibrous tissue (*tunica adventitia*).

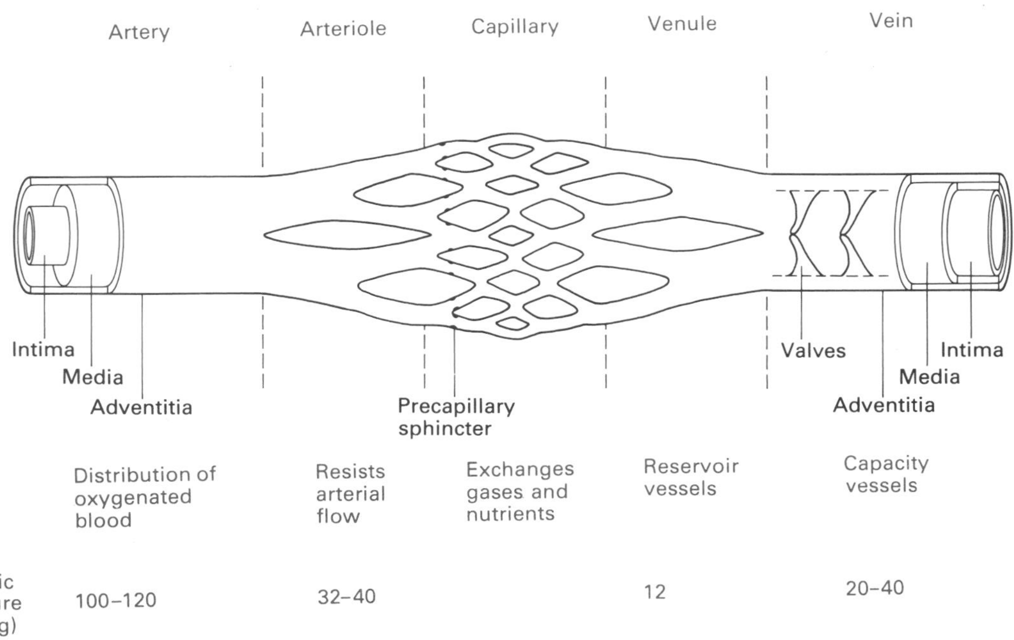

Fig. 28.1 Types of blood vessel.

A **middle layer** composed of smooth muscle arranged in circular fibres, within which are elastic tissue fibres enabling the vessel to recoil and relax in rhythm with the heart beat. Small arteries only have smooth muscle and these are innervated with specialised nerve cells which allow the vessels to dilate or constrict according to the body's needs (*tunica media*).

The **inner coat** is composed of endothelial tissue, the cells arranged within elastic tissue and providing a perfectly smooth surface over which the blood can travel without undue turbulence (*tunica intima*).

The principal function of arteries is the distribution of oxygenated blood by their ability to relax and recoil in sympathy with the heart beat. In many parts of the body there are arterial anastomoses which provide alternative routes for the blood supply to a given area or organ, e.g., the joints, muscles, intestine, and base of brain have such a system of alternative routes. Certain structures, however, possess 'end arteries' which imply that there is only one vessel or route by which oxygenated blood can reach its target organ or structure. Examples of end arteries include the coronary, retinal, cerebral, renal and appendicular arteries. If these single arteries become blocked or obstructed there is no alternative route and diseases such as appendicitis, renal thrombosis, cerebrovascular accident, retinal haemorrhage and coronary thrombosis can prove difficult, if not fatal, entities.

Arterioles

Arterioles are the end divisions of arteries. Their structure is similar to smaller arteries but they have no elastic tissue and the coats are much thinner. Their ability to constrict and dilate resembles a water-tap system regulating the flow of arterial blood to its target site. The control of blood flow is by autoregulation, depending on the oxygen and metabolic activity at any one time.

Subserving this autoregulation are locally released chemicals and neurotransmitters, e.g., histamine, bradykinin, adrenaline, noradrenaline and angiotensin. The ultimate control of arteriole diameter is via the vasomotor centre located in the medulla oblongata. This centre responds to stimuli received from specialised nerve tissue known as baroreceptors located in the carotid artery and in the right atrium.

This autonomic control of the arterioles depends on a wide variety of stimuli, e.g., temperature, emotion, blood pressure, and exercise. Being of a narrower diameter than the artery and coupled with autoregulation, the arteriole resists the flow of blood and contributes to maintenance of blood pressure. Resistance to arterial flow is increased in shock, haemorrhage, trauma, and surgery, when the arterioles are shut down to ensure a shift of arterial blood to those vital areas where it is needed most, e.g., the brain, heart and kidneys. Innervation of the arterioles is either via α or β receptors. The heart and muscle arterioles are innervated by β receptors (dilation) while the remaining arterioles are innervated by α receptors (constriction). Blocking drugs are commonly used to influence either α or β receptors in the control of hypertension.

Capillaries

Capillaries are single-layered endothelial cells with a diameter of about 7 μ and are arranged as a semipermeable membrane. Their main function is the exchange of oxygen and nutrients with carbon dioxide and waste materials at tissue level. The entry to each capillary is guarded by a precapillary sphincter. At the arteriole end of the capillary the pressure is about 32 mmHg; this decreases to 12 mmHg at the venule end of the capillary. Opposing this internal capillary pressure is the external tissue pressure created by water and proteins, i.e., osmosis and hydrostatic pressure. This counterbalance is essential if gases and nutrients are to cross the semipermeable membrane of the capillary. Permeability and the filtration ability of the capillaries varies throughout the body. It is extremely high in the kidneys, being four hundred times greater than that for muscles.

Apart from the mechanical exchange of materials due to the counterbalancing pressures, the capillary wall is also influenced by neurochemical transmitters, e.g., adrenaline, histamine, acetylcholine, and carbon dioxide. They all tend to dilate the capillary.

Venules and Veins

Venules have a similar structure to the larger veins, but since they have less smooth muscle they have a natural ability to pool blood and hold it in reserve. The larger veins with their thicker muscle coat can also expand to hold a great volume of blood. When the individual is at rest almost 85% of the total blood volume is within the veins. Only the veins of the internal jugular and lower limbs have cusps or biconcave valves arising from their inner endothelial lining. Spaced along the veins at regular intervals, the valves ensure the flow of venous blood upwards against gravity to ensure that the blood reaches the right atrium of the heart. In addition to the mechanical closing and opening of the valves, the physiological mechanisms of the muscle pump of the legs and inhalation of air acting as a suction pump also draws venous blood towards the heart.

In summary, the arteries *distribute* oxygenated blood due to their autoregulation, the arterioles *resist* arterial blood flow maintaining the blood pressure, the capillaries are *exchange* vessels, while the venules and veins tend to act as *reservoir* and *capacity* vessels.

Symptoms of a diseased blood vessel may remain localised to within a minor circulation such as the coronary circulation, cerebral circulation, pulmonary circulation or portal circulation but ultimately the effects are felt and experienced throughout the systemic circulation.

PRELIMINARY INVESTIGATIONS

Symptoms of peripheral vascular disease tend at first to be localised and many of the preliminary investigations are completed in the out-patients department of the hospital.

On physical examination careful note is made of the peripheral pulses, e.g., radial and dorsalis pedis. It is always worthwhile comparing the pulse of the right and left limbs to denote if there is a marked comparison in the pulse obtained. Colour and temperature of the skin should be noted at the peripheries. If the skin is slightly cyanosed it may imply there is an obliterative disease within the vessels supplying the limb. If there are distended blood vessels on the body surface these are usually veins as the arteries tend to be placed more deeply.

The blood pressure is always assessed but is only of value if the systolic and diastolic pressures are recorded when the patient is in the dorsal position, sitting position and standing position, especially if investigating postural hypotension. Readings will be inaccurate if the patient is excited or has just arrived at the department or ward after a long journey. Standard assessments of blood pressure require the nurse to chart the patient's measurements every 4 hours for at least 24 to 48 hours. A true assessment would be recorded if no drugs had been administered for at least 1 week prior to the investigation. Conversely the effect of antihypertensive drugs can be assessed only by noting the blood pressure at frequent intervals.

Radiological investigations such as arteriograms of the arteries, e.g., aortograms and angiography, where an opaque dye is injected into the vessel and then followed by rapid filming, may indicate if a specific artery is partially obstructed or is pursuing an abnormal course, if there is an aneurysm present or if the vessel has a filling defect. Venograms can be used to highlight specialised areas, e.g., the kidney (renogram), the liver (portal-hepatic venogram), or the spleen. Isotope tracers may be used to follow the course of blood through a particular vessel. Lymphangiograms may be combined with arteriograms or venograms if there is suspicion of a tumour blocking the flow of blood to a particular area.

Blood screening is invariably quite extensive, not only to exclude such obvious things as anaemia, infection and diabetes but to measure coagulation factors, e.g. the prothrombin time, and the level of lipids which often are the basis of obstructive arterial disease. Grouping and cross-matching of blood is also a routine measure if surgery is being contemplated. Cardiac function is invariably tested when there is arterial obliterative disease and the patient may have several electrocardiograms to ascertain if the heart is affected in any way before treatment is prescribed.

Social factors such as smoking, dietary habit, alcohol intake, type of employment and psychological profile are also assessed as many stresses and disorders of the vascular system are directly attributable to social behaviours and circumstances.

Chapter 29
Arterial Peripheral Vascular Disease

A few examples of obliterative arterial disorders include: Buerger's disease, Raynaud's disease, atheroma, arteriosclerosis and hypertension. The first 4 examples have several factors in common in that they all exhibit a decreased and disturbed blood supply to a local area and induce:

Local ischaemia and pain due to decreased tissue oxygenation

Inadequate cellular nutrition and therefore poor tissue regeneration and healing

Increased levels of carbon dioxide, urea, and uric acid within the ischaemic area

Disturbed electrolyte distribution within the affected area

BUERGER'S DISEASE

The definition of Buerger's disease is that of a segmental obliteration to the arterial blood flow of the lower limbs. It occurs more readily in males between the ages of 20 and 40 years of age and has an incidence of 1 in every 5000 of the adult male population. Those who suffer from the obliterative disease tend to be smokers, the nicotine in the cigarette being the most likely cause as it acts as a vasoconstrictor on the smaller arteries.

Signs and Symptoms

Initially the patient may complain of pain in the calf muscles and the arches of the foot when walking; this is also known as **intermittent claudication**. The pain recedes within 2 or 3 minutes of rest after the walk but in time the arterial constriction becomes progressively worse and the distance walked before the pain occurs gradually decreases. When a distance of between 300 and 400 yards is walked with the occurrence of pain, clinical investigation and treatment is required. The degree of pain becomes quite intense so that any contemplated walking or even standing for short periods of time becomes a major undertaking and the patient alters his or her working and lifestyle patterns accordingly.

On examination the area of ischaemia is cold to the touch and skin colour can be almost cyanotic, the distal part of the lower limb being most commonly affected, i.e., the toes and feet. A typical history will show that these patients prefer warm woollen socks, automatically put their feet up when resting and are intolerant of cold weather. These may be taken as early signs of obliterative arterial disease. Closer inspection of the skin may reveal a scaly appearance and there may be a clear demarcation line circling the limb identifying the area of ischaemia. More seriously, complications such as skin ulceration, cellulitis, pitting oedema and gangrene may be the first indication that the patient is suffering from an obliterative disease.

Arteriograms of the lower limbs show the poor filling defect of the peripheral arteries; this combined with the obvious symptoms leads to a quick diagnosis.

Patient Counselling

Conservative measures are usually strictly enforced to minimise the risk of further obliteration. If the patient smokes, this must stop **immediately** otherwise other active forms of treatment will prove useless. Vasodilator drugs will be used to improve the local blood supply and if there is gangrene it is usual to refer the patient to an orthopaedic surgeon for an elective amputation. In other cases it may be decided to do a sympathectomy operation.

Until decisions are made about the treatment plan the patient should be given specific advice particularly on the care of the feet. Direct heat should never be used to warm the extremities as this is more likely to cause a minor burn which will not heal very well.

Patients with ischaemic limbs also have reduced sensations of touch, heat and cold and may not be aware that they are actually burning themselves, hence the advice never to apply a hot water bottle directly to an ischaemic limb. Warm wool socks or stockings worn with a well-fitted low-heeled shoe are essential and constrictive garments such as garters should never be worn around the lower limb. Care of the toenails is best performed by a chiropodist and attention to bunions, calluses and ingrowing toenails must be dealt with only by a highly trained expert.

The patient should be encouraged to elevate the limbs at night on several pillows so that the limbs are higher than the waistline. Many patients find it beneficial to take an alcoholic beverage before retiring to bed since the alcohol acts as a vasodilator relieving the symptoms of pain. Patients should be advised to exclude animal fats from their diet as the lipids will only tend to increase the gradual obliteration of the arteries. In all cases of obliterative arterial disease, diabetes mellitus must be excluded by rigorous testing of both the urine for glycosuria and the blood for its glucose level.

RAYNAUD'S DISEASE

More commonly found in the younger female population, Raynaud's disease is characterised by extreme pallor or cyanosis of the fingers or toes when exposed to cold temperatures. Usually the digits of the hands are more commonly affected than the feet and the disease is usually bilateral. Even in warm climates the fingers appear and feel cold. In the winter months the skin of the fingers is prone to chilblains and superficial ulceration and protective gloves have to be worn. If there is ulceration it will heal slowly.

Although the cause is unknown the mechanism is believed to be due to the dominance of the sympathetic system which keeps the local blood vessels of the hands in vasoconstriction. Vasodilator drugs such as tolazoline (Priscol) and nicotinyl tartrate

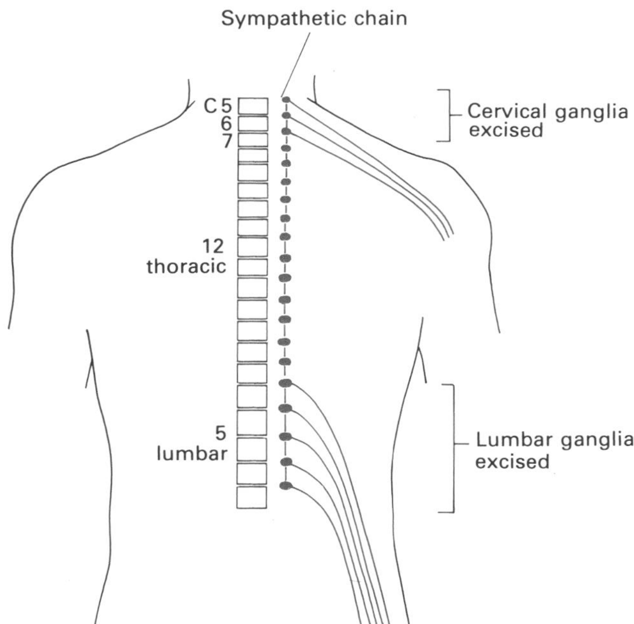

Fig. 29.1 Sites of sympathectomy.

(Ronicol) are usually prescribed and the operation of sympathectomy may be offered in the more serious cases of Raynaud's disease.

Sympathectomy

The intention of a sympathectomy operation is to cut and excise the nerve ganglion along the sympathetic chain running alongside the spinal cord (Fig. 29.1). The nerves travelling from these ganglions are sympathetic in action, i.e., they cause vasoconstriction. Removing the sympathetic ganglion either at the cervical or lumbar regions will allow the parasympathetic system to become dominant permitting vasodilation of the affected arteries. The site of incision is indicated by the surgeon, usually being a *cervical* sympathectomy for Raynaud's disease and a *lumbar* sympathectomy for Buerger's disease.

In the case of cervical sympathectomy it is usually done only if the preoperative vasodilation test is positive. In this the patient has direct heat applied to the hands and the arteries should partially dilate, then following local or regional anaesthesia the hand arteries should once again dilate. If both criteria are met the operation may be recommended.

Preoperative Care

Specific preoperative care for sympathectomy includes the following points:

The patient must **not** smoke at all. Apart from the obvious reasons such as the respiratory disadvantages in arterial disease the nurse may have to give more detailed reasons. It should be explained to the more receptive patient that nicotine in a cigarette causes the smaller arteries to remain constricted since it is a drug which stimulates the sympathetic nervous system. It also increases the fatty acids in the blood in addition to making the blood platelets more sticky, i.e., increased platelet viscosity. All these factors risk the success of the operation.

The affected limb although not operated upon requires to be kept warm, clean and dry. It should be free of any risk of trauma from pressure. It may prove useful to install a bedcradle to prevent any heavy pressure on the toes. If it is the hands that are affected, they should be protected by warm woollen mittens or gloves. Although the bed should be warm, hot water bottles should never be used in an attempt to warm a specific part of a limb. Constrictive clothing, e.g., elasticated sleeved garments, should **not** be worn.

Cervical Sympathectomy

If a cervical sympathectomy is to be performed, the patient may have an underwater seal pleural drainage system since the incision is through the posterior thorax. Counselling and postoperative care will be specifically related to the type of sympathectomy performed.

Postoperative Care

For a cervical sympathectomy patient, the nurse should expect to plan and provide care for a patient with an underwater seal pleural drainage that will be in place for at least 24 hours. To determine whether the surgery has been successful, repeated observations of the radial pulses and the skin temperature of either hand are taken. The complications to be expected are mainly those resulting from a thoracic incision, e.g., pneumothorax or internal haemorrhage from a ruptured intercostal artery.

Lumbar Sympathectomy

A lumbar sympathectomy will involve an incision into the lumbar region. This may lead to many complications because of the effect this may have on the neighbouring nerve fibres. Vigilant nursing observation will be required to determine when surgical opinion and intervention is necessary. The potentially more complex complications which may occur after a lumbar sympathectomy are:

Urinary retention, more probably the result of a disturbed parasympathetic nerve pathway. If the patient has not passed urine in the 8–12 hours after the operation, the surgeon should be informed and permission sought to pass a urinary catheter.

Paralytic ileus may occur due to a disturbed parasympathetic nerve pathway. Until bowel sounds spontaneously return, it may be necessary to aspirate the stomach every hour or to leave the nasogastric tube on free drainage.

Ureteric haemorrhage is a possibility. Because of its proximity to the site of the incision, observations for the signs of shock and low blood pressure should be continued for at least 24 hours.

Femoral nerve damage, intense pain of the hip and the anterior thigh of the affected leg, requires frequent administration of analgesia and bedrest for at least 48 hours.

Postoperative Care

If at all possible the patient should be allowed out of bed the day following surgery for a short period of time. The dressing is left intact for 48 hours and any drains can then be removed. Sutures are usually removed between the fifth and seventh postoperative day.

Patient Counselling

Postoperative advice prior to convalescence is the same as that given in the preoperative phase of conservative care. Patients should continue to care for the limb in the same manner until they are reviewed in the outpatients department on their first appointment. The affected limb should begin to feel warmer, joint movements become easier, skin colour and temperature should also improve but the results are not immediate.

Exercise tolerance for patients with Buerger's disease should be graduated so that they can walk increasingly longer distances without any pain, but when at rest they should keep the legs elevated.

ATHEROMA

The term *atheroma* defines the deposit of fatty plaques within the endothelial cells of the arterial intima. The fats implicated tend to be lipids and are mostly derived from dairy produce. They enter the vessel wall as cholesterol or its esters. Localised focal swelling occurs from the reaction between fat and endothelial tissue, and this results in a fibrosis of the vessel wall. Fibrosis roughens what was once a smooth surface, and the blood travelling over any patch of roughened tissue will be subjected to more turbulence than previously experienced. There are 4 main predisposing factors to atheromatous changes of the intima of the arterial wall:

1. **Arteriosclerosis**, or hardening of the arterial walls, is due to natural ageing. With the loss of elasticity the arteries harden making it easier for the lipids to attach to the intima.

2. With **smoking**, the nicotine induces persistent vasoconstriction of the smaller arteries and makes it easier for the lipids to invade the arterial intima. Smoking also increases the levels of fatty acids in the blood.

3. A **high cholesterol dietary intake**, excessive amounts of **white sugar** or too many **carbohydrates**, all tend to raise the blood fatty acid levels, thus increasing the risk of atheroma. In surveys carried out over the last decade, the younger population were more prone to atheroma because of current dietary trends and habits.

4. An increased **cardiopulmonary peripheral resistance**, i.e., pulmonary hypertension coupled with a high lipid intake, doubles the risk of atheroma. Hyperlipidaemia can be proven by measuring the blood lipid level. It is possible for individuals of normal weight to have hyperlipidaemia, therefore its association with obesity is not always the case.

The risk of thrombi developing is high if the endothelium has ulcerated as the result of lipid deposit. If calcium is also deposited during fibrosis this risk is even greater. Large plaques tend to reduce the blood circulation to neighbouring tissues and organs creating an obliterative arterial disease. The vessels most prone to artheromatous changes include the:

External iliac arteries branching from the aorta, especially at the point where they immediately branch off

Coronary arteries, in particular the left coronary artery

Cerebral arteries, notably the middle cerebral artery which supplies the motor-sensory area of the cerebral cortex.

Effects

The physiological effects consequent to developing atheroma follow a classical pattern. Narrowing of the arterial lumen reduces the blood flow and elastic recoil of the smooth muscle is lost. The effect of these two changes is to reduce the blood supply to the affected area when ischaemia occurs due to the lack of oxygen. Complicating the ischaemia can be ulceration of the arterial intima where the plaque is deposited, an obliterative thrombus or an embolus detaching itself from the thrombus, which if impacting into a smaller artery can lead to an infarction. Infarctions can be compensated for by collateral circulations or end artery anastomosis, but this takes some time, usually after the ischaemic area has undergone replacement fibrosis. Clinical examples of these conditions are myocardial infarction, cerebrovascular accident and intermittent claudication of the lower limbs.

Health Education

Health education in the prevention of atheroma especially for the younger age group emphasises the need to stop smoking, to eat foods with the minimum of saturated or animal fats and to exercise regularly. These are positive steps in preventing a clinical atheroma.

HYPERTENSION

Hypertension is said to exist when the diastolic pressure is persistently raised above 90 mmHg. Although the systolic pressure is also raised, the importance about the diastolic pressure is that it records the pressure when the heart is at rest. If the resting pressure is high then the heart is being overtaxed and the left ventricle may go into failure. Hypertension affects about 10% of the adult population in the UK of which the greater number belong to the Negroid races. The high diastolic pressure is the result of increased resistance to the flow of arterial blood through the arterioles. Such a persistent vasoconstriction of these vessels arises from a variety of causes.

Causes

Specific

Disorders of any of the factors which contribute to maintaining the normal blood pressure may result in increased resistance to flow. These are:

A decrease in circulating volume of blood, on average 5 litres in the adult.

An increase in viscosity or stickiness of the blood due to the plasma protein, albumin.

A decrease in elastic recoil of the arterial wall; such elasticity is lost as age advances.

A decrease in cardiac output of the left ventricle which is approximately 70 ml of blood on each contraction of the heart.

General

Everyday changes and conditions can influence the normal blood pressure:

Age. As one grows older the elasticity of the arterial walls is lost and the vessels become harder, i.e., arteriosclerosis.

Gender. Males are more prone to hypertension than are females, and this may be related to the difference in hormonal levels of oestrogen and progesterone.

Emotional stress of a persistent nature raises the adrenaline level to unacceptably high levels and keeps the arterioles in vasoconstriction. In normal health transient rises and falls of blood pressure are a common experience due to emotional changes.

Postural changes of the body which mean a shift of blood, i.e. on rising from a seated position, the blood pressure must rise because the cardiac output increases and the arterioles constrict. If it fails to rise the individual tends to faint. This is what may happen after a prolonged period of bedrest.

Body weight at the normal range for a given height does imply a normal average blood pressure. With obesity, several factors raise the blood pressure: a possible high serum cholesterol threatens an early atheroma, and an increased blood viscosity is not compensated for by an improved heart beat. In fact it will be the reverse as the heart has extra work to do to keep the excess weight oxygenated.

Climatic conditions influence the blood pressure. In warm climates the vessels are dilated tending to keep the blood pressure low; while in cold climates the arterioles remain constricted pushing the blood pressure up to keep the vital organs well oxygenated.

Social habits are of major importance as they more than most factors influence the actual health of the blood vessels. Smoking causes persistent vasoconstriction of the arterioles. Although alcohol does dilate blood vessels, alcohol abuse can cause early arteriosclerotic changes. Dietary custom wherein the individual has a large intake of saturated fats, white sugar and salt, all proven harmful to the arterial intima, can cause either atheroma or early arteriosclerotic changes. The individual's occupation if it means irregular hours, constant wining and dining, and high anxiety levels will also bring on early arteriosclerotic changes due to persistent high levels of adrenaline.

Other

Excess secretion of the hormones adrenaline and noradrenaline, and the enzymes renin and angiotension from diseased endocrine glands or disorders of the kidney will influence the blood pressure.

CLINICAL HYPERTENSION

Clinical hypertension is classified as being primary, secondary or malignant.

Primary

Primary, essential or idiopathic hypertension means that the cause is unknown. It is the more common type of hypertension, often being asymptomatic and discovered only on routine medical examination. It tends to affect males more than females and can often be traced as being familial. The underlying mechanism seems to be related to increased secretion of renal renin. This combined with angiotensin increases the release of aldosterone. The effect of this hormone-enzyme interaction is to cause persistent vasoconstriction of the arterioles. It is for this reason that the kidneys are extensively investigated in all cases of clinical hypertension.

Secondary

Secondary hypertension as the term implies is due to or consequent upon a primary disease. If patients are admitted to hospital with diabetes, renal disease, pituitary or adrenal tumours, coarctation of the aorta, atheroma, or toxaemia of pregnancy, the nurse should routinely screen their blood pressure at 4-hourly intervals unless otherwise instructed.

Malignant

Malignant hypertension refers to a persistent diastolic pressure exceeding 130 mmHg and usually accompanied by renal failure and papilloedema. Such a hypertension is a medical emergency requiring immediate hospital admission, and investigation and treatment.

Signs and Symptoms

The possible early manifestations of hypertension which would cause sufficient stress to cause a patient to seek medical help may include:

Headaches of a generalised nature which are persistent and often associated with dizzy spells and nausea

Memory impairment for simple routine things and irritability of manner

Although physically tired the individual finds it **impossible to rest**, being always on the go and suffering from insomnia and restlessness

Later effects include **dyspnoea**, **angina pectoris** and **odd chest pain** as the heart tries to compensate

Visual changes such as 'haloes' and fundal exudates impair vision. It is possible that the patient may first come to consultation with a retinal artery haemorrhage.

The vessels at greatest risk from hypertension include the coronary, cerebral and retinal arteries since their organs all suffer from ischaemia. It is possible the patient may be admitted to hospital with a heart attack, a cerebrovascular accident, or retinal haemorrhage.

Investigations

Investigations to determine the degree and cause of hypertension are often extensive requiring the patient to be hospitalised for several days. Initially a careful social history is taken to denote if there is a familial tendency and to highlight any behaviours which may be contributing to the hypertension, e.g., smoking, diet, alcohol and occupation. A complete physical examination with especial concentration on the pulses, blood pressure and cardiac efficiency is followed by more exacting tests. These may include:

A **chest X-ray** to outline the size and shape of the heart and aorta. If indicated cardiac arteriography may be requested.

Electrocardiograms are studied to note if there are marked changes to the PQRST wave patterns.

Blood pressure readings are usually taken every 4 hours. The doctor may request that the readings are taken with the patient in the dorsal, sitting and standing positions on each occasion, in which case the results should be noted in different colours on the blood pressure chart for easy comparison.

Apex beat and **radial pulses** may be requested every 4 hours to detect the difference between heart rate and pulse rate.

Detailed **ophthalmology examination** may be requested. The examination of the fundus may be used to assess the degree of hypertension by noting for the presence of exudates and the health of the retinal arteries.

Renal investigations may include 24-hour urinary collections to assay for catecholamines, i.e., waste products of adrenaline and noradrenaline. Assay for other hormones may also be done in further 24-hour urine collections. Estimations of the protein excreted may be measured either by 24-hour urinary collections or by the daily Esbach's test. Routine urinalysis for sugar, protein, albumen, and blood are made each day on the ward and the results accurately charted. An intravenous pyelogram or renal arteriography is quite usual in cases of hypertension to determine if the structure and arterial flow to the kidney are normal.

Haematology screening is very extensive. The basic tests for haemoglobin, urea levels, leucocyte and erythrocyte counts, and the electrolyte levels, especially for sodium, may be made every 48 hours and then again for comparison once treatment has been prescribed.

Nursing Care

The principles of treatment are also the basis for creating a nursing care plan. Several principles which are well-established can be employed by the nurse for giving care.

The degree of restricted activity or otherwise **must** be determined. If the diastolic pressure remains over 90 mmHg the patient should be on bedrest, being assisted with the basic activities of daily living. Ambulation is considered when the pressure remains below 90 mmHg for 48 hours.

Psychological reactions to stress, insomnia, restlessness and irritability will in the first instance usually require sedative or tranquillising drugs but their use is in the short-term only. Therefore, counselling sessions are planned for, as an altered lifestyle is an essential component of treatment.

Patient Counselling

Counselling sessions regarding behaviours which contribute to hypertension must be part of the treatment plan. It is important that the patients understand the need to review the habits of a lifetime such as their customary diet, their occupation and their level of drinking or smoking. It is not only the change of a lifestyle but a change of attitude that may prove the stumbling block. The nurse, however, can begin by keeping in mind a brief list of what the patient should be trying to achieve:

Restricting sodium from the cooking and at table

Eliminating cholesterol and saturated fats from the daily diet

Reducing the intake of white sugar

Abandoning the smoking habit

Exercising regularly which will reduce the serum cholesterol levels

When counselling a nurse should remember that the uniform can add to the role of educator. Emphasis should be placed on the positive benefit to be gained if the patient follows a prudent and sensible lifestyle. While encouraging the patient to read pamphlets, the nurse should follow up with further discussions and clarify any misunderstanding the patient may have.

Drug Regimens

Antihypertensive agents which are available act mainly by reducing the peripheral arteriole resistance by blocking the sympathetic innervation of either the α or β receptors located in the arteriole wall, i.e., they are blocking agents (Fig. 29.2). The more common of these drugs are:

Methyldopa (Aldomet) displaces and reduces the effect of noradrenaline, a hormone which vasoconstricts the arterioles.

Propranolol hydrochloride (Inderal) re-

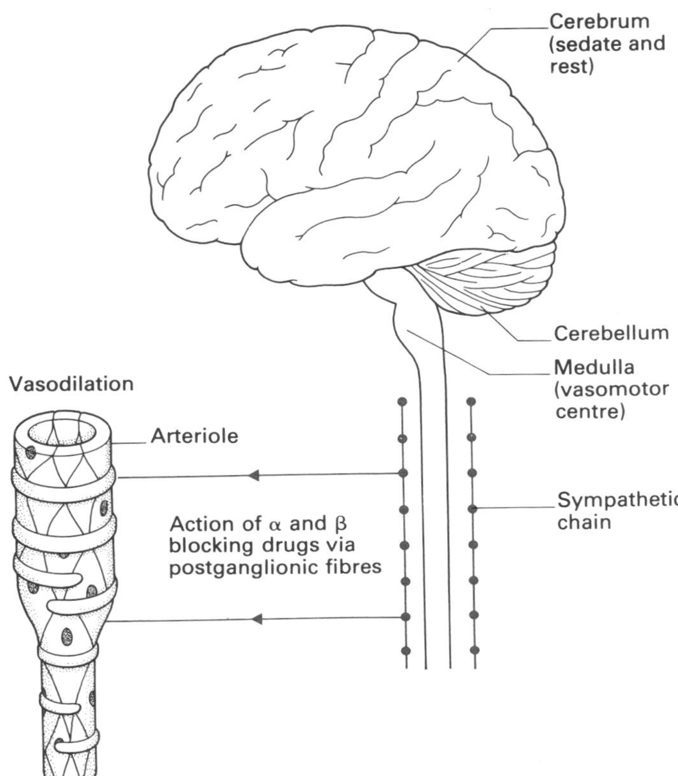

Fig. 29.2 Action of α and β blocking drugs.

duces the cardiac output particularly of the left ventricle by acting on the β adrenergic receptors.

Spironolactone (Aldactone A) inhibits the production of the hormone aldosterone and aids increased excretion of sodium in the urine without affecting the levels of potassium in the body.

Guanethidine monosulphate (Ismelin) blocks the release of noradrenaline from the nerve fibre terminals allowing the arterioles to relax thereby reducing peripheral resistance.

Combined with these drugs, the doctor may also prescribe a diuretic such as frusemide (Lasix) to reduce the total blood volume by ridding the body of excess fluid.

ANEURYSMS

A localised dilation or bulging of an arterial vessel wall is referred to as an *aneurysm*. This tends to occur at the weakest point in the structure of arteries, and such a point is wherever a main artery bifurcates or divides into two sub-branches, the actual point of branching being the weakest point. It should also be noted that in this area the arterial intima is most likely to be invaded by lipids. There are 4 main types of aneurysm (Fig. 29.3) which aim to define their size:

Mycotic, i.e., the dilation is very small and may be asymptomatic

Saccular aneurysm is a localised but large dilation which is located to one side of a main artery

Fusiform refers to the shape which is a spindle-like dilation involving the circular wall of the vessel

Dissecting aneurysm implies that the intima and medial coats are torn apart by blood escaping from the arterial lumen through a structural defect. This type of aneurysm is large, tends to pulsate and is at

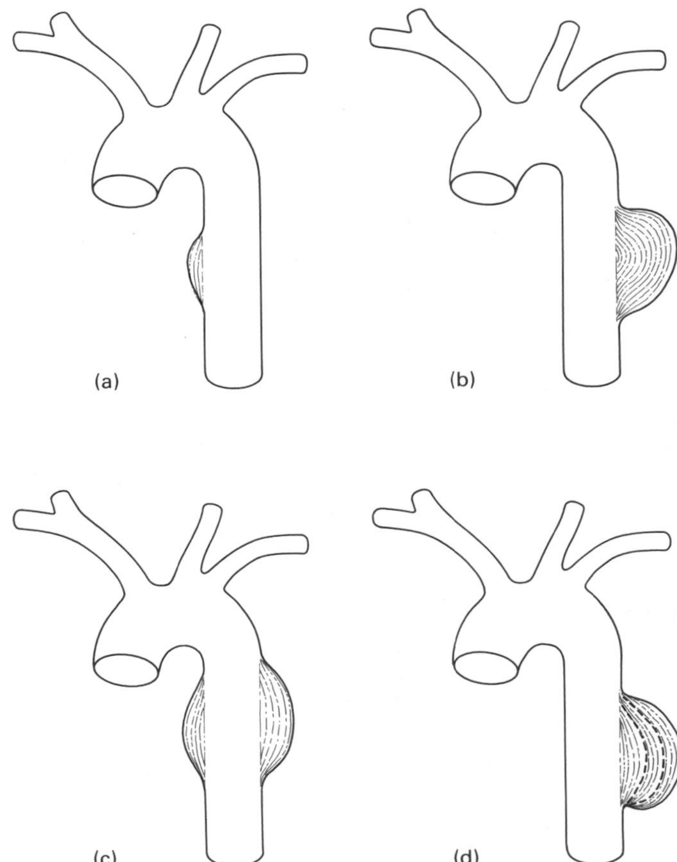

Fig. 29.3 Types of aneurysm: mycotic (a); saccular (b); fusiform (c); dissecting (d).

risk of rupture at any time, representing a true surgical emergency.

Within the arterial system aneurysms tend to occur readily at specific sites (Fig. 29.4). These dilations if present are found at the:

Cerebral anterior arteries at their junction with the circle of Willis

Internal carotid artery at its junction from the arch of the aorta

Arch of the aorta

Abdominal aorta below the level of the renal arteries

Point where the common iliac artery bifurcates

Iliac-femoral junction, **or** at the

Femoral-popliteal junction immediately behind the knee

The cause of aneurysms when a clinical diagnosis has been made is usually due to arteriosclerotic changes occurring over many years, to atheromatous changes in the arterial intima, to a traumatic injury or to a previous infection of the blood vessels. Aneurysms may develop as a secondary feature to hypertension, untreated thyrotoxicosis, and more rarely today late stage syphillis. Asymptomatic aneurysms tend to exist where there is a congenital weakness of the arterial wall without any clinical manifestations. The individual may reach 40 or 50 years of age before the first signs appear.

Symptoms

Symptomology of aneurysms depends on the site affected. For many years the arterial bulging can exist without causing any discomfort. Once it becomes large enough to cause pressure on neighbouring structures and nerves, the oddity of the symptoms will

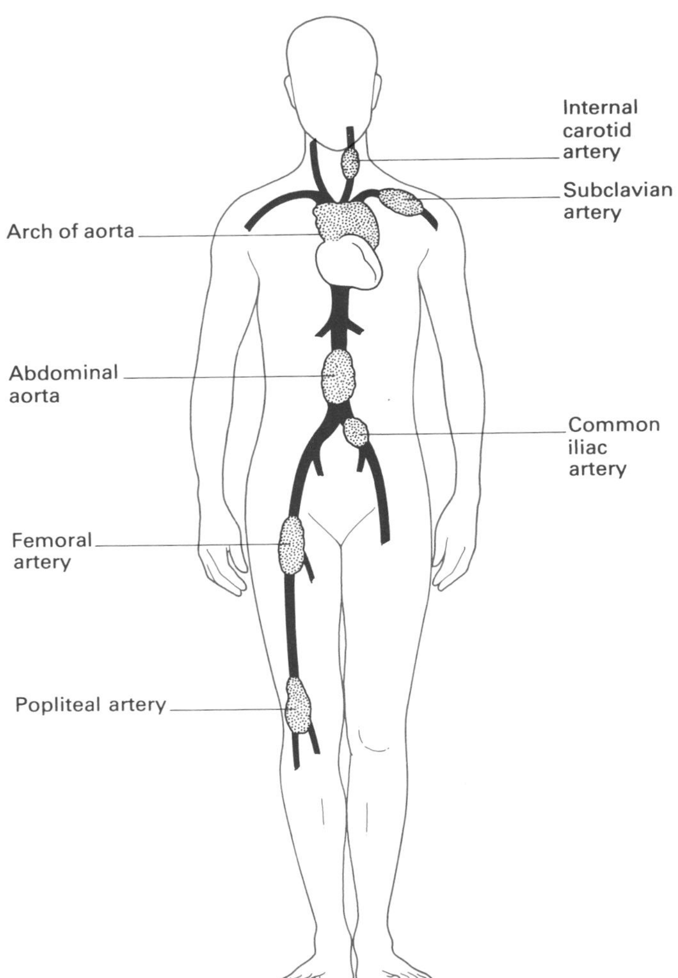

Fig. 29.4 Common sites of aneurysm.

be sufficient to encourage the patient to seek medical advice. Aneurysms of the anterior cerebral vessels and the internal carotid artery cause a vast array of neurological signs as the result of pressure on the cranial nerves. A focal headache very similar in its features to a classical migraine may be the earliest sign. Pressure on one or several cranial nerves gives rise to ophthalmic and facial nerve disturbances, e.g., third nerve palsy. If the anterior cerebral artery ruptures the individual may be admitted suffering from a subarachnoid haemorrhage. This may happen if the individual has taken even a mild blow to the skull resulting in a congenital aneurysm of the anterior cerebral vessels spontaneously rupturing. The outlook for a patient with this type of aneurysm is rather bleak.

Aneurysms of the arch of the aorta may first present as a congestive cardiac failure with accompanying dilation of the superficial veins of the neck, face, arms, and thorax. When compared, the left and radial pulses show a marked difference due to the low pressure in the left subclavian artery. Pain can resemble that of myocardial infarction and electrocardiograph readings may look similar, in addition the serum enzymes of glutamic oxalate and pyruvate transaminases can also give a high reading. Hypertension if present is

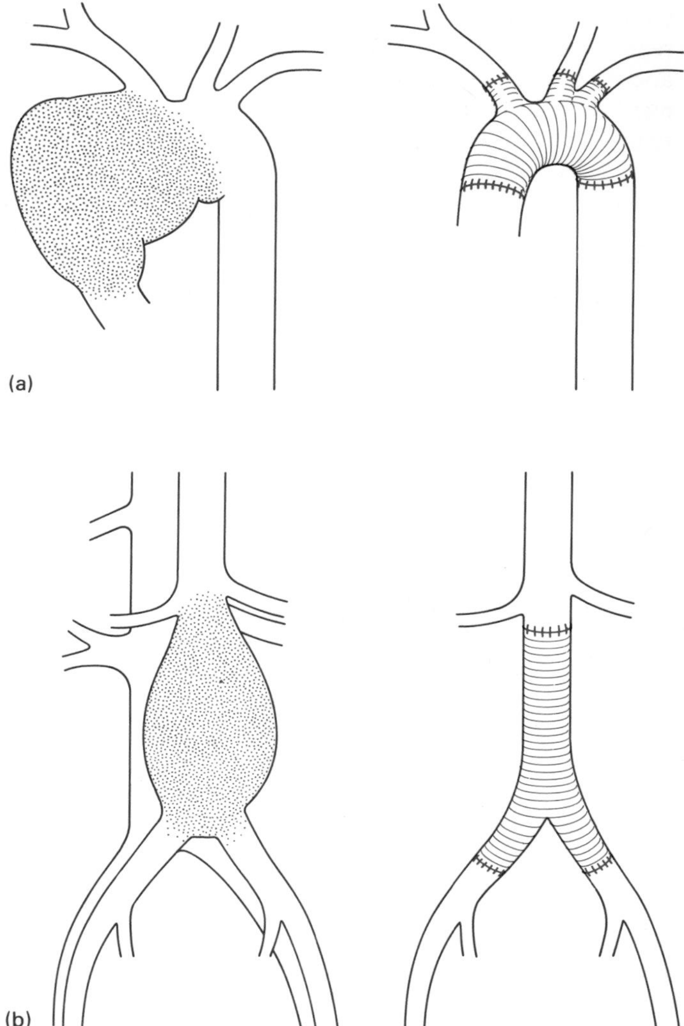

Fig. 29.5 Aneurysmectomy: an aortic aneurysm (a) and an abdominal aortic arm (b) before surgery (left, stippled) and after a replacement graft (right, hatched).

more than likely due to any arteriosclerotic changes. Aortic arch bulging however would be obvious on a routine chest X-ray and would prove the difference between aneurysm and myocardial infarction.

Abdominal aneurysms invariably develop below the level of the renal artery and can extend downwards to involve the arterial wall until it reaches the common iliac artery. Initially the pressure symptoms cause referred abdominal pain, but on palpation the doctor may be able to detect a pulsating abdominal mass. Pain is an unfavourable sign as it implies the aneurysm is about to rupture or *dissect*. If ruptured, the aneurysm will cause intense abdominal pain, circulatory collapse and deep shock, and arterial bleeding of such intensity that the patient has a poor prognosis without emergency surgery.

Femoral and popliteal aneurysms cause localised symptoms of an obliterative nature as the arterial blood flow is impeded and venous return may prove inadequate. In all types of aneurysm the diagnosis is made and confirmed by fluoroscopy and arteriography.

Treatment

The treatment of aneurysms is mainly with by-pass or replacement arterial surgery. A variety of operations have been designed to remove atheromatous plaques or replace aneuryitic arteries by grafting with replacement flexible, impervious, nonallergic materials such as synthetics.

Endarterectomy is an incision into an artery for the removal of an artheromatous plaque with the possibility of using grafting material to replace part of an artery.

Aneurysmectomy (Fig. 29.5) refers to the replacement of the aneuryitic part of either the arch of the aorta or abdominal aorta by synthetic material.

Femoral or **popliteal by-pass surgery** refers to the anastomosis of the principal artery to a collateral artery to by-pass the aneurysm.

Craniotomy may be done to ligature an aneuryitic vessel within the skull if it has been diagnosed at an early stage.

Chapter 30
The Variscosities

As a group of disorders, the variscosities refer to dilation of the veins beyond their normal capacity and to such an extent that the vessel cannot empty completely of venous blood. They are partially obliterative and the veins most commonly affected tend to be:

The veins of the lower limbs, i.e., varicose veins

The anal canal, i.e., the haemorrhoidal veins

Within the testes, i.e., varicocele minor

At the oesophageal-gastric junction, i.e., oesophageal varices

VARICOSE VEINS

The exact reason why the submucosal layer of the veins of the lower limbs remains dilated is unknown, and the condition is referred to as being idiopathic. The veins most commonly affected are shown in Fig. 30.1. Primary factors which contribute to the occurrence of varicose veins are well-established. Statistically, the evidence is that 10% or 20% of the Western hemisphere's population is suffering from varicose veins.

Pregnancy and obesity, which increase the intra-abdominal pressure, reduce the venous return from the lower limbs causing a marked venous dilation. Those occupations where the individual has to stand still for long periods also reduce effective venous return, e.g., theatre nurses, hairdressers, soldiers on sentry duty. Coupled with standing still for long periods there is an added problem if the individual works in a warm temperature as a

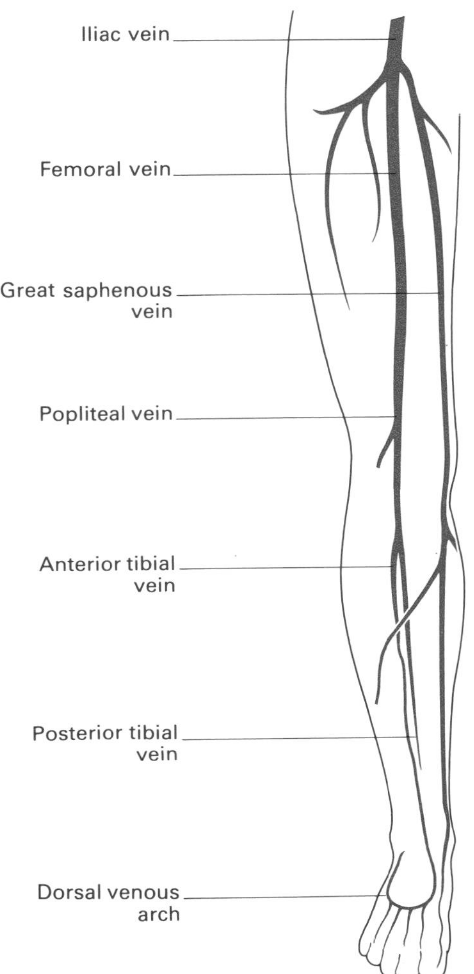

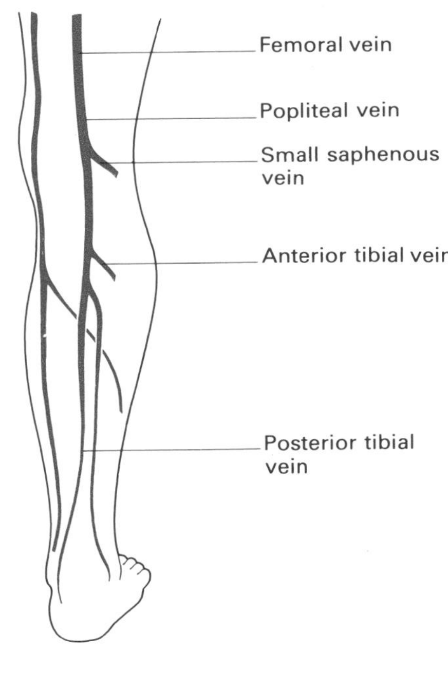

Fig. 30.1 Veins of the lower limb: anterior view (*left*) and posterior view (*right*).

warm climate in itself will dilate the superficial veins.

Women are affected five times more often than males are, the left leg tends to be more varicosed than the right lower limb, and branches and tributaries of the greater saphenous vein are more prone to dilation than the branches of the short saphenous vein. There does seem to be strong statistical evidence for a familial incidence.

Dilation of the submucosal layer of the veins results in defects of the valves. If unable to close effectively the venous pump becomes inadequate and superficial veins remain filled with blood. These superficial veins enlarge becoming visible at the back of the leg and extending from the calf to the thigh in serious cases.

In appearance they are tortuous but they are painless and easily compressed. A typical history shows that patients are more concerned by their disfigurement. If there is an ache or localised pain it is more pronounced in women in the immediate premenstrual period. As the condition worsens the ache becomes more problematical and there may be mild ankle oedema. Advanced varicose veins may cause a localised ankle eczema, skin ulceration, pigmentation, phlebitis, i.e., an infection, or rupture with severe venous haemorrhage.

Diagnosis

Initially the diagnosis is by the appearance of visible, tortuous disfiguring superficial veins. The degree of varicosity can be assessed by the Trendelenburg's test. In this the patient is asked to lie down and the affected leg is raised. The venous flow is then occluded by thumb compression at the groin. When the patient stands, the venous flow is seen to travel from the groin downwards to the foot proving that the valves of the long saphenous vein are **ineffective**, i.e., incompetent sapheno-femoral valves and communicating veins. Venography and phlebography using Conray (280) 60% contrast medium can demonstrate if there is a filling defect in the veins of the lower limb.

Treatment

The treatment of varicose veins may follow 1 of 3 alternatives:

Conservative advice which must be followed for the individual's lifetime

Sclerotherapy to obliterate the varicosed veins

Surgery to strip or ligate the affected veins.

Conservative Advice

It is important to stress that the advice given must be followed for the patient's lifetime and there are 4 basic rules to follow to control the veins from becoming worse.

1. The majority of experts recommend **daily exercise**. The patient should walk a minimum of 3 km each day to encourage the calf muscles to act as an effective pump. This exercise should be done wearing sensible low-heeled shoes.

2. The lower limbs should be **elevated** higher than the waist for at least 20 minutes each day to empty the long saphenous vein automatically.

3. The patient must achieve the correct **weight** for his or her height. These can be learned from standard charts held in the outpatients department. Many surgeons will not consider any form of treatment until the correct weight has been achieved.

4. **Elasticated hosiery** should be worn during the day. These stockings are available in a wide variety of styles from which the patient can choose a preferred fashion. They act by compressing the superficial veins keeping them empty of venous blood and so aid venous return. They are necessary in those patients who may be obese, pregnant or elderly. The stocking should fit from the toes to the groin; half-length stockings are preferred by many but in the long-term are inefficient. Several pairs are required as they need daily changing and frequent washing. It should be pointed out that the elastic becomes inefficient with washing, and frequent replacements are necessary.

If the patient tends to suffer from eczema, oedema or pigmentation these should resolve as a consequence of wearing the elasticated hosiery. **Venous ulcers,** however, are a more protracted problem. The ulcer is caused by ischaemia; therefore, the only remedy is to restore arterial circulation and ensure good venous return. The ulcer itself should be kept as clean as possible, dressed with nonadherent sterile material over which a full-leg-length bandage (Tubigrip) is applied and over this is worn elasticated hosiery.

The patient must be persuaded to abandon all commercial creams, lotions, ointments and pastes. Antibiotics are only of value if the venous ulcer has become infected, otherwise the nurse and patient should persist with a daily clean dressing and effective compression bandaging. Some ulcers are notoriously difficult to heal and repeated and constant explanation of the underlying principle of good circulation is required to overcome the patient's anxieties about the delay in healing.

Sclerotherapy

The principle underlying schlerotherapy is that by injecting a sclerosing agent directly into the dilated vein the agent will cause an inflammation and coagulation thus inducing a permanent obliteration of the varicosed vein. Collateral veins are then used by the body to drain the limb of venous blood. Examples of sclerosing agents in common use are:

Ethanolamine oleate
Hypertonic saline
Sodium tetradecyl sulphate in alcohol solution

These injections are given at weekly intervals usually in the out-patient clinic of the hospital. The site to be injected is marked with a skin pencil while the patient is in a standing position. The amount of solution is decided by the surgeon and with the patient at rest the agent is injected into the region of the failed valve. After a few moments the affected limb is then dressed with elasticated hosiery. This treatment has a fair success rate providing the patient wears elasticated hosiery for at least 5 weeks after the treatment, elevates the lower limbs each evening for about 20 minutes and walks at least 3 km each day.

Recurrence of varicose veins near to the site of the injection is quite common because of re-channelling of other venous tributaries. In fairness to the patient, the recurrence is more likely if the attending nurses have not advised the patient correctly following the first treatment.

Surgery

When varicose veins are severe, extending for the whole length of the leg and are visible at the back of the thigh, the surgeon may elect to offer to correct these by one of two techniques. The long saphenous vein is stripped using a long flexible wire and the main venous tributaries are tied off, alternatively the identified incompetent vein(s) are tied off at either extremity and treated by schlerotherapy at the same time or at a later date.

There is no specific preoperative care other than that the affected limb be absolutely clean and that the toenails have been trimmed to the contour of each digit. The skin is shaved for the whole length of the leg. Since there is little in the way of specific preoperative preparation the patient is usually admitted the day preceding surgery and routinely prepared as for any surgery.

Postoperative Care

On recovery from anaesthesia the pain of varicose stripping can be quite severe and therefore analgesia should be routinely offered every 6 hours for the first 24 hours postoperatively. On the first postoperative day the patient should be sat out of bed and allowed to stand by the side of the bed for a few minutes. Some surgeons will request that the patient walks for a short distance.

For the best results a compression bandage should be worn for at least 3 or 4 weeks, being reapplied daily for comfort and integrity. It is necessary therefore to teach the patient how to reapply a crepe bandage from toe to thigh. Once any oedema of the limb has resolved the patient would then wear elasticated hosiery and the fitting of a fashionable stocking **must** be exacting if it is to compress the superficial veins effectively.

Postoperative Complications

During recovery the nurse should check for postoperative problems.

There may be a **haematoma** over the site of incision. Apart from being disfiguring it is also quite painful and may require to be incised to drain the area of old blood.

Infection at the incision site below the suture line is a second possibility and should be checked for at each reapplication of the bandages.

Phlebitis or inflammation of the vein may occur as a result of surgical technique and requires to be brought to the attention of the surgeon.

A fourth complication which is long-term is that of **recurrence** of varicose veins. Usually 20% of cases recur within 5 years of operation.

Patient Counselling

The patient on discharge from hospital requires to be referred to the district nurse for the removal of sutures within 5 or 7 days and to follow up the correct application of bandages. The patient should be issued a supply of bandages so that he or she has at least 3 in hand: one to wear, one in the wash and a third in reserve.

The nurse should ensure that the patient is given the same advice as that for conservative treatment of varicose veins. Car driving can be quite painful if the affected foot is used. It is best to avoid driving for 2 weeks.

The return to work depends on the type of employment. For sedentary work the patient can assume his or her normal work routine within 2 weeks so long as the limb is elevated at frequent periods during the day. With other types of work, the patient should have at least 3 weeks's sick leave to allow the venous flow of the operated limb to re-establish itself.

For some patients the surgeon may require them to return to the outpatients department for further treatment with sclerotherapy.

HAEMORRHOIDS

The veins within the submucosa of the anal canal if they become dilated are referred to as *internal* haemorrhoids. When they prolapse through the anal sphincter they are referred to as *external* haemorrhoids, or piles (Fig. 30.2). Prolapsed veins are covered by a layer of squamous epithelium and are invariably thrombosed which accounts for their bluish colour. The associated risks with thrombosed haemorrhoids are infection of the surrounding perineal tissues and possibly gangrene. If the dilated veins are near the anal sphincter and are small they may cause a perineal haematoma.

A primary cause of haemorrhoids is venous congestion induced by increased 'mechanical' intra-abdominal pressures. Chronic constipation, straining at defaecation, the misuse of powerful purgatives, pregnancy, obesity, and portal hypertension all raise the pressures within the abdomen. This pressure affects the veins where they join the portal circulation either at the oesophagus or the anal canal and distend as the result of the abnormally high pressure. Haemorrhoids may be secondary to other diseases such as cancer of the distal bowel, ulcerative colitis, severe anaemia and hepatic disease such as portal hypertension. For these reasons, haemorrhoids may be extensively investigated to exclude a primary disease before they are treated.

Conservative management

Conservative management of haemorrhoids is always tried first and the advised measures are simple to carry out if the patient has first been reassured and any initial embarrassment has been overcome by a tactful approach.

Daily hot water baths to which salt has been added will shrink external haemorroids and relieve the intense itching associated with the condition and reduce local oedema. The perineum will also be cleansed thoroughly, reducing the risk of infection. Nupercaine ointment applied with gauze will relieve the

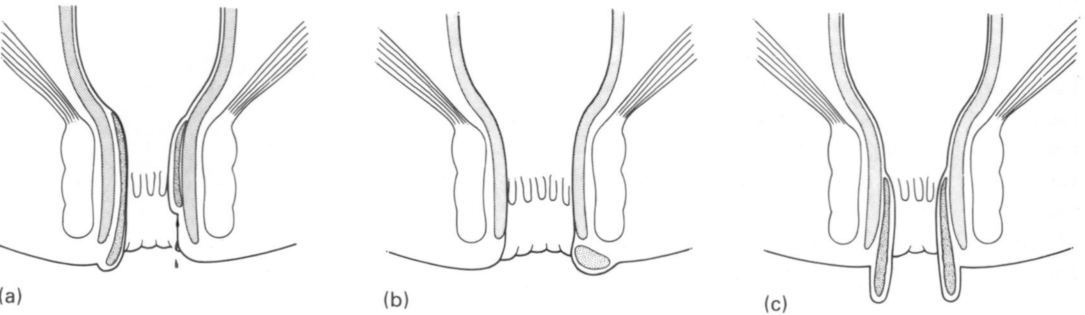

Fig. 30.2 Sites of haematoma: internal haemorrhoids (a); perianal haematoma (b); and external haemorrhoids (c).

pain not only of the prolapsed haemorrhoid but also around the anal sphincter.

High fibre foods especially fruit and a liberal fluid intake will soften the faeces making defaecation that much easier and less painful. If used, aperients should be mild and only taken by the oral route. Suppositories should **not** be used on a patient with haemorroids.

With this conservative approach the haemorrhoids should naturally thrombose. As they heal by fibrosis a small tag of tissue is the only remnant and this will recede back into the anal canal causing no further trouble.

If haemorrhoids remain a persistent problem the surgeon may then recommend sclerotherapy. In this treatment the haemorrhoid is injected with 5% phenol in almond oil and should sclerose and obliterate the dilated vein. Prior to this injection, the surgeon usually carries out a proctoscopy to exclude other bowel diseases. Apart from sclerotherapy of external haemorrhoids the surgeon may induce thrombosis of the internal haemorrhoids by applying tight rubber bands at the base of each dilated vein. These elastic rubber bands are so constrictive that the vein naturally thromboses and heals by fibrosis. The elastic bands are evacuated by bowel motion in due course.

Surgery

Haemorroidectomy, or surgical excision of the varicosed veins, requires that the patient has a completely emptied sigmoid colon and rectum. The surgeon's preferred method of achieving this **must** be known. Some will ask that the patient receives rigorous cleansing with enemas to enable a sigmoidoscopy to be done before the actual operation. Other surgeons have a more gentle approach recommending the use of mild aperients and a soft diet with plenty of oral fluids to achieve the same result. The basic rule, however, is that the lower colon **must** be empty and absolutely clean. Apart from this specific need the patient has routine preoperative care.

Postoperative Care

A main postoperative difficulty following recovery from anaesthesia is for the patient to achieve a comfortable position. Many patients adopt a supine position, i.e., lying on their abdomen, to avoid the discomfort of direct pressure against the perineum. Haemorrhoidectomy is quite a painful operation as the many nerves supplying the anal canal and sphincter have been dramatically stretched by instrumentation. Analgesia therefore is a prerequisite to ensure rest and pain-free first 48 hours postoperative care.

When the patient is sitting out of bed or resting in an armchair, an air-ring is a vital nursing aid to avoid direct pressure on the perineum.

As it is a pelvic operation, retention of urine is a potential problem. This has to be assessed and if remaining persistent, despite nursing techniques, then the surgeon may allow for a urinary catheter to be passed to empty the bladder. This should be a last resort. If the surgeon has placed a pressure pack within the anal canal to control possible bleeding, it is generally removed within 48–72 hours of surgery. Prior to doing this the patient should be given sedation 30 minutes before the procedure as it can be painful and distressing.

To keep the external perineal dressing in place it is useful to cut out a pair of modesty underpants from the large diameter Tubigrip bandaging. In addition to wearing modesty underpants, a male patient should also be offered a suspensory bandage to support the testes. After surgery the scrotal sac not only is painful but can be slightly swollen.

On the third postoperative day the patient should be encouraged to have a bowel motion. In the more difficult cases an olive oil retention enema followed 30 minutes later by a cleansing soap and water enema may prove the only method to achieve defaecation. Liberal oral fluids, a very soft diet and mild aperients are the more usual way of achieving the first preoperative bowel motion.

Postoperative Complications

Two complications following this operation which should be observed for are **haemorrhaging** and **stricture**. The first is noted if the perineal dressing is obviously stained with fresh blood and by monitoring the pulse and blood pressure for the first few postoperative hours.

The second complication is the more long-term problem. Stricture of the anal sphincter, if it occurs, is due to fibrosis as the result of healing. If this is noted the sphincter requires stretching by the use of a St Mark's dilator. The procedure is done in the outpatients department and may have to be repeated every few days as anal sphincter stricture is long term. It may be necessary to teach the patient how to use the dilator immediately before defaecation.

VARICOCELE MINOR

Dilation of the veins of the pampiniform plexus of the spermatic cord which drain the testes (Fig. 30.3) occurs from an unknown cause. The patient is aware of a dragging and aching type of pain, but apart from this the condition is asymptomatic. On palpation the testes contain a soft elastic swelling which feel like a collection or bag of worms, i.e., the dilated veins. When diagnosed the surgeon may decide to investigate to determine if the patient is subfertile or has a defect in spermatogenesis.

The treatment plan is to advise the patient to wear a suspensory testicular bandage which will relieve the pain and dragging feeling. If there is an associated oedema the surgeon may elect to drain this fluid by trocar and cannula (as for a hydrocele). The actual varicocele itself may be injected as for schlerotherapy, or excised while the patient is under the effects of a general anaesthetic.

A major problem following excision is the great difficulty the patient has in passing urine, and this should be relieved by catheter if the patient has not micturated within 12 hours of surgery.

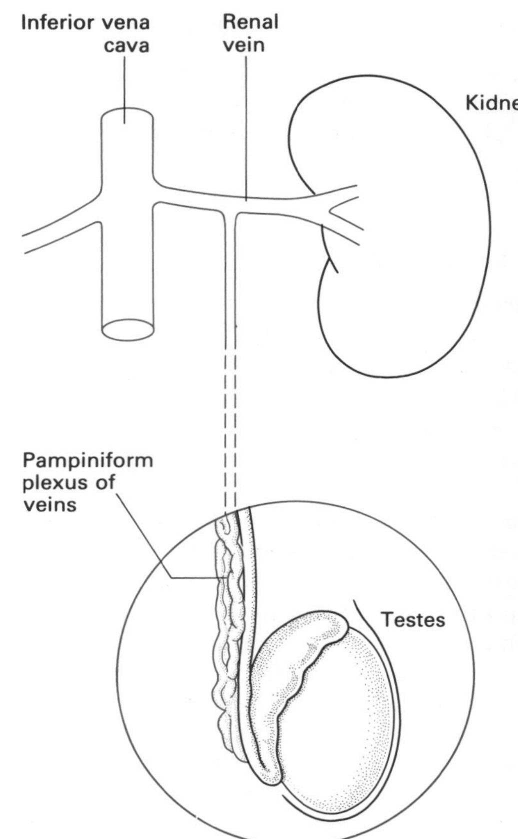

Fig. 30.3 Dilation of the veins of the pampiniform plexus of the spermatic cord.

OESOPHAGEAL VARICES

The portal circulation anastomoses with the systemic circulation at the oesophageal-gastric junction. When this junction suffers any increased pressure between the two systems, the azygos veins at the base of the oesophagus may dilate and become engorged with blood. If there is portal hypertension from any cause and subsequent varices at the oesophagus, these veins are subject to the trauma of food passing over their dilation with a high risk of haemorrhage. Bleeding therefore from these varices may result in a painless *haematemesis* (vomiting of blood) or a massive *melaena* (passing blood per rectum).

Haematemesis

A painless haematemesis which can be of a large volume leading to severe shock and circulatory collapse requires emergency conservative treatment.

Immediate Treatment

Treatment of haematemesis will involve:

1. Massive blood transfusions at first using the universal donor blood group, i.e., Group O, until such time as the patient's own blood has been grouped and cross-matched.

2. Sedating to control restlessness which is always a feature of haemorrhage. This is obtained with one of the morphine group of drugs and is continued until the blood pressure remains stable for at least 12 hours.

3. A special tube, the Sengstaken–Blakemore oesophageal tube, is passed intranasally into the stomach (Fig. 30.4). This is a triple lumen tube with two balloons at its distal end. The first balloon anchors the tube within the stomach, and the second balloon when inflated presses against the oesophageal veins. By this compression the bleeding is controlled. The third lumen is used to aspirate the stomach of any contents, usually partially digested blood. The oesophageal balloon has to be deflated at regular intervals to avoid necrosis of the oesophageal mucosa, and when it is reflated it is to a pressure of 40 mmHg. Associated with the care of the tube is the need to maintain accurate fluid intake and urinary output.

4. Drugs such as antibiotics are employed to counter the risk of abdominal infection due to stagnating blood. Vitamin K_I is also

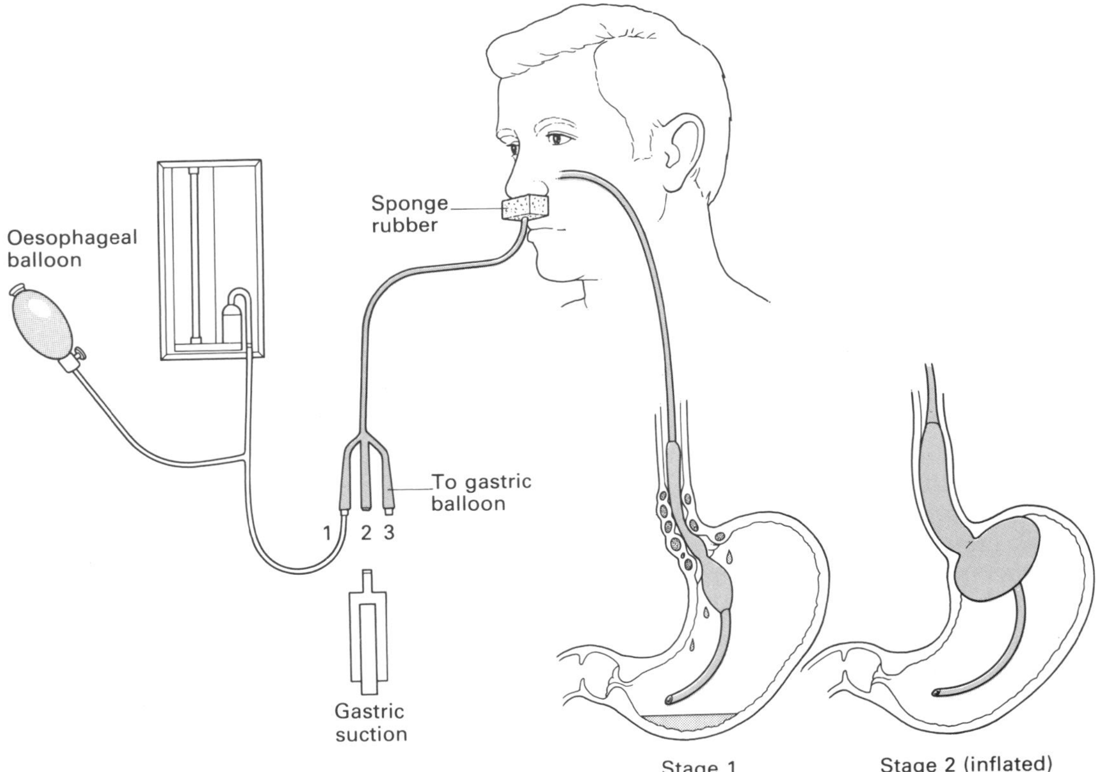

Fig. 30.4 Sengstaken-Blakemore tube (triple lumen) for the treatment of oesophageal varices. Stage 1 the tube is in place in the stomach. Stage 2 the tube is inflated compressing the veins.

used to raise the prothrombin time of blood and vasopressin (Pitresin) may be used to reduce the portal blood pressure if the varices are due to portal hypertension.

5. Haemodialysis may be requested if the patient is threatened by hepatic coma. The coma is usually due to increased levels of nitrogen being released by the decomposing blood trapped in the intestines. The haemodialysis would be used to remove excessive levels of nitrogen from the blood.

6. Linked to this emergency treatment for oesophageal varices are the intensive nursing observations of blood pressure, radial pulses, cardiac monitoring, electrocardiograph readings, and central venous pressure. These are monitored and checked regularly every 15 or 30 minutes until the immediate crisis is under control. Fine detail to the patient's comfort during this type of crisis will undoubtedly promote a positive psychological outlook in the patient to help combat this life threatening situation. Frequent oral toilet, assisted by frequent washes, and giving constant verbal reassurances that everything that can be done is being done will all help until the immediate crisis is over. During the giving of physical care it is better to lift, rather than roll, the patient.

Investigations

Associated with the intensive treatment are many investigations which are carried out to confirm the diagnosis. These include extensive screening of the blood for the electrolyte balance, serum bilirubin and albumen levels, prothrombin time, haemoglobin, leucocyte count, and grouping and cross-matching for multiple units of donor blood.

Radiography of the spleen and liver may demonstrate enlargement of both structures. A barium swallow if performed would show the dilated area at the base of the oesophagus and a portal venography will confirm if the portal circulation is hypertensive. A gastroscopy is a traumatic procedure at this time and may be reserved for the immediate period prior to the surgical by-pass operation. Depending on the cause of the portal hypertension a liver biopsy may be requested.

Causes of Portal Hypertension

Investigations will serve to confirm the cause of portal hypertension, which may be:

Cirrhosis of the liver
Infective Hepatitis
Bile duct stricture
Pancreatitis
Hepatic poisoning from heavy metals
Schistosomiasis
Late stage syphilis

All these diseases cause obstruction to the blood flow through the intralobular veins and their tributaries throughout the liver. Extrahepatic conditions which may raise the portal blood pressure include abdominal tumours, trauma to the liver area, and mesenteric thrombosis with an extension thrombus. Whether the cause of portal hypertension is intrahepatic or extrahepatic it may be associated with ascites, enlarged spleen, a marked anaemia, and jaundice. The preceding 4 problems in their turn require specific nursing care plans to relieve the patient's discomforts of abdominal distension, correction of the haemoglobin levels, bedrest, and calamine lotion to relieve the pruritis caused by the jaundice.

Surgery

Once the conservative measures have controlled the haematemesis and the diagnosis has been confirmed, the surgeon may elect to perform a by-pass surgical procedure to relieve the portal hypertension. By-pass surgery refers to a short circuiting of the blood flow by the anastomosis of one of the principal veins leading into the portal circulation to another principal vein (Fig. 30.5). Several possibilities are considered, these being:

1. Splenic-renal anastomosis; the spleen is removed and the splenic vein is joined to the left renal vein.

2. Portal-cava anastomosis; the portal vein is joined to the inferior vena cava.

3. Devascularisation; a splenectomy

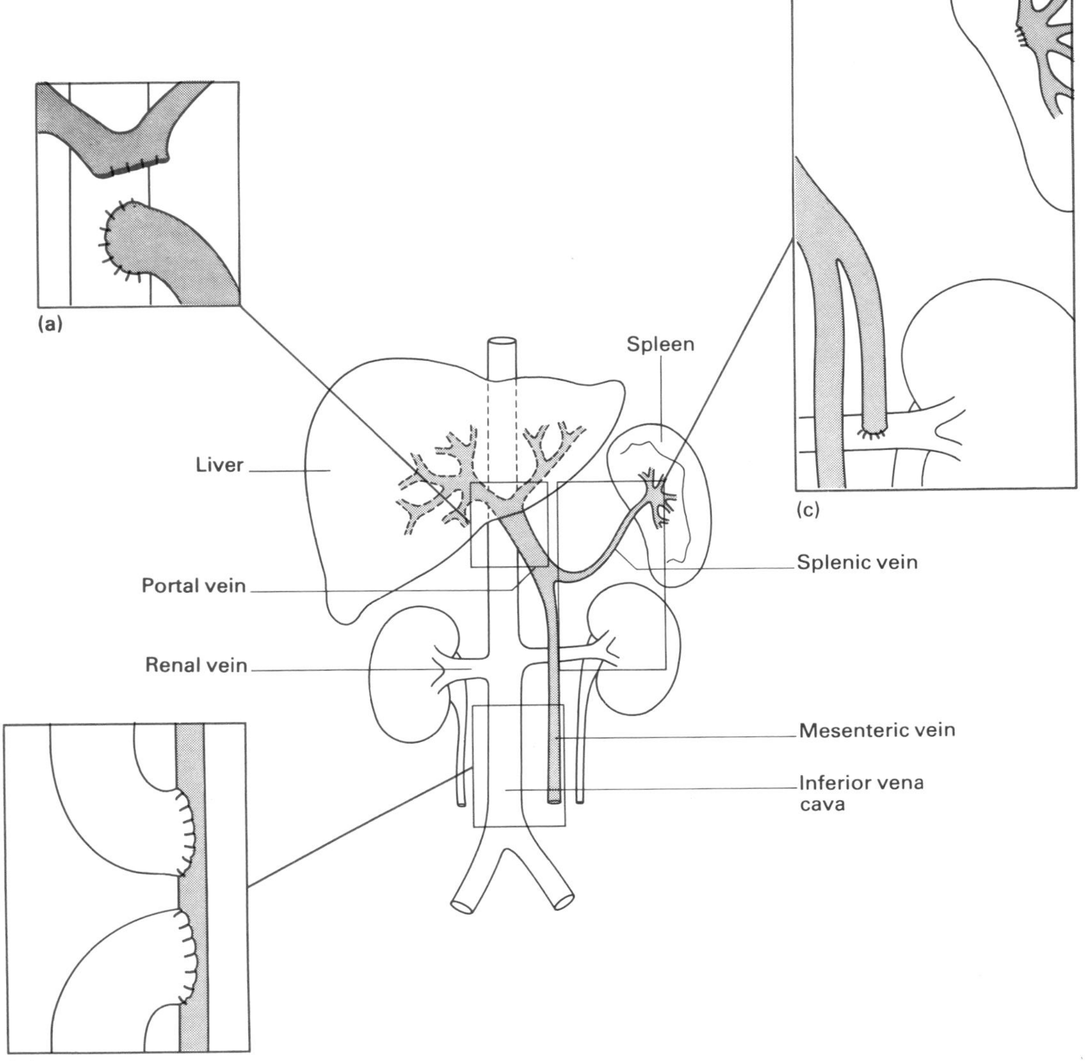

Fig. 30.5 Bypass surgical procedure for portal hypertension and oesophageal varices: portal-cava shunt (a); caval-mesenteric shunt (b); and splenic-renal shunt (c).

combined with excision of the oesophageal and upper gastric veins to remove the varices.

4. Liver transplant; a last resort, but is increasingly a successful operation. There are still problems of meeting the natural functions of purifying the recipient's blood in the postoperative period.

All these surgical procedures are exceptional steps, but they remain the only life-saving measures if the oesophageal varices cannot be controlled by conservative treatment.

It is impossible to predict specific nursing care plans until the type of operation is known except to say that common to all these operations is the risk that the anastomosis will break down or rupture within the first 48 hours of surgery. Throughout this risk interval, intensive nursing observations are made every 15 minutes to assess the danger of internal haemorrhage. Assessment of the patient's progress is made every 4 hours by the surgical team who will be carefully monitoring the state of the blood and electrolyte balance and intervene at a moment's notice should anything go adversely wrong.

Hepatic Coma

Should the patient as the result of oesophageal varices or by-pass surgery suffer from an hepatic coma, a baseline guide will be followed in an attempt to restore the patient to consciousness and maintain homeostasis.

Dietary protein is totally avoided for at least 7 days to keep to a minimum the level of waste products of proteins or nitrogen.

A calorie intake of 1600 calories per day via either nasogastric or intravenous feeding is ensured by supplying carbohydrates in the form of dextran.

Electrolyte and fluid balance requirements are maintained by intravenous solution, the actual volumes being determined by repeated blood tests and assessing the urinary output.

Neomycin antibiotics are usually prescribed to reduce intestinal enzyme activity and to control the risk of peritonitis from any decomposing stagnant blood.

Vitamin K_I and vitamin B complex are usually prescribed being administered either via the intragastric tube or intravenously.

Magnesium sulphate 15 ml given daily as an enema may help to rid the lower colon of any decomposing stagnant blood.

Haemodialysis is now frequently used to rid the blood of both high levels of urea and nitrogen reducing the period of unconsciousness quite considerably.

Cortisone 100 mg once daily may be given to bolster the systemic circulation if oseophageal bleeding continues despite compression from the Sengstaken-Blakemore tube.

Should the hepatic coma remain prolonged and become protracted the surgeon may elect to perform a tracheostomy or ask the anaesthetist to pass an endotracheal tube to keep the patient on intermittent positive pressure ventilation.

Fifty per cent of all patients recover from hepatic coma, therefore the intensive and complicated nursing and medical regimen are very worthwhile.

Chapter 31
Overview of the Respiratory System

The respiratory system is artificially divided into the upper and lower respiratory tracts. While the upper tract is *extrathoracic*, the lower tract refers to structures below the level of the trachea or *intrathoracic*. Structures combining to form the upper tract (Fig. 31.1) include the:

Nose
Paranasal sinuses
Oral, nasal and laryngeal pharynx
Larynx, vocal cords and laryngeal cartilages
Upper trachea

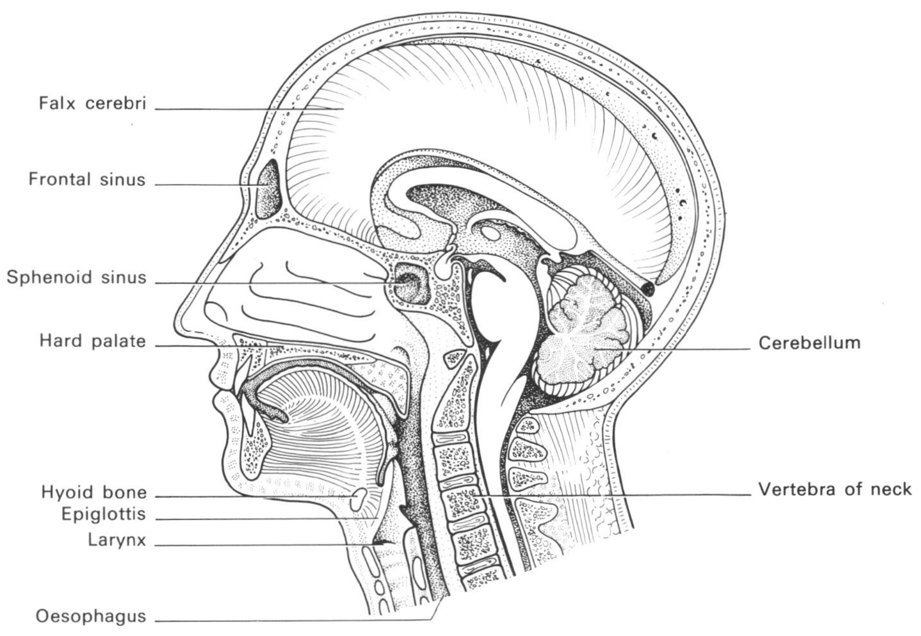

Fig. 31.1 Upper respiratory tract.

LOWER RESPIRATORY TRACT

The lower respiratory tract commences at the termination of the trachea, which is a flexible tubular structure, being about 10 cm in length and 2.5 cm in diameter. It extends from the cricoid cartilage and terminates at the level of the sterno-manubrial junction, i.e., at the base of the sternum. At this point the trachea divides into the right and left bronchus, entering the right and left lung at an area called the *hilum*. The tubular arrangements of the trachea and the bronchi are interrupted at regular intervals by C-shaped cartilages connected to the trachea and each other by fibrous tissue. This cartilagenous arrangement ensures that the trachea always remains open, regardless of the position of the body or head.

The Bronchi

Each bronchus is composed of several layers. Starting with the surface layer, they are:

A mucous layer containing a small number of goblet cells which secrete *mucin*, also known as sputum. In normal health the volume of mucin is minimal.

Hair-like projections emerging as the ciliated epithelium which sweep debris and unwanted small particles upwards, from the bronchus towards the pharynx for expectoration.

A submucosal layer of connective tissue through which the bronchial arteries and veins convey the oxygen supply for the bronchi and permit venous drainage.

Involuntary muscle which determines the diameter of the bronchial lumen and also its contractility.

As the bronchi enter the lung they immediately divide and subdivide, as lobar bronchi (3 to the left lung, and 2 to the right lung). Within each lobe the main bronchi further subdivide into segmental bronchi. At this point the bronchi begin to lose their supporting cartilage and are anatomically referred to as *bronchioles*.

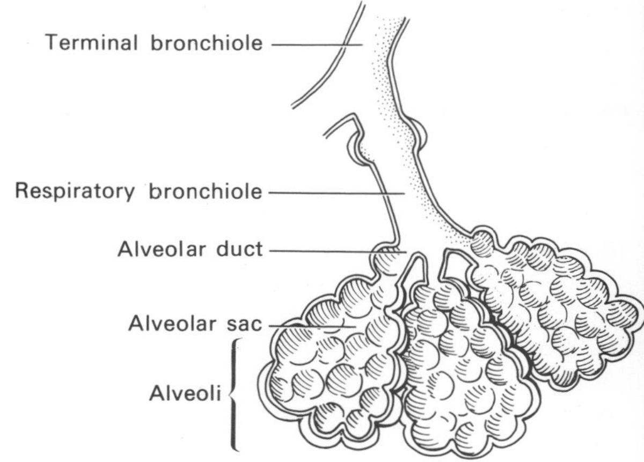

Fig. 31.2 A bronchiole.

The Bronchioles

As finer tubes of much narrower diameter, the bronchioles (Fig. 31.2) eventually lose their involuntary muscle before terminating as the alveolar ducts and alveoli.

The basic functional unit of the lower respiratory system is the bronchiole with its cluster of alveoli, a single alveoli being referred to as an alveolus.

Invested around each cluster of alveoli are the pulmonary capillaries. It is between the semipermeable membrane of these two structures that gaseous exchange takes place. The alveoli remain expanded due to a semiviscous fluid manufactured and secreted from within the alveolus itself, contributing to surface tension. This fluid is referred to as *surfactant*.

The Lungs

Each lung is conical-shaped and has 4 anatomical surfaces:

The **apex**, or apical surface, which extends from the clavicle and enters at the neck

The **costovertebral** surface, which is moulded to the shape of the inner chest wall

A **mediastinal** surface into which the pericardium and great vessels are placed

A **basal** surface, which rests on the diaphragm

The right lung is divided into 3 lobes by 2

fissures creating an upper, middle and lower lobe, and the left lung is divided into an upper and lower lobe by a single fissure. Each lobe is further subdivided into segments, each segment being wedge-shaped and independently supplied by its own bronchi and blood vessels. The right lung has 10 segments while the left has only 9. This segmental structuring of the lungs is an important concept towards understanding thoracic surgery.

Structures other than the bronchi which enter the lung at the hilum include the pulmonary arteries and veins, the lymphatic ducts, and the branches of the autonomic nervous system. The right and left pulmonary arteries convey venous blood to the lungs from the right ventricle of the heart. Like the bronchi the pulmonary arteries continuously subdivide branching ever smaller until they become capillaries surrounding each cluster of alveoli. After the exchange of gases the capillaries unite to form 2 pulmonary veins, a pair from each lung conveying oxygenated blood to the left atrium of the heart. The lung itself receives its own blood supply via the bronchial arteries emerging from the thoracic aorta, and venous drainage of the lungs is via the bronchial veins pouring their contents into the superior vena cava.

Lymphatic ducts enter and leave the hilum of the lung pouring their contents into the large grouping of lymph nodes located at the bifurcation of the trachea, and from there the lymph is taken to the glands positioned in the upper trachea and mediastinum. The lung is innervated by both the tenth cranial nerve (vagus) and branches of the sympathetic nervous system.

Each lung is covered by a thin double membrane known as the *pleura*. The inner or visceral layer is in immediate contact with the lung surface, while the outer or parietal layer is in contact with the chest wall. A potential space exists between these 2 layers, i.e., the pleural cavity, except at the root of each lung where they come into direct contact. A minimal amount of serous fluid is secreted into this space to permit smooth and quiet expansion of the lungs during respiration.

The lower respiratory tract is housed in the thoracic cavity, the design of which allows for expansion and contraction of the lungs. The thorax contains the heart, both lungs, the great vessels, the trachea and oesophagus. A sheet of muscle called the *diaphragm* separates the thoracic cavity from the abdomen. The walls of the thoracic cavity are bounded by the ribs and sternum at the front, the ribs and intercostal muscles laterally and posteriorly. The thoracic vertebra articulate with the ribs posteriorly and permit attachment for the musculature. Both the sternum and the ribs are primary sites for the manufacture and production of erythrocytes from their bone marrow.

Respiration

Respiratory movements are determined by the contractions of the diaphragm and the intercostal muscles via a stimulus from the phrenic, intercostal and vagus nerves. A contraction of these muscles causes the thorax to expand, drawing atmospheric air into the lungs. After filling with air each lung and the intercostal muscles passively recoil forcing air out of the lungs. The main influence on respiratory movements is the combined effects of nervous and chemical controls (Fig. 31.3).

The principal mechanism which determines the rate at which an individual breathes is to be found in the respiratory centre located within the medulla oblongata at the base of the brain. This centre is influenced by the arterial blood gas tensions, in particular the pressure of oxygen (PO_2) and the pressure of carbon dioxide (PCO_2). The pressure exerted by these 2 gases in the arterial blood determines the pH of blood (between 7.35 and 7.45) which in turn is often determined by the current metabolic state of the individual. Both the pH and the arterial blood gas tensions contribute to a chemical-nervous respiratory control.

Baroreceptors (nerve tissue) located on the aortic and carotid arches are sensitive to the blood pH while specialised nerve tissue at the base of the fourth ventricle is sensitive to the CO_2 levels. Both factors influence the res-

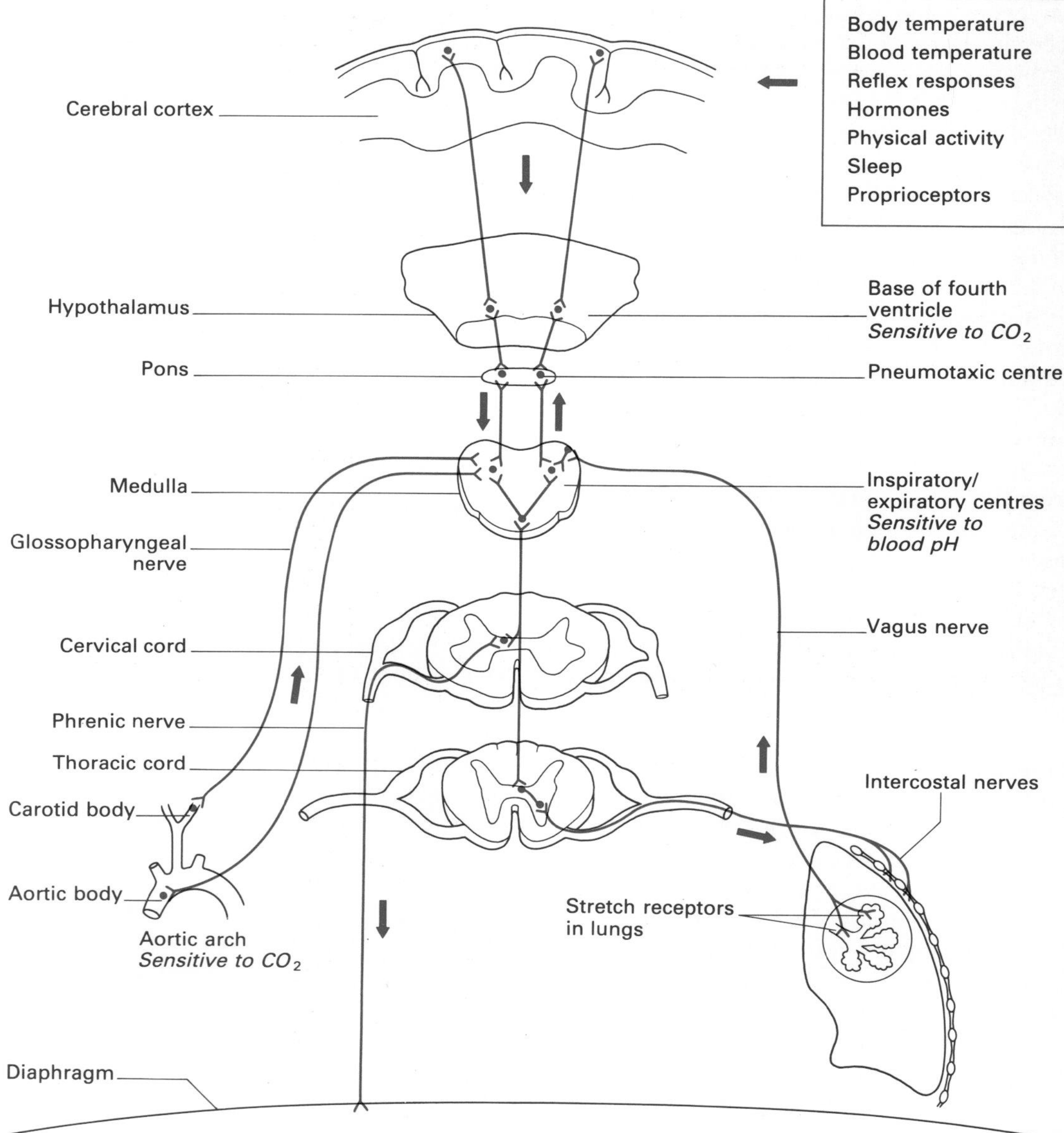

Fig. 31.3 Chemical-nervous respiratory control.

piratory centre which in turn innervates the intercostal, phrenic and vagus nerves which cause the diaphragm and intercostal muscles to contract thus expanding the thoracic cavity. These controls are further influenced by body temperature, endocrine function, and the blood pressure. The most sensitive determinant of respiratory rate is the level of CO_2 in the blood. This gas readily alters the pH of blood, setting off a chain reaction to ensure that the respiration rate satisfies the oxygen needs of the individual.

External respiration involves the mechanical expansion and recoil of the thorax and lungs which enable pulmonary ventilation to take place (Fig. 31.4). The exchange of gases at the alveoli will only be efficient if the existing pressures within the lungs are correct. O_2

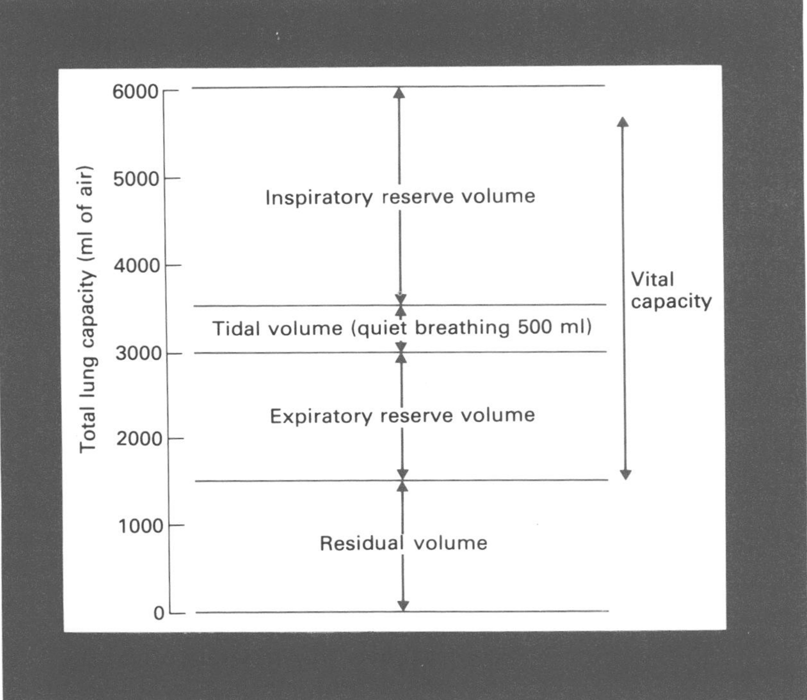

Fig. 31.4 Variable lung capacity.

Table 31.1. Composition of expired and inspired air

Contents	Inspired air (%)	Expired air (%)
Nitrogen	78	78
Oxygen	21	17
Carbon dioxide	0.4	4
Inert gases	1	1
Water	Minimal	Saturated

Each respiration exchanges about 4% of oxygen for 4% of carbon dioxide between 1 and 5 litres of air for respiration.

diffuses from the alveoli to the capillaries and the O_2 molecules attach themselves to a molecule of haemoglobin within an erythrocyte. Haemoglobin contains iron which has a natural affinity for O_2. One molecule of haemoglobin attracts up to 6 molecules of O_2 to itself. Haemoglobin saturated with O_2 is referred to as oxyhaemoglobin.

Internal respiration refers to the transportation of O_2 from the lungs via the arterial system to the peripheral tissues and organs. When it reaches the periphery, the O_2 is surrendered by diffusion to the receiving tissues where it will combine with glucose to produce energy and engage in cellular metabolism. At the end of each respiratory cycle the body utilises 4% of O_2 for 4% of CO_2 from between 1 and 5 litres of air per respiration (Table 31.1). The demand for cellular oxygen is extremely variable depending on such factors as body temperature, blood pH, blood pressure, cardiac output, exercise and rest.

NURSING ASSESSMENT

Respiration

On meeting a patient for the first time, the nurse can visually assess a person's respiratory condition by looking for any sign of cyanosis of the hands or face. Without indicating that the nurse is doing so, a patient's respiratory rate can be quickly assessed by watching the rise and fall of the chest wall and noting if there is any degree of dyspnoea. Even more precisely the nurse should be able to say whether the patient has exertional, inspiratory or expiratory dyspnoea.

Pattern

The pattern of respiration should also be considered. If the patient is solely dependent on mouth breathing it would suggest some difficulty with the upper respiratory tract. Nasal or nasal and mouth breathing are both normal. If the patient is obese it can be assumed that pulmonary ventilation will be inefficient. Equally if it is visually obvious that there is oedema, then again pulmonary ventilation is invariably affected. Clubbing of the fingers is a late sign of advanced lung disease.

Sounds

By listening to the patient's speech one can often detect if there is nasal obstruction or sinusitis. Hoarseness of speech should always be pursued to find out how long the patient has endured such a discomfort, as it may indicate serious problems with the vocal cords. Whether speaking or sitting quietly the nurse should be alert to odd respiratory noises made by the patient. Noises such as broncho-vesicular sounds are audible as 'rattles' from the chest; such noises indicate an excess fluid in the lungs.

Rate

When counting the rate of respiration, the nurse should **not** advise the patient that it is being done. It is a common experience that anyone, even the extremely ill, can alter his or her respiration rate if aware that respiratory observations are being made. Note should be made if the patient purses the lips with the effort of breathing and if the nares are dilated with the effort.

Posture

During respiratory effort the patient will adopt a posture which is the most beneficial for gaining the maximal air. While it is usual to allow patients to take up their preferred adopted position, bunching of the shoulders will decrease ventilation of the upper lobes and the position may have to be corrected for the benefit of the patient. The particular groups of muscles being employed during inhalation should be noted. Use of the shoulder girdle and abdominal muscles, i.e., accessory muscles of respiration, does indicate excessive effort to obtain minimal amounts of air, and suggests advanced disease of the lungs.

Sputum

The production of sputum indicates that the number of goblet cells in the bronchial mucosa has increased, probably due to chronic inflammation of the bronchi. The amount of sputum expectorated, its colour, viscosity and odour require to be reported upon and a sample retained for the doctor's inspection.

Patient History

When taking a history some specific questions should be asked of the patients to ascertain how they see and understand their own difficulties. It is surprising how much knowledge they have of their own disabling respiratory condition and the coping skills they have developed to minimise the effects of their illness.

Prior to a physical examination of the patient, the nurse should not only have made a basic assessment of the patient's respiratory function but should also have recorded the temperature, pulse, blood pressure and, if thought necessary, taken the apex beat, and made these records available to the doctor.

Terminology

Several commonly employed terms relating to the respiratory system should be understood by the nurse so that the medical findings and intentions are more readily understood and interpreted and the nursing care plan more meaningful.

Hyperventilation refers to an increased pulmonary ventilation causing a reduction of the arterial CO_2 content. This can lead to a respiratory alkalosis often seen in hysteria or extreme physical exertion.

Hypoventilation is reduced alveolar ventilation seen in the unconscious patient or in hypothermia, in which case there may be retention of CO_2.

Hyperinflation is excessive expansion of the chest wall in an effort to ventilate the lungs. This is often seen in advanced emphysema when the patient may have developed what is colloquially known as "pigeon's chest". The sternum is thrust forwards and the ribs recede into the intercostal muscles.

Hypercapnia is an excessive level of CO_2 in the lungs, the true measurement of which can only be assessed by analysis of the blood gases. An extreme case of this would cause the patient to present with warm hands, bounding pulse, distended peripheral veins, dilated conjunctival vessels, headache and mental confusion. Cyanosis of the lips and mouth indicates a central cyanosis as opposed to just a peripheral oxygen lack. It implies that 56% of the existing haemoglobin is without oxygen, presuming there is no anaemia. If hypercapnia exists without dyspnoea it implies a disease of a chronic obstructive nature, e.g., bronchitis, or a depressed central nervous system.

Cheyne–Stokes respiration, or periodic respiration, is characterised by a waxing and waning of respiratory depth punctuated by regular periods of apnoea. The periods of apnoea can be quite prolonged and would indicate a disturbed CO_2 level, usually very low, hence a temporary lack of respiratory stimulus.

Kausmaul–Kein respiration describes air hunger or sighing respiration. This is a distressing dyspnoea occurring in paroxysm and may be associated with metabolic acidosis as seen in ketoacidosis.

Tachypnoea an excessively rapid rate of respiration.

Respiratory failure is defined as being an arterial O_2 tension below 60 mmHg (8.0 Kpa) and an arterial CO_2 tension more than 49 mmHg (6.5 Kpa) requiring the patient to have assisted mechanical ventilation.

Chapter 32 Investigations and Procedures

Many of the respiratory diseases encountered by the hospital-based nurse are often medically diagnosed on the clinical findings alone, with the subsequent investigations being used to confirm the doctor's provisional diagnosis. Investigations are also used to determine the course of any proposed therapy and of course to note the patient's response to the prescribed therapy. Experienced nurses would from previous studies be already aware of their role and responsibilities to the patient and to the doctor during and after the investigations.

Respiratory investigations can be summarised thus:

- Radiology
- Bacteriology
- Haematology
- Endoscopy
- Lung function tests

RADIOLOGY

The simple straightforward *chest X-ray* remains one of the cornerstones of diagnostic technique. Views taken of the chest from the anterior, posterior or lateral aspects can demonstrate the shape, size and position of the heart. Enlargement of the heart may displace the great vessels within the mediastinum as they enter and leave the heart. Calcification of the aorta can be noted and it implies that the natural recoil of this great vessel is partially or completely lost. Oedema of the lungs can be demonstrated by looking for certain shadows and the displacement of the diaphragm. The peripheral contours of the thoracic boundaries may reveal calcified areas or shadows which may raise the suspicion of effusion of fluid within the pleural cavity.

Tomography is a less frequently used technique today, but it involves the filming of sections of the lungs at different depths by moving the X-ray tube a short distance between each film. It is a useful investigation in tuberculosis and cancer of the lung.

Fluoroscopy of the diaphragm is employed to visualise the effects of a pericardial effusion, phrenic nerve paralysis, cancer of the bronchus, or the movements of the diaphragm during respiration.

Bronchogram is an invasive technique where a contrast medium is introduced into the bronchial tree, either via a needle puncture of the cricothyroid cartilage or via an intranasal catheter. It is mainly used to determine the degree of airway obstructive disease, e.g., bronchiectasis, which is the narrowing of the lumen of the bronchioles.

A **barium meal** is normally employed to outline the shape and diameter of the oesophagus and stomach. It will also reveal if the trachea is dilated when its shape is compared to that of the oesophagus.

Angiography of the pulmonary blood flow between the right side of the heart and either lung is achieved by injecting a contrast medium into the pulmonary vessels. Aberration in the anatomy of the blood vessels or altered pulmonary pressures will affect the diameter and therefore the blood flow through the lungs.

Mass X-rays are still occasionally used as a means of screening large populations to detect random cases of tuberculosis or cancer. It is still customary for industrial populations who are at risk of respiratory disease to be mass screened, e.g., coal miners, asbestos workers and those at risk from radiation hazards.

Computerised axial tomography (CAT Scan) employs the principle of tomography but is linked to a computer with a memory bank and screen display. The soft tissues of the body are scanned to detect any unusual densities which would not normally be present. Such scanning would detect early tumours, either benign or malignant.

Obtaining a sputum specimen is a common nursing procedure which the senior learner should be familiar with. Regardless of the type of request, the nurse should always inspect and report on the colour, viscosity, volume and odour of the specimen and immediately report if there are any streaks or flecks of blood in the sputum. This may be an early sign of cancer or of a pulmonary embolus. Apart from collecting specimens for culture of organisms and sensitivity testing to antibiotics the nurse may be asked to collect a specimen for cancer cells. A special container to which has been added a preservative called Bouin's fluid has to be used for this test.

Pleural Aspiration and Biopsy

Fluid for bacteriology obtained from pleural aspirate may be requested, if the patient has a pleural effusion. This collection of serous fluid in the pleural cavity may be as much as 500–1000 ml. It will cause pressure on the lung tissue and be accompanied by a severe dyspnoea. Pleural effusions may occur as a consequence of lung cancer, tuberculosis, thoracic injury or surgery. Plain X-rays of the thorax are taken to outline the exact position of the fluid levels, usually between the middle and lower lobes of the lung. These films aid the doctor in deciding where to insert the aspirate needle, usually at the lowest point of the fluid accumulation.

Procedure

Pleural tapping is an aseptic technique which requires two nurses, one to assist the doctor and the other to remain with and reassure the patient during and after the procedure. The nurse accompanying the patient would ensure that toilet facilities have been offered and that sedation has been given, if prescribed, 30 minutes before the procedure is started.

Positioning the Patient

One preferred position in which to place the patient is sitting upright on a firm chair which

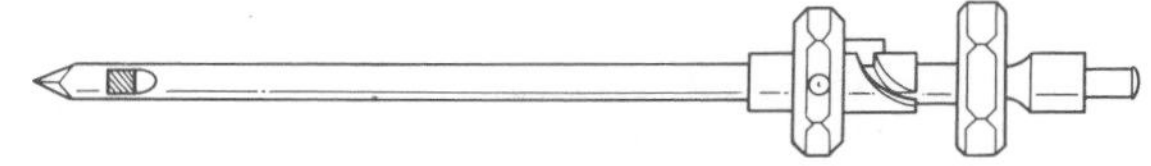

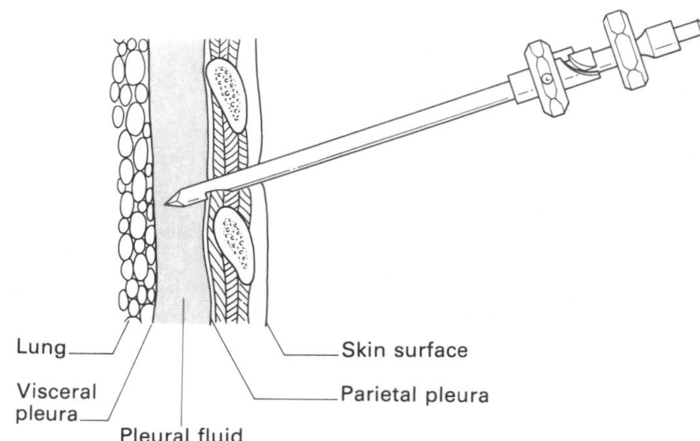

Fig. 32.1 Pleural biopsy using the Abrams' needle.

is facing into the side of the bed. This enables the patient to lean forwards and to stretch the spaces between the ribs, i.e., exaggerate the intercostal spaces. Alternatively, the patient can lie on the unaffected side with the use of a firm pillow placed below the thorax to once again help stretch the spaces between the ribs. It should be borne in mind that a dyspnoeic patient cannot take or hold a deep breath, hence the need to exaggerate the intercostal spaces during the actual procedure.

After the skin and underlying muscles have been cleansed and locally anaesthetised the doctor will advance an Abrams' needle through the tissues of the selected intercostal space until the point of the needle gives, when it reaches the parietal pleura (Fig. 32.1). The stylette of the needle is removed and a 2-way or 3-way tap is applied to the hub of the needle. This tap controls the volume of fluid which is permitted to escape. Several samples are collected into specimen jars and then the remaining fluid drained into a calibrated jug or disposable plastic bag, to ensure that the volume of fluid is accurately measured.

Observations

Throughout the procedure the nurse accompanying the patient keeps a continuous observation for any signs of shock. This may be noted by sudden *breathlessness* or severe *pallor*. The doctor must be told at once so that the procedure can be temporarily halted while the patient regains composure. Prior to the needle being removed a seal dressing is prepared and immediately applied to the site once the tip of the needle is removed.

Nursing Care

After the procedure the patient is nursed in the semirecumbent position for at least 30 minutes with observations made of the pulse and blood pressure. These should be taken and recorded at 10 minute intervals for at least 1 hour. A poor needling technique may cause bleeding into the lung if the visceral pleura has been breached accidentally, but symptoms may not be obvious for some time; hence the need to monitor for shock for at least an hour.

HAEMATOLOGY

It is quite usual for the patient with respiratory disease to have a full screening of all the routine blood tests.

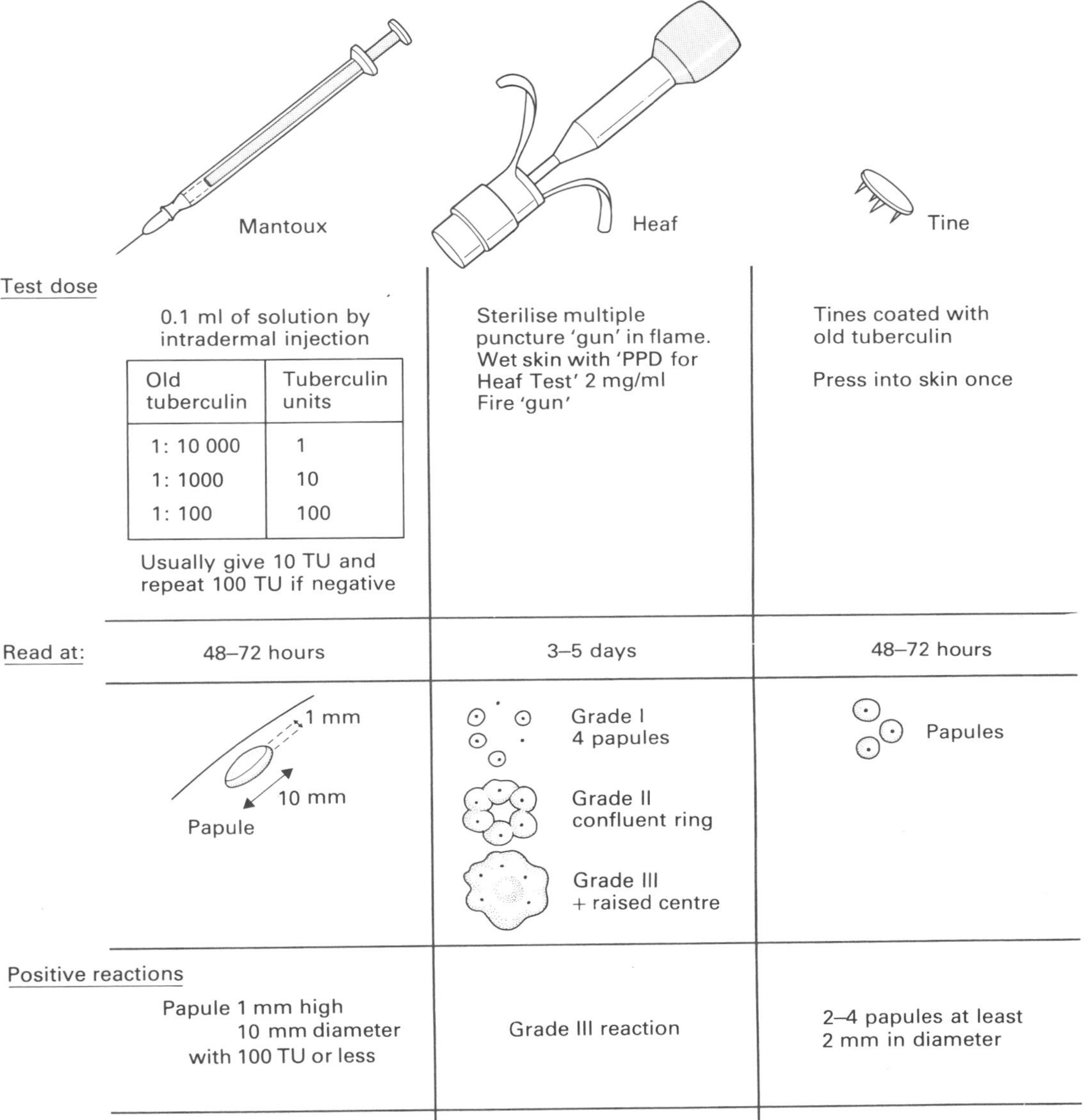

Fig. 32.2 Tuberculin testing.

Leucocyte count

The leucocyte (white blood cells) count is usually raised as the result of pyogenic, viral, or tubercle infections. In an allergic respiratory attack, e.g., asthma, the eosinophils are usually raised while the basophils and neutrophils remain at normal levels.

Erythrocyte and Haemoglobin Count

Erythrocytes (red blood cells) and the haemoglobin count while routinely tested are of some significance in respiratory disease. An anaemia would not only cause circulatory symptoms but because of reduced O_2 uptake there is the implication of an equally reduced cellular metabolic activity.

Electrolyte Levels

Electrolyte levels are always estimated if the patient has any type of oedema and this includes a pulmonary oedema.

Tuberculin Testing

Tuberculin testing may be done to prove whether the patient has a resistance or is susceptible to tuberculosis (Fig. 32.2). A small volume of tuberculin is inoculated subcutaneously, usually into the forearm. If there is no reaction to the tuberculin within 3–5 days, it is assumed that the patient has a potential susceptibility to tuberculosis. With a positive reaction, i.e., a raised inflammatory lesion over the inoculated site, it implies that the patient is naturally resistant to the tubercle bacillus, the causative organism of tuberculosis.

Arterial blood gas analysis

Arterial blood gas analysis is a useful and valued haematology test in those patients who are unconscious from an unknown cause and require assisted mechanical ventilation. They may be suffering from a respiratory or metabolic acidosis or alkalosis which is being corrected. A specimen of arterial blood is taken from the brachial, the radial or the femoral artery and the blood subjected to extremely sensitive electrodes which can distinguish between the pressures exerted by the O_2 and CO_2 in the blood sample. The normal range of blood gas pressures are:

Oxygen (PO_2) 90–100 mmHg.

Carbon Dioxide (PCO_2) 34–44 mmHg.

Since the pressure of these gases determines the rate at which an individual breathes each minute, it is obvious that the blood pH will have to be measured at the same time. It is also usual for the serum bicarbonate to be measured as this also has a bearing on the alkalinity of the blood at any instant in time.

Blood Culture

Blood culture may occasionally be requested if a respiratory disease is associated with a septicaemia. A specimen of blood is added to a prepared solution of nutrients and then incubated for 48 hours before it is subjected to culture and sensitivity testing.

ENDOSCOPY EXAMINATION

Bronchoscopy

Bronchoscopy is the direct visual examination of the trachea, bronchus and bronchi to determine the patency of the airway (Fig. 32.3). Simultaneously a biopsy of tissue is usually obtained for histology studies. The procedure

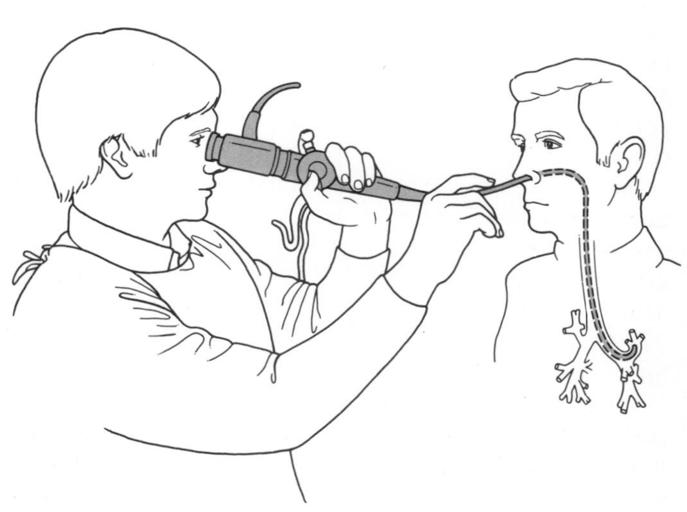

Fig. 32.3 Bronchoscopy using the flexible (fibreoptic) bronchoscope.

is requested if the patient has suffered from a bout of haemoptysis, a symptom suggestive of cancer of the lung or bronchus. Bronchoscopy may help to determine if the tumour is amenable to surgical removal. Apart from being investigative, bronchoscopy may also be therapeutic in visualising an impacted foreign body to enable its removal, e.g., a fishbone.

Rigid tubular bronchoscopes are still in use, e.g., the Negus, Jackson or Albert models, but these are gradually being overtaken by the use of the fibreoptic bronchoscopes, i.e., the Olympus. There are many advantages with the fibreoptic type: it is much slimmer, it is flexible, easier and safer to use, it causes minimal tissue trauma and requires less investigative time. With its second eye piece 2 doctors may examine the airway together. This allows for improved teaching of the medical student and student nurse.

Preparing the Patient

The nurse should spend a great deal of time explaining to the patient the reasons for such an investigation and providing reassurance that it is not painful although it may be uncomfortable. Much of the discomfort, however, will be reduced by the use of local anaesthesia. Prior to any discussion with the patient, the nurse should establish whether the doctor wishes to use a local or general anaesthetic.

Some sedation may be administered 30 minutes before the procedure, especially if a local anaesthetic is being used. A routine premedication would be necessary if general anaesthesia is being employed, e.g., in children and the elderly.

On the day previous to the examination, the nurse should give detailed attention to the patient's oral hygiene, perhaps offering 4-hourly antiseptic mouthwashes. Any tendency in the patient to cough may require a cough suppressant being prescribed for the 24 hours previous to the procedure.

Toilet facilities should be offered to the patient immediately before the examination. If the patient has dentures, these are removed and stored safely in a dental carton. The patient is dressed in a tie-back loose operating gown with no restrictions or jewellery around the neck. A local anaesthetic such as amethocaine hydrochloride (Decicain) may have been prescribed for the patient and this is given 30 minutes before the procedure. As the patient sucks on the tablet, the tissues of the mouth and throat are made insensitive to sensory stimuli. This is further reinforced with Nupercaine throat spray immediately before the operation.

If the bronchoscope is to be inserted via the mouth, the patient is placed in the dorsal position with the head extended. Should the bronchoscope be passed intranasally, the patient is sat upright well-supported on a firm mattress and the back supported by firm pillows. Inadequate local anaesthesia does mean the patient will be unable to co-operate since the cough reflex will prevent any invasion of the trachea.

Nursing Care

After the procedure has been completed by the doctor, and it may have included a laryngoscopy, the patient is sat and nursed in the upright sitting position and allowed to rest for 30 minutes. Suction should be available so that any excess mucus can be removed mechanically since the patient will not have a cough reflex to enable natural expectoration. During the following 2 hours the patient cannot be allowed anything to drink until the local anaesthetic has lost its effect. After this, only sips of sterile water are offered until the patient has completely regained both the swallow and cough reflex.

When a general anaesthetic and a rigid type bronchoscope have been used, the nurse should make these observations immediately following the procedure. Bruising of the patient's lips will need soothing applications of crushed ice. A persistant irritating cough may respond to a cough suppressant. When the patient recovers from anaesthesia, any sign of haemoptysis must be reported immediately. Should a biopsy have been taken, the patient should be nursed on that side. Expectorated sputum containing blood should be retained for the doctor's inspection. Pulse and blood pressure records must be kept, being taken at 30-minute intervals for at least 4–6 hours. A continuous small bleed from the biopsy site into the lungs may not be detectable for several hours and it will eventually reveal itself with early signs of shock and haemoptysis.

Mediastinoscopy

Mediastinoscopy is an aseptic technique to visualise the lymph nodes by fibreoptic illumination of the mediastinal lymph nodes. It is routine to take a biopsy at the same time. Usually the procedure is reserved for those patients with a proven malignant lesion of the lung or bronchus which may be metastasizing from its primary site via the mediastinal lymph nodes.

An incision is made into the anaesthetised skin at the supramediastinal notch and the tip of a Carlin's mediastinoscope is inserted to illuminate the cluster of lymph nodes. The biopsied node is quickly examined to detect for cancer cells. A rapid diagnosis is possible thereby guiding the type of treatment that the patient will require to contain the spread of cancer cells.

The preparation will be for a general anaesthesia and the patient will need much reassurance due to the implications of the possible outcome.

LUNG FUNCTION TESTS

Lung function tests upon the respiratory system can be carried out by subjecting the patient to expiratory stress measurements using spirometers or peak-flow meters, e.g., the Wright peak-flow meter. These meters measure the volume of exhaled air under controlled conditions. The figures obtained are always an average as some allowance has to be made for exercise tolerance levels, height, weight, age, sex, and whether the patient is sitting or standing throughout the test. For these reasons the patient may have the test serialised over a period of several days or weeks and the average figure over a whole series of tests is then used to determine lung function. The tests have to be measured against a known background of any regularly taken prescribed medication. If possible the patient should not have taken any drugs for the previous 48 hours if it is a primary investigation.

Assessments can be made of several features of respiratory function:

Tidal volume (TV) is the volume of air inspired and expired during normal quiet respiration. Adults usually respire 500 ml of air in one respiratory cycle. Of this volume about 150 ml can be substracted as being "dead air" as this volume would occupy the space between the nasal cavity and bronchioles, in which gaseous exchange does not take place.

Functional residual capacity (FRC) is the total volume of air remaining in the lungs after a quiet respiration.

Residual volume (RV) is the volume of air remaining in the lungs after a maximal exhalation.

Total lung capacity (TLC) is the volume of air accommodated within the lungs after a maximal inhalation.

Forced vital capacity (FVC) is the maximal volume of air that can be exhaled after a forced maximal inhalation. It is usually measured over a defined period of time, i.e., 1 second.

These measurements can be visually recorded on a vitalograph showing the precise volumes inhaled or exhaled. The forced vital capacity is a useful measurement as it can indicate the approximate amount of surface area lost from the alveolar surface area due to chronic respiratory diseases. This is usually measured by figures obtained from the forced expiratory volume in 1 second, i.e., FEV 1 second with the forced vital capacity. A difference of less than 70% suggests that there is airway obstructive disease of a chronic nature.

The portable lightweight peak-flow meters with the disposable mouthpieces are commonly employed on the general hospital wards to measure instantaneous forced maximal expiratory volume in 1 minute. The apparatus measures the forced exhaled air flow rate in litres, an average healthy adult has a volume between 400 and 650 litres of forced air flow in 1 minute. With a few experimental trials patients soon become familiar with the apparatus and can measure their own forced vital capacity before and after inhaled aerosol therapy and can monitor their own progress.

The **diffusion gas test** is sometimes used to determine the ability of the lung to diffuse the gas carbon monoxide. The patient is given an inhalation of a prepared gas mixture containing a trace of carbon monoxide, usually for no longer than 10 seconds. A specimen of blood is then collected and examined for the presence of the carbon monoxide. In emphysema the values of carbon monoxide are extremely low proving that the alveolar surface area has lost a considerable surface area for the diffusion of gases.

Chapter 33
Care of the Patient with a Respiratory Disorder

From 1961 to date the mortality rate from all types of respiratory disease equally affecting males and females, particularly after the age of 40 years, has remained persistent at 20% of all causes of death. Currently, respiratory disease is the second greatest cause of death after accidents and violence. It can be readily appreciated that a combination of damp climate, industrial pollution, poverty and certain types of employment contribute to disease of the respiratory system. Certain social behaviours such as smoking, drug abuse and alcoholism have a proven link in the incidence of respiratory disease. Less directly, there is an acknowledged incidence of hospital acquired respiratory infections following major surgery, or in those instances when resistance or immunity is low. Conversely, respiratory disease as a consequence of notifiable infectious diseases, especially in children, has fallen dramatically in the last 20 years.

A few of the more common respiratory diseases with which the learner nurse would be involved in creating and implementing a care plan in a general hospital are highlighted.

HAY FEVER

Between 2 and 10% of the adult population of the UK are effected by *hay fever*, an allergy of the respiratory tissues. It was the cause of 1500 deaths in 1982.

Generally speaking it is a 'seasonal' occurrence when grass pollens are freely released from a wide variety of grasses and trees, between May and August. The pollen grains tend to be released during the late afternoon and early evening and conveyed to distant areas on wind currents. In the UK the grasses most frequently cited as being the cause of allergy are Timothy, Cocksfoot and Rye grasses. The types of tree releasing pollen grains which have been cited include the Silver Birch, Hazel, Elder and Yew. A non-seasonal allergy can be attributed to some other factor such as weed pollens.

Symptoms

The intensity of the symptoms can be at marked variance from individual to individual; much will depend upon the person's immunological status. The severity can vary from a mild rhinitis to a severe bronchial spasm and unconsciousness. After the pollen grains have been inhaled their irritation of the respiratory mucosa causes the release of damaging toxins such as histamines and mast cells. These toxic agents induce a sneezing bout, a degree of rhinitis, rhinorrhoea, mucosal oedema of the nasal passages, conjunctival weeping and intense itching of the upper palate and inner ears. The mucosal oedema may block the Eustachian tube and cause a temporary bilateral deafness.

As the pollen count falls the symptoms tend to resolve but this is of little help to the patient who is seeking some way of preventing the attacks from occurring in the first place. Severe attacks can be quite disabling necessitating periods of time off work, or away from school, and disrupting the social life of an individual during the summer months.

To help identify the causative pollen, the patient may be asked to maintain a personal chart during the course of 1 year. In this personal assessment of their attacks, the patient is asked to state on the chart the exact date and time the allergy starts, and to describe if the attack was 'nuisance only', 'moderately bad', 'severely incapacitating'. Corresponding with this information gathering, the Asthma Research Council completes a pollen count each day during the pollen season. The figures are broadcast or published and quoted in grains/mm^3 of air, the higher the count the more risk of an allergy. Each day the air is sampled and the pollen grains collected and examined microscopically to identify which grass or tree pollen has the highest incidence.

Treatment

Two pieces of information, i.e., the patient's personal assessment and the Asthma Research Council's figures are compared. In this first analysis the doctor has a reasonable picture of which drugs would be most effective in preventing an attack at a given time of the year. The next step that is usually taken is to offer the patient a skin patch test to confirm if the suspected pollen or several pollens are in fact the cause of this seasonal allergy. Pollen immunotherapy can then be considered though it is seldom offered to patients under 10 years of age. It consists of an annual injection for three years; given before the pollen season starts. In effect, it gradually desensitises the patient to the pollen causing the allergy.

As an intermediate therapy, several anti-allergic medications may be prescribed to control the worst of the symptoms.

Antihistamine drugs such as chlorpheniramine (Piriton) 1 to 4 mg orally, if prescribed, should carry the warning that the tablets tend to make the patient sleepy and tired since they contain a sedative action.

Beclomethasone (Beconase) is a nasal spray which reduces the oedema of the mucosa permitting normal nasal breathing.

Predosol eyedrops, if prescribed, help to counter intense conjunctival irritation and reduce any tendency to tear overspill due to a blocked lacrimal duct.

Sodium chromoglycate (Intal) is an inhalant in powder form. If prescribed, it is meant to be taken before an attack actually begins, therefore the patient has to know of the early warning signs. When inhaled the drug Intal prevents the release of toxic amines from damaged respiratory tissues aggravated by pollen grains.

Patient Counselling

During the pollen season, patients can increase their comfort by taking certain precautions. When out they should wear either spectacles or sunglasses to protect the conjunctiva. It is best for them to stay indoors during the late afternoon with the windows and doors shut unless it has been raining, in which case the pollen count is always very low. Lawn mowing should always be done in the morning when the grass still has its dew.

Commercial nasal drops are not to be recommended as their prolonged use without medical supervision may induce a chronic chemical inflammation of the nasal mucosa leading to irreversible loss of the ciliated epithelium.

Recent work on a portable filtering mechanism, i.e., the head glasshouse, which can be worn when outdoors would suggest one preventative technique, but has yet to complete clinical trials.

ASTHMA (*See also* Nursing 1)

Asthma is an airway obstructive disease characterised by 3 main features:

The **lumen** of the bronchi becomes narrowed due to an involuntary muscle spasm caused by the release of damaging amines from the lung tissues.

A localised **mucosal oedema** which further contributes to the narrowing of the bronchial lumen.

The **goblet cells** lining the bronchi secrete excessive amounts of tenacious mucus which blocks the bronchial lumen, i.e., mucus plugs.

While mainly a disease occurring in children with all the clinical features appearing before adolescence it occasionally occurs in adults for the first time as a late onset attack and is invariably due to a chest infection. In the absence of chest infection it may be due to an extrinsic allergen and in a minority of cases the attack may be triggered by psychological stress.

Immediately preceding the attack the patient is aware of increasing respiratory difficulty associated with respiratory wheezing. The wheezing or whistling intrathoracic noise is due to air being forcibly inhaled and exhaled over the mucus plugs blocking the bronchi. As the attack proceeds the patient experiences great difficulty in exhaling completely and in compensation takes short sharp inhalations, i.e., gasps and pants. This difficulty leads to frightening sensations of suffocation and choking with a pronounced peripheral cyanosis, physical agitation and fear.

Observations

Observations made during such an attack would show:

peripheral and central cyanosis

marked tachycardia, the faster and weaker the pulse becomes the more serious the attack

should there be drowsiness with breathlessness and tachycardia, it is evidence of cerebral hypoxia and is an extreme medical emergency

the degree of anxiety and literal fear cannot be overstated being a major feature of the generalised shock

As a first aid measure the patient should be sat upright and inclined slightly forward so that the accessory muscles of respiration can be used to their maximum effect. These muscles will help the patient overcome some of the problems of adequate exhalation until drugs can be used to relax the bronchial spasm. Loosening tight clothing around the neck, chest wall and waist will also remove feelings of constriction. Remaining with the patient is the greatest act of reassurance. Asthmatic patients should never be left alone during an attack, even adult patients who have experienced such attacks before.

Treatment

The principles of medical therapy with which the nurse will have to help include:

administering bronchodilator drugs by an intravenous route

increasing the pulmonary ventilation by oxygen therapy. It should be noted that this is of no value until after the bronchodilator drugs have become effective

counteracting the generalised physiological shock and correcting the hypotension

Drugs such as ephedrine, isoprenaline, salbutamol and aminophylline if given intravenously act within several minutes of their administration, relaxing the bronchial muscle and permitting the patient to exhale properly. It will, however, be some time before the patient stops gasping for air and even longer before the peripheral cyanosis begins to recede. Oxygen therapy of high volume and concentration, e.g., 6–8 litres at 30–40% concentration via a sealed mask, is continued until the cyanosis has completely receded. This would imply that any central cyanosis will also be receding.

Generalised shock may respond to an intravenous injection of adrenaline 1 in 1000. If tachycardia or hypotension persist as noted from the nurse's frequent recordings every 15 minutes then hydrocortisone succinate may be used to increase the systemic blood pressure.

On immediate recovery the patient will remain in a state of psychological shock for some time. The patient will respond to reassurance from medical and nursing staff that the asthma attack is now under control, but it also indicates the need for a period of rest in a calm atmosphere and under nursing supervision. The fear of being left alone should never be overlooked and asthmatic patients will not rest adequately unless given this assurance by the nurse.

Tests

Initial attacks of asthma associated with a pulmonary infection may in fact confuse the clinical signs and symptoms of a typical attack. Antibiotics are invariably prescribed to treat or act as a prophylaxis in case of pulmonary infection.

To determine if an infection exists a sputum specimen should be despatched for culture and sensitivity of any pathogenic organisms. Chest X-rays are usually requested along with requests for an assessment of the basic blood picture, and blood gases. If the cause of the asthma is due to an allergen the eosinophils are usually raised. Peak flow rate readings of the lungs' respiratory vital capacity can be taken and recorded every 4 hours and an improvement should be noted if the treatment and rest are effective.

At a later time forced expiratory volume and forced vital capacity tests can also be made to measure the patient's pulmonary capacity. The family and social history of the patient when taken may highlight if the patient has any existing allergic diseases such as hay fever, eczema, or rhinitis. If there is a history of any allergy the patient may be referred to the dermatology department for skin patch testing to identify the causative allergen. Grass pollens and house dust mites are the most frequent causative allergens in the UK.

Further treatment

On the patient's recovery from the asthma attack and following a medical review, the doctor may continue medication by prescribing one of the following drugs:

Salbutamol (Ventolin) or terbutaline for the relief of mild bronchial constriction

Choline theophyllinate (Choledyl) or aminophylline suppositories for persistent bronchial constriction

Sodium chromoglycate (Intal) may be prescribed as an inhalant for prophylactic use if an allergen has been identified. This drug when inhaled prevents the release of toxic amines from the lung tissues.

Corticosteroid drugs, e.g., prednisone may be prescribed for a prolonged period if the patient has a history of repeated pulmonary infections due to persistent inflammation of the bronchi. Beclomethasone (Becotide) is a corticosteroid inhalant drug which may be given as an alternative.

Desensitisation to the causative allergen may be possible by offering a small amount of it to the patient in an annual subcutaneous injection usually during the spring months.

Complimenting the medical regimen the

patient will also require a review of his or her lifestyle and employment to assess those risk factors which may contribute to a second or third asthmatic attack. Simple measures such as dust control in the home, avoiding wherever possible the causative allergen and remaining loyal to any drug regimen will reduce attacks.

STATUS ASTHMATICUS

One asthmatic attack quickly succeeded by others is now a rare medical emergency with modern therapy. However it can and still does occur. It is a most urgent medical emergency requiring immediate hospital admission usually to the intensive therapy unit. The risk of death from respiratory failure is high hence the need for oxygen via intermittent positive pressure respiration using a Bird's ventilator. Large doses of steroid therapy are also required to counteract the generalised shock, e.g., hydrocortisone succinate 200–300 mg intravenously along with aminophylline 250–500 mg as a bolus injection. Aminophylline may be continued thereafter, 500 mg every 8 hours via an intravenous infusion. Once the patient's condition is stable the oxygen therapy is continued via a face mask and the patient can then be transferred to a general ward for the underlying causes to be pursued and for prophylactic therapy.

BRONCHITIS AND EMPHYSEMA

Acute Bronchitis

An attack of acute bronchitis is usually a singular event and often follows upon an upper respiratory tract infection or exposure to an atmospheric bronchial irritant. The acute inflammatory response involves the ciliated epithelium lining the bronchial tree and trachea. Initially the patient complains of dysphagia, hoarse speech, mild pyrexia, headaches, and muscular fatigue. Typical of acute bronchitis is the very painful dry cough which gradually becomes productive, i.e., infected mucus can be more readily expectorated.

Nursing Care

Treatment and nursing care centres upon dealing with the symptoms until the acute inflammation resolves. Bedrest alternating with armchair rest is advised until the pyrexia abates, this being noted by 4-hourly recordings of the body temperature.

A cough suppressant, e.g., Gee's linctus, is advised in the early stages while the cough remains painful and dry. Persistent coughing if not overcome will exhaust the patient. Medicated steam inhalations, e.g., Friars' Balsam should be offered every 4 hours during the daytime. Not only will it help to soothe the irritated trachea and bronchus but will help liquify any tenacious sputum.

It is usual for the patient to be prescribed a 5–7 days course of broad spectrum antibiotics to deal with the causative pathogenic organism.

The illness generally runs a course of about 7 days. During this time the nurse should ensure the patient's further comfort by giving detailed attention to the patient's oral and personal hygiene and meeting his or her toilet needs. Lightweight cotton bedwear should be used to absorb the perspiration caused by the pyrexia, and bedclothing should also be light and free. If possible the atmosphere should not only be warm and well-ventilated but slightly humidified as this will also help to liquify the bronchial secretions.

A copious fluid intake and a light but nutritious diet are all that the patient can normally cope with during the acute state of the illness. Both smoking and alcohol should be forbidden until the course of antibiotics is completed.

Chronic Bronchitis

Chronic bronchitis is a symptomatic disease and implies irreversible changes to the peripheral bronchioles. The classical symptom of the disease is a productive cough during the last 3 months of the year and suffered for at least 2 years. This symptom alone with no other established disease indicates the presence of a chronic inflammation of the bronchioles.

The incidence of chronic bronchitis is twenty times greater in cigarette smokers than in nonsmokers. All the research of the last 20 years conclusively points to the tar of cigarettes as being the bronchial irritant causing the chronic inflammation. Industrial atmospheric pollution is also a major contributing factor, however, the pollution has to be persistent and severe. The best example is sulphur dioxide fumes combined with persistent damp foggy weather. This latter example is increasingly unlikely due to the legislation controlling pollution of the atmosphere by industrial smokes and fumes.

Over a period of several years the patient suffers mild respiratory tract infections, each succeeding attack being more prolonged in duration and severity. The infections are exacerbated by the cold damp conditions of a typical winter, when viral influenza is also at its peak incidence. With each infection there is a gradual impairment of respiratory function. At first there is loss of the protective ciliated epithelium; such a loss means that mucoid secretions can no longer be swept upwards towards the pharynx for expectoration. The stagnant mucus therefore makes the bronchi even more prone to infection and inflammation.

With time and continuing irritation of the bronchial mucosa the goblet cells enlarge and become more numerous, increasing their secretion of mucus. In an effort to rid the bronchial tree of these excessive secretions the patient has to cough a great deal more, usually in the early morning on first awakening. It should be noted that persistent coughing makes the patient more than usually prone to a hernia. As the chronic nature of the inflammation progresses the peripheral bronchioles begin to become scarred and fibrotic, reducing the ability of the lung to naturally recoil.

Clinical Signs

It is at this late stage that the patient begins to show clinical signs other than a persistent morning cough. There is evidence of:

Exertional dyspnoea which is increasingly obvious on physical activity which was formerly well within the patient's abilities. Some patients ignore the symptom believing it to be due to advancing age.

Audible pulmonary wheezing due to the air being inhaled over plugs of mucus trapped in the smaller bronchioles.

Lung function tests show a reduced pulmonary ventilation.

Inadequate gaseous exchange may give the first signs of peripheral hypoxia, i.e., cyanosis of the extremities.

Blood gas analysis may show a raised PCO_2 level. If this is so, the patient will be suffering from a respiratory acidosis which means respiration will be rapid but shallow.

Emphysema

Emphysema often coexists with chronic bronchitis or asthma. It implies that the alveolar walls are gradually being destroyed. Emphysema is more common among men, and especially after the age of 70. With a heavy smoker, it is seen between the ages of 50 and 70. There is an increase in the overall size of the terminal air spaces at the alveoli and a loss of their surrounding supportive tissue. In addition a lubricating substance within the alveoli, i.e., surfactant, is no longer produced. This substance would normally protect the surface tension of the alveoli.

The total effect of these changes means that on exhalation the alveoli wall will collapse, being unable to participate in gaseous exchange. Gradually but inexorably, the total surface area available for gaseous exchange is irreversibly reduced which has obvious connotations for the oxygenation of the peripheral tissues. Other changes occurring include the thickening and distortion of the bronchial walls with excessive secretion from the goblet cells. Such changes lead to a narrowing of the bronchial lumen requiring increased muscular effort to exhale since the lung has lost its natural recoil, i.e., chronic obstructive airway disease or COPD. The remorseless progressive nature of emphysema means that the blood flow between the lungs and the right side of the heart becomes congested leading to a right-sided heart failure, or cor pulmonale.

Both chronic bronchitis and emphysema are irreversible changes which means that any treatment will be aimed at minimising the severity of any symptoms.

Patient Counselling

A major part of therapy is counselling patients about adaptations which will have to be made to enable them to cope with the crippling effects of the disease. One of the most positive steps to take would be to discourage the patient from cigarette smoking, though this is easier said than done. Few commercially available antismoking preparations actually help with the withdrawal symptoms, especially the craving for a cigarette. In the last analysis it is the patient's own determination and self-will which needs to be encouraged.

Joining a self-help group may provide the necessary motivation in the early stages to promote self-discipline from within a peer group. Some patients respond if during the early stages of giving up the habit they are given light sedation, but this is not popular among doctors since it is merely exchanging one habit with another. On the other hand the desperate craving which the patient feels does require sympathetic handling. Often patients are encouraged by how well they feel, enjoying a renewed vigor, with a restored appetite, and some money saved. These feelings when achieved may be enough to encourage the patient to abandon the habit altogether. Some research does suggest that giving up smoking for at least 2 years does restore some of the previously lost pulmonary ventilatory function.

Drug Regimens

Exertional dyspnoea can be temporarily overcome by a variety of medications but all have a limited effect on the actual disease process. Many patients gain some temporary benefit in the short term. Commonly prescribed medications include:

Mucolytic Agents

Mucolytic agents reduce the viscosity of tenacious sputum thus aiding easier expectoration, but they do not necessarily improve pulmonary ventilation:

Bromhexine (Bisolvon) 8–16 mg orally 4 times daily may be used with those patients who have a mild bronchitis and moderate airway obstruction.

Acetylcysteine (Airbron), methylcysteine (Visclair) and carbocisteine (Mucodyne) may be given as an inhalant if the viscousness of the sputum prevents adequate expectoration.

Simple steam medicated inhalations should not be overlooked as an effective but cheap way of keeping the sputum moist and watery.

Bronchodilators

Bronchodilators principally act on the involuntary muscle of the bronchioles by relaxing the muscle fibres and thereby increasing the bronchial lumen:

Isoprenaline (Isoproterenol, Isopropylnoradrenaline) may be given in small oral dosage because of its vigorous effect on the heart. It is dissolved sublingually in tablets of 10 or 20 mg and repeated as needed. It can also be prescribed in a sustained release tablet (Saventrine). If supplied as an aerosol inhalant it has a beneficial effect within 30 seconds and is therefore used in the more severe forms of bronchitis and emphysema.

Ephedrine sulphate tablets 25 mg twice daily can be used as a bronchodilator but are gradually being replaced by more effective drugs which produce fewer side-effects.

Salbutamol (Ventolin) can be prescribed in tablet or inhalant aerosol form. It is effective for up to 4 hours without any unwanted side-effects on the heart. Terbulatine (Bricanyl) has a similar effect.

Aminophylline (Cardophyllin) rectal suppositories are rapidly absorbed by the gut mucosa reaching a bronchodilator effect within 30 minutes to 2 hours. If used, aminophylline has to achieve a plasma level of between 5 and 20 μg/ml for its best effect, otherwise the patient will continue to remain breathless. A derivative of aminophylline is choline theophyllinate which when given orally produces a longer bronchodilator effect without any serious toxic effects. Suppositories are usually administered about 2 hours before the usual bedtime to ensure a reasonable night's sleep.

Inflammatory Suppressants

Inflammatory suppressants such as the corticosteroids may be used to suppress the bronchial inflammation. If the combined effect of other drugs is proving ineffective in dealing with the symptoms then steroids may be tried. It is normal practice to give steroid drugs as a short course and on a reducing sliding scale, e.g., prednisone 5–10 mg daily for 5 days, thereafter reducing the dose every few days until the patient is weaned off the drug altogether. Prolonged use of steroid drugs is unusual.

Antibiotics

Antibiotics may be used either as a long-term or short-term therapy, especially during the winter months when the patient is generally prone to chest infections. In addition to antibiotic therapy the patient may be advised to also have an injection of influenza vaccine every year as an added precaution.

Patient Education

Educating the patient in one of several physiotherapy techniques should help to improve pulmonary ventilation. Such techniques include intermittent positive pressure breathing and postural drainage. Intermittent positive breathing involves the patient in exhaling slowly by small grunting noises from the diaphragm while pressing downwards on the anterior abdomen. As the air is exhaled it is forced out through pursed lips. If done at regular intervals, e.g., a few minutes in every hour, the patient should find that the lungs are emptied more effectively and it also helps with the expectoration of sputum. The underlying principle of this technique is that the patient has lost natural recoil of the lung and therefore requires more muscular effort to empty the lungs adequately. Controlled expiratory effort reduces the need to use accessory muscles of respiration.

Postural drainage of the lungs employs gravity to assist in draining individual lobes or segments of the lungs towards the main bronchi. This in turn aids expectoration of stagnant mucoid material. The anatomy of the bronchial tree is such that merely tipping the patient into a head down position is of no practical value. Both the patient and the nurse must be aware of the particular part of either lung which requires draining and then use the appropriate position to promote adequate pulmonary drainage (Fig. 33.1).

The upper lobes or apices are in constant drainage so long as the patient is sitting upright. When the patient is in the dorsal position excess mucus will accumulate. After a period of sleep these upper lobes are easily drained by merely sitting the patient upright for several minutes. If the middle lobes require to be drained the patient is placed into the lateral position and two firm pillows placed beneath the pelvis so that it is tilted higher than the shoulders. To drain the lower lobes the patient is placed in the head down position with the foot of the bed raised by at least 50 cm. The abdomen is then raised by placing 2 pillows under the abdomen.

When introducing postural drainage, the nurse should only permit its use for 5-minute intervals twice a day. A dyspnoeic patient will be frightened and any emotional distress will only worsen the existing dyspnoea. As the patient adapts to the technique and begins to gain some benefit, the intervals can be extended up to 30 minutes. This is the most beneficial time interval for complete drainage of excess mucus from the lungs.

Postural drainage is enhanced if prior to it being carried out the patient has a 10-minute steam inhalation. During the period of drainage further benefit is gained if the rib cage over the affected lobe or lung segment is

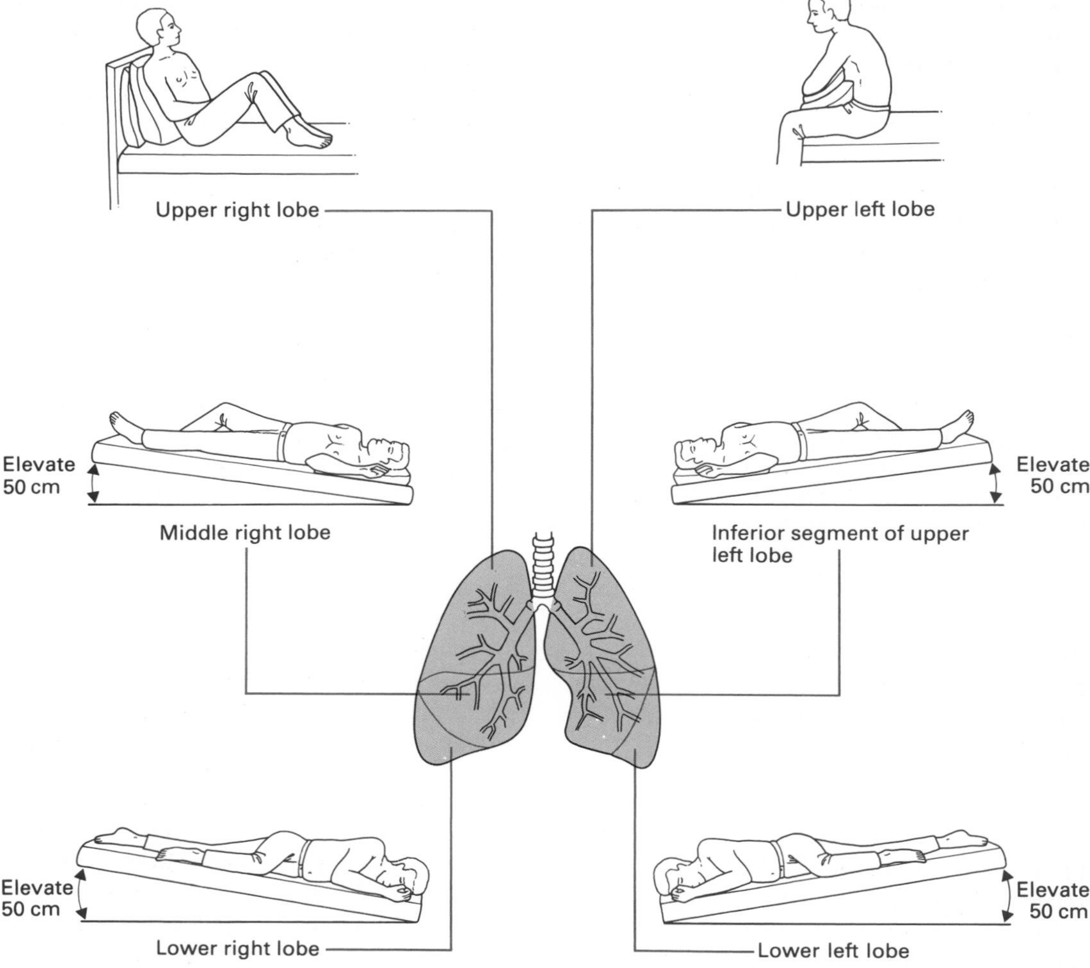

Fig. 33.1 Positions for postural drainage.

manually vibrated by either cupping or clapping methods. This does vibrate the underlying structures and moves the mucus towards the bronchus.

Postural drainage has to be used with caution and is inadvisable in certain groups: the elderly, those with cardiac conditions, the obese, the hypertensive, those with abdominal surgery, and psychiatric patients. Should the patient report benefit from the technique the nurse should then consider if the relatives should also be taught the method so that they can encourage and supervise the patient at home.

Counselling for Discharge

Assessment of daily activities should be made before the patient is discharged home from hospital. The crippling nature of chronic bronchitis and emphysema is such that a great deal of thought and discussion should be given in search for those ideas which will enhance the patient's coping skills. A few ideas which may lend themselves as a basis for discussion include:

Any kind of emotional distress or excitement worsens the dyspnoea, making the breathlessness a major handicap and a frightening experience for both the patient and any witness. A calm approach to a family crisis is absolutely essential.

Within the patient's day, a defined period of rest should be agreed with the relatives and this should take into account the patient's preferred sleep pattern. Within this agreed time there should be minimal disturbance to the patient.

Physical tolerance levels are notoriously difficult to assess in the domestic situation, but a respiratory disease patient tires easily, and, if attempting any kind of persistent physical work, can quickly be overcome by exhaustion. If the patient is mentally orientated to 'work' behaviour patterns, then serious psychological problems can occur if early retirement is necessary.

PNEUMONIA

An acute inflammation of the lung, *pneumonia*, mainly affects the alveoli within either a single lobe or involves several segments of one lobe, in which case the inflammation tends to spread rapidly throughout the lung. *Bronchial pneumonia* implies that the inflammation is extending from the alveoli towards the bronchioles and bronchi. *Double pneumonia* refers to the fact that both lungs are inflamed.

In times before antibiotics were used on a wide scale, pneumonia was known as 'the old man's friend'. The inflammation and purulent material were so extensive but insidious in their spread throughout the lungs that although the patient became increasingly breathless, there was not too much pain or suffering as the patient passed into a coma and died. With the advent of antibiotics the course of pneumonia rarely runs its natural course, but there are exceptions to this rule.

The causes of pneumonia can be grouped as being due to a primary pathogen, secondary to another disease, atypical if it does not conform to a normal pattern, and predispositional to certain circumstances (Table 33.1).

The early clinical features of pneumonia can be regarded as problems which the nurse can assess by their degree of severity and plan nursing measures to improve the patient's comfort and to develop coping skills with the illness.

Dyspnoea

Increasing dyspnoea or difficulty with respiration is due to the accumulation of purulent exudate combined with pulmonary oedema and pleuritic pain. Correct upright positioning, supporting the small of the back with firm pillows and the shoulders with soft pillows, will help the patient use what respiratory muscle is required to ventilate the lungs without causing too much effort or pain. The shallow respirations are rapid and gasping, usually via the mouth, and a low percentage oxygen may have been prescribed to aid in the oxygenation of the peripheral tissues.

Table 33.1. Causes of pneumonia

a Primary bacterial infections	d Predisposition if there is
Streptococcal pneumococcus Staphylococcal pneumococcus Mycobacterium bacillus	Hypothermia Reduced immunity states Alcoholism Drug dependence Chronic bronchitis Tracheal aspiration e.g., vomitus Cancer of the lung
b Secondary to upper respiratory tract infections	
c Atypical pneumonia	
Mycoplasma pneumonia Respiratory syncitical virus	

Persistent Cough

A persistent cough is the body's first defence in ridding the bronchial tree of purulent exudate from the inflammed alveoli. Although an excellent defence mechanism in the early stages of pneumonia, the cough is dry and painful, with the constant racking nature of the cough contributing to utter exhaustion. If possible the cough should be suppressed with a cough linctus in the early stages of pneumonia. Later, when the purulent exudate is less viscous and easier to expectorate, the linctus can be discontinued, and the patient given an abundant supply of disposable tissues and a disposable sputum carton in which to expectorate. The oral mucosa will appear dry and cracked and this will be accompanied by a foul breath odour. Liberal mild antiseptic mouthwashes and sips of lemon or barley water will do a great deal to freshen the mouth and remove any foul taste.

Purulent Sputum

The purulent sputum when produced should be observed for colour, odour, and viscosity. Blood streaks are quite common in atypical viral pneumonia. In bacterial pneumonia the sputum often appears a rust colour. A specimen should be collected and despatched for culture and sensitivity preferably before any antibiotics are administered; in any event a broad spectrum antibiotic, e.g., tetracycline, is usually commenced pending pathology results and if indicated a specific antibiotic can be prescribed at a later date.

Physiotherapy

Physiotherapy techniques are not introduced until the inflammation of the lungs has started to resolve and the exudate is being expectorated. Apart from deep breathing exercises the physiotherapist may use percussion techniques over the lower chest wall and the back to vibrate the tissues which will help to loosen the exudate within the lungs, making it easier to expectorate. Such techniques should be used with caution as the patient can be readily exhausted and feel very frightened if it is done too aggressively. If the patient is not responding to either antibiotics or to physiotherapy a blood culture may then be requested to establish if the patient has a generalised subclinical septicaemia. Repeated chest X-rays are taken to monitor if the shadows on the lung caused by the consolidated exudate are being resolved with treatment and bedrest. Blood is routinely assessed for both the haemoglobin and erythrocyte levels.

Pleuritic Pain

Pleuritic pain arising from any part of the chest wall will inhibit the patient from taking a reasonable inhalation of air. Generally this type of pain should respond to a mild analgesic, e.g., codeine or aspirin, though it is unusual to give anything stronger. At regular intervals, about every 4 hours, the nurse should specifically ask the patient about the level of pain. Many patients expect that pain will occur anyway and with this expectation they may not realise it can be relieved by a mild analgesia which is usually prescribed on an 'as required' basis.

Other Symptoms

Tachycardia, headache and muscular lethargy are all quite pronounced in viral pneumonia requiring the patient to have a defined period of bedrest in a quiet well-ventilated part of the ward until the symptoms resolve from their intensity. The basic but all important skills of planning and meeting the patient's need for cleanliness, toilet facilities, and copious amounts of clear fluids to drink cannot be overstated. If there is a persistent pyrexia noted by the 4-hourly recording of body temperature, simple measures should be tried to help the patient keep cool but without any draughts. A rigor may require the nurse to seek medical permission before doing a tepid sponge bedbath. With a pyrexia or rigor the patient should remain on bedrest until the temperature has been normal for at least 48 hours.

Treatment

Antibiotics which may be prescribed include:

Benzylpenicillin 2–8 million units intramuscularly daily for pneumococcal pneumonia

Cloxacillin 2–4 gm orally each day, either as capsule or syrup for staphylococcal pneumonia

Tetracycline 500 mg in syrup or tablet form 4 times daily for mycoplasma pneumonia

Resolution of a pneumonia may take between 10 and 14 days leaving the patient both tired and anaemic. A further period of convalescence may be required until the patient recovers his or her former health. If the anaemia is very marked a short course of iron compounds may be prescribed. The complications of an untreated pneumonia include lung abscesses which can perforate through the pleura giving rise to a pneumohaemothorax. This sometimes occurs in staphylococcal pneumonia. Pleural effusion may arise if the pulmonary oedema acts as a transudate leaving the lung and crossing into the pleural cavity. If cancer is a predispositional cause of the pneumonia, it usually does not resolve even with the use of the most powerful antibiotics.

PNEUMOTHORAX

A pneumothorax refers to the presence of air in the intrapleural space. As the visceral and parietal layers are pushed apart by an increasing volume of air the effect would be to compress the underlying lung inwards and downwards resulting in dyspnoea. In normal health the pressure exerted in the pleural cavity is about 5 mmHg, i.e., negative to the intrathoracic pressure which is about 755 mmHg. These figures added together equal the pressure within the lungs, i.e., 760 mmHg or atmospheric pressure at sea level. This lung pressure is necessary for the natural recoil of the lungs during exhalation. In pneumothorax the pressures are reversed and quickly lead to painful breathlessness. Pneumothorax can either occur *spontaneously* or arise from trauma being an *open* or *tension* pneumothorax (Fig. 33.2).

Spontaneous Pneumothorax

A spontaneous pneumothorax may be either a primary condition or a secondary condition to an existing disease.

A primary spontaneous pneumothorax can be due to the rupture of a symptomless bulla, a pulmonary bleb, or a cyst within the lung which in rupturing tears a hole in the visceral pleura. These bullae and pulmonary blebs are usually congenital, and tend to be located in the upper lobes of the lung and quite near the pleura. The typical patient is a young adult male enjoying good health, and is quite fit. At the time of the spontaneous rupture a slight chest pain is experienced which is at first ignored. As time passes more air escapes into the pleura from the lung causing an increasingly marked and painful dyspnoea at the slightest exertion. A chest X-ray is the most define means of confirming the diagnosis and shows the inward compression outline around the lung.

A secondary spontaneous pneumothorax is consequent to a primary existing disease such as cancer of the lung, tuberculosis, recurrent pneumonia, pulmonary abscess and chronic bronchitis, or follows cardiac resuscitation. The symptoms are similar to those of primary pneumothorax as is the diagnosis.

Treatment

In some instances the pneumothorax is so small that the air will eventually be reabsorbed without any ill effects, merely requiring the patient to remain on bedrest for several days and be given analgesia as required.

A larger pneumothorax may require the doctor to perform a needle thoracotomy. After a local anaesthetic has been injected into the skin over the needling site a large bore needle is inserted between either the second or fifth intercostal space at the sternoclavicular midline and air allowed to escape from the pleura. When the needle is removed the assisting nurse must be ready with a seal

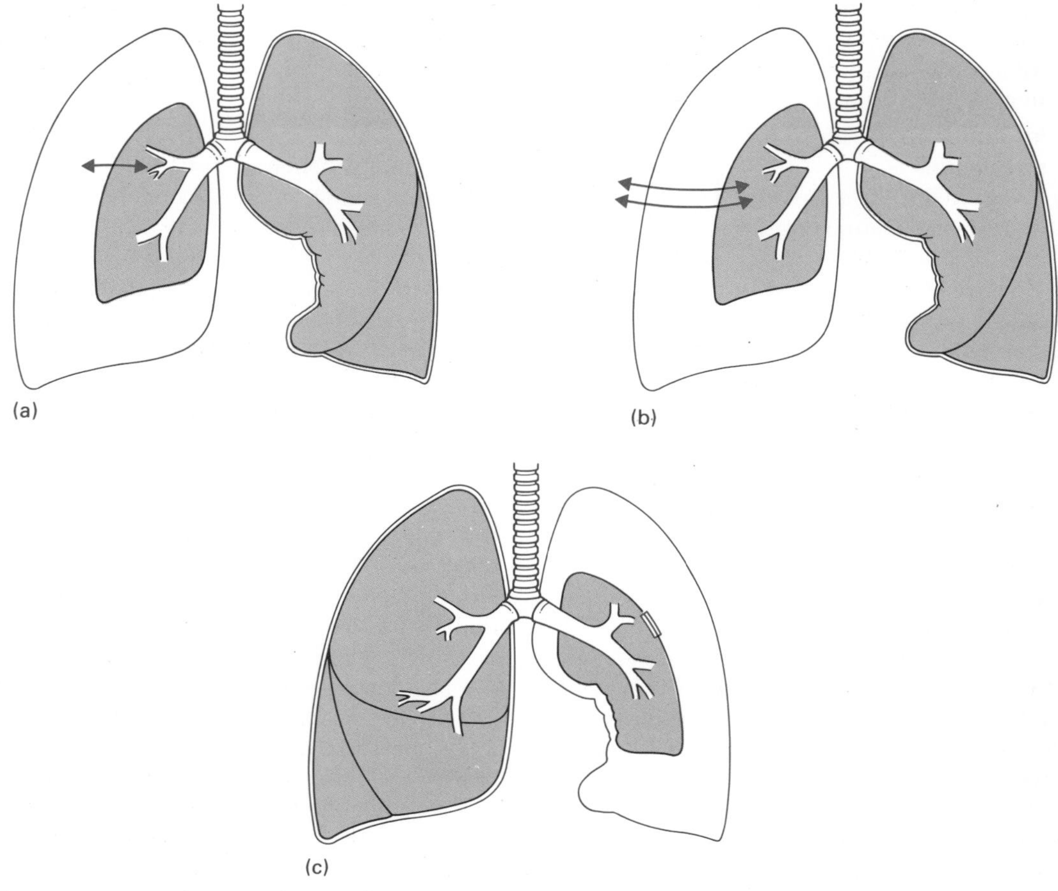

Fig. 33.2 Types of pneumothorax: closed or spontaneous (a); open (b); with sucking chest wound, and tension (c).

dressing which is immediately applied over the operated site.

Open or Tension Pneumothorax

Open and tension pneumothorax arise as the result of chest injury. With an open pneumothorax there is a sucking wound of the chest wall. Air is directly drawn in to the pleural space through an open chest wound and each time the patient inhales the rush of air causes a sucking sound. It should be noted that some of this air will be expelled as the patient exhales.

In tension pneumothorax, the chest injury is usually caused by a penetrating wound which has left a flap of tissue over the torn pleura. This flap of tissue acts as a one-way valve, on inhalation the patient draws air into the pleura but on exhalation the flap of tissue seals over the torn pleura. In this way the tension between the pleural layers becomes ever larger compressing the lung and causing a mediastinal shift. This midline shift of the heart, trachea and great vessels towards the opposite lung affects venous return to the right side of the heart. The blood flow of both the inferior and superior vena cava is drastically impeded.

Emergency Treatment

Both open and tension pneumothorax require emergency medical intervention and there are basic principles of emergency medical care with which the nurse has to assist.

1. Administration of oxygen at a high concentration and fast flow, not less than 28% concentration at a rate of 4 litre/minute. In serious cases the oxygen is given via positive pressure.

2. Needle thoracotomy is usually done to remove as much air as possible from the pleural cavity.

3. Intravenous therapy is established as quickly as possible, either with Ringer's lactate or dextrose 5%.

4. Insertion of a chest tube into the pleural space to permit continuous underwater seal drainage, thus permitting gradual re-expansion of the lung. This mechanism will also allow the pleural tear to heal naturally.

5. Continuous monitoring of the cardiac output by observing the pulse, blood pressure, cardiac monitor, renal function and general physical condition.

Persuading the patient to remain calm and rested is impossible without both sedation and analgesia being prescribed and administered. The patient will be unable to speak, will be experiencing severe choking sensations and will be extremely frightened, therefore reassurance will only be meaningful if it is combined with action to positively relieve the respiratory distress. Lifting and moving the patient is a critical manoeuvre, any rough or quick handling may risk a further tear of an already damaged pleural wall. The desired position for a patient with pneumothorax is to have him or her sitting upright with applied support over the site of injury. Once the degree of the pneumothorax is established by chest X-rays the doctor will urgently establish chest drainage.

Underwater Seal Pleural Drainage

To obtain an underwater seal pleural drainage (Fig. 33.3), a needle thoracotomy is performed either between the second or the fifth intercostal space over the affected lung usually in the sternoclavicular midline. The tip of a catheter or drain is inserted into the pleural space and secured there by a skin suture to the chest wall. A second suture thread is sewn over the drain site and its ends left loose. This 'purse' suture will be required when the chest drain is eventually removed. The drainage tubing from the chest drain to the drainage bottle is secured firmly. Within the drainage bottle a volume of sterile distilled water should cover the long glass rod for at least 2.5 cm. This water acts as a seal and prevents air travelling back up into the pleural space so long as its glass rod tip is covered by water. The drainage bottle should also have an air outlet so that excess air can escape from the bottle. When the patient exhales, air bubbles appearing in the water imply there is still air in the pleural space.

The connecting tubing between the chest drain and bottle tends to be heavy and should be secured to the bedclothing with a heavy duty safety pin to avoid any tension at the connection points. The doctor's wishes should be known with regard to the use of clamps, i.e., 2 artery forceps. Where their use is advised, each clamp is applied to either end of the connecting tubing when the nurse wishes to move the patient for nursing procedures, otherwise the clamps will remain at the bedside at all times, in case of emergency. If the clamps are not recommended then the nurse must be extra careful when moving or attending to the patient so that no tension is exerted on the connecting tubing.

On occasions the chest drain may dislodge from the chest wound. Should this occur the nurse **must immediately** apply palm pressure over the wound and summon help by pressing the emergency bell with the free hand. The drainage bottle should never be higher than the mattress level at any time. Its floor position should be known to everyone and if necessary it should be secured to the floor with adhesive tape to avoid accidents.

Observations

Observations to be continuously made during underwater seal drainage include noting if the fluid level in the long glass rod within the bottle is rising on inspiration and falling on expiration. This 'swinging' of the fluid level means that no air is entering the pleural cavity

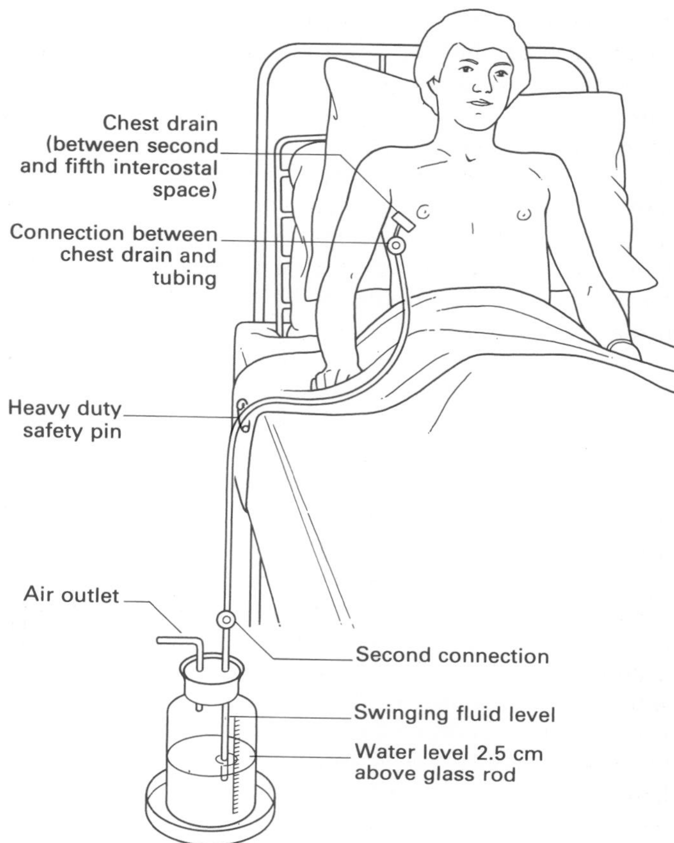

Fig. 33.3 Underwater seal drainage.

either from the wound or up the drainage tube and is taken as a good sign. The absence of the 'swing' in the fluid level should be reported immediately to a senior colleague, and as a safety measure the clamps applied to both ends of the connecting tubing. Other observations of pulse, temperature, fluid balance, and physical condition are routinely completed to obtain a total picture of the patient's responses to therapy.

When the chest drain is being used to remove pleural fluid, e.g., a haemopneumothorax, it will be necessary to change the drainage bottle at frequent intervals. This is a sterile procedure requiring the nurse to check that the replacement drainage bottle is sterile, that the bung and glass rods are not broken and that the sterile seal is within its expiry date. The bung is removed aseptically, i.e., without contaminating the inner surface of the drainage bottle, and a measured amount of distilled sterile water is poured into the drainage bottle. After the bung has been replaced firmly, the long glass rod is checked to ensure that its tip is below the level of water by at least 2.5 cm. Both clamps are then applied to the connecting tubing before the actual exchange of bottles takes place. The reconnection at the drainage bottle must be firm and secure before the clamps are removed. The nurse should remain with the patient for at least 2 minutes to check that no adverse reactions are occurring. Finally the fluid level in the old bottle is measured to calculate how much fluid has been drained from the pleural cavity.

Therapy

During the time the chest drain is in position it is usual for the patient to have a course of antibiotics as a prophylactic measure. Modified physiotherapy may be commenced but this should be matched up with the gradual re-expansion of the lung as determined by chest X-rays taken each day. The presence of the chest drain and tubing has a limiting effect on the patient's ability to move; often the patient is naturally very frightened of moving for fear of upsetting the equipment, but there is no reason why the patient cannot sit out for armchair rest so long as the integrity of the closed drainage system remains intact.

Drain Removal

When the time comes for the chest drain to be removed it should be carried out preferably by the doctor who inserted the drain. It is a useful hint to ask for and give the patient a mild sedative 30 minutes before the procedure since it may require a strong pull to actually disengage the chest tube. When the wound is exposed there should be 2 sutures. One skin suture to hold the drain in place, and a second suture with long threads. Both have to be identified before the skin suture is cut. The long ends of the purse string suture are held by the assisting nurse and when the chest drain is disengaged, while the patient exhales, the suture ends are tied off immediately as the patient inhales. This procedure can be alarming for the patient especially if the chest drain is adherent to the underlying tissues requiring a vigorous pull by the doctor, therefore a second nurse should be available to reassure the patient. After the procedure the patient should be allowed an uninterrupted period of rest.

PNEUMOCONIOSIS

Pneumoconiosis is generic in that it describes a wide ranging group of diseases induced by the effects of inhaling industrial dusts over a long period of time. They have as their common feature a progressive scarring and fibrosis of the lung tissue and a gradual loss of pulmonary function. There tends to be a higher incidence in males and invariably the specific disease refers to the industrial dusts of a specific industry. Some examples are:

Silica dust causes silicosis

Dust from asbestos mineral ore causes asbestosis

Industrial processing of talc, mica, and kaolin can induce pneumoconiosis

Coal Miner's pneumoconiosis is self-explanatory

Inorganic dusts from iron (siderosis), barium (barytosis), tin (stannosis), aluminium, carborundum, and berylium

Inhalation of decomposed vegetable matter such as dried sugar cane (bagossis), spore rich dust (farmer's lung) and yarn dust (weaver's cough)

Asbestosis

Asbestosis and silicosis are similar in symptomology, and asbestosis will be concentrated on here to give the reader some insights into how the dust of this mineral ore can ultimately lead to pneumoconiosis and highlight the necessary preventive measures taken by industry to protect the worker.

Asbestos is a naturally occurring silicate mineral ore which can be mined. It occurs in 3 states:

Blue asbestos or crocidolite
White asbestos or crysolite
Brown asbestos or amosite

The ore was used extensively in the textile, shipbuilding and car industries for both its sound proofing and fire retardant qualities. During its industrial processing random fibres released into the air can be inhaled or ingested. Sufficient exposure to this risk over a period of years will cause a progressive scarring of the lung tissues as the inhaled fibres induce a chronic inflammatory response. Such damage from the inflammation and scarring eventually reduces pulmonary ventilation with bronchial obstruction. Asbestosis is known as a precancerous disease and therefore the risks of lung, peritoneal and pancreatic cancer have a higher than usual incidence in asbestos workers.

Apart from inhaling or ingesting the asbestos fibres, the worker's family is also at risk from the dust from the worker's clothing. Those living on housing estates neighbouring onto asbestos factories or asbestos dumps are equally at risk from random atmospheric pollution. Do-it-yourself enthusiasts handling asbestos in its natural state are also at risk.

The Asbestos Research Council (1971) persuaded Parliament to bring in legislation which insisted on stringent controls during asbestos mining and manufacture. In fact blue asbestos has been withdrawn from use since 1971. Dust sampling of the air requires that the random fibres should not exceed half a fibre in 1 ml of air. Great emphasis is given to substitution fabrics wherever possible to replace asbestos, in addition to dust control by wet drilling techniques and exhaust ventilation during handling and manufacture. The individual worker is also required to wear both protective clothing and filter face masks to reduce the risk of dust inhalation.

When the precautions for control of any industrial dust are ignored it means the progressive nature of pneumoconiosis will lead to a marked exertional dyspnoea, extreme lethargy from hypoxia, recurrent pleuritic pain, and persistent coughing with slight haemophysis. Repeated chest X-rays show a gradual thickening of the pleura and diaphragm which further embarrasses respiratory effort.

Unfortunately there is no medical therapy for any of the pneumoconiosis disease entities, except palliative measures to control the worst of the symptoms of these crippling diseases. In addition the medical interest would continue to monitor for the high risk of cancer. The true answer lies in prevention and for the managers and workers to insist on safe working practice in the spirit as well as in the letter of the law.

CANCER OF THE LUNG AND BRONCHUS

The ironic and sad fact about cancer of the lung and bronchus is that in the majority of cases the disease is preventable. Of the reported annual deaths from cancer, 40% in men and 10% in women are due to lung cancer. The primary cause of this form of cancer is due to cigarette smoking; occasionally it is attributed to atmospheric pollution, e.g., asbestosis and chronic bronchitis are said to be precancerous diseases. In recent times an increasing number of cases have been attributed to exposure to radiation hazards from atomic bomb explosion fallout. A typical patient is male (8:1 ratio with women) aged between 50 and 70 years; usually an urban dweller who has been smoking cigarettes for about 20 years.

Signs and Symptoms

Lung cancer has an insidious onset with the signs and symptoms spread over a number of years. The sheer multiplicity of symptoms and their unobtrusive nature does not make the patient suspect anything is wrong until the cancer is well established.

In the early stages the patient may be aware of a slight dry cough early in the morning, but this is usually dismissed as the typical 'smoker's cough'. A slight haemoptysis is an alarming sign which may bring the patient to the doctor for the first time. Odd intermittent pleuritic and chest wall pains associated with bouts of breathlessness may be ignored since the pain may be in fact referred well away from the actual primary site of the growing cancer. For these reasons the patient may not present for help until the cancer is well advanced. This highlights the need to find a screening technique for the vulnerable population of those who smoke heavily. Such a screening technique has yet to be devised. Later symptoms which are almost diagnostic include pleural effusions, marked dyspnoea, anorexia, significant weight loss, and persistent lassitude. When taken together they add up to the classical pattern of lung cancer.

The dangers of metastasis cannot be lightly dismissed as the symptoms of a secondary cancer may be the first sign of a primary lung tumour. From the primary lung site the malignant cells penetrate through the semi-permeable pulmonary capillary walls to travel throughout the whole pulmonary circulation into the systemic blood stream. The lungs have a rich lymphatic supply and malignant cells can also travel throughout the body to deposit and commence a secondary tumour elsewhere. Intrathoracic metastasis may cause a segmental or lobar collapse and give rise to lung abscess, pleural effusion, pneumonia, pericardial effusion, and cardiac arrhythmias. The tumour can metastasize directly into the pleura and then onwards into the musculature of the chest wall.

Extrathoracic metastasis may be by the blood stream, the lymphatic system, or via the nerve tracts. Vocal cord and diaphragm paralysis may be the first obvious extrathoracic sign to be followed by peripheral neuropathy, spinal cord compression and cerebral cancer. Occasionally the lung tumour may secrete a hormone like substance which is inappropriate to the lung and induce hormonal changes mimicking an endocrine disease. With this potential to present either with a single vague symptom or a multiplicity of signs, the nurse should begin to appreciate why it is that a given patient may be subjected to a battery of tests and investigations which at first glance bear no relationship to the disease. Equally it is why some symptoms if not thoroughly pursued may leave a patient undiagnosed until it is too late.

Investigations

Non-invasive techniques of simple chest X-rays may be the first investigation to suggest the presence of a tumour by highlighting the odd shadow or contour of a tumour or a pleural fluid level.

Sputum specimens for cytology if requested should be collected in a specimen jar containing Bouin's fluid, preferably first thing in the morning when the patient's sputum is most abundant. Bronchoscopy and biopsy are usually combined, a fibreoptic bronchoscope being used on a sedated or anaesthetised patient.

Histology studies of the biopsy specimen are undertaken to identify the type of cancer cell. This is important as it may indicate the type of treatment the patient should be offered.

Squamous cell carcinoma (47% incidence) has a slow type of growth and responds well to surgical removal.

OAT cell carcinoma (17% incidence) has a rapid growth rate with a high risk of metastasis and carries a very poor prognosis.

Adenocarcinoma (16.5%), undifferentiated (16.5%) and other (3%) all carry a risk of metastasis but are amenable to other forms of treatment.

These figures suggest that over 50% of lung cancers if not diagnosed at an early stage are inoperable. Apart from being due to the cancer cell type other factors such as age, any secondary tumours, inadequate respiratory function, recurrent pneumonia, and recurrent pleural effusions may preclude surgery as the best option.

In addition to these basic investigations the patient may have extensive biochemical tests on both the blood and urine, skeletal scanning and hormonal assay in a determined effort to pinpoint the sites of any metastasis before treatment of the primary site is decided upon.

The various forms of therapy are outlined in detail in the chapter dealing with Oncology. Briefly these treatments are:

Surgery employing a thoracotomy to complete a lobectomy with the patient having a 46% survival rate after 2 years and a 29% survival rate after 5 years, or a pneumonectomy with a survival rate of 36% and 25% after 2 and 5 years respectively.

Radical radiotherapy directed at the tumour site and the associated lymphatic drainage.

Chemotherapy with the anticarcinogenic drugs possibly combined with steroids and/or immunosuppressive agents.

Palliative therapy and nursing care to control the symptoms of pain, respiratory distress and associated discomforts.

Any nursing plan for such a patient presents a challenge as the problems will be unique and different in a more dramatic way than for other types of patient. The particular physical and psychological discomforts cannot be anticipated, except to say that should the patient be admitted to hospital for palliative care then the nurse should bear in mind that the nursing plan must meet the particular needs of the dying patient.

Chapter 34
Care of the Patient for Thoracic Surgery

COMMON THORACIC OPERATIONS

The most common thoracic operations following an exploratory thoracotomy include:

Wedge resection of the peripheral part of one lung where a lesion is localised to the edge of the surrounding pleura.

Segmental resection where each lobe is built up from anatomical segments with an independant blood supply. It is therefore possible to remove one or several segments from one lobe if for example the segment has a chronic lung abscess which did not respond to conservative therapy.

Lobectomy or the removal of one lobe may be undertaken if there is a diagnosed cyst, benign tumour or a localised cancer.

Pneumonectomy is the removal of a lung and such major surgery is usually reserved for bronchial cancer or if there is a unilateral bronchiectasis.

Basic Preparation

For each operation the nurse should appreciate that the patient will have to be prepared for a thoracotomy, i.e., an incision into and through the intercostal muscles with resection of one or several ribs. The operations are of course designed to cure intractable symptoms of respiratory distress and remove the source or cause. The emphasis for the nurse, therefore, is on being positive during the preparation and following the surgery.

It is usual to admit the patient at least 48 hours before the operation is scheduled to take place to prepare the patient physically and psychologically, and to take into account the social background into which the patient will be returned. An initial step in planning the patient's care is to study the investigations which have already been completed by the out-patients department and to gather together all known results. Further investigations required by the surgeon during this planning stage can be integrated into the care plan.

Investigations

Electrocardiograms to detect any cardiac abnormality.

Bronchoscopy and biopsy would have normally been done on an out-patient basis but the histology studies should be available to the surgeon.

Repeat X-rays of the chest are normally requested for comparison with the most recent to note if there are any further radiological changes, and to preclude lung infection.

Culture and sensitivity tests on specimens of sputum are routinely requested to note if there is any current chest infection.

Blood specimens are taken for grouping and cross-matching of at least 2 units of blood, which should be available to the theatre department for use during surgery.

Pulmonary function tests have invariably been completed in the out-patients department.

Specific points which the nurse should ensure are completed in the physical preparation of the patient and can be generally applied to all thoracotomy patients involve:

1. A complete physical examination by the anaesthetist in the expectation of a prolonged anaesthetic time and its effect on both the heart and the unaffected lung.
2. Prophylactic antibiotics are commenced as soon as possible to subordinate any risk of postoperative infection.
3. To improve upon the existing pulmonary ventilation, bronchodilator drugs either in tablet or nebulized form may be prescribed.

It is important that the patient's oral and dental hygiene are of the highest standard, and these should be assessed in detail. Mild antiseptic mouthwashes offered every 4 hours should be part of the preoperative routine and frequent brushing of teeth should be encouraged in the patient to reduce the real risk of postoperative chest infection arising from an infected mouth or throat. If necessary the patient may have to undergo a dental clearance if the teeth are obviously in a decayed state. A throat swab may be requested to exclude oropharyngeal infection. The nurse should also inspect the outer ear canal for signs of infection. If present, it should be drawn to the attention of the surgeon.

Postural drainage is normally done twice a day, in the morning and evening, to drain particular segments and lobes of the lung for at least 20 minutes in each session. The correct method of coughing may have to be demonstrated to the patient as in the postoperative phase deep coughing is used to keep the bronchi clear of excess mucus. The patient is asked to take as deep a breath as possible and while pressing into and on the abdominal muscles with both hands he or she coughs from the diaphragm.

For 5 minutes in every hour the patient should be supervised doing deep breathing exercises. This involves inhaling to the maximum holding the breath for the count of 5 and then exhaling slowly. These physiotherapy techniques will improve the existing pulmonary function and also reduce the risk of postoperative infection. Incidentally the patient is also learning what to expect in the postoperative period as the deep coughing and deep breathing are continued after the initial recovery period.

Physiotherapy

Since the incision will extend from the anterior chest midline to the posterior thoracic midline the underlying musculature strength of the shoulder girdle and the intercostal muscles of the affected lung can be expected to lose their strength and tone. With a rib resection included, the patient's posture is altered slightly. To counteract these risks the patient is shown a series of exercises for the arms and shoulder girdle. The exercises include extension, flexion, and circumduction movements of part and then the whole limb. These exercises are also included in the postoperative care plan.

The patient can be expected to be thin and rather emaciated as a result of the prolonged illness. An appraisal of weight, haemoglobin count, and hydration level may determine specific dietary needs. However, the patient should be encouraged to select a high protein, high carbohydrate diet from the menu choice with vitamin and mineral supplements added if required. The desired fluid intake should be at least 2500 ml per 24 hours to achieve a good renal output.

Additional to the specific physical points already mentioned the nurse is responsible for ensuring that basic procedures are completed such as skin cleanliness, shaving, urinalysis, consent to surgery and the correct identity of the patient and operation site.

Patient Counselling

Psychological fears regarding the proposed operation and the eventual outcome affect both the patient and family. The nurse should spend some time with them offering counselling sessions to discuss what will happen and take the opportunity of exploring the patient's fears. The following guidelines will help the nurse plan for and carry out the necessary counselling while also giving the patient reassurance.

Postoperative Pain

Postoperative pain can be quite severe and is the result of the nerve fibres running along each rib being cut. The surgeon and anaesthetist will usually prescribe a definite programme of analgesic drugs to be administered for the first 48 hours after surgery. Despite this, the patient may still have pain and should be encouraged to tell the nurse rather than suffer in silence. From the nurse's point of view postoperative thoracic pain may indicate a complication of surgery. Equally pain control is in everybody's interest to obtain the maximum co-operation for the essential physiotherapy.

Disorientation

On recovery from surgery the patient may be either in the recovery room or in the intensive therapy unit for the first 24 hours of care. The patient may be nursed by someone he or she does not know. This can lead to a minor disorientation if the patient is not warned about a strange environment.

Equipment

Additional to details about the wound, the patient needs to know a little about the various pieces of equipment to which he or she will be attached. The surgeon may be able to be specific about the types of chest drain or tubing intended for postoperative use. Usually there will be an intravenous infusion, an oxygen mask, and possibly a cardiac monitor. If not advised of this equipment the patient may inadvertently struggle against the awkwardly placed items risking his or her own well-being.

Frequent Observations

During the first 6–12 hours after the operation, the patient should not be alarmed by being frequently disturbed as the nurse is making and recording essential observations to ensure that everything is going according to plan. It does mean, however, that the patient will have little chance to rest during this very critical time. If this point is not explained many patients believe themselves to be far more critically ill than otherwise and the resulting anxiety will delay their expected progress, and incidentally lower their physical pain threshold.

Visitors

It is preferred if the family or close friends can confine their visits to very short periods during the first 48 hours after surgery and to rely on the nursing staff for details of the patient's progress. Each visit should be for no more than 10 minutes and only the next-of-kin permitted to visit in this time.

Home Assessment

There are many more points which emerge during the counselling with the individual patient and many of these relate to the social dynamics of the patient's own domestic situation. Often it is advisable to delve into the home conditions to ensure that the patient has a reasonable chance to convalesce and make a full recovery. While the surgery may be successful, the actual recovery may be hindered by circumstances outside of the surgeon's remit and for this a home assessment may be useful to highlight social difficulties.

Preoperative Care

One hour before surgery it is usual to give the patient a premedication with a higher than usual amount of atropine which ensures any bronchial secretions are inhibited completely. The type of anaesthesia used is usually administered via an endotracheal tube after an intravenous injection to thoroughly relax the voluntary muscles.

Postoperative Care

In preparing to receive the patient back from theatre, the nurse should have in mind that the patient will need a firm mattress supported by either wooden boards or a metal-based framework. Both the oxygen and suction equipment should be checked and functional, and ready with the appropriate masks and catheters. The surgeon will normally indicate if underwater seal drainage is to be expected and it may be necessary to anticipate a tracheostomy on some occasions. In some units a thoracocentesis pack, i.e., pleural aspiration pack, is held as an emergency standby. Intravenous therapy is invariably used and a cardiac monitor should be available as an option. Observation charts should be prepared and the necessary equipment immediately available at the bedside with which to carry out basic observations.

A specific plan of postoperative care should include several features.

Immediate Phase

Correct positioning of the patient's head to the right or left maintains the airway while the anaesthetic drugs remain effective and this may be for several hours after the initial recovery of the swallow reflex.

Observations of the pulse, blood pressure and respiration are taken every 15 minutes for the first 3 hours and then every 30 minutes for the following 3 hours. At this point the patient should be reviewed by the surgeon for further instructions.

Oxygen is administered at the prescribed flow rate continuously until otherwise instructed. The drying effect of this gas is not desirable and it may be humidified if oxygen is being given for a prolonged interval.

The flow drip rate of the intravenous infusion should not exceed 50 drops/minute to prevent pulmonary oedema should there be any risk of overtransfusion. Removal of part or a whole lung removes a considerable amount of blood vessel surface area and therefore the risk of overtransfusion is correspondingly increased. Accurate fluid balance charting and observations for bubbling chest noises or dependant oedema should continue for as long as the patient is having an intravenous infusion.

Patency and security of the chest drain and chest tubing attached to an underwater seal drainage system should be checked frequently in the first few hours of postoperative care. The chest drain should be monitored for haemorrhage and the chest tubing for 'swinging' of the fluid level to detect the risk of pneumothorax.

Intermediate Phase

The intermediate phase involves the period 6–12 hours after the operation. Control of the rib cage pain is absolutely vital and the prescribed analgesia **should** have been commenced and **must** be administered.

Minimal oral fluids should now be commenced and gradually increased in volume each hour until the patient can tolerate 120 ml each hour.

The turning and movement of the patient is related to the surgery. It is usual for the head of the bed to be raised or tilted to an angle of between 30° and 45° to correct the position of the diaphragm so that it will fall into its natural alignment on the operated side.

For pneumonectomy the patient should never be turned onto the unaffected side. If this is allowed to happen and the suture line of the operated lung ruptures, the healthy lung may be flooded with blood, or be affected by a mediastinal shift.

For segmental and wedge resection surgery the patient should not be turned onto the affected side, otherwise the operated lung may not expand adequately.

For lobectomy patients the alternative positions of care are without any danger, being limited only by the presence of chest drains and tubes.

Physiotherapy should commence 30 minutes after the first analgesic injection. It is best if the patient commences with a few deep breaths each hour and then the nurse supporting the patient at the front and back will ask him or her to make a deep cough. This will be painful for the patient but is made somewhat easier if the patient is supported firmly. Arm and shoulder exercises are also commenced, very gently at first and if need be aided by the nurse, i.e., passive physiotherapy.

Comforting measures such as care of the skin, changing bedwear, attending to the patient's toilet needs and appearance, will improve the patient's morale before being settled for a defined period of rest if the observations are reduced in their frequency.

Late Phase

The late phase involves care of the patient 24 hours after the operation.

The amount of bedrest is determined by the type of operation. For a lobectomy it may be possible to ambulate the patient in a bedside chair in 24–48 hours. For a pneumonectomy it may be 5 days before the patient is allowed out of bed. Wedge and segmental resection surgery requires only a short period of bedrest for the patient, e.g., 24 hours.

The care of the wound is minimal, leaving the covering dressing intact for as long as possible and confining the care to observing for staining with fresh blood, in which case the surgeon must be informed immediately. The chest drain is usually secured to the midline of the incision and drains any wound exudate. This tube is shortened by 2.5 cm after 48 hours and thereafter shortened daily until it is finally removed. The chest tube is usually secured at the base of the incision and remains attached to the underwater seal drainage until the chest X-rays taken each day determine when and if the pleura is free of any fluid or air; the tube can then be removed. Should the pleura suffer either a pneumothorax or hydrothorax a pleural aspiration may be completed as an emergency measure.

Observations

During the recovery phase the nursing observations should centre upon noting if any of the following adverse combinations of symptoms are occurring indicating specific complications of thoractomy surgery:

Cardiac arrhythmias on the cardiac monitor imply that the nurse should increase the recordings of the radial pulse, noting not only the pulse rate but the volume and rhythm. It is possible that it is an early indication of mediastinal shift.

Cyanosis, **dyspnoea** and **sudden chest pain** if combined may suggest a postoperative atelectasis or a tension pneumothorax requiring immediate surgical intervention.

Pallor, **tachycardia** and **hypotension** are indicative of internal haemorrhage. The chest wound dressings should also be checked for any bloodstaining. Immediate surgical intervention is required as the anastomosis within the lung is possibly rupturing or breaking down and would require the patient to go back to theatre as soon as possible.

Pyrexia, foul breath and **increased amounts of sputum** may indicate a chest infection, e.g., pneumonia, which requires vigorous treatment with antibiotics and intensive physiotherapy.

Counselling for Discharge

As the patient makes satisfactory progress to recovery the nurse should increasingly turn attention to assessing and planning for the patient's discharge from hospital. Postoperative counselling should take into account the following:

Those patients with a pneumonectomy should be instructed not to sleep on the affected side for at least a further 6 months to allow for complete healing of the area. The main danger is mediastinal shift.

Deep breathing exercises should become part of the patient's everyday routine, perhaps setting aside 5 or 10 minutes each morning and afternoon for the exercises.

Body alignment exercises done in front of a full-length mirror should help the patient with correct posture, especially the tendency of the affected shoulder to tilt downwards and the rib cage to recede a little taking with it the spinal cord.

To minimise the risk of infection the patient should avoid smoky or dust-polluted atmospheres and continue with a high standard of oral and dental hygiene. He or she should also be more than usually careful about coming into contact with upper respiratory tract infections, especially during the winter months.

The advised period of convalescence is a period of at least 2–3 weeks for wedge and segmental resection and up to 8 weeks for lobectomy or pneumonectomy. The patient, who has probably never enjoyed a good tolerance physical stress level, may find some improvement, but this is limited by the operation. It will be about 8 weeks before he or she knows the true potential of physical endurance, and in a subtle way this advice has implications for the patient's own body image. If the nurse is in any way negative, the patient may not reach their true potential.

As with all surgery these patients should be advised to take specific periods of rest each day until they feel they have reached their maximal independent health status.

DISORDERS OF THE OESOPHAGUS

Fortunately, disease and disorder of the oesophagus is rare but, since the principal symptom is invariably dysphagia or difficulty in swallowing, the patient may be referred for treatment from many specialists. Access to the oesophagus is mainly by thoracotomy, and it is for this reason that it is placed in this section of the book (Fig. 34.1).

The oesophagus is a hollow muscular tube about 25 cm in length extending from the pharynx to the cardiac junction of the stomach. At its terminal portion it penetrates the crura or hiatus opening of the diaphragm. In its descent through the thorax, it slightly inclines to the left in its posterior position to the trachea. Normally the muscular walls remain flattened unless involved in deglutination or peristalsis, its two main functions. Similar to the other parts of the gastrointestinal tract, it has 3 main coats:

An **inner lining** of mucous membrane composed of keratinised squamous epithelium.

A **submucosal layer** containing goblet cells which secrete a small amount of mucus to lubricate the inner wall and ease the passage of food.

Its **muscular wall** which consists of fibres that travel in both a longitudinal and circular direction to perform efficient peristalsis. The upper third of the oesophagus is composed of voluntary muscle, which means the individual still retains some control over swallowing, but the middle and lower third is composed of involuntary muscle, i.e., the control is exercised via the autonomic nervous system. Within the muscular fibres are nerve plexus (Aurbach's) which relay nerve impulses to and from the muscle fibres. Peristaltic movement of the oesophagus is similar to

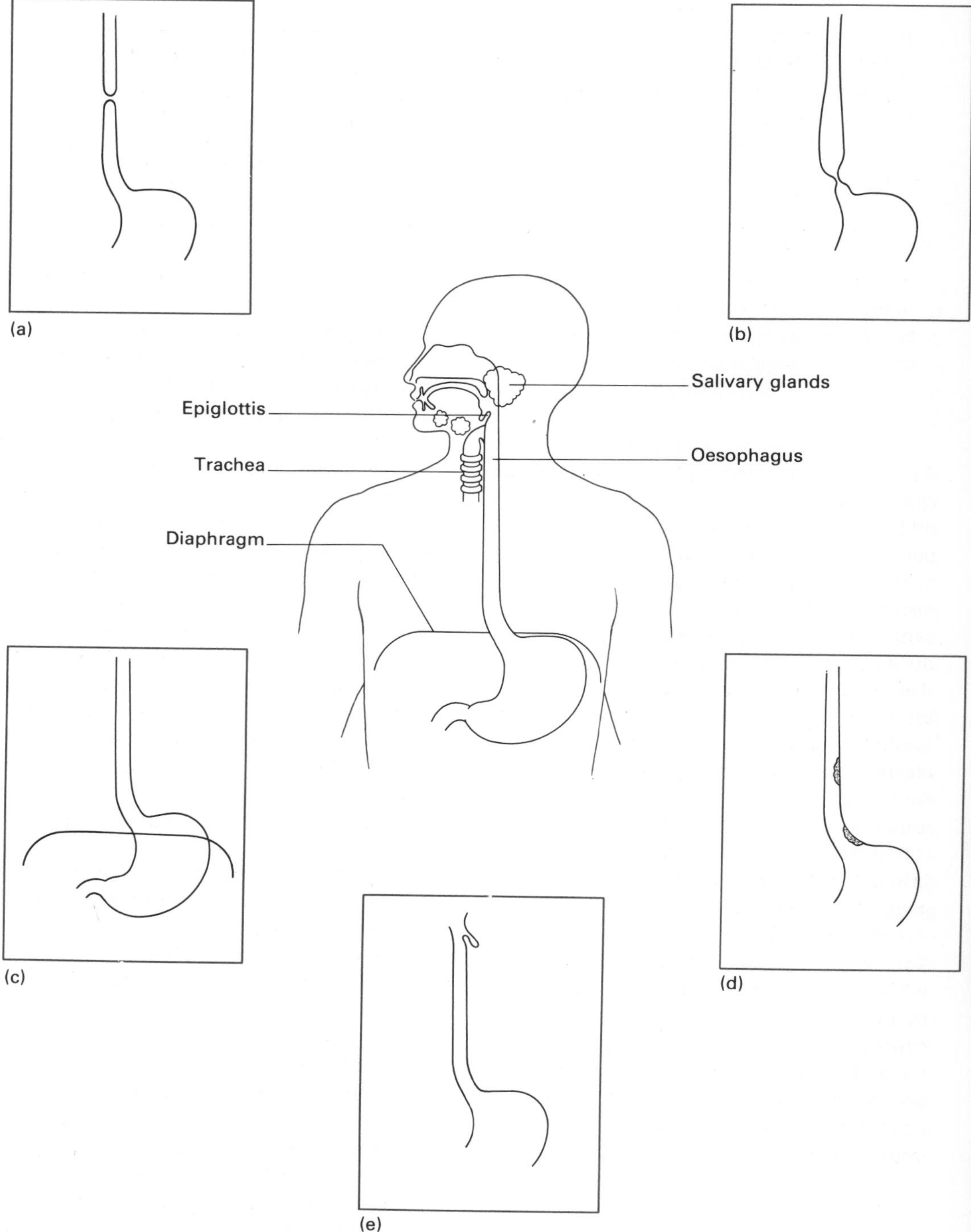

Fig. 34.1 Disorders of the oesophagus; atresia (a); achalasia (b); hiatus hernia (c); cancer (d); diverticulum (e).

Table 34.1. Causes of dysphagia

Nerve supply aberration	Extrinsic causes	Intrinsic factors
Diphtheria Myasthenia gravis Globus hystericus Achalasia Oesophageal spasm	Compression of mediastinal structures	Congenital atresia Oesophagitis Diverticulitis Hiatus hernia Plummer-Vinson syndrome Carcinoma

the movements of a worm, contracting and relaxing each section until the bolus of food being swallowed is forced through the cardiac sphincter into the stomach.

Dysphagia

As mentioned, dysphagia is the cardinal symptom of disorders of the oesophagus. This difficulty in swallowing can often be pinpointed to the exact section if the patient is asked to fingerpoint to the location of discomfort. Dysphagia does not occur as a symptom on its own, perhaps because there is an associated loss of body weight, anaemia, dehydration, excess salivation, difficulty with speech and pressure on the trachea which all hinder respiration. These associated problems require a nursing assessment and an applied care plan to relieve physical distress. Correct nursing positioning, tube feeding, communication charts and a balanced fluid intake and urinary output may be a few of the nursing points to be implemented.

The causes of dysphagia are listed in Table 34.1 and it is proposed to deal only with those with which the nurse may come into contact in his or her general experience. Common causes of dysphagia, (e.g., tonsillitis, quinsy, stomatitis and pharyngolaryngeal pouching) are readily identified on an ENT physical examination and are amenable to conservative treatment.

Achalasia

The abnormal dilation of the oesophagus is associated with poor motility due to the absence of innervation of Auerbach's nerve plexus in the muscular wall of the oesophagus. The lack of innervation means that the muscle layers will atrophy and become increasingly dilated until eventually the oesophagus adopts a funnel shape with a narrow tip at the oesophageal cardiac junction. In an extreme case, food remains trapped in this dilated tube and will stagnate. The putrified food may then spill over from the oesophagus into the trachea and enter the bronchi. This is more likely to happen if the cardiac region of the oesophageal junction remains in tonic contraction and the nerve ganglion cells are few and scant within the muscular wall. The patient will suffer reflex vomiting, severe halitosis, marked weight loss and dehydration, and a pneumonia is a very real risk. Once invasive investigations begin, the nurse is usually requested to prepare the patient for a barium swallow and possibly an oesophagoscopy.

The treatment of achalasia is usually by surgery. An oesophagomyotomy, or Heller's operation, if done, will mean that the circular fibres at the base of the oesophagus are cut leaving the longitudinal fibres intact. This should widen the oesophageal-cardiac junction, permitting food to enter the stomach.

Oesophagitis

Inflammation of the oesophagus is always chemical in origin; either by swallowing corrosive substances accidentally or, more commonly, as the result of gastric juice reflux. The constant bathing of the oesophageal mucosa by gastric juice, which is very acid, will eventually cause a chronic inflammation and fibrosis of the lower third of the oesophagus.

Oesophagitis is more commonly associated

with those who are obese and when the intra-abdominal pressure is raised, such as in pregnancy. In both these conditions, the cardiac sphincter is forced open, which results in gastric juice reflux. Sometimes the pain of oesophagitis is so severe and located retrosternally that it can be similar to a myocardial infarction.

A third cause can be hiatus hernia; the upper portion of the stomach rolls upwards through the hiatus, or opening in the diaphragm, and comes to rest in the thorax. Gastric juice is then trapped in a U-shaped loop at the oesophageal-cardiac junction. If the inflammatory condition does lead to a fibrosis, the possible complication would be oesophageal stricture and eventually complete dysphagia.

Treatment

After the diagnosis has been confirmed by a detailed medical history, barium swallow and oesophagoscopy, treatment may follow one of several avenues:

Conservative advice to reduce weight, sleeping in an upright sitting position, and avoiding excessive stooping or bending should help to diminish gastric juice reflux, and thus help natural healing.

Conservative medication, such as antacids, should be taken regularly to buffer the effects of the gastric acid juices.

Surgical procedures to correct gastric reflux, which include:

1. Oesophagoscopy and dilation of the oesophagus with bougies, if a stricture due to fibrosis is present.

2. Repair of a hiatus hernia, either via the abdomen or a thoracotomy, providing the patient has reduced their weight to ensure the cardiac sphincter can naturally close.

3. A partial gastrectomy or a vagotomy and pyloroplasty may be done if the patient has an associated peptic ulcer; these operations reduce gastric acidity by removing the gastric cells or reducing their secretion.

Cancer of the Oesophagus

The type of cancer most frequently found by biopsy is the *squamous cell carcinoma*, i.e., a slow growth with limited metastasis. It tends to occur in the mid-section of the oesophagus. If it spreads, it usually does so in a downward direction and involves the lower third of the oesophagus. While this type of cancer mostly affects males over 40 years old, when it occurs in women it may present as the Vinson Plummer syndrome.

A series of symptoms, if grouped and occurring together, i.e., iron deficiency anaemia, dysphagia, glossitis, and mucosal oedema of the postcricoid space, are strongly suggestive of oesophageal cancer. The local mediastinal lymph nodes are usually enlarged. If asked, the patient can usually fingerpoint the precise location of the tumour.

Radiology of the oesophagus and endoscopy with biopsy will clarify if the obstruction is actually a malignant tumour; a few are benign. The treatment of choice for an individual patient will depend on all factors when taken together.

Radiotherapy has a 10% success rate, either with radiation therapy or insertion of radium needles.

Surgical resection of the oesophageal tumour via a thoracotomy with anastomosis between the remaining oesophagus and stomach poses a major problem in that the anastomosis remains a structural weakness for a long time. Any rupture of this delicate junction implies a leakage of oesophageal contents into the thorax.

Palliative therapy for an inoperable tumour is to insert a polyvinyl inert oesophageal tube, i.e., a tube prosthesis such as the Celestin or Mourau Barbin tubes. The oesophagus is initially bougied to allow for the tube to be comfortably passed. The tube allows for the taking of food with reasonable comfort, but can become readily blocked. The patient has to be taught how to cleanse the tube, both before and after taking a meal of softened or liquified food. A solution of either sodium bicarbonate, or a weakened solution of hydrogen peroxide, is frequently used to remove particles of food obstructing the lower end of the tube.

In addition to correcting the patient's nutritional status, it should be remembered that the majority of these patients are also terminally ill; the nursing care plan will need to take this into account.

Part 4
Endocrinology Nursing

Chapter 35
Overview of the Endocrine System

Endocrine means within but separate. It refers to one gland producing substances within its structure but when the substance is secreted it has its effect on a separate structure.

Hormones

The substance secreted, a *hormone* (to excite), is in effect a chemical messenger, transported via the blood from its production gland to have its effect on a specific target tissue. Hormones are quite specific to their target tissues, locking on to the cell wall in a very specific manner, i.e., the *lock and key theory*. A hormone always stimulates its target site towards increased activity, and the hormone itself can be utilised from 1 of 3 sources. The majority are short or long chain polypeptides, i.e., amino acids; several are derived from amines, while a third group are derived from steroids.

Hormones are secreted from 2 main sites:

Ductless glands—the hormone passes directly from the gland structure into the blood stream

Humoral sites—tissues or organs other than the endocrine glands

Whatever their original source, the hormones control or influence many physiological functions, working in harmony with the autonomic and central nervous system to achieve a biological balance.

The Hypothalamus and Pituitary Gland

Exerting an overall influence on the body's functions is the hypothalamus. This area of the brain is increasingly regarded as a form of biological clock. Its functions are to influence sleep pattern, temperature regulation, thirst, appetite, sodium regulation, and it is the main centre for responding to emotional states. Given these functions, many of which are rhythmic in nature, and its sensitivity to the cerebral neurotransmitters noradrenaline, dopamine, and serotonin, it is immediately feasible that it exerts an overall influence on the endocrine system.

In response to the cerebral neurotransmitters the hypothalamus automatically secretes *releasing* factors or *inhibiting* factors which influence the acknowledged main endocrine gland the pituitary gland. In its turn the pituitary gland releases or inhibits stimulating hormones to the various endocrine glands.

FEEDBACK MECHANISMS

The stimulus for hormone secretion is by one of several feedback mechanisms; negative feedback (direct and indirect), short feedback, positive feedback, open loop control and the autonomic and central nervous system influence.

Negative Feedback

Direct

Direct negative feedback refers to the relationship between hormone release and the existing plasma level of the substance it controls, e.g., insulin release and blood glucose levels (Fig. 35.1). It is a negative system because nothing else is required to maintain blood glucose level.

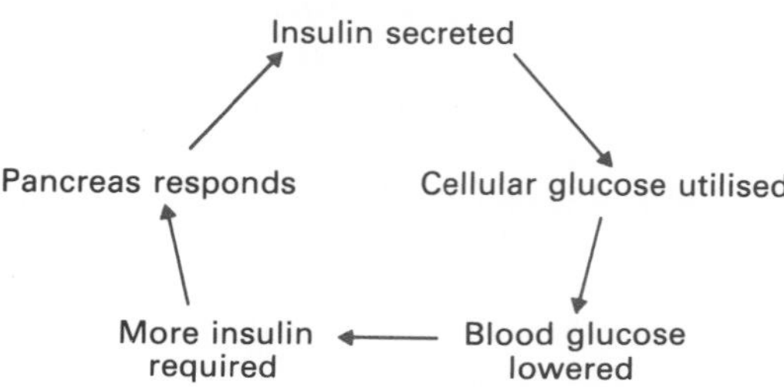

Fig. 35.1 Direct negative feedback system.

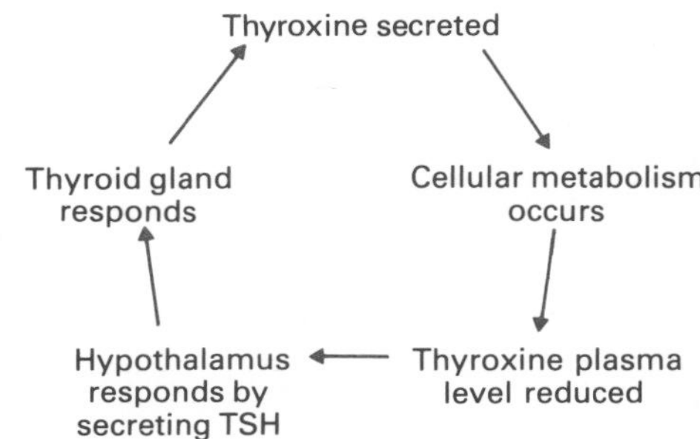

Fig. 35.2 Indirect negative feedback system.

Indirect

Indirect negative feedback refers to the fact that further hormone release depends on the releasing factors secreted by the hypothalamus, e.g., the thyroid gland (Fig. 35.2).

Short Feedback

A short feedback system refers to the relationship between the hypothalamus and the pituitary system only (Fig. 35.3 and Table 35.1).

Positive Feedback

Positive feedback is when a hormone has a direct effect on the pituitary in stimulating further release regardless of the existing plasma level. It is exerting a positive effect. This can be dangerous and usually requires secondary controlling mechanisms to keep the plasma levels within a normal range, e.g., oestrogens (Fig. 35.4).

Open Loop Control System

The open loop control system refers to the many external stimuli influencing the higher centres of the brain, e.g., the cerebellum and medulla oblongata. These in turn transmit neurochemical messages to the hypothalamus. The hypothalamus will either secrete releasing factors or inhibiting substances to adjust the needs of the body in its response to external stimuli.

Table 35.1 Examples of short feedback system

Target organ	Hormone secreted	Activity stimulated
Thyroid gland	Thyroxine	Cellular activity regulated
	Tri-iodothyronine	Quick acting cellular metabolism
	Calcitonin	Opposes the effect of parathormone
Parathyroid glands	Parathormone	Maintains calcium level in the blood
Adrenal glands	Aldosterone	Assists in regulating sodium levels
	Cortisone	Multiple effect on carbohydrate and protein
	Adrenaline	Stimulates autonomic nervous system
	Noradrenaline	Stimulates autonomic and central nervous system
Ovaries and uterus	Oestrogen	Menstrual cycle and female characteristics
	Progesterone	Stimulate endometrium for pregnancy
	Oxytocin	Uterine contraction in third stage of labour
Testes	Testosterone	Male secondary sexual characteristics
Pancreas	Insulin	Permits glucose through cell walls
	Glucagon	Promotes glucose release from liver
	Somatostatin	Inhibits production of growth hormone
Gut	Gastrin	Maintains secretion of hydrochloric acid
	Secretin	Increases secretion of pancreatic juice
	Cholecystokinin-pancreozymin	Contracts gall bladder
	Glucagon	Stimulates pancreatic secretion
Kidney	Renin	Stimulates secretion of aldosterone
	Erythropoietin	Stimulates production of erythrocytes
	Antidiuretic hormone	Regulates absorption of water in renal tubules

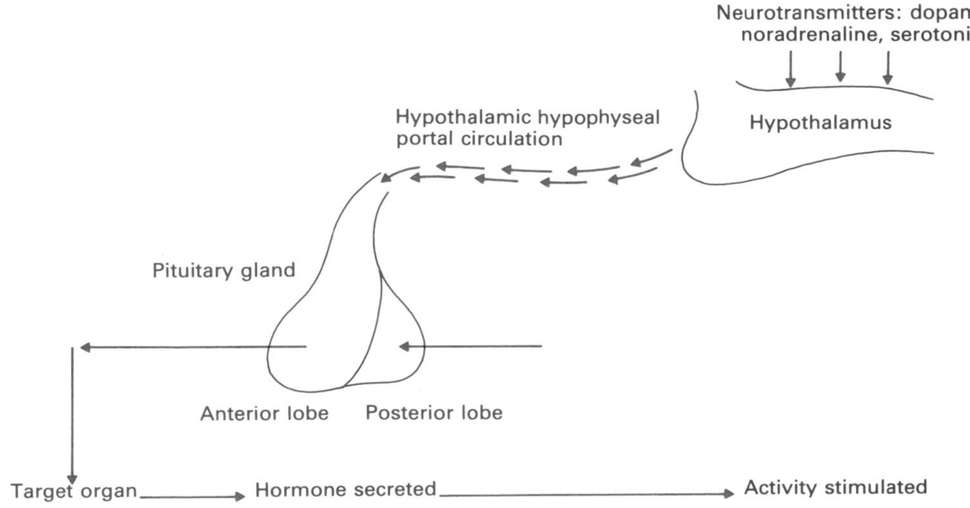

Fig. 35.3 Short feedback system.

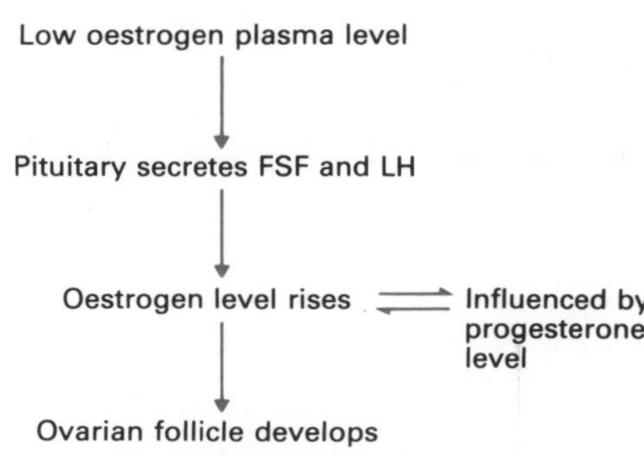

Fig. 35.4 Positive feedback system.

Autonomic and Central Nervous System

The autonomic and central nervous system influence is notably the posterior lobe of the pituitary and the adrenal medulla which are both directly controlled by nerve impulses originating from the hypothalamus. In each case their response is mediated by the neurotransmitter, acetylcholine. The eventual hormone release from the posterior lobe and adrenal medulla is regulated and controlled by autonomic reflex responses, e.g., antidiuretic hormone control.

Chapter 36
Pituitary Gland Disorders

The pituitary gland is a pea-sized structure weighing less than 1 g. It is located in the sella turcica, a depression in the sphenoid bone, immediately behind but slightly above the nasal cavity and below the optic chiasma. The gland is attached by a neural stalk to the third ventricle of the brain; this stalk (the infundibulum) conveys blood vessels from the hypothalamus to the pituitary gland.

The gland is divided into two distinct lobes and the anterior and posterior lobes are separated by the pars intermedia (Fig. 36.1). The **anterior** lobe is purely secretory being

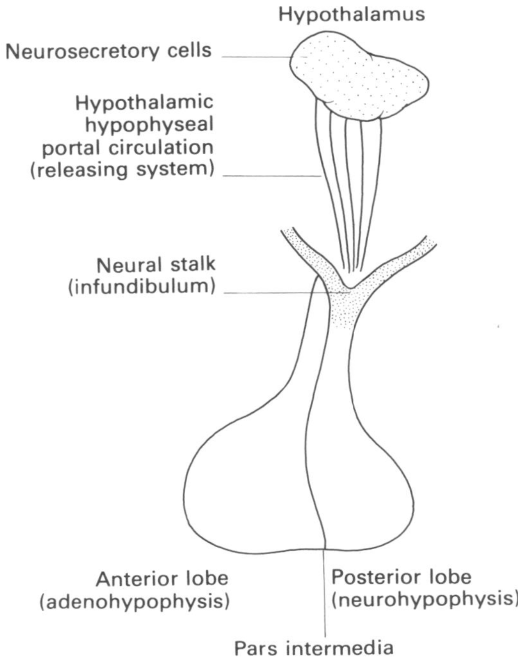

Fig. 36.1 The hypothalamic-hypophyseal system.

influenced by releasing hormones from the hypothalamus. There are 3 cell types: basophil, acidophil, and chromophobe. These cells secrete:

Growth hormone (somatotrophin)
Thyroid stimulating hormone
Adrenocorticotrophic hormone
Melanocyte stimulating hormone
Prolactin (lactogenic hormone)
Follicular stimulating hormone } gonadotrophins
Luteinizing hormone }

The **posterior** lobe, also referred to as the *neurohyphosis*, is a storehouse for 2 hormones manufactured and secreted by the neurosecretory cells of the hypothalamus.

Antidiuretic hormone (vasopressin) acts on the renal tubules to increase water reabsorption. The controlling mechanism is by the neurone receptors in the hypothalamus which are sensitive to plasma osmolality. Nicotine and morphia are also known to stimulate antidiuretic hormone (ADH) release, while alcohol opposes the effect of ADH causing the typical diuretic effect after a spell of drinking. In excessive secretion ADH causes a transient syndrome referred to as an *inappropriate* ADH secretion, while a deficiency causes cranial diabetes insipidus.

Oxytocin is released for the contraction of uterine muscle during labour. Its synthetic preparation is used therapeutically during the third stage of labour. This hormone also establishes milk secretion when the newborn infant is first put to suckle. Excess oxytocin secretion is unknown, a deficiency may occur in association with cranial diabetes insipidus, and while a deficiency would delay the third stage of labour, it does not affect milk secretion.

Over- or under-production of growth hormone from the anterior lobe and lack of antidiuretic hormone from the posterior lobe are 2 examples of pituitary gland disorders.

GROWTH HORMONE

Growth hormone is species specific. This implies that growth hormone extracts from animals are inappropriate for treatment of human growth disorders.

Its release from the pituitary gland is dependant on releasing hormone from the hypothalamus. Surprisingly the plasma levels remain proportionate to size even after puberty when perhaps the human has reached maximal linear growth. The adult output is on average 1–4 mg per day.

The specific functions of this large molecular hormone are to:

1. Promote linear growth of bone until epiphyseal union is complete.
2. Develop the subcutaneous tissues.
3. Assist in the synthesis of protein for cellular repair and growth.
4. Assist in the breakdown of fat.
5. Oppose the effects of insulin.
6. Stimulate the parathyroid glands to secrete parathormone.

Growth hormone plasma levels when measured are known to be raised during sleep, and at their lowest immediately after a meal. Apart from the demands of growth, the hormone is also released when there is a prolonged emotional stress, traumatic injury, major surgery, extremes of heat or cold, severe exercise, hypoglycaemia, and prolonged malnutrition. There is now evidence to show that it is inhibited in children suffering from maternal deprivation. The effects of growth hormone are opposed by hyperglycaemia (diabetes mellitus) and by the drugs somatostatin and bromocriptine (Fig. 36.2).

Oversecretion

Acromegaly

Acromegaly is a chronic disease and occurs in 1 in 50000 persons. Due to the oversecretion of growth hormone there is progressive enlargement of the bones of the head, face, hands, feet and thorax. It is most often seen during the late stages, when diagnosis is easy but treatment far more difficult. The cause of the oversecretion is usually due to a tumour arising from one of the cell types in the anterior lobe, e.g., basophil adenoma. Alternatively, a tumour arising immediately in the

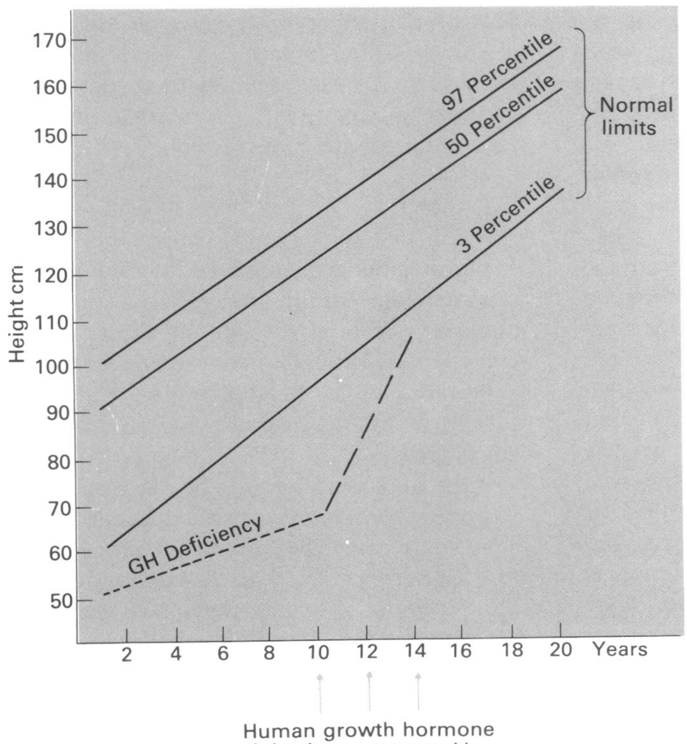

Fig. 36.2 Effects of growth hormone.

vicinity of the sella turcica can be pressing inwards into the pituitary fossa. Occasionally it is seen in patients suffering from a hormone-secreting tumour, e.g., cancer of the bronchus or stomach, but in these instances the cancer symptoms will have dominance over the acromegaly.

Signs and Symptoms

Should acromegaly occur before puberty the linear growth rate will be phenomenal, but there will be poor development of the secondary sexual characteristics, i.e., *gigantism*. In adults, however, the bones will have fused at the epiphyseal junction and therefore linear growth is no longer possible. The effect will be seen on the thickening of the bones of the face and skull. The nasal bridge becomes wider and deeper and the orbital margins protrude outwards as does the lower mandible. Simultaneously the subcutaneous tissues thicken giving the skin a coarse texture. The cartilage tissue increases around and between joints, especially of the hands and feet. The fingers in particular become enlarged and adopt a tubular shape limiting the flexibility of hand movements. This affects the cartilages of other joints causing early osteoarthritic changes, notably of the spine, hip, and knees. The tissues of the blood vessels also thicken causing a rise in blood pressure and ischaemic heart disease. Protein synthesis and fat breakdown are increased and this upsurge in metabolic activity causes the patient to perspire heavily with a constantly raised temperature.

An oversecretion of growth hormone affects the release of the remaining hormones from both lobes in the pituitary. In general terms, it tends to reduce the level of other hormones. In addition to the direct physical changes, the patient may suffer from hypothyroidism, amenorrhoea or impotence, and if the antidiuretic hormone is also affected, persistent diuresis, i.e., diabetes insipidus.

Since the disease is of a progressive nature, the patient may not realise that physical changes are occurring. It is only when involved in everyday activities such as dressing, washing, and working, that odd occurrences may draw the patient's attention to his or her changing physique. Clothes such as socks and gloves no longer fit, jewellery, i.e., rings, have to be removed because they are too tight. Spectacle frames no longer fit over the bridge of the nose or are too short to fit over the ear. Shoe sizes are odd and ever increasing. Handling cutlery or fine manipulative movements become increasingly difficult and frustrating. The patient may suffer from a headache but it is of a nonspecific nature and the patient may not be too alarmed about it until visual changes coincide with the headache. It may be then that the tumour is now pressing upwards against the optic chiasma.

Diagnosis

The investigations by X-ray confirm the enlargement of the bones of the face, skull, and further skeletal scanning may show changes in the joints due to thickening of cartilaginous tissues. If possible photographs from the patient taken over a period of years may highlight the structural changes particularly of the face and thorax. Regardless of whether there is a history of headaches, visual perimetry tests and those for visual acuity are performed. If either has deteriorated and there is a proven bilateral hemianopia, it indicates that the tumour is pressing on the optic chiasma and may suggest the need for surgical removal of the tumour.

Due to the growth hormone's anti-insulin effect, it is usual to do a blood glucose test and at the same time take blood to measure the plasma growth hormone level. It is important that no stress factors are occurring during this test, and for this reason the venous cannula may be left in position for 1 hour before sampling the blood. If the hormone level remains above 5 μg/l despite the glucose then it is regarded as a positive indication of excess growth hormone. In addition the plasma levels for other pituitary secreted hormones are assayed, and in general these results tend to be low. An electrocardiograph and blood pressure measurements are taken to indicate heart changes and hypertension.

Treatment

In some patients the disease may burn itself out leaving behind the altered physical changes but otherwise no ill effect. When there is a continuous over-secretion, the life expectancy of the patient is threatened. For this reason one of several treatments may be considered.

If the tumour is found to be extra-pituitary as proven by X-ray studies then a *transfrontal craniotomy* may be done to remove the tumour. If successful then the compression on the pituitary is immediately relieved with excellent results.

When the pituitary fossa (sella turcica) is expanded from an intra-pituitary tumour either a *transphenoidal* or *transethmoidal craniotomy* may be planned, to complete a hypophysectomy. Either operation implies that the incision will be made either through a facial sinus, or at the junction of the nose and eye. For several days following surgery the patient will have severe bruising of the face. Immediately after surgery the hormone levels are carefully monitored and nursing care is designed to anticipate reactions to low hormone levels. Once these levels are stabilised by replacement therapy and the patient recovers from the surgery, a second assessment is made. This is to decide the maintenance level of hormone replacement which the patient will require for the rest of his or her life. It is also usual to combine surgery with a short course of postoperative radiotherapy to irradiate the area of residual tumour cells.

With an uncomplicated case of acromegaly, i.e., no visual disturbances, the patient may be given a course of *radiotherapy* spread out over 2–4 years. During radiotherapy the head is carefully protected with a plastic mould, which has been individually designed for the patient. When worn it restrains the head so that no movement can take place while the pituitary gland is bombarded with atomic radiation from a cyclotron. Alternatively radioactive seeds in the form of Yttrium are implanted into the pituitary via a transphenoidal burr hole and guided into place via X-ray techniques.

Drugs such as somatostatin (growth hormone releasing inhibiting hormone, GHRIH) and bromocriptine which is derived from ergot, both lower the plasma levels of growth hormone. The most recent trials suggest that bromocriptine would have to be given for life at doses of 10–30 mg every day to maintain its suppressive effect.

If these treatments are successful the thickening of bone and cartilage spontaneously recede and the patient becomes quickly aware of physical and physiological functions returning to normal. This includes a return of menstruation, increased sexual libido, a normal metabolic rate, and an improved psychological outlook.

Undersecretion

Hypopituitarism

The undersecretion of growth hormone is only one of several causes of small stature in children. The others are: genetic, metabolic, orthopaedic, chromosomal, and chronic diseases.

Signs and Symptoms

When dwarfism is due to an undersecretion of growth hormone, the failure to grow is not immediately obvious for several months. The gonadotrophins also seem to be linked with growth hormone undersecretion causing poor development of the gonads and failure of puberty with the absence of secondary sexual characteristics. The body configuration remains that of prepuberty with the height never exceeding 135 cm.

Diagnosis

To gauge if the child is developing linear growth proportionate to age, his or her existing height is matched against a percentile chart and if it remains on the lowest line it indicates dwarfism (Fig. 36.2). X-rays of the wrists are taken to calculate bone age and compare this with chronological age. This is another indication of small stature or dwarfism.

All the pituitary hormones have to be measured from the blood plasma and since patients with hypopituitarism tend to suffer from hypoglycaemia, the blood glucose levels are carefully monitored. X-rays of the pituitary fossa may reveal a compression tumour invading the sella turcica or a chromophobe adenoma within the pituitary. Otherwise the cause of undersecretion is not known.

Treatment

After a firm diagnosis is made the child may be given injections of human growth hormone 6–18 mg once-weekly for several years which will promote growth. It seems to be a limited treatment, however, as the body eventually develops antibodies against the drug.

Panhypopituitarism

In adults, undersecretion of growth hormone is more likely to be accompanied by an undersecretion of all pituitary hormones, i.e., *panhypopituitarism*, and is often referred to as *Simmonds' disease*. The causes of panhypopituitarism in adults are grouped as being:

- Tumours or granulomas of the pituitary gland
- Postpartum haemorrhage causing pituitary necrosis (Sheehan's syndrome)
- Head injuries
- Surgical removal
- Irradiation therapy
- Infection reaching the pituitary via the paranasal sinuses, e.g., tuberculosis, syphilis

Sheehan's syndrome, which is now rare, follows upon severe haemorrhage after the delivery of a newborn baby. During the patient's pregnancy the pituitary gland is enlarged. With a massive loss of blood the gland suffers an infarction and necrosis with a subsequent loss of the pituitary hormones. With ample blood available for immediate transfusion this emergency situation is only rarely seen today.

Since all the hormones are affected a complete assay of plasma levels should be done and their replacement given rapidly. For hypothyroidism, thyroxine is required. Adrenocortical failure will only respond to cortisone. Amenorrhoea, impotence, and infertility require replacement gonadotrophins. Lactation failure requires prolactin. Diabetes insipidus will respond to vasopressin.

INAPPROPRIATE ADH SECRETION

There are many diseases which cause a temporary excess of ADH. These include: meningitis; head injury; cerebral tumours; bronchopneumonia in the elderly; undersecretion of the adrenal, pituitary and thyroid glands; cirrhosis of the liver, and as a side effect of some drugs, e.g., clofibrate. Because the total water content of the body is raised, the patient suffers from nausea, malaise, general muscular weakness, vomiting, slight confusional states, and abnormal reflex responses.

When urine osmolality is measured it is seen to be greater than that of plasma, i.e. hyponatraemia. There is not an obvious oedema and renal function is unimpaired. A true hyponatraemia, if confirmed by assay of the blood levels of ADH, is treated by restricting the fluid intake to 500 ml per day plus the same quantity from the previous day's output, and dealing with the underlying cause. Drugs such as cortisone would in effect worsen the condition since they tend to further retain body fluids as does normal saline intravenous therapy.

Diabetes Insipidus

Cranial diabetes insipidus (posterior pituitary) is so termed to distinguish it from nephrogenic diabetes insipidus when the renal tubules are insensitive to ADH. Apart from disorders of the posterior lobe of the pituitary gland, disorders of the hypothalamus may also cause this condition. Other causes include head injury, craniopharyngioma (tumours) of any type which affect the pituitary and include the pars intermedia. In over one third of patients no cause can be elicited, except to suggest that these patients may be suffering from an enzyme defect in hormone synthesis.

Signs and Symptoms

Gradually there is a need for the patient to increase the intake of water to relieve a persistent and raging thirst, and this is contrasted with an excessive polyuria, perhaps as much as 14–20 l of urine per day. The urine is pale, dilute, of very low specific gravity (similar to water). So long as the polyuria matches the volume of fluid consumed there is little effect on the electrolyte balance in a temperate climate. In those patients who have undergone cranial surgery, who are unconscious, or who are infants, a marked polyuria without a corresponding intake should alert the vigilant nurse to the real danger of rapid dehydration.

Diagnosis

The blood urea level, electrolyte levels, and a full blood count would determine if in fact there is a degree of dehydration. Specific investigations to establish a deficiency of ADH are the vasopressin test and water deprivation test.

Vasopressin Test

The vasopressin test is used to stimulate the posterior lobe of the pituitary and then to measure the ability of the kidneys to reabsorb water by noting the concentration of urine. If the drug, vasopressin, is administered intravenously then the patient must also be catheterised so that the urinary output can be accurately measured. The vasopressin is given as 100 μu followed by further injections of 5 μu every 5 minutes for 1 hour. The urine collected at the end of this period should show an increase in its osmolality from

100 mOsm/kgH_2O to over 600 mOsm/kgH_2O, meaning that it has increased in concentration. Alternatively, intramuscular aqueous vasopressin is given as 5 units at 19.00 hours and then the patient is asked to void the bladder. For the next 12 hours the urine is collected and the following morning it is despatched for osmolality concentration measurement. In this second test the patient does not require to be catheterised.

Water Deprivation Test

The patient is deprived of water and during the period of deprivation is weighed accurately every 30 minutes. During the course of deprivation all urine passed is collected in a specially marked container. When the patient has lost 3–4% of his or her original body weight the test is stopped.

When osmolality measurements are made, if the urinary osmolality remains low despite being deprived of water, it confirms the deficiency of ADH. The nurse supervising this test must be vigilant to note and report the first signs of dehydration. If it does occur the dehydration will be rapid in its effect requiring immediate medical intervention. It is best to stop the test if there is no medical supervision at the bedside during the test.

It may be necessary to exclude the possible diagnosis that the patient is an hysterical personality or a compulsive water drinker. Instead of vasopressin, a placebo drug may be employed which will in fact show normal osmolality levels.

Replacement therapy for ADH deficiency is by the administration of an analogue of ADH. This drug is known as DDAVP or to give its full title 1-desamine 8-D-arginine vasopressin. It is taken by intranasal spray in volumes of 0.1–2 ml once or twice daily. If the diabetes insipidus is due to nephrogenic insensitivity, the diuretics of the thiazide group are given to create a paradoxical control over the diuresis.

Chapter 37 Thyroid and Parathyroid Gland Disorders

The thyroid gland is a bilateral lobed endocrine structure, the lobes being connected by a bridge of tissue lying in front of the trachea. The total gland is contained within a fibrous capsule. It lies at the level of the second and third cartilaginous tracheal ring immediately below the cricoid cartilage of the larynx. A pronounced vascular blood supply arises from the right and left thyroid arteries. It is in close anatomical relationship with the recurrent laryngeal nerves which innervate the vocal cords for speech. Immediately behind and tending to be invested in the thyroid gland lie the 4 parathyroid glands which secrete parathormone.

THE THYROID GLAND

In function the thyroid gland secretes 3 hormones from the vesicles or sacs which contain the *colloid*, the storehouses of the hormones. The secretion of thyroxine (T4), tri-iodothyronine (T3), and calcitonin is dependent on the thyroid stimulating hormone (TSH) secreted from the anterior lobe of the pituitary gland. This, in turn, is dependent on the releasing factors from the hypothalamus, i.e., positive biofeedback. The thyroid gland can also be stimulated by a gamma globulin, the *long acting thyroid stimulator* (LATS) which is derived from the lymphocytes.

Both thyroxine and tri-iodothyronine are derived from tyrosine and iodine, which are available in any normal diet. Since iodine is now added to commercially manufactured table salt, a dietary deficiency of iodine is very rare. Both hormones are responsible for the rate at which the body metabolises its energy resources at cellular level. Tri-iodothyronine is a quick acting hormone with a short duration effect, while thyroxine is more slowly released with a more durable effect. Calcitonin is closely related and helps control the level of blood calcium, by depressing the level of parathormone.

The common disorders affecting the thyroid gland include: enlargement of the gland, oversecretion and undersecretion of thyroxine.

Enlargement

Enlargement of the gland may occur in either oversecretion or undersecretion of thyroxine and its more common name is goitre. Such enlargement may be due to:

Absolute dietary lack of iodine (rare today)

Overeating of the brassica family of vegetables, e.g., cabbage (rare today)

Excessive levels of blood calcium preventing the absorption of dietary iodine

Hereditary absence of enzymes necessary for thyroxine synthesis

Excess dose of antithyroid drugs

Toxic effects of drugs, e.g., sulphonamides, para-aminosalicylic acid, resorcinol

Toxic thyrotoxicosis

The thyroid epithelial cells become hyperplasic and at the same time the pituitary gland continues to stimulate the production of thyroxine, the combined effect being to enlarge the gland, i.e., goitre. Apart from the obvious visible enlargement of the gland at the neck, there may be pressure symptoms onto the trachea and the recurrent laryngeal nerve, and also affecting the facial nerve.

It is unusual for a goitre to occur before the age of puberty. Once the cause has been determined effective treatment can be prescribed, e.g., potassium iodide 0.1 g daily to compensate for reduced thyroxine levels. If thyrotoxicosis is present then either conservative treatment or surgery may be proposed.

Oversecretion of Thyroxine

Excessive secretion of thyroxine has been described by Graves, Parry, and Basedow and the disorders of thyrotoxicosis is often named after one of these doctors, e.g., Graves' disease. The disorder is also classified as being either toxic or exophthalmic. The disease occurs more commonly in women; a ratio of 5 : 1 is the current figure. The acute form tends to occur in early adult life, while a milder form occurs in the mature and later years of life.

The exact reason why thyroxine should become excessive is not yet known but the underlying features are:

It tends to be familial suggesting a genetic factor

In some cases long acting thyroid stimulator (LATS) may be responsible and since LATS is derived from lymphocytes, it suggests an auto-immune process

Nodules or adenomas may develop within the gland creating a 'hot' area in one or both lobes which oversecretes thyroxine in response

As a consequence of excessive secretion the vesicles empty their colloid rapidly, the right and left thyroid arteries become widely dilated and the gland may be felt to pulsate.

Signs and Symptoms

Classically the signs and symptoms of thyrotoxicosis correspond with an increased metabolic rate.

The pulse rate is very rapid, a tachycardia of a persistent nature may complicate to give the patient palpitations, cardiac arrhythmias, especially atrial fibrillation, and in the older patient heart failure may be an early feature of thyrotoxicosis. The systolic blood pressure is raised which may further contribute to a cardiac complication.

There is an intolerance to heat, coupled with excessive perspiration. Even on a cold day the patient wears cool clothing, and at night prefers very light bedclothing. While the appetite is increased there is no weight gain, but rather a weight loss. There is a tendency to have frequent bowel motions which are diarrhoetic in nature. The hands and feet are always moist, and when outstretched the fingers and hand have a noticeable tremor.

There is a pronounced restlessness, with brisk reflexes, although in fact the muscles are weak. Insomnia is often a feature of this restlessness as is the appearance of anxiety or nervousness. Thyrotoxicosis and anxiety resemble each other closely but there are two major differences. The hands of an anxious person are usually cold not hot and moist, and the sleeping pulse remains high in thyrotoxicosis, but falls in a true anxiety state. The female patient will usually report a disturbance of the menstrual cycle and it is usually amenorrhoea.

A rare but important sign is exophthalmos when the eyes bulge forward with a staring appearance. This eyeball protrusion is due to the loss of orbital fat and ocular oedema. If it is accompanied by degeneration of the extrinsic eye muscle the eyelid will not close properly, i.e., lid lag, or Horner's syndrome. The risk of corneal ulceration becomes very high, and therefore this sign requires careful nursing assessment.

Diagnosis

Along with the clinical features, tests usually confirm the diagnosis very quickly.

A measured amount of radioactive iodine (I^{131}) is given to the patient to take orally. Its uptake by the thyroid gland is then measured by a scintilloscope using a Geiger counter. In thyrotoxicosis the uptake is very rapid.

The blood level of tri-iodothyronine is raised, although thyroxine levels may be normal.

A 24-hour urine sample may be assayed to estimate the level of excreted radioactive iodine; the level will be low.

The sleeping pulse is about the only noninvasive method of assessing the basal metabolic rate, and as mentioned earlier it is also useful to differentiate between anxiety and thyrotoxicosis.

Treatment

The treatment of thyrotoxicosis may follow one of 3 courses:

- Antithyroid drugs
- Radioactive iodine
- Surgery

Antithyroid Drugs

Carbimazole suppresses the secretion of thyroxine, and after an initial high dose it is reduced to a daily maintenance level. Alternatively methylthiouracil combined with thyroxine may be prescribed to reduce the thyroid stimulating hormone from the pituitary gland. With antithyroid drugs there are 2 main hazards. The side effects are serious and include agranulocytosis, which means the patient becomes prone to infections. Secondly, the incidence of relapses into thyrotoxicosis after a short remission are quite frequent. If after 12 months of a drug regimen the treatment is not fully effective, surgery is usually proposed.

Radioactive Iodine

The first treatment of choice for an elderly patient with thyrotoxicosis and heart failure is radioactive iodine. The iodine, having been taken by mouth and absorbed, irradiates the thyroid tissue and destroys hyperactive secreting cells. The major problem remaining is the accurate calculation of the amount of radioactive iodine which should be prescribed.

Surgery

Thyroidectomy usually consists of removing five-sixths of the hyperactive gland, and is considered when:

- The enlargement (goitre) is due to a 'hot' nodule or an adenoma of the thyroid
- If the enlargement is causing pressure symptoms of dyspnoea, dysphagia or persistent hoarseness
- To resolve cosmetic disfigurement at the request of the patient
- If the enlargement or thyrotoxicosis suggests a malignancy

If a conservative medical regimen has failed after 12 months

If atrial fibrillation persists during the conservative drug regimen

Thyroidectomy

The majority of the investigations are usually completed prior to the patient's admission for the thyroidectomy. The nurse should however carefully assess the drugs which are normally prescribed for a fortnight preceding hospital admission.

Previous Drug Therapy

Drugs prescribed to the patient prior to admission may include any of the following:

Carbimazole (Neo-mercazole) to reduce thyroxin secretion for about 10 days, possibly followed by *potassium perchlorate* (800 mg daily in divided doses) to continue the effect of carbimazole until the patient's date of admission to hospital.

Lugol's solution (0.3–0.9 ml in milk) to reduce the vascularity of the thyroid gland, taken for 5 days before admission.

Phenobarbitone sodium (30 to 60 mg three times daily) to act as a sedative.

Propranolol for 10 days prior to admission if there is a marked hypertension.

Digitalis therapy if there is atrial fibrillation.

Following admission to hospital the drug regimen must be reviewed by both the surgeon and the anaesthetist and further prescribed therapy determined. This will take the patient up to and beyond the operation.

Nursing Care Plan

Nursing assessment is made of those particular problems from which the patient is suffering and are included in the specific care plan for thyrotoxicosis.

If the symptoms are severe enough then bedrest is essential for the patient until after surgery. This would apply if the patient was suffering from atrial fibrillation, extreme restlessness and dyspnoea.

A record should be made of the patient's sleeping pulse and body weight. Many surgeons decide to operate when the sleeping pulse is stable at about 80 beats per minute. Also the apex beat may be requested by some surgeons if the heart has or is fibrillating. Body weight must be known before surgery so that it can be contrasted with postoperative expected body weight gain.

The patient will have a preference for very light bedclothing, and a cool well ventilated area of the ward is essential to decrease the discomforts of a high body temperature and perspiration. Personal bedwear will usually be of a light loose cotton material.

Sometimes visitors should be limited if it is seen that they are making the patient overexcited and restless. Strong sedation may be required for several nights to overcome the problem of insomnia.

Preparation of the skin may necessitate shaving the axilla. Hair should certainly be clean and since it will have to be tied back and up away from the neck it may be advisable to have it trimmed or cut at the patient's discretion.

Specific advice about the operation should include a discussion about the horizontal incision made into a skin crease at the front of the neck and reassurance that this scar heals without any cosmetic disfigurement. A warning should be given about the difficulties the patient will experience for a few days after the operation. These include having a sore throat, painful shoulders, difficulty with speech and swallowing. The experienced nurse will be able to deal and help with these problems.

In addition to the specific and general preparation for surgery, the nurse will assist and organise with further specific investigations usually completed before surgery. These may include:

An electrocardiogram to demonstrate any cardiac arrhythmias

A chest X-ray to show the size of the heart and any pressure being exerted on related structures to the thyroid

Blood grouping and cross-matching of blood

Prior to the patient's return to the ward from

the recovery area, the nurse in addition to preparing the postoperative bed and area, should prepare a small tray containing a Michel's suture clip remover, 10 ml syringe and needle, and an ampoule of calcium gluconate. This tray should remain on the patient's locker for the first 48 hours of postoperative care.

On regaining the swallowing reflex and recovery from anaesthesia the patient should be sat upright, well supported at the shoulders and neck by pillows. The incision line and drains should be checked at frequent intervals, especially for haematoma, and the volume of wound exudate if suction drainage has been applied. If haematoma or respiratory distress should occur it indicates that there is bleeding into the soft tissues of the neck and that several suture clips need immediate removal. Hence the suture clip remover is maintained at the bedside. If this occurs it means that there is a blood vessel requiring ligature and the patient will need to return to theatre, for evacuation of the haematoma and vessel ligature.

To prevent pain, anxiety, or restlessness the prescribed analgesic and antiemetic should be administered at the prescribed intervals, promoting both sleep and rest.

Some surgeons will request a 1-hourly pulse rate and a 2-hourly temperature chart to be maintained for at least 48 hours to anticipate the event of a postoperative thyroid crisis. In the absence of instructions both pulse and temperature should be recorded and charted at frequent intervals during the first 24 hours on a decreasing frequency scale if they remain stable. Pyrexia should be expected, but not a tachycardia.

It is usual for Lugol's solution, and if prescribed digoxin, to be continued for several days following surgery.

As soon as it is feasible the patient should be encouraged to swallow, clear fluids at first. If the throat remains sore, making swallowing and speech difficult, an aspirin mucilage (preferably flavoured) should be offered at 4-hourly intervals. If speech remains a difficulty a pad and pencil should be supplied, but only for a short period.

During the first postoperative night, the night nurse must remain vigilant in observing for any sign of haematoma, respiratory distress, restlessness, tachycardia, and to see that the analgesia and sedation are effective.

Forty-eight hours after surgery the wound drains are usually removed, and on the fourth or fifth day the sutures are removed. Within a week of surgery the patient should notice feeling more calm and becoming increasingly sensitive to cold, usually asking for an extra blanket. The patient's appetite remains healthy and now there should be some increase in body weight. These features are more correctly assessed 3 months after surgery and in the out-patient's department.

Complications of Thyroidectomy

Many of the observations specified in the first 48 hours after surgery are aimed at detecting potential complications at the earliest opportunity. In addition to haematoma and haemorrhage other complications may arise.

Thyrotoxic Crisis

Thyrotoxic crisis is a rare occurrence. If it happens it will do so in 6–24 hours following surgery. There is a sudden upsurge in the secretion of thyroxin from the remaining gland for reasons which are not clear and this causes an immediate toxic thyrotoxicosis. The pulse becomes extremely rapid, hyperpyrexia supervenes, extreme agitation and restlessness precede a coma due to an intense metabolic crisis. The immediate regimen consists of administering:

Morphia 20 mg every 4 hours. **NB** It is excreted very rapidly due to the crisis

Intravenous digoxin to correct cardiac fibrillation

Intravenous normal saline to correct dehydration

High concentrations of oxygen (an oxygen tent may be required)

Lugol's solution 20 ml of 10% solution intravenously

Tepid sponging to reduce the hyperpyrexia

It must be emphasised that this is a rare occurrence but should it happen it requires an immediate medical response with intensive nursing skills and care to correct the crisis.

Tetany

Tetany is due to the accidental removal or surgical injury of the parathyroid glands. The secreted parathormone is responsible for calcium metabolism, and in tetany parathormone levels are reduced.

It is first felt as a tingling sensation of the face and limbs which develops into spasmodic twitching of the muscles of the hands and feet, i.e., carpopedal spasm. A combination of these features may be assessed by testing for Chvostek's sign. The treatment is by replacement therapy with calcium gluconate 10%, hence the need to keep the ampoule, syringe and needle by the bedside. Parathormone may be used, and large doses of vitamin D also increase the uptake of calcium from the intestine.

Persistent Hoarseness

Within 48–72 hours following surgery the patient should show signs of returning to a normal speech pattern. If the hoarseness persists, however, then the vocal chords will need to be examined to see if they both open and close in unison. If either is nonfunctioning then one of the laryngeal recurrent nerves has been surgically damaged. The recurrent laryngeal nerves are located behind the thyroid gland. Since the vocal chord is nonfunctioning there may be an associated respiratory difficulty. If both vocal chords are damaged then there will be respiratory obstruction which will be evident immediately the anaesthetic airway is removed, but this is an extremely rare cause of respiratory difficulty.

Hypothyroidism

Hypothyroidism occurs in about 36% of patients and is not immediately noticeable in the postoperative period. It implies too much of the gland has been removed and a small maintenance dose of thyroxine will be required for the rest of the patient's life.

Persisting Thyrotoxicosis

Persisting thyrotoxicosis occurs in about 6% of patients and the recurrence develops at a later time following discharge from hospital. It implies that not enough of the gland has been removed during surgery.

Undersecretion of Thyroxine

Myxoedema literally means mucus swelling and refers to the thick dry skin and nonpitting oedema patients suffering from it acquire. The undersecretion of thyroxine from a nonfunctioning gland may be due to:

1. A tumour of the pituitary gland (craniopharyngioma) which arrests the secretion of the thyroid stimulating hormone.
2. The end result of an auto-immune process such as Hashimoto's disease in which the thyroid cells are attacked by the individual's own antibodies.
3. Over-irradiation of the thyroid gland with radioactive iodine.
4. Excess tissue being removed at thyroidectomy.
5. Viral thyroiditis.

In the newborn child a nonfunctioning gland or an absent gland if undetected gives rise to *cretinism*. It is usually recognised during the first 2 weeks of life when the infant fails to thrive. Cretinism can be prevented by a life-long maintenance dose of small amounts of thyroxine. More frequently however it occurs in females during the middle years of life.

Signs and Symptoms

Without adequate levels of thyroxine there is a pronounced defect in the metabolic rate and the presenting features are exactly opposite to those of thyrotoxicosis.

Such features as increasing physical lassitude with a pronounced psychological lethargy and failing memory present. The patient becomes disinterested in every day activities and gradually withdraws totally, remaining indoors and out of social contact. An increasing weight quickly proceeds towards obesity but there is a marked loss of appetite with constipation.

The skin becomes coarse in texture, appears thicker and there is a puffiness around the eyes and face which is not oedema. The hair gradually thins, lacks lustre, and is very dry. While the speech becomes slower, the tone of the voice becomes hoarse.

The patient is extremely sensitive to cold, requiring a considerable amount of house heat and many clothes to keep warm even on a hot day. The elderly patient who is myxoedematous is a prime candidate for hypothermia.

The pulse rate is slow but the blood pressure rises and this may develop into heart enlargement or angina. About 10% of myxoedematous patients have an accompanying pernicious anaemia and many have an iron deficiency anaemia. There is invariably a disturbance of the menstrual cycle. A serious development is that of *myxoedematous madness* in which the patient suffers from hallucinations and paranoia.

Myxoedematous patients rarely seek out medical advice as the changes are slow and progressive. It is more usual to find that a close relative or friend comments on a swelling around the neck, or that speech and thinking skills are altering to such a degree that a medical opinion is required.

Diagnosis

The clinical features combined with the results of the following investigations quickly confirm the diagnosis. These investigations may include:

An electrocardiograph to demonstrate reduced cardiac output

A chest X-ray to show heart enlargement

Radioactive iodine uptake test which shows little concentration in the thyroid gland

Tests for an increased blood cholesterol level

Tests for a raised blood thyroid stimulating hormone level

Tests for pernicious and iron deficiency anaemia

Treatment

The treatment of myxoedema is to initially administer prescribed low doses of thyroxine and at the same time monitor the pulse for any sudden tachycardia. The more obvious features of the disease should resolve in several days and a maintenance level of thyroxine 0.1–0.3 mg daily is then usually prescribed. This is a life-long therapy.

Severe myxoedema may require an initial regimen of hydrocortisone together with the thyroxine to combat adverse reactions. The patient's condition is reviewed each month for the following 6 months, especially so for persisting cardiac abnormalities and any possible ischaemic changes.

Patients recovering from myxoedema are prone to coronary thrombosis because of the changes in the heart. If the blood pressure remains high propranolol may be prescribed to be taken twice daily. Both psychologically and physically the improvement can only be described as dramatic and pleasing as the patient takes up the strands of his or her life once more with renewed vigour and a positive outlook.

THE PARATHYROID GLANDS

Measuring 3–4 mm in diameter each of these 4 glands are arranged in 2 pairs immediately behind the right and left lobes of the thyroid gland. The secreted hormone, *parathormone*, maintains the plasma calcium level within the normal range, 8.5–9.2 mg per 100 ml of blood and phosphorus at 6 mg per 100 ml of blood. The parathyroid glands do not rely on the pituitary gland for their stimulation, but rather react to the circulating level of plasma calcium, i.e., it is an example of negative biofeedback.

To maintain the plasma calcium levels, parathormone acts on 3 main sites;

1. It transfers calcium from the bone reserves to the blood.

2. It increases calcium reabsorption from the renal tubules back into the blood but allowing the excretion of excess phosphate.

3. It renders dietary calcium to be absorbed via the intestine into the blood. To prevent calcium levels reaching too high a level, the hormone calcitonin, secreted from the thyroid gland, depresses the action of parathormone and essentially prevents calcium being transferred from the bone to the blood. An adequate intake of calcium is about 1.5 g per day for an adult but this intake must be increased during pregnancy and in childhood to allow for growth.

Calcium metabolism in combination with vitamin D is essential for the structure and growth of bone and teeth. This vitamin also increases the absorption of calcium from the intestine. Calcium contributes to the control of the excitability of nerve impulses, especially to the voluntary muscles, and is also a vital factor in the natural coagulation of blood.

Undersecretion

Hypoparathyroidism

The lack of parathormone is rare. No obvious cause has been accurately identified with the exception of the accidental removal or surgical injury to the parathyroid glands during thyroidectomy. A plasma calcium level below 6 mg per 100 ml of blood is regarded as being hypoparathyroidic.

Signs and Symptoms

Irritability of nerve impulses accompanied by painful spasms and cramps of the hands and feet are the earliest signs of hypocalcaemia, also referred to as tetany. The joints within the hand flex while those in the fingers extend and the thumb is drawn into the palm of the hand. A similar pattern also happens to the feet, i.e., carpopedal spasm. If the facial nerve is tapped with a reflex hammer it produces facial twitching, i.e. Chvostek's sign. Spasm of the larynx may occur leading to respiratory difficulty, e.g., crowing respiration. This type of respiration leads to a reduced carbon dioxide level and respiratory alkalosis usually follows. If the patient is predisposed to epilepsy then convulsions may occur.

Treatment

The most effective emergency treatment is the immediate intravenous administration of calcium gluconate. This is followed by a maintenance level dose of vitamin D, e.g., calciferol, to promote calcium absorption from the intestine. Parathormone is available orally but it is an expensive and unreliable therapeutic regimen.

Oversecretion

Hyperparathyroidism

In over 90% of cases the cause of excess parathormone secretion is due to a benign tumour or an adenoma. Malignancy is rarely if ever present. If the disorder is referred to as *primary* it implies the disorder is combined with another endocrine disease. Should the term *secondary* hyperparathyroidism be used it implies the glands are enlarged, possibly due to renal disease, intestinal malabsorption syndrome, or an inadequate diet of calcium-containing foods.

Signs and Symptoms

Excess parathormone removes too much calcium from the bone reserves and this gives rise to muscular weakness, constipation, anorexia, polyuria and thirst. The polyuria and thirst are due to increased calcium urinary excretion, and renal calculi. In the longer-term a continued depletion of bone calcium leads to an osteoporosis or weakness in the structure of the bone matrix, and a tendency to fractures, e.g., von Recklinghausen's disease. Calcium depletion also leads to duodenal ulceration.

These wide ranging symptoms may involve the nurse in organising and arranging for the patient to have a series of tests.

Diagnosis

If the provisional diagnosis is correct the results of tests may show that:

Serum calcium levels are raised

Urinary calcium levels are raised about 250 mg in a 24-hour urine specimen

Blood parathormone levels are increased

If there is osteoporosis, the alkaline phosphatase is increased and the patient will probably have a skeletal scan to see if there are any linear fractures

As part of the investigations the history would determine if in fact the patient has a diet rich in either vitamin D or milk which may account for the symptoms. Equally important it is essential to know if the patient is taking any of the hydrocortisone group of drugs, as these lower plasma calcium levels and may in fact be masking the symptoms.

Treatment

The main treatment is surgery, i.e., parathyroidectomy. The nursing care plan for this surgery parallels that for thyroidectomy with the major exception that the incision is more extensive and postoperatively the calcium plasma levels are monitored very closely in addition to the observations for tetany.

Chapter 38
Adrenal Gland Disorders

Each adrenal gland caps the upper pole of each kidney being separated from the renal structure by perirenal fat. Weighing about 3–4 g each, the adrenal glands have a complex arterial blood supply derived from the aorta, the phrenic and renal arteries. The amount of vitamin C and cholesterol stored in each gland is quite considerable and contributes to the synthesis of the hormones which are secreted from the glands.

The inner portion of each gland known as the *medulla* is innervated by the sympathetic branch of the autonomic nervous system to secrete 2 major catecholamines, i.e., adrenaline and noradrenaline. These hormones are synthesised in the chromaffin cells and are secreted by the stimulus of acetylcholine, a neurotransmitter from the sympathetic nerve endings. Although influenced by releasing factors from the hypothalamus, the adrenal glands are not influenced by the pituitary gland. This is an important point to appreciate when the symptoms of either pituitary or adrenal medulla disorders are being scrutinised.

The medulla is particularly prone to acetylcholine stimulus when the hypothalamus is influenced by any of these states: anger, cerebral anoxia, cold, fear, hypoglycaemia or hypotension.

When adrenaline and noradrenaline are secreted directly into the blood stream they have a stimulus effect on both A and B receptors located on the walls of the blood vessels and Table 38.1 indicates the typical response of the body. These responses,

Table 38.1. Effect of adrenaline and noradrenaline stimulus on body systems

Systemic change	Adrenaline only	Adrenaline and noradrenaline	Summation of effect
Cardiovascular			
Increased heart rate		√	Increases blood pressure
Increased heart contraction		√	
Increased coronary flow		√	
Increased erythrocyte count	√		Overall increased haemoconcentration
Increased haemoglobin concentration	√		
Increased plasma protein concentration	√		
Decreased blood flow to			Peripheral blood flow shutdown, i.e., patient is cold and clammy
skin		√	
mucous membranes		√	
splanchnic area		√	
skeletal muscle	√		
Decreased coagulation time	√		
Respiratory			
Dilation of			
bronchi		√	Increased rate and depth of respiration
bronchioles		√	
Gastrointestinal			
Decreased smooth muscle tone		√	Creates feelings of nausea, vomiting and may cause diarrhoea
Inhibition of peristalsis		√	
Contraction of sphincters		√	
Conversion of liver glycogen to blood glucose	√		Increase in energy
Increased lipolytic activity		√	
Increased internal tissue respiration	√		Increased basal metabolic rate
Nervous System			
Inducement of arousal	√		Coping mechanism for flight or fright
Increased anxiety	√		
Inducement of exocrine activity	√		
Dilation of pupils of the eyes		√	

however, are only temporary and are considerably modified and in some cases cancelled out by local reflexes of the central nervous system. The table also gives a reasonable insight into what is happening to an individual when frightened. Fear is all too commonly the experience of those who are ill or who are admitted for surgery. It also demonstrates what happens when adrenaline is given as a drug.

Surrounding the medulla is the adrenal cortex. The secretory cells of the cortex are arranged in 3 distinct layers or zones. The hormones secreted from these zones are synthesised from the cholesterol stored in the gland. If required, extra cholesterol can be taken directly from the blood for further hormone synthesis. With the exception of one zone, the releasing factors from the hypothalamus and the stimulating hormone adrenocorticotrophic hormone (ACTH) from the pituitary are required to initiate cortical secretion (Fig. 38.1). The hormone aldosterone is directly influenced by the hypothalamus, mainly by the concentration of plasma osmolality.

If plasma osmolality is low, i.e., dehydration, a given sequence of events should occur. The

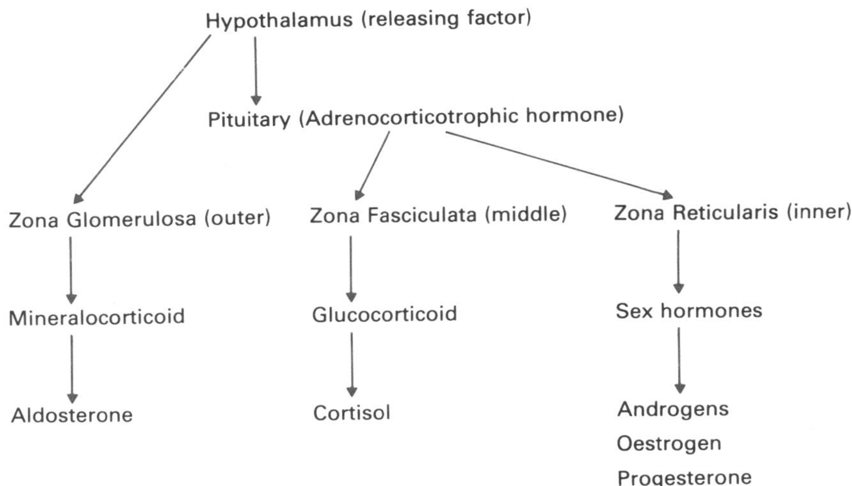

Fig. 38.1 Chain of hormone secretion.

renal glomerulus produces the hormone *renin* which converts *angiotensin 1* to *angiotensin 2*. This then stimulates the secretion of *aldosterone* from the zona glomerulus of the adrenal cortex. This acts on the pituitary gland to secrete *antidiuretic* hormone. Both hormones then act on the distal convoluted tubule of the nephron to reabsorb sodium and water. This in effect corrects dehydration and helps to restore blood pressure.

The *middle zone* or the *zona fasciculata* secretes the glucocorticoid hormone cortisol. This hormone has a wide ranging influence on a number of factors. It antagonises the effect of insulin permitting both amino acids and fat to be converted and stored, e.g., amino acids to glycogen; animal or vegetable fat to human fat deposit. Fat is mobilised for breakdown in the liver to ketone bodies. The development of cartilage is impeded. Cortisol also controls the overabsorption of calcium from the intestine by antagonising vitamin D. It is both anti-inflammatory and anti-infective from its influence on eosinophils and tends to retain both sodium and water. It controls and influences the contractility of vascular smooth muscle.

These functions taken together enable the body to cope with stress, especially the influence on long-term body metabolism. Another application is to consider the effects of synthetic hormones which are given as part of a drug regimen, e.g., hydrocortisone. A prolonged use of cortisone-based drugs can induce glycosuria, osteoporosis and spontaneous fractures, a poor response to infection, and oedema.

The *inner zone* or *zona reticularis* secretes 3 main hormones: the androgens, oestrogen and progesterone. These hormones produce the sexual characteristics. The hormones testosterone, from the testes, and oestrogen, from the ovaries, are far more important in determining the totality of masculinity or feminity.

HORMONES FROM THE ADRENAL CORTEX

A deficiency of the hormones secreted from the zones of the adrenal cortex leads to Addison's disease while an excess leads to either Cushing's syndrome or aldosteronism.

Undersecretion

Addison's Disease

The primary cause of a reduced secretion from the adrenocortical zones is due to the atrophy of the cells. Tuberculosis used to be the main cause of such atrophy, but with the eradication programme, Addison's disease is now much more rare. Atrophy can be caused by:

Amyloidosis
Metastatic malignancy
Syphilis
Auto-immunity disease

Should the adrenal glands be removed to correct Cushing's syndrome, then obviously there will be no hormones to be secreted. An important cause of adrenal deficiency today is the prolonged used of cortisone therapy for a wide range of inflammatory and allergic disorders. Such therapy tends to reduce the stimulation hormones being secreted from the pituitary gland. Without such stimulation the adrenal glands will atrophy, i.e., hypopituitarism.

Signs and Symptoms

In the early stages of the disease the clinical features have an insidious onset with the deficiency occurring most frequently between the ages of 30–50 years old. The patient may not relate the early symptoms of weight loss and an ill-defined anaemia to a serious illness. Fainting spells (hypotension) accompanied by tachycardia will alarm the patient into seeking medical advice at this point. Investigations aimed at monitoring the blood pressure of the patient while he or she is sitting, lying, and standing, usually reveal a postural hypotension.

The accumulation of melanocytes causes pigmentation on the creases in the palms of the hands and also in the mucous membrane of the mouth. This is more readily seen on a pale skinned individual. There is a disturbance in the bowel habit which veers from diarrhoea to constipation perhaps accompanied by vomiting and is a main cause of severe agitation. Stress in the form of infection, pyrexia, or trauma when combined with the chronic features of the illness can induce a *cortical crisis*. Such a crisis is a medical emergency necessitating the patient's immediate admission to hospital. The crisis takes the form of a sudden hypoglycaemia, marked hypotension, severe dehydration, and a severe exacerbation of existing chronic symptoms.

Investigations

In the chronic form of Addison's disease several investigations apart from monitoring the blood pressure usually include a careful scrutiny of the patient's electrolyte levels. This involves water excretion tests. These latter tests show a reduced secretion rate of aldosterone if the excretion of water is below 70%.

Treatment

The treatment is by replacement therapy with cortisol usually 10–40 mg daily for life. If aldosterone is also deficient this is replaced by fluorohydrocortisone which should correct the tendency to oedema. The cortisone group of drugs may reduce the patient's normal response to infection by inhibiting the normal body defence mechanisms. For this reason patients must be advised to report to their personal doctor if they contract any type of infection so that the cortisol can be adjusted. When patients attend the outpatients department for their checks on blood pressure and for oedema, the nurse should check that they are carrying their steroid card or alternatively are wearing a 'medicare bracelet' in the case of emergency treatment being required.

Corticol Crisis

The treatment of corticol crisis is the immediate infusion of normal saline/sodium chloride with hydrocortisone. Both should correct dehydration and restore the blood pressure. The nursing observations of the patient are absolutely vital, and consist of:

Hourly recording of blood pressure and pulse

Reporting any decline in conscious level immediately

Maintaining a strict fluid balance report

Routinely testing every specimen of urine for any abnormality (reagent test)

Reagent test on blood samples for glucose level

If hypoglycaemia is present then dextrose will be infused intravenously

Oversecretion

Cushing's Syndrome

Oversecretion of the hormones from the adrenal cortex may be due to an overactive pituitary which is secreting too much adrenocorticotrophic hormone influencing the zona fasciculata and reticularis. The zona glomerulosa is **not** affected in this instance therefore there is no disturbance of electrolyte or water levels since aldosterone is not affected. If, however, the cause is due to an adenoma or tumour within the adrenal cortex then all the zones will be affected. Cancer of the bronchus and the ovary tends to promote synthesis of ACTH and to promote excess secretion of the adrenal cortex. Children born with congenital adrenal hyperplasia give rise to the phenomena of precocious sexual virilism or alternatively the andrenogenital syndrome when there is overt masculinisation of the anatomical female and the overt feminisation of the anatomical male.

Signs and Symptoms

The classical features of someone suffering from Cushing's syndrome is firstly that it affects mostly females, and they are obese due to the redistribution of body fat. This redistribution is particularly noticeable around the face and trunk but sparing the limbs; the effect is often summarised as 'an orange on sticks'. The face is described as being moon-shaped. With the abdominal obesity the skin develops striae which are purple in colour. The thin limbs show marked wasting of the muscles and the bones when X-rayed demonstrate osteoporotic changes. This is especially so of the vertebral column which lead to backache and kyphosis. All these changes are due to excess glucocorticoid.

If aldosterone is also in excess then further changes involving oedema and potassium depletion will occur. The excess sex hormones, notably the androgens, cause loss of feminity with hair loss, amenorrhoea, and a deepening tone of voice. Continued oversecretion leads to hypertension, diabetes, and protein deficiency. Less specifically the patient is prone to infection and tends to bruise easily.

These many discomforts are best understood by returning to the functions of the adrenal cortex where it can be noticed how closely the symptoms match the disordered function. From this the nurse can create a nursing plan which deals with each discomfort in priority order as the patient describes them.

Investigations

Investigations are designed to find out the circulating cortisol level and whether the cause is the pituitary gland or if it is primary, i.e., in the adrenal gland. The nurse may be involved in these investigations and may be requested to:

1. Record the patient's blood pressure frequently with the patient in the sitting, lying, and standing positions.
2. Test the patient's urine every 4 hours for glycosuria.
3. Collect 24-hour specimens of urine for a series of assays, e.g., free cortisol levels, vanillylmandelic acid (VMA), 17-oxygenic and 17-oxysteroids.
4. Assist with the dexamethasone suppression test. This drug is given every 6 hours for 48 hours and then measurements made of the cortisol plasma levels. Since the drug suppresses the secretion of adrenocorticotrophic stimulating hormone from the pituitary gland the cortisol levels should be low. If they remain raised, however, the disorder of Cushing's syndrome may be originating in the adrenal gland or be from an ectopic source, e.g., cancer of the bronchus or ovary.
5. Assist and prepare the patient for a series of X-ray examinations. A straight abdominal X-ray may show calcification of the adrenal gland. Intravenous pyelography may reveal displacement of the kidney due to such calcification. X-rays of the skull may show enlargement of the pituitary fossa (sella turcica). Arteriography of the adrenal gland may be attempted if the disorder is thought to originate from there.

A simple chest X-ray may show a tumour of the bronchus. Defects of vision may occur if the pituitary gland is compressing the optic chiasma though this is rare.

Treatment

The results of these many tests will determine one of several possible treatments. The nursing care plan cannot be created until there is a medical decision.

For oversecretion of the adrenocorticotrophic hormone (ACTH) either irradiation of the anterior lobe of the pituitary gland with implants of yttrium or gold, or proton bombardment.

Anterior hypophysectomy will be performed if there is a tumour extending from the anterior lobe into the optic chiasma. Such surgery is always followed by hormone replacement therapy for life.

For tumours of the adrenal gland surgical removal is the treatment of choice. At the time of surgery both adrenals are carefully examined to decide if one or both glands are to be removed. In this type of surgery careful monitoring of steroid therapy immediately after surgery and beyond is required.

Carcinoma of the adrenal glands is invariably a metastatic tumour. Such tumours are known to synthesise cortisol which leads to an excess. The synthesis of excess cortisol may be blocked by the use of drugs, e.g., metyrapone and aminoglutethimide, combined with the cortisol needs of the patient. Since the tumour is usually secondary, investigations and treatment for the primary tumour are completed before decisions are made on treatment for the adrenal tumour.

Aldosteronism

Excess secretion of aldosterone from the zona glomerulosa of either one or both adrenal glands is rare. It is classified as being either primary or secondary aldosteronism. *Primary aldosteronism* (Conn's syndrome) is when the secretory cells of the zona glomerulosa are hyperplastic or the zone has a single or multiple adenoma, usually benign. *Secondary aldosteronism* is due to the overactivity of the renin angiotensin system which in normal circumstances is the biofeedback system controlling hydration, but for a variety of reasons becomes overactive, and overstimulates the zona glomerulosa.

Signs and Symptoms

The main feature is hypertension due to fluid and electrolyte imbalance. The disturbed potassium levels give rise to feelings of weakness in the muscles, and if at a very low serum level may cause cardiac changes.

Investigations

The investigations centre upon determining the plasma levels of aldosterone and plasma angiotensial renin levels. Since both of these are affected by dietary intake of sodium and protein, the doctor may request the patient has a low sodium, low protein diet for several days before taking any blood samples. If adenoma is suspected the patient may undergo adrenal vein sampling under the effects of a general anaesthetic to establish if one or other glands are affected. The main cause of secondary aldosteronism is established diuretic therapy for the control of oedema. It follows that the history of the patient becomes vital when assessing past drug regimens prior to hospital admission.

Treatment

The treatment of choice for adrenal adenoma is surgical removal. Prior to this the patient may be prescribed the drug spironolactone which is an aldosterone protagonist and usually lowers the blood pressure to good effect. If surgery is not possible then spironolactone may be offered as a long-term therapy and apart from its side effects gives satisfactory results. Secondary aldosteronism is treated by assessing its many causes, which include cardiac failure, cirrhosis of the liver, nephrotic syndrome, renal artery damage, and renin secreting tumours.

HORMONES FROM THE ADRENAL MEDULLA

The inner portion or centre, the *medulla*, of the adrenal gland secretes the catecholamines: noradrenaline and adrenaline.

Tumours

When disorders of the medulla occur, which is rare, it is due to one of several types of tumour. *Neuroblastoma*, or a tumour of the sympathetic nerve secreting cells, is a variable tumour ranging from the highly malignant to the benign. *Phaeochromocytoma* is a type of tumour mainly found in the adrenal medulla but can also occur in any part of the sympathetic ganglia in the trunk. It tends to be familial and is usually detected between the ages of 25–55 years. One or both adrenal medullas may be involved.

Signs and Symptoms

Both tumours cause an excess secretion of adrenaline and noradrenaline. Both catecholamines cause the main feature of this excess which is hypertension. The high blood pressure may be intermittent or be persistent. During a hypertensive phase the severe pounding within the skull causes intense headache of a most crippling nature. Perspiration and pallor are marked and contrast with the severe agitation which keeps the patient on the move, being persistently restless. The pressure in the thorax and intestine gives rise to duodenal and thoracic pain. These attacks often follow on from emotional stress or physical exercise, and when they conclude leave the patient physically exhausted. Should the hypertension persist, the blood pressure when recorded may actually be low, this being due to a loss of circulating fluid.

Investigations

The easiest investigation is the collection of a 24-hour specimen of urine to estimate the level of the waste product of the catecholamines which is vanillymandelic acid (VMA). Blood pressure recordings taken at frequent intervals and charted accurately are part of the nursing duty. Radioisotope tracing of the enzymes involved in plasma noradrenaline are increasingly used to estimate the levels of the catecholamines. Occasionally the doctor may use an alpha blocking drug and then take frequent recordings of the blood pressure, which in adrenal tumours will remain high.

Treatment

The treatment of choice is surgical removal of the adrenal tumour. It is one of the most successful treatments for the hypertension. Prior to surgery the surgeon will usually prescribe sedation for the previous 48 hours to surgery, and the nurse should parallel this with creating an atmosphere of calm and quiet to reduce the patient's anxiety and restlessness. The blood pressure will also be reduced for the preceding 48 hours to surgery and an alpha blocking drug, e.g., phenoxybenzamine, may be given in divided doses.

The surgical handling of the gland may cause a sudden release of catecholamines with adverse effects on the blood pressure, or alternatively a marked hypotension. The postoperative monitoring of blood pressure may be as frequent as every 15 minutes. A single unit of blood is usually transfused after surgery to correct hypovolaemia and this is followed by an infusion of normal saline mainly to keep the vein open in case of the need for noradrenaline. This is a most successful operation and the outlook for the future is extremely good with the blood pressure returning to normal levels very quickly.

Chapter 39
Testes Disorders

About the sixth week of fetal life the testes (Fig. 39.1) develop and suppress the female system (Müllerian system). The germ cells develop into the seminiferous tubules which will produce the spermatozoa, while the developing interstitial cells which are interspersed within the tubules secrete the main androgen, testosterone.

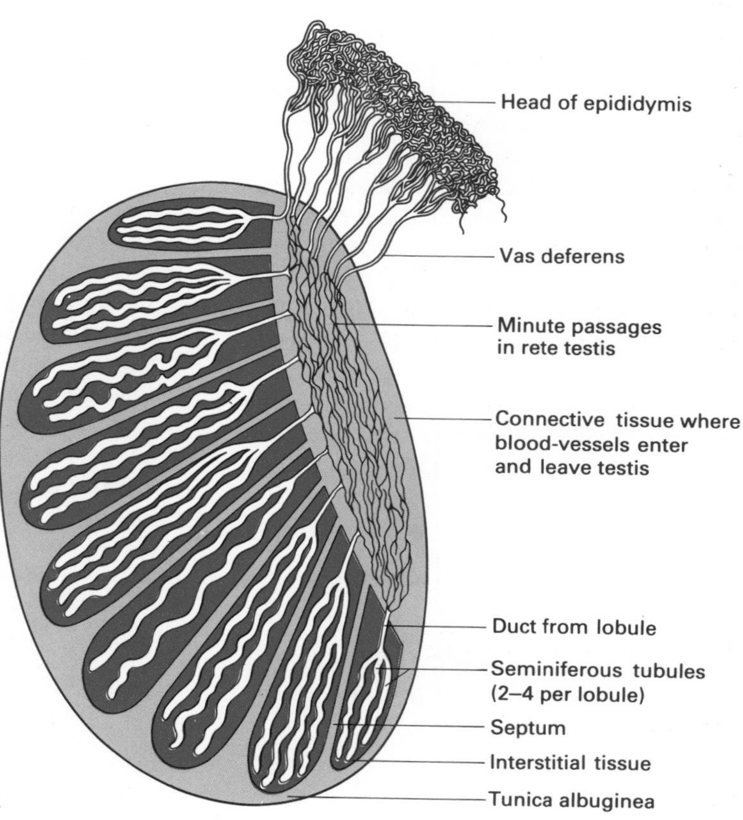

Fig. 39.1 Diagrammatic vertical section of the testis.

The initial secretion during fetal life stimulates the development of the vas deferens. When this is completed about the seventh to eighth month of fetal life, the testes descend from the posterior abdominal wall to lie outside the body in the scrotal sac.

The present theory is that the testes will only produce spermatozoa in a temperature range which is 2° C below the core temperature of the body. The testes are ovoid in shape, measuring 4 cm by 2 cm and encased in a fibrous capsule called the *tunica albuginea*. The outer serous membrane, a double coat, is known as the *tunica vaginalis*. The rich blood supply to the testes is directed through a fine mesh of vessels known as the *tunica vasculosa*. Within the testes the coiled seminiferous tubules are composed of layers of spermatogenic cells within which are interspersed the interstitial cells of Leydig. The coiled seminiferous tubules lead into ducts which convey the spermatozoa into the epididymis where it is stored until maturation. When ejaculated the sperm leaves the epididymis via the vas deferens to reach the urethra.

Testosterone

Testosterone is secreted directly into the blood stream from the interstitial cells where it is both manufactured and stored until required. It is released from the interstitial cells on a negative feedback mechanism (Fig. 39.2).

Testosterone like other androgens is manufactured from cholesterol and once secreted influences many functions in the body.

1. It stimulates growth of the seminiferous tubules in the testes.
2. It regulates the rate of spermatogenesis.
3. It develops and maintains the accessory male sexual organs, i.e., the penis, prostate gland, seminal vesicles, bulbourethral glands, and scrotal capacity.
4. At puberty testosterone develops the secondary sexual characteristics of masculinity:

   Increased muscular mass and strength

   Increased facial and body hair

   Thickening of vocal cords to deepen the pitch of voice

   Along with other androgens increased sebum secretion

   NB Masculine aggression may be due more to social learning than testosterone secretion levels.
5. Stimulates epiphyseal bone growth and eventual epiphyseal fusion, i.e. growth spurt at puberty. Puberty in the male is defined as the point at which the testes produce both testosterone and mature spermatogenesis.

Secretion

Excess testosterone secretion is unknown as a natural phenomenon, the exception being when someone takes androgens as a deliberate

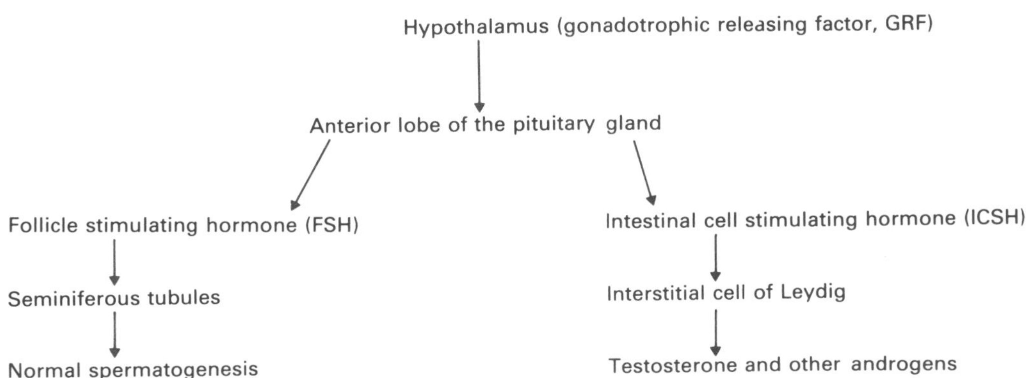

Fig. 39.2 Negative feedback mechanism.

means of improving their physique and strength especially for sports.

Deficiency of testosterone may occur either from a primary disease of the testes or as a secondary manifestation from impaired secretion from the hypothalamus, the pituitary gland, or related to adrenal cortex deficiency.

Reduced Secretion

There are many conditions which lead to a reduced secretion of testosterone. It should be appreciated that prolonged psychological stress of itself does produce a reduction in libido and therefore a reduction in sexual drive. Conversely a true male infertility or an impotence also causes psychological stress. For this reason counselling should only be done by experts, and only after a thorough physical assessment by an endocrinologist to exclude several disorders.

Klinefelter's Syndrome

Seminiferous tubule dysgenesis or Klinefelter's syndrome is the most common of the genetically determined testicular disorders in which there is an additional X chromosome to the normal 46. In physical appearance, the patient may range from normal to eunuchoid; frequently the intelligence is impaired with the patient suffering from behavioural problems. There is both infertility and impotence. In some patients there may be bilateral breast development.

This condition is clinically diagnosed using a buccal smear test which shows the extra chromosome. In addition, the trophic hormone (luteinising hormone) and testosterone blood levels are estimated, the former being raised but the latter being low.

The treatment is the administration of testosterone proprionate (Testoral) 10 mg three times daily in combination with Sustanon 250 mg once or twice monthly.

Testicular Feminising Syndrome

When the body cells fail to respond to secreted testosterone this condition is known as testicular feminising syndrome. At birth the genitalia are female but the female reproductive organs are absent and the testes are usully lying intra-abdominally. The child grows as a girl developing breasts until it is noted there is amenorrhoea with scant pubic hair. Often these patients are not referred until puberty and in some cases until after marriage when they are worried about their infertility.

The investigations require the patient to be genotyped, which is male, and the testosterone levels are normal as for the male. The testes (either intra-abdominal or within the inguinal canal) are surgically removed and on recovery from this surgery the patient is commenced on oestrogen to prevent menopausal symptoms.

Severe Bilateral Orchitis

As a complication of mumps, severe bilateral orchitis affects about 20% of the male population who suffered from mumps. As a consequence of the inflammation of the testes (orchitis) the patient may develop infertility, and if occurring before puberty, hypogonadism. The investigations for infertility are the the same as for Klinefelter's syndrome. This complication may possibly be prevented by the administration of cortisone therapy during the acute stage of the mumps. If, however, eunuchoidism occurs the treatment is that for Klinefelter's syndrome.

Undescended Testicle (*see also* Nursing 1)

If the testes have not descended into the scrotal sac during intra-auterine life, they may do so by the end of the first year of life. It is possible to manipulate the testes to descend into their natural position if they are retractile. It is usual for only one testis to be undescended, i.e., unilateral (Fig. 39.3), and because of the intra-abdominal higher temperature it will affect spermatogenesis of the trapped testis.

Treatment may be by giving chorionic gonadotrophin in the early years. If the testis has not descended by the seventh year then surgery may be offered to place the testis in

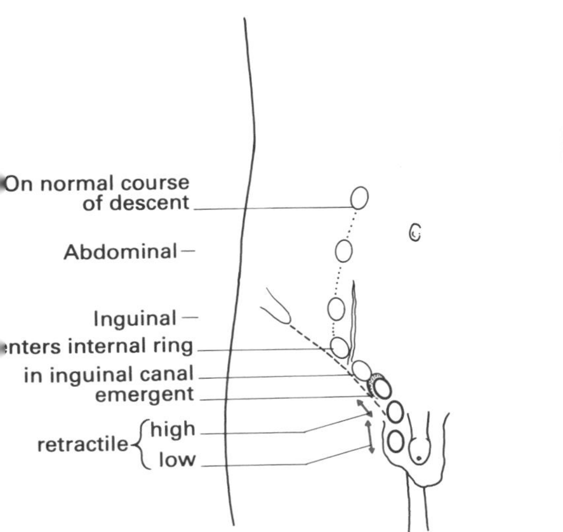

Fig. 39.3 Undescended testicle.

the scrotal sac. The later the treatment the more likelihood of malignant changes.

Malignant Tumour of the Testes

Malignant tumours secrete oestrogens or androgens and depending on the type of cell they originate from they are classified as *seminoma* or *teratoma* if they occur from the germ cells and *interstitial* if they originate from the interstitial cells.

In the early stages they are noticed as painless swellings or inflammation of the scrotum. If the patient comes forward for advice and help the only safe method seems to be surgical exploration of the testes to determine if the hard mass is a tumour. Biopsy of the testicular tissue will show what type of tissue is affected and careful exploration will determine the stage of spread.

Stage 1 the tumour is confined to the testes. If it has spread to the tunica vaginalis the patient may have a hydrocele (Fig. 39.4).

Stage 2 the tumour has invaded into the para-aortic lymph vessels.

Stage 3 the tumour has spread to the mediastinal lymph vessels and beyond.

The treatment depends on the stage of spread. Simple orchidectomy followed by retroperineal irradiation is completed for stages 1 and 2. For more advanced stages chemotherapy is the treatment of choice.

CAUSES OF INFERTILITY

Azoospermia

Azoospermia or absence of spermatozoa in the semen may be due to organic damage to the testes, or to a reduced secretion of testosterone. Full physical examination and screening tests are completed to exclude endocrine disease. The personal details of previous sexual ability are carefully assessed and this means noting if the patient has had an erection, can penetrate the vagina, and can ejaculate. In most cases

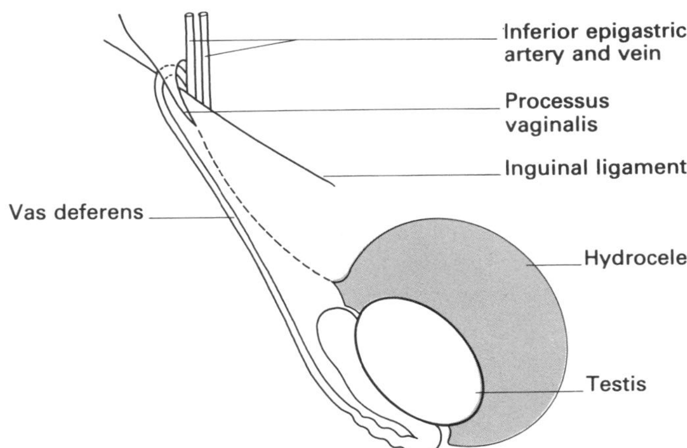

Fig. 39.4 Hydrocele.

it is essential to do a sperm count, the normal values being 50×10^6 sperm/ml of semen. If below 50% of this figure, the patient is usually diagnosed as being infertile. Assessment is also made of the blood concentration of both gonadotrophic hormone and testosterone.

Several conclusions are possible. The sperm may be normal in number and morphology, but for some unknown reason cannot penetrate the female egg. If there are fewer than normal sperms (*oligospermia*), it may be possible to increase their density by prescribing one of the androgens. If there are no sperm at all then testicular exploration may be done to see if there is a mechanical blockage of the epididymis, vas deferens, or the ejaculatory duct. As a last resort testicular biopsy may be done to identify if the seminiferous tubules are normal in their structure.

It is usual practice to counsel the patient and his partner together about the results of all these tests and to advise on whether artificial insemination is feasible or if they should consider adopting a child.

Impotence

Impotence is more precisely defined as a problem with erection or ejaculation. A complete physical examination is undertaken to exclude endocrine and genitourinary disorders, and disease of the lower lumbar sympathetic ganglion. In the absence of organic disorders, i.e., diabetes, vascular problems or neurogenic lesions, there is little that can be done except to refer the patient for psychosexual counselling. If there is an obvious depression then psychiatric help is more useful. Sometimes androgen therapy may be attempted but this is unusual.

Part 5
Oncology Nursing

Chapter 40 Nursing Role and Social Implications

THE ROLE OF THE NURSE

Patients suffering from cancer are nursed in a wide variety of clinical situations. Acute medical, surgical, paediatric, and geriatric wards always have a small number of patients with one or other form of cancer. Although they are referred to radiotherapy units and oncology centres for opinion and treatment, there are inadequate facilities within these units to cope with the numbers requiring inpatient specialist care. From these specialist centres a deep and ever-increasing body of nursing knowledge can be extrapolated for applied use in the general situation, and highlights specific roles for the nurse caring for a patient with cancer.

In manner and approach the nurse should always be cautiously optimistic and encouraging towards the patient. This positive approach can be based on current research which indicates an ever-increasing remission rate over prolonged periods of time for a wide variety of cancer types. The term *cure* must be used with caution; periods of 5–10 years without recurrence of the original cancer are being achieved in a high proportion of patients. Diagnosis is quicker and more accurate than in former times. Investigations also take far less time and with the recent sophistication in new techniques there is far more precision in the results. When taken together, a rapid diagnosis based upon exacting investigations means more rapid decisions being made about the most appropriate therapy.

The techniques now employed to control

pain, which is a major fear for the patient, are achieved with adept and flexible use of analgesics. This is most reassuring to the patient when the severe pain of metastatic cancer is being effectively controlled. The nurse should note that the early stages of cancer are painless. It is when the tumour becomes invasive to neighbouring tissues and structures which contain pain receptors that pain becomes a dreaded reality. Once pain is controlled it is the nursing duty to administer the very necessary drugs, and to report any subtleties of the pain recurring. The control of the patient's pain is vital to ensure a dignity, quality and quantity of life tolerable to both the patient and the nurse.

Nurses caring for cancer patients are those with a highly developed sense of detail and are skilled in observing the most minor of changes. This is combined with an unsurpassed expertise in the most basic of bedside nursing skills. The cancer itself does not respond to nursing care but rather to the effects of prescribed treatment. The problems of prolonged bedrest, nutrition, insomnia, altered body image, psychological distress and many other physical alterations induced by the cancer do respond to nursing interventions. A major problem of cancer is that it must not be seen in isolation occurring to one person, but rather it affects a whole family and the hospital nurse must have a sense of trying to assuage some of the difficulties which a family goes through when their relative is hospitalised.

Empathetic Objectivity

A degree of **empathetic objectivity** is essential if the nurse is to avoid emotional involvement. It has to be agreed that the nurses' emotional responses are a prime motive for their caring attitude and indeed are part of the joy and rewards in nursing job satisfaction. These emotional responses, however, have to be conserved if the nurse is to avoid the increasing phenomena of *emotional burnout* which occurs most frequently in specialised units. The danger to the nurses is that by involving themselves overemotionally in a cancer patient's care, they become physically and mentally exhausted. This exhaustion is soon reflected in errors and incompetent nursing practice. Such a state of affairs can be minimised if nurses develop a sense of objectivity. Emotional involvement can readily be appreciated when the patient is of a young age.

Sharing Problems

An attitude of **sharing** the problem with the patient is of paramount importance. This sharing is a two-way process between nurse and patient. How often it is remarked that many nursing observations are irrelevant to the patient but vital for the nurse. Equally, how often the patient's remarks and conversations have no bearing on the treatment plan or nursing aims, yet, these very remarks highlight what is of greatest concern to the patient. When both observations and patient's comments are brought together they make a much better basis for a positive nursing care plan, which the patient sees as being of direct benefit. This is arrived at if the nurse is willing to share.

Sharing problems with the caring team requires the team to be structured on democratic lines, so that every viewpoint is valid and equal among peers. The clinician is head of the caring team, but relies on the skills of nurses, physiotherapists, the dietician, social worker, spiritual adviser, and the family, to achieve a total balance of care. The nurse's role is to act as the liaison person between all these professional specialists and with the family. **Liaison skills** are an essential component of communication ability, and they should be a part of the nurse's persona. A good communicator promotes the feeling in others of **approachability**, and without this skill many of the aims of clinical therapy and nursing plans will not achieve the individual care plan so vital for the cancer patient.

Communication Skills

An attitude of mind which hinders many nurses is their often expressed anxiety: 'Who is responsible for telling patients they have cancer?' The reality is that many patients know they have cancer, often deduced from wary attitudes of doctors and nurses, the environment in which they are being nursed, and from their general knowledge.

More positively the nurse should consider how do you confirm the patient's worst fears. Once again we return to the **communication skills** of the clinician or nurse. The correct moment to sit down and discuss with the patient the diagnosis and prognosis is arrived at by assessing the verbal and nonverbal cues given by the patient as to when he or she would be most receptive to counselling. The decision to counsel is a very personal judgement. The majority of medical opinion is that the patient has the right to know and that the best person to do the initial counselling is the doctor in charge of the patient's treatment. Thereafter counselling can be continued by any member of the caring team depending on the patient's needs. The major figure in this supportive counselling is the nurse.

It is the nursing role to act as the 'patient's advocate', especially so in circumstances when the physical and psychological distresses of the patient are so great they would antagonise any benefits to be derived from ordered investigations, prescribed therapy or resuscitation. In defending the patient's interests it must be done professionally and discreetly, out of hearing of the patient, and in confidence with the professional colleagues affected. An important rule to remember in nursing cancer patients is that their emotional distress must be considered and their interests should be advocated away from their presence so as not to increase their anxiety.

Clinical Skills

The oncology nurse should develop applied clinical skills which encompass the various therapeutic measures to treat the cancer. These methods include:

Surgical excision of malignant tumours
Radiotherapy techniques
Hormone therapy
Chemotherapy (cytotoxic and antineoplastic drugs)
Immunosuppressive therapy
Palliative therapy for the terminally ill (*see* Nursing 1)
Radioactive implants via surgery

These treatments may be prescribed individually or in combination. Assessing the patient's response to these therapies is a component of the clinical expertise. For example, chemotherapy requires a supreme knowledge of the drugs prescribed, their interactions, possible side effects, methods of administration and hazards. With this knowledge ongoing clinical assessments can be made with confidence and accuracy. Complementary to these particular clinical skills is the mastery of basic nursing procedures adapted to the needs of the individual patient. Careful assessment is required at frequent intervals of the patient's physical needs. Such an assessment may be done by working through the body systems or by assessing the activities of daily living. The most basic nursing skill must never be taken for granted. Moving or lifting a cancer patient without causing pain may seem a simple task, but it is one of the most cherished skills appreciated by the patient in pain.

Professionalism

A nurse can by example influence the sensitivity of colleagues and the general public. Smoking cigarettes while in uniform or when on duty sets an extremely bad example. This lack of professionalism can indicate to an onlooker that all the publicity about cancer is so much nonsense when the professional person is seen to be smoking a cigarette.

Senior students should remember that they by their behaviour are the models for their junior colleagues.

Nurses are often asked their opinion on topics related to cancer and this type of question requires a great deal of thought to avoid creating alarm and despondency. One of the best ways to cope with such a question is to refer to and emphasise the preventative aspects of cancer. Professional journals are widely available and carry many articles on the topic of cancer. Needless to say there is an overabundance of related research to which the nurse can refer in the professional library of the hospital. Local and national organisations, whether statutory or charitable, issue pamphlets, booklets, and advertising material which provide a fruitful resource when trying to communicate with a difficult patient. Patients themselves often gain a great deal by being put in direct contact with these agencies. They provide the help the patient may need when discharged from hospital.

The current medical philosophy when dealing with cancer patients is that investigations, and treatment, are always preferably completed on an outpatient basis while keeping the patient in his or her personal environment, for the duration of any therapy.

Hospital admission is reserved for those cancer patients who require:

Invasive investigations, e.g., endoscopy or biopsy

Invasive therapeutic measures, e.g., surgery, implants

Transfusions of blood or blood fractions

Control of a serious infectious risk

Palliative therapy, if the family cannot cope with a dying relative

SOCIAL IMPLICATIONS

The increasing cure (remission) rate of patients suffering from cancers implies that the nurse must have a close liaison with the medical social worker. Working together, the patient, nurse, and social worker can identify those problems which are beyond the scope of the patient or the family to resolve. A working knowledge of what help is available to a cancer victim is essential for the nurse to direct the patient to the correct social agency. It is not enough to depend entirely on the medical social worker to set the wheels in motion. A few of the more important agencies are the primary health care team, the Social Services Department, the Department of Health and Social Security, and voluntary and research organisations.

Social Agencies

Primary Health Care Team

The GP will continue medical supervision. The community nursing services will deal with physical and other direct care. A speech therapist will be needed if the patient has had a laryngectomy. An ostomy nurse will provide care if the patient has a colostomy or ileostomy, while a mastectomy nurse will supervise and counsel the patient on the use of prostheses.

Social Services Department

The Social Services Department can provide help in many ways. Home helps can be arranged to visit the patient's house to help with cleaning and shopping for several hours each week at a small charge. Social workers can investigate and support the patient if there are difficulties in the home conditions, or with claiming benefits. An occupational therapist can visit the home to suggest some pursuits or activities if the patient is confined to the home.

If adaptations are needed to the house to accommodate aids and appliances, e.g., wheelchairs, or major alterations are necessary such as an indoor toilet, these adaptations can be made by the housing department of the local authority. Meals on Wheels prepared by the catering department of the local authority can be delivered by one of the local voluntary agencies.

Department of Health and Social Security

The Department of Health and Social Security will pay any benefits or pensions due to those over 16 years of age, and will make *exceptional needs payments* to relatives of a cancer victim requiring 24-hour nursing care.

Voluntary Organisations

The patient's denomination may give a clue as to which church or religious group to approach for spiritual support. Aids to daily living are supplied for a small rental fee from the British Red Cross in most major cities. These range from hoists and beds to wheelchairs and commodes. In many instances the equipment is delivered and collected to and from the home.

St John's Ambulance Association should also be approached as they undertake many voluntary duties to help patients in need. Local voluntary groups often take an interest in a particular disabling disease, of which cancer is only one. A quick check with the local information bureau often highlights unpublicised resources.

The National Society for Cancer Relief will consider giving various kinds of help: financial, equipment, and booklet information, if they are approached.

Research Organisations

The Madame Curie Foundation is both a charitable and a research foundation. They provide a night-nursing service to help relatives obtain some sleep and also have rest homes for the long-term care of cancer patients.

The Imperial Cancer Research Fund and The Co-ordinating Committee on Cancer Research, although depending on public subscription for their work, do issue pamphlets and booklets containing useful information for the professionally interested.

Social Dimensions

In the wider social context the nurse should be aware of social dimensions of cancer. The most lethal cancers are those of the stomach, bowel, breast and lung. These 4 taken together account for 110,000–120,000 premature deaths each year. To counter this toll of unnecessary death the Health Education Council's campaign in the media, funded by the Government, is to warn the ordinary citizens of the preventative measures which as individuals they can take on their own initiative.

Research indicates that the modifying of certain behaviours, e.g., smoking cigarettes, drinking strong alcohol, and sexual promiscuity, would reduce the incidence of lung cancer, cancer of the head of pancreas and cervical cancer. It should also be noted that smoking and alcohol also contribute to an even greater killer—cardiovascular disease.

Health Screening

Health screening of those employed in many industries is a requirement of The Health and Safety Act 1974. It would apply particularly to those industries based on the hydrocarbons, where there is persistent exposure to coal, tar, oil, benzene, soot, pitch, and paint. A urine test is all that is usually required to exclude the main risk which is cancer of the bladder. Certain industries require their employees to wear protective clothing, e.g., if working with asbestos, or with radiation, either in the atomic industry or in hospitals. It is worthy of observation that some carcinogens are found in foods and cosmetics, with much depending on their source and basis.

Voluntary attendance at health screening clinics, e.g., Well Woman Clinics, every 2 years after the age of 40 is also to be recommended for the early detection of cancers. Cervical cytology tests available from GPs on a regular basis will detect precancerous cervical states which can now be treated successfully with laser therapy. Blood sampling tests, chest X-rays, and endoscopic examination are routinely done to exclude the possibility of cancer of the lung, bowel or stomach.

Of increasing social significance is the treatment of early detected cancers with laser therapy.

Laser Therapy

The full meaning of the word laser is *light amplification stimulated emission radiation*. In medical use it consists of a concentrated form of electric light which has been intensified by passing it through a second source of energy. Such a light ray is of a single wavelength and can be focused to concentrate its energy on an area no greater than a pinhead. The energy emitted from such a light ray does not usually exceed the heat given off by an average lightbulb, i.e., 1 W. The second source of energy can be variable depending on the type of cell being treated. In the treatment of cancer or tumours the 2 forms of laser which have been successful are: *Neodymium YAG*, which is four times more powerful than the argon laser and when directed through a fibreoptic endoscope can treat tumours of the bladder; and the *carbon dioxide* laser beams which are absorbed by water. This means that this type of laser is an excellent 'scalpel' in those tissues which are composed of 75–90% water. When the laser light is beamed onto the target tissue to within 1 mm and then electronically triggered to last only a few seconds, the energy focus literally vapourises the cells within that area. This therapy is being used successfully in precancerous tumours of the cervix.

The *argon* laser light is being used to coagulate haemorrhaging blood vessels, e.g., the retinal blood vessels, gastric ulcers and birth marks, while the *ruby* laser light is being used to repair detached retinae.

Advantages

There are many advantages to this form of therapy for the patient:

1. It is quick.
2. The infection risk is minimal.
3. Since laser light carries a coagulation effect the risk of post-therapeutic haemorrhage is minimal.
4. Pretherapeutic sedation may be required but the risks of full general anaesthesia and postoperative analgesia have been eliminated since there is little pain.
5. Hospitalisation, if required, would be as a day patient, releasing the resources of the hospital for those in greater need of these facilities.
6. The healing time of laser therapy is extremely rapid.

Nursing Role

The nursing role remains the same. The patient still requires reassurance and guidance as to what to expect and what is expected of them. They need to be comforted while they are being treated and maintained in the desired position.

Chapter 41
Oncology Defined and Classified

Cancer when translated means 'crab', while the term oncology means 'study of tumours'. To overcome emotive responses, *oncology* has been coined in recent times to refer to the study and care of cancer and is now preferred to the single term *cancer*.

All human cells are liable to malignant change, at any age, and the causative factors of such a change are set out in Table 41.1. For this reason any definition of cancer can only be of a general nature. A working definition which can be applied to most types of cancer is the *unrestrained proliferation of a mutant cell due to an irreversible physiological change in the deoxyribonucleic acid, or DNA.*

Table 41.1 Established causes of cancer

*Exogenous**	*Endogenous*
Hydrocarbons from	Steroids
coal	Oestrogens
tar	
oil	
Aniline dyes from rubber	*Hereditary* (rare)
Fluorine compounds in insecticides	Polyposis coli
Arsenical compounds	Retinoblastoma
Asbestos dust	Neurofibromatosis
Tar content of cigarettes	
Cholesterol in diet	*Premalignant states*
Radiation hazards from	Keratosis
ultraviolet light	Leukoplakia
gamma X-rays	Pernicious anaemia
strontium^{90}	Ulcerative colitis
luminous paints	Chronic bronchitis

* 90% of registered cancers are due to exogenous causes.

Table 41.2. Terminology to classify tumours

Tissue affected	Classification	
	Benign	Malignant
Epithelial	Epithelioma	
Skin, mouth, lung		Squamous cell sarcoma
Skin, face		Basal cell sarcoma
Urinary tract, bladder		Transitional cell sarcoma
Bone	Osteoma	Osteosarcoma
Muscle	Myoma	Myosarcoma
Cartilaginous	Chondroma	Chondrosarcoma
Lymphatic	Lymphoma	Lymphosarcoma
Nerve	Neuroma	Neurosarcoma

CELL MUTATION AND GROWTH

How this physiological change in the DNA of the cell actually occurs has not been accurately determined. One postulation is that the endoreticular membrane oxidises the causative carcinogen. Following this the DNA in the cell breaks down, and the genetic code carried by the DNA becomes damaged, mutating the orderly structure of the intracellular organisation. The mutated cell has at first a slow reproductive rate, but a prolific metabolism. To meet this need it relies on the sugars of the glycoproteins. A typical cancer cell doubles every 100 days, implying a prolonged period before the resulting tumour grows and reaches a detectable size.

At 0.25 cm the tumour can be detected with modern techniques, e.g., body scan

At 1 cm the tumour can be felt on palpation, e.g., breast cancer

At 2 cm symptoms will be present

As the malignant tumour grows, parts, or individual cells may break off and spread to adjacent or distant structures well removed from its primary site. This spread, or metastasis, is aided by:

Infiltration of a neighbouring structure by direct spread

Entering the circulatory system to be conveyed to a new site

Travelling via the lymphatic system

Transcoelemically, i.e., across the peritoneal membranes in the abdomen

CLASSIFICATION

The classification of malignant tumours is based upon the name of the originating tissue, and to mark the difference between malignant and benign tumours. The suffix *sarcoma* is added to the tissue named in the prefix and implies malignancy, while the suffix *oma* is used to identify benign tumours. Examples of the terminology used are given in Table 41.2.

Once the muscle and nerve tissues have matured, i.e., after full growth has been reached, the cells of these tissues do not reproduce. The incidence of cancer, therefore, in these tissues is much rarer than in any other type of tissue. The differences between a benign and malignant tumour are outlined in Table 41.3 and some emphasis should be given to the fact the majority of tumours are benign, e.g., only 10% of all breast tumours are malignant.

CAUSES

The known causes of cancer are grouped under the subheadings outlined in Table 41.1. Exogenous causes are by far the greatest, i.e., approximately 90%, highlighting the importance of various industries such as the chemical, rubber, asbestos, and nuclear organisations. The Health and Safety at Work Act 1974 acknowledges the risks to which these workers are exposed and the working environment is so structured as to protect the individual employee from the handling,

Table 41.3. Pathological differences of malignant and benign tumours

Structure	Benign tumour	Malignant tumour
Gross	Encapsulated Defined border edge Minimal vascularity Localised to area Surrounding tissue unaffected	Without a capsule Irregular border edge Tendency to ulcerate and bleed Rapid spread in soft tissues Surrounding tissues infiltrated
Microscopic	Slow growth Normal DNA Normal cellular chemistry Normal nucleus Normal morphology	Rapid growth after a slow start Mutated genes on damaged DNA Rapid abnormal metabolism Abnormal nucleus Irregular shape
Comparison with parent cell	Similar characteristics of parent cell, i.e., poorly differentiated	Dissimilar to parent cell, i.e., well differentiated Mitosis of the cell is independent of the initiating carcinogen

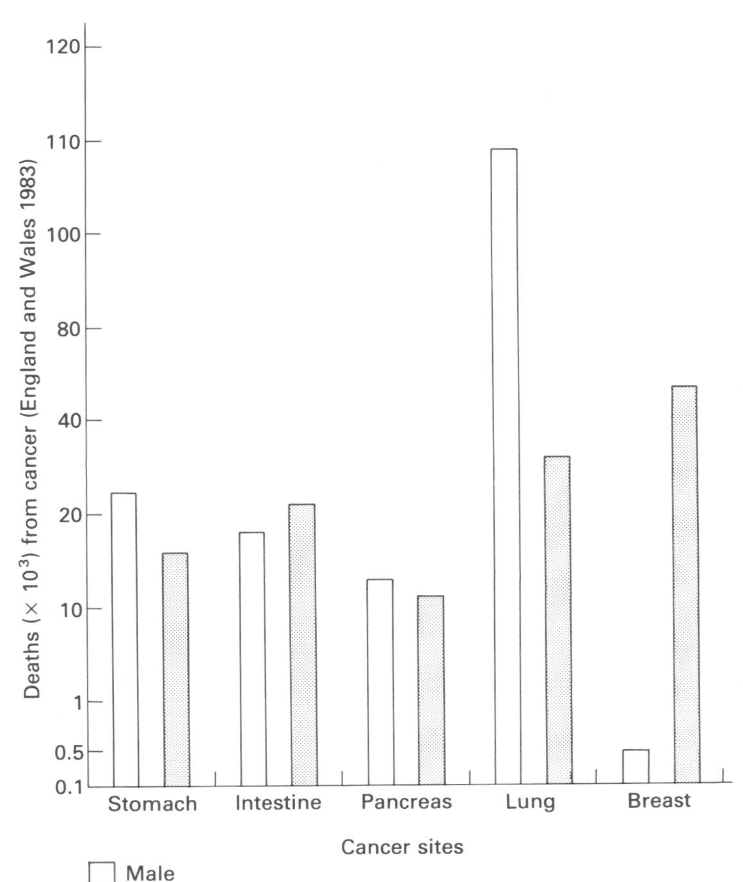

Fig. 41.1 Comparison of number of male and female deaths occurring from different types of cancer.

inhaling, or exposure to the known carcinogens.

The greatest exogenous cause is the habit of smoking cigarettes; the relationship between cause and effect is too great to ignore. The Royal College of Physicians state that there are 90 000 premature deaths every year in the UK as the result of smoking, of which cancer of the lung is a leading cause. In addition 50 million working days per annum are lost from the illnesses arising from this habit.

Experimentally it is proven that the Rous virus can cause cancer in animals, and research continues to attempt to show that this or a similar virus can cause cancer in man. More recently nutritional research indicated refined white sugar and excess cholesterol in the diet as not only contributing to vascular disease but also as being carcinogenic initiating agents. Emphasis has been placed on what has become known as the *prudent diet*. In this the dietetic intake of these particular foodstuffs is reduced while a greater amount of fibre (roughage) taken in the daily diet is encouraged, to reduce the risk of intestinal cancer. Studies from Africa show that the indigenous population rarely suffer from cancer of the bowel crediting this to their high intake of fibre foods. In Japan the incidence of cancer of the stomach has the highest rate internationally and is said to be due to the culturally accepted method of eating semicooked or raw fish. Scottish culture and social habit on the other hand shows a relationship between the high cholesterol diet and the considerable smoking incidence. It correlates with the statistical evidence that Scots have the highest rate of cancer of the lung.

While there are few endogenous causes, that is arising from within the body, it illustrates the importance of not abusing drugs, e.g., steroids and oestrogens. The former are used for many chronic inflammatory conditions while the latter are used in contraceptive pills. Prolonged chronic diseases with an associated inflammatory process may be the initiating carcinogen, and the incidence of cancer following these diseases is too high to ignore. Figure 41.1 indicates several differences between the incidence of cancer in males and females. Males have an extremely high propensity to lung cancer, while females have a propensity for breast cancer.

Chapter 42
Radiotherapy Nursing

A means of disrupting and ultimately destroying a cell is to radiate it with either particulate or electromagnetic rays. These rays when emitted from a controlled source upset the cell by altering both the molecular and biochemical structures. This is known as *ionisation* since ions are added to the cell's existing structure.

PARTICULATE RAYS

The more commonly used particulate rays are alpha, beta, neutrons and protons. Alpha rays have limited power of penetration; much of the kinetic energy is lost when the ray is emitted. Beta rays are directed through a cathode tube and have good powers of penetration. The kinetic energy however depends on the radioactive material being used, e.g., ^{32}P, ^{14}C, or ^{131}I. In effect they only modify the cells' biochemical structure. Neutrons and protons are negative particulates, but when set on a collision course with any other atoms they have a high reactivity, which allows them to penetrate the nucleus of the atom. The result is that the nucleus of the cell body becomes modified.

ELECTROMAGNETIC RAYS

Electromagnetic rays such as X-ray and gamma rays are derived from high voltage electricity and their effect is to disturb the electrons surrounding an atom, causing them to become detached. When directed at cells they upset the electrical neutrality of the solution surrounding the cell. If of sufficient power, e.g., a Van de Graaff machine will give

13000 volts while a linear accelerator machine will emit 6 million volts, the effect on a malignant cell would be that the cell:

Dies outright
Dies during cell division
Is rendered incapable of reproduction
Has a reduced blood supply
Becomes amenable to the body's immune system

Radiation

Radiation is also given off from certain elements, e.g., radium, caesium, cobalt and yttrium. Radium, although an unstable source, is used in radium needles for implanting into body cavities or tissues which are malignant. Caesium, when enclosed in specially designed applicators and implanted into body cavities, can emit sufficient radiation to completely disrupt a malignant cell. Cobalt radiation is directed through a cathode tube and used for superficial penetration of malignant tumours on the body surface. Yttrium is enclosed in needles or grains for implant into tumour sites.

THERAPEUTIC USES

Teletherapy can be used in many situations as:

Deep X-ray therapy to radiate tumours not amenable to surgery
Superficial X-ray therapy for skin and surface lesions
Implants either into a body cavity, interstitially or as a surface mould
An aid to diagnosis using X-rays and gamma rays
Tracers when radioactive isotopes are injected into the body

The types of teletherapy that are used therapeutically to treat cancers are graded as being radical, preoperative or palliative. Treatment is *radical* if the radiation dose is between 6000 and 7000 rad in a series of treatments over 6–7 weeks. Following each 2000 rad dose the patient is usually given a week's rest period. *Preoperative* treatment is when the radiation dose is up to 4000 rad over a period of 4 weeks which is then followed by a rest period before being admitted for surgery. *Palliative* doses of radiation up to 2000 rad over a 2-week interval will induce some resolution of the severity of the symptoms from which the patient is suffering and should improve the quality of the patient's life.

Planning and Investigations

The majority of patients receive the teletherapy regimen as outpatients, but before the treatment begins there is a period of planning and pretherapeutic investigations. Haematology screening is completed to exclude any hint of infections or anaemia both of which would be treated first. The patient is counselled to expect repeated blood investigations throughout the course of treatment perhaps as often as twice a week. This is to ensure that anaemia is not being caused by the treatment. Some patients will require during the course of the teletherapy to be admitted for blood transfusions and if on combined chemotherapy are usually admitted as a day patient.

The planning involves detailed measurements of the site to be irradiated. Precise calculations are made to allow for body contours to enable the technicians to design and make a protective mould which will protect healthy tissues during the actual radiation treatment. The skin of the tumour site is marked with indelible ink or pencil and the patient is advised that on no account must it be washed off or altered.

Advising the Patient

Psychologically many patients have difficulty in coping with what is to them an abstract treatment, since they cannot see anything other than space-age type machines which are confusing in their complexity. To overcome the many diverse emotional responses to teletherapy that patients may experience, most radiotherapy departments issue information booklets giving advice on the dos and don'ts for patients during their course of treatment.

Skin Care

The skin over the treatment area will invariably have a reaction. The present sophistication of teletherapy, especially of the linear accelerator, is described as being *skin sparing*. Generally, however, the following guidelines in the care of the skin should be followed unless the nurse is otherwise instructed:

1. The irradiated skin area should be washed with plain tap water only, and patted dry, not rubbed.
2. Soaps, cosmetics, perfumes, powders, and adhesives are not to be used if they are known to be zinc or lead based as both increase the sensitivity of the skin during a course of teletherapy. Since the average person does not know the base of these compounds they are best avoided altogether.
3. Skin folds and creases are particularly vulnerable to excoriation when the combined effects of teletherapy, moisture from perspiration and body heat take their toll on these areas, e.g., the breast folds, groin crease and perineum. These areas must be kept absolutely clean and as dry as possible at all times.
4. Clothing worn over the treatment area should be lightweight, worn loosely, and be of a smooth texture, e.g., silk-type materials.

Nursing Care

When giving care to the skin the nurse should observe for certain reactions:

1. Erythema or a red discolouration. If very pronounced a steroid cream may be prescribed to promote healing
2. Dry desquamation or epithelial shedding. This will usually respond to applications of gentian violet
3. Moist desquamation which requires the teletherapy to be temporarily cancelled until the skin heals. The area is dressed with nonabsorbent sterile dressings secured to the skin with light bandaging. Adhesive tape should not be used, and this includes the nonallergic type

Diet

Whether as an inpatient or an outpatient, advice will be required by the patient about diet as some loss of appetite is to be expected. The patient should persist with a high protein bland diet supplemented with milk and prescribed vitamins. If the patient has difficulty with swallowing then foods should be liquidised and flavoured to the patient's preference. The drinking of extra fluids by the patient is to be encouraged, up to a volume of 2–3 litres per day if possible. Feelings of nausea and episodes of vomiting should also be expected and to anticipate this prescribed drugs such as Stemetil will normally be available for the nurse to administer as and when required. This is particularly true when the abdomen and mediastinum are being irradiated.

Lethargy

The patient should be warned to expect increased tiredness and to accordingly plan to have more rest periods and to prolong the normal sleeping pattern. If anxiety is causing insomnia or restlessness then sedative drugs are employed to encourage the necessary periods of rest. Equally important for outpatients is for them to reduce their working commitment to a minimum but at the same time retain some interests or hobbies which do not involve heavy physical activity.

Localised Reactions

Local teletherapy will create localised reactions and the nurse should include within the nursing plan specific observations to be made for the area being treated.

Brain—observe for the signs and symptoms of cerebral oedema and alopecia.

Head and neck—daily observation of the mucous membranes for any reactions. Inspect the mouth daily for any sign of infection and dental decay.

Eyes—check the conjunctiva for signs of inflammation and the cornea for abrasions.

Implement eye toilet on a routine basis and consider if eye pads would help.

Oesophagus—if dysphagia occurs, liquidised food of the correct nutritional calorific value may either be offered orally or be administered via a nasogastric tube. If the patient is able to swallow a Mucaine mucilage given 30 minutes before meals, it will decrease the patient's difficulties with swallowing.

Lung and trachea—note if there is a persistent dry cough, any sign of breathlessness and carefully monitor the risk of lung infection. Often prophylactic antibiotics, steriods, and inhalations are prescribed to deal with these anticipated difficulties, but such prescriptions do not come with any guarantees.

Abdomen—anorexia, vomiting, and diarrhoea are to be expected but they must not be confused with radiation sickness. They are the end result of toxic metabolites released when the malignant cells are destroyed. Urinary frequency, bladder infections, and haematuria can be expected if the pelvic region is being treated and often this is anticipated by the use of an indwelling urinary catheter. Tenesmus, mucoid diarrhoea, proctitis and rectal bleeding must be reported even if the preventive treatment of prednisolone (Predsol) enema is being used. There is a danger of a localised fibrosis if the local teletherapy is of a prolonged nature. Note and report on the condition of the perineum and groin creases which are liable to excoriation.

Bones—expect the patient to complain of localised severe pain which will require analgesia. Take precautions when lifting or moving the patient to avoid the risk of pathological fractures as the bones are prone to breakage.

RADIOACTIVE IMPLANTS

Caesium (^{137}CS) is one of the more commonly used radioactive substances to irradiate a tumour of the vagina, cervix, and body of the uterus. The amount of caesium, measured in millicuries, required to destroy the tumour is calculated and ordered by the radiotherapist from the caesium curator of the medical physics department. Planning, preimplant fitness and haematology screening are all completed before admission to hospital.

Nursing Care

Several days before the implant is placed in position under the effects of a general anaesthetic, the patient will be admitted to hospital. This 2–3 day interval is used by the medical and nursing staff to counsel and orientate the patient to her nursing environment and to obtain her co-operation during the course of therapy. Particular points which must be explained to the patient include:

1. The anticipated period of bedrest may extend from 40 hours to 10 days. During this time she will have to remain on bedrest in the dorsal position being allowed only 2 pillows. The implant and its position invariably excludes any other position of care.

2. Her bed area will be screened with half-body height, portable lead screens. Anyone approaching the bed must stand behind these screens, especially the nurse when giving care of any type to the patient. They are so positioned to protect the nursing staff from being irradiated during the giving of care.

3. Family visitors will be discouraged during the period of irradiation. If it is to be a prolonged period of therapy, visitors may be allowed at the bedside for no more than 5 minutes per day and they too must be shielded by the lead screen.

4. Nursing care will be planned to be given in the minimum of time with the maximum comfort achieved. This is necessary because of the radiation being emitted from the caesium implant.

5. The evening before and the morning of the operation an enema will be given to completely evacuate and cleanse the lower colon. This does make it easier for the radiotherapist to implant the caesium applicator.

6. While the implant is in position the

patient will receive a low residue diet to eliminate the need for defaecation. This type of diet may have to be continued if the caesium treatment is to be followed by teletherapy. Relatives should be asked not to bring foods or chocolates as the patient may not be allowed to have them.

7. To eliminate the need for micturition an indwelling urinary catheter will be in position and continuously draining, into a 12-hour collection bag.

8. The perineum and vagina will need to be shaved because the majority of patients have a dilatation and curettage of the uretus and a cystoscopy of the bladder before the implant is secured into position. This is usually done for all patients having a first implant.

Preoperative Care Plan

A specific preoperative care plan should take into account the patient's postoperative needs. Bathing the patient and the care of her hair will be more difficult than usual during this period. Suitable personal bedwear should be available for the postoperative period.

Premedication is usually atropine 0.6 mg given 1 hour before the scheduled time of surgery.

Application of Caesium

Depending on the type of applicator being used to house the caesium, of which the nurse will be advised, the following may have to be done:

1. A Blomfields applicator which can house sufficient caesium to emit 350 mCi of radiation is made out of perspex and moulded to fit the uterine body. To help secure the applicator in place the patient is fitted with a gynaecological harness. This is made of a lightweight linen and consists of 2 shoulder straps connected to a waistband. From the back of the waistband 2 lengths of rubber are brought forward and downwards and connected to the applicator. After the applicator is in place the rubber bands are tightened and secured at the waistband and remain so until the applicator is due for removal.

2. Uterine tube applicators are also moulded from perspex and are held in place by packs.

3. Heyman's beads which are for cervical implant are housed in a perspex mould. There are usually 6 in number. Each bead has a thread and coloured numbered disc which are visible and should be checked each day.

4. Radioactive needles housing radium, gold or yttrium are implanted into the vagina. These too have visible threads emerging and require to be checked each day.

Postoperative Care

On return from theatre the nurse must visually check that the implant is safely in place, checking the number of threads and comparing this check with that recorded on the caesium treatment chart. The intended time and date of removal is noted on the patient care plan. The nursing plan of physical care must be strictly adhered to and is usually designed to give direct care every 8 hours and, whenever possible, to coincide with the administration of drugs such as antiemetics, analgesics, and sedation.

Therapeutic Plan

The therapeutic plan depends on the site of the tumour. For the body of the uterus, patients may have 2 caesium implants, each insertion being interrupted by an interval of 3 weeks. In addition to the frequent haematology screening, blood sugar estimations are also done as are liver function tests prior to the treatment. For treatment of the cervix, 1 caesium implant is usually followed by 3 weeks of high energy teletherapy on an outpatient basis. After a rest interval the patient is readmitted for a second caesium implant. Prior to this planned therapy the patient normally would have a chest X-ray, intravenous pyelography, and a Wassermann reaction test.

Caesium Removal

When the caesium is due for removal a very strict procedure is followed by a qualified nurse. A double check is made with a nursing colleague on the removal date and time, and the type and amount of caesium to be removed.

One hour before the implant is removed a powerful prescribed analgesic is administered, e.g., Cyclomorphine 10 mg. Several minutes before the applicator is withdrawn the urinary catheter is disconnected and removed. When a gynaecological harness is being used the rubber attachments are slackened off and disengaged. Sterile rubber gloves must be worn throughout these procedures. First remove any packs and then the applicators. These are removed in reverse order if they are threaded with numbered discs, i.e., number 6 disc first then 5, 4, 3, 2, and finally number 1. When released from the body cavity, long-handled forceps should be used to transfer the caesium applicator to a lead container filled with tap water. These lead containers must be immediately sealed and returned to the caesium safe in the medical physics department as soon as possible.

Following removal of the applicators, vulval toilet is a prerequisite to enhance the patient's personal comfort. The patient should however remain in the dorsal position for a few hours more, being raised to the semirecumbent position gradually. This is due to postural changes in the blood pressure, which can be expected following a period of prolonged bed-rest in one position.

Premature or accidental removal of the implants is most unusual. In the unlikely event of this happening, the radiotherapist must be informed immediately, the time noted, and check X-rays organised. Used linen may have to be double checked if radioactive needles become displaced, or when the disc or thread count does not tally with the caesium treatment chart.

HEALTH AND SAFETY

Nurses working with patients receiving radiotherapy, especially with implants, should have regard to their own health and safety. They will be issued with a radiation detection badge which should be worn at all times when on duty. This badge contains a disc which will be Geiger countered to assess the amount of radiation the nurse has been exposed to over a period of 1 month. If the exposure level exceeds the internationally agreed safety level, the nurse should be temporarily transferred to another type of nursing duty. Then once checks have been completed and cleared on the nurse's haemoglobin and leucocyte count, she or he can return to previous duties.

Chapter 43
Chemotherapy Nursing

Should a cancer not prove amenable to either teletherapy or surgical treatment then the chemotherapeutic group of drugs known as *cytotoxic agents* may be prescribed to destroy the malignant cells. Cancers amenable to chemotherapy are shown in Table 43.1. These are supplemented by other drugs, e.g., hormones, vitamins, and immunosuppressive agents.

CYTOTOXIC AGENTS

Cytotoxic agents are in an ever-increasing range of drugs used primarily to:

- Prolong life by inducing a remission
- Relieve the worst of the symptoms including pain
- Be curative, which in many cases they are
- Prevent micrometastases in early diagnosed primary cancers.

Their method of action is to penetrate the malignant cells' nuclei and disrupt the genetic code of the cell which is carried by the genes along the double helix strand of the DNA (deoxyribonucleic acid). Cytotoxic agents perform this task in a variety of ways depending on the group from which they are derived.

Table 43.1. Cancers amenable to chemotherapy

Acute or chronic leukaemia	Ovarian cancer
Breast cancer	Choriocarcinoma (fetus in utero)
Retinoblastoma (eye)	Wilms' tumour (kidney)
Lymphoma (Hodgkin's disease)	Small cell lung cancer
Ewing's sarcoma (long bone)	Neuroblastoma (brain)
Seminoma (testes)	Rhabdomyosarcoma (muscle)

This grouping is artificial as many cytotoxic drugs are in fact combined to achieve the best effect.

Plant alkaloids are obtained from the tropical periwinkle plant and interrupt the division of the malignant cell. Of itself this would not rid the body of the malignant cell but limits its potential to multiply. *Alkylating agents* interact with the DNA to break or cross strand the double helix preventing further cell reproduction. *Antimetabolite* drugs compete with the existing cellular metabolites. They oppose the cell's ability to utilise both purines and folic acid. In addition they antagonise the malignant cell's ability to synthesise intracellular enzymes. *Antibiotics* lock onto the DNA and interfere with DNA–RNA synthesis thus disrupting cellular reproduction.

Drug Prescription

Cytotoxic drugs may be prescribed as a single agent, combination or adjuvant therapy. **Single agent therapy** is when only one drug is prescribed and administered. **Combination therapy**, or the grouping of several of these drugs is the most prevalent form of chemotherapy. **Adjuvant therapy** usually follows or precedes radiotherapy or surgery in the treatment of cancer.

Limiting Factors

Cytotoxic drugs have limiting factors. Tolerance to the drugs can be very low before serious side effects are seen. Careful calculations of dosage, assessment of course duration and screening of the patient's blood for anaemia are made before a course of therapy is embarked upon. Toxicity to healthy tissues, cells and organs can also produce serious side effects, e.g., nephrotoxicity, hepatotoxicity, and encephalotoxicity.

Care on Handling

Nurses involved in the preparation and administration of cytotoxic drugs must take additional precautions beyond those used with other drugs. Several of the cytotoxic agents are corrosive to the skin and potentially they can be absorbed through the mucosa of the eyes and mouth. It is strongly recommended that all such drugs being prepared for intravenous injection should be drawn up in a quiet, well-ventilated area away from the busy mainstream of the ward.

Ampoules or containers should only be handled with the gloved hand, preferably with the 'triplex' type of glove being worn. A mask and close-fitting disposable gown with full length sleeves should be worn. For protection of the eyes from an inadvertent spray from the syringe and needle, eye goggles are available and should be worn. When opening ampoules they should be held away from the eyes and face.

In combination therapy several drugs will be drawn up at the same time. It is advisable to label each prepared syringe with the name of the drug which will ensure that they are administered in the correct order and to the correct patient. Several of these drugs cannot be mixed in the same syringe and for this reason they should **never** be mixed during preparation. The checking of cytotoxic drugs **must** always be done by a registered nurse who may *only* give these drugs if she or he has had extended training in intravenous therapy, otherwise they must be given by a doctor. After the drug has been administered all items used should be sealed in a disposable plastic bag and despatched for incineration. If spillage should occur the drug must be diluted with ample amounts of water before the contaminated surface is wiped dry. Wherever possible the drugs should be prepared by the pharmacy department.

Side Effects

The side effects of cytotoxic drugs are numerous and are varied in their intensity. The nursing care plan must take into account the potential of these drugs to increase the patient's physical distress and psychological anxieties. Many of the side effects only last for several days beyond the completion of the course but this is of little help to the patient while these discomforts are endured. The sophistication of drug dosage has meant a decline in the more ferocious of the side effects.

Systems Affected

Gastrointestinal Tract

Stomach—nausea and vomiting which can be minimised with the use of antiemetics, e.g., prochlorperazine (Stemetil), and a careful choice of menu.
Colon—diarrhoea and intestinal hurry are a major problem for the patient in that unexpected 'accidents' lead to a great deal of embarrassment. Codeine phosphate reduces intestinal hurry and Kaolin et Morphia may be prescribed for the diarrhoea.

Haemopoietic Tissues

Bone marrow—some drugs depress the blood cell forming marrow giving rise to leucopenia. This will lower the patient's resistance to infection. Thrombocytopenia may cause minor haemorrhagic episodes which take the form of petechia of the skin. Careful lifting and moving of the patient will be essential. Anaemia of the iron deficiency type may necessitate the patient having a blood transfusion during the course of therapy. A serious agranulocytosis often requires a temporary cessation of therapy to rest and restore the patient.

Reproductive Organs

Testes—sterility but not impotence may be the long-term effect.
Ovaries—menstrual cycle is arrested with early menopause.

Integumentum

Scalp—hair loss in moderate amounts from the scalp and other hair bearing areas can be expected. Wigs are available from the NHS for a small fee, and are vital for the 'cosmetic' dignity of the patient.
Skin—excoriation of the skin can be prevented by careful nursing. Rashes and altered pigmentation may require the use of steroid creams and soothing lotions.

Renal System

Kidney—fluid balance charting is required for certain drugs and daily testing of urine should be done as a routine screening for any abnormality.
Bladder—urinary tract infections can be detected by despatching at regular intervals samples of urine for culture and sensitivity.

Central Nervous System

Periphery—if the patient complains of pins and needles or muscular weakness then neurotoxicity to the drugs may be developing. Careful lifting, moving, and positioning of the patient becomes increasingly important because of muscular weakness.

Advising the Patient

Many patients have their course of cytotoxic drugs as an outpatient and in these instances there is usually little change to their daily life. A normal well-balanced diet but with easily digested foods is normally recommended with some increase in the fluid intake. Alcohol, however, is best avoided until the course of treatment is concluded.

Medicines other than the cytotoxic drugs can only be taken with the consent of the treating physician; this equally applies to inpatients. The majority can continue with their normal employment, but should they require temporary admission they are advised to bring along some form of diversional therapy with which to occupy themselves until they are again discharged from hospital. Leisure activities, e.g., sport, must be reviewed in the light of the particular drugs being prescribed. In all cases patients will be screened twice- or once-weekly to check on their blood counts to assess the degree, if any, of anaemia, as this is a potential side effect of cytotoxic drugs.

Chapter 44
Breast Cancer

During a woman's life there are frequent changes occurring within the breast tissue and structure. At puberty the natural enlargement of the mammary glands is influenced by the hormones oestrogen and progesterone. At each menstrual period the breasts slightly increase in size and may be painful. During pregnancy the breasts enlarge by one third in preparation for lactation and breastfeeding. If there is a gain or loss in weight this is reflected in the amount of adipose tissue contained within the breast capsule. Fig. 12.8 (p. 99) illustrates healthy breast tissue.

At the menopause the Cooper's ligaments lose their former elasticity causing the density and firmness of the breast tissue to sag with some atrophy. These are normal changes and may confuse some individuals when the change is concurrent with a 'tumour'. Correctly used, the word *tumour* means a swelling which may be entirely benign. For many people 'tumour' is synonymous with 'cancer' and therefore a careful choice of words is required by the nurse. Until the type of tumour is firmly diagnosed the word 'swelling' is more accurate and without the threats implied in the word cancer. The majority of these swellings are benign, i.e., 90%; it is the remaining 10% of patients who are at risk that their swelling is a cancer.

For a malignant tumour to be felt or palpated it has to be at least 2 cm in size, which means that the cancer cells have been in the breast tissue for some time. A visual swelling of the part of the breast affected which does not recede before or after

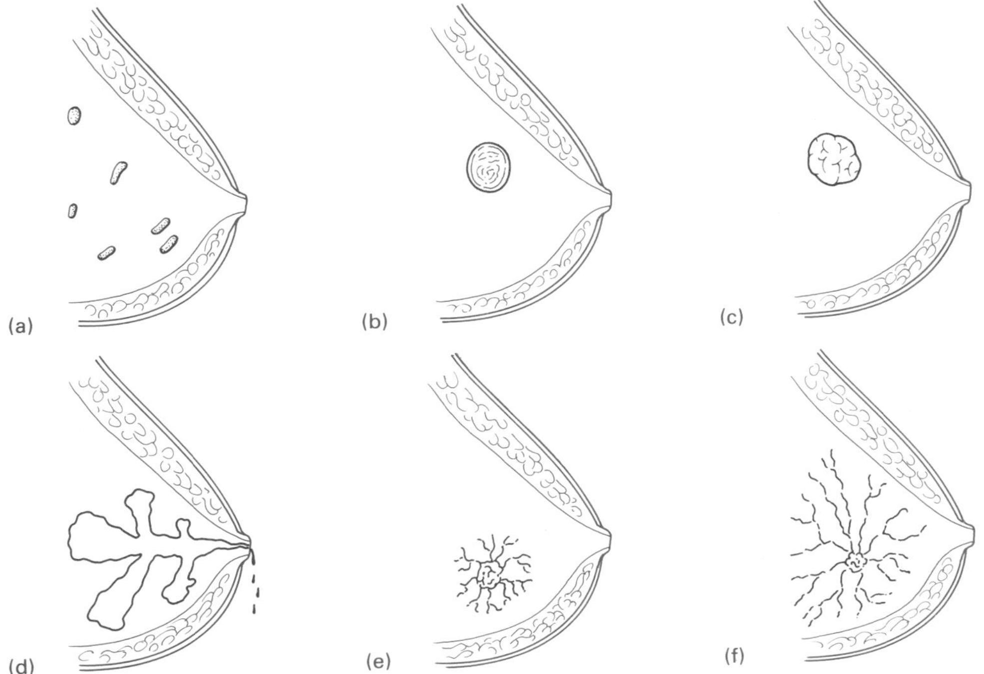

Fig. 44.1 Breast tumours: fibrocystic disease (a); simple cyst (b); fibro-adenoma (c); papilloma (d); early malignant tumour (e); malignant tumour (f).

menstruation is highly suspect. The malignant tumour at this stage is painless and this is a most important concept since other types of swellings, in general, cause some degree of discomfort. Any of these 3 signs, palpable lump, obvious enlargement, which is painless, are sufficient grounds for a doctor to request a biopsy of breast tissue to confirm or exclude a breast cancer. Different types of tumours are illustrated in Fig. 44.1. Without exception most GPs refer their patients directly to local breast clinics or oncology centres for further investigations.

POSSIBLE CAUSES

The causes of breast cancer can only be speculated upon, and from the tremendous amount of research, recurring themes suggest that:

1. There is a geographical distribution which is comparatively higher in the western, well-developed countries in comparison to a low incidence in third world and under-developed countries. The implications being that there is some factor in diet, industry, or culture which causes breast cancer.
2. Those countries adopting a western style culture, notably Japan, are showing an increasing incidence of breast cancer.
3. Lactation and childbearing under the age of 25 years seems to confer a protection against breast cancer, while childbearing over the age of 30 and older does not exclude the possibility of developing breast cancer.
4. A short interval between the first menarche and the first pregnancy seems to confer a natural protection.
5. The Bittner virus can produce breast cancer during experimental research on mice but has only been isolated in some women in Iraq who had breast cancer.
6. Ionising radiation, e.g., as at Hiroshoma, increases the incidence of breast cancer.
7. Prolonged use of hormones may

influence changes in the breast tissue which might initiate a cancer.

INCIDENCE

In the UK the current mortality rate is 12 000 deaths per annum from advanced breast cancer, mainly affecting the female population aged 35–55 years old. It is calculated that 1 in every 14 females in the UK is at risk of developing a breast cancer. The younger the patient the more rapid the dissemination of the tumour, the older female tends to have a slowly growing tumour with a reduced risk of metastases.

With these facts and figures it is not to be wondered at that the female patient can be in panic and dread if she discovers a lump in her breast. The initial reaction of many patients is one of 'denial'. Some patients tend to laugh it off, others suppress their knowledge from their family, while others experience a reactive depression which prevents them from communicating their fear and anxiety. The converse fact is that with an early diagnosis and treatment, the curative rate is 50% without a recurrence in the following 10 years. If this fact were known more generally by the lay public it would do much to encourage patients that if they come forward quickly they can look forward to quick and positive steps to deal with any type of 'lump'.

DETECTION

The nurse by example and advice can advocate that the single most effective method of detecting early changes in the breast tissue is by regular self-examination: on the day following the end of each menstrual period, *or* the first day of each month for postmenopausal women.

By looking at the breast in a mirror and palpating each breast in a clockwise direction, any of these four signs should be noted if present:

1. A lump which was not there the previous month.
2. Pain in or of the breast which is not related to the menstrual cycle.
3. Discharge from the nipple.
4. Alteration of the colour or texture of the breast between each examination.

With any of these signs patients should ask for an immediate appointment to see their GP, and it is always wise to state why the appointment is required to avoid delay if an appointment system is in operation. This method of self-screening is far more reliable than any other form of screening yet devised and does much to reduce anxieties that would otherwise plague the mind of the uncertain individual.

INVESTIGATIONS

The investigations which may be undertaken to confirm the patient's suspicions and the doctor's provisional diagnosis are:

Mammography—a specialised technique of X-raying the mammary glands. It can detect tiny calcified areas which occur within a malignant tumour. It is also used on a widespread scale as a 'screening technique' for the general public.

Xerography—using a selenium X-ray sensitive film the dark and light areas of soft tissues of the breast are dramatically pronounced, a small malignant tumour may be detected by its density against the shaded areas.

Thermography—malignant tumours emit infra-red rays from the tumour site because of their increased metabolism, and higher temperature, and these rays can be detected by special photography.

Cytology—microscopic study will be undertaken for nipple discharge, if it is present, aspirated breast fluid and cervical smear to detect for metastasis.

Skeletal scan—the painless nature of breast cancer may mean that before localised symptoms occur the cancer may already have spread to deposits in the bones.

Biopsy of tissue—this is usually performed under a general anaesthetic in hospital and immediately precedes surgery upon the breast. The biopsy sample when taken is immediately frozen. The pathologist examines sections of the specimen under the microscope and confirms or excludes the cancer diagnosis and indicates to the surgeon the type of operation necessary.

TUMOUR STAGES

From the investigations and their results the surgeon in charge of the patient may stage the progress of the cancer, that is, how far it has developed. Staging the tumour will indicate to the surgeon the type of treatment best suited for the patient and it also permits a prognosis to be constructed. Two methods of staging are in current use: The Manchester method and the Union Internationale contre le Cancer method (IUCC).

Manchester Method

Manchester method classifies the tumour into 4 stages.

Stage 1—the tumour is confined to within the breast capsule and is curable by surgery.

Stage 2—the tumour has infiltrated down to the muscle or up to the skin and is curable by surgery.

Stage 3—the tumour is fixed to the pectoralis major muscle or the skin and is invasive to the regional lymph nodes. Surgery and radiotherapy are the treatments of choice.

Stage 4—the tumour is invasive locally with distant dissemination. The treatment involves radiotherapy, chemotherapy, and systemic therapy.

Union Internationale Contre le Cancer Method

Using the symbols **T** which means tumour, **N** meaning lymph nodes, and **M** meaning distant metastasis, the 3 aspects of breast cancer can be tabulated (see Table 44.1).

THERAPEUTIC REGIMENS

Once the tumour has been staged (Fig. 44.2), the therapeutic regimen is decided upon. The various regimens include surgery, chemotherapy, hormone therapy and radiotherapy.

Surgery

Often the decision as to which type of operation is not made until after the result of a frozen biopsy is known. The operation may involve a partial, simple, modified or radical mastectomy.

A *partial mastectomy* is also known as a *lumpectomy* and refers to the excision of the tumour only. Normally the wound would not have a drain in position.

A *simple mastectomy* involves the removal of the breast tissue as far as the axilla and a sample of the axillary lymph nodes may be

Table 44.1. UICC method of staging breast cancer

Tumour status (T)	T. 0	T. 1	T. 2	T. 3	T. 4
Description of tumour	Not palpable	Size: $\leq$ 2 cm Not fixed	Size: 2–5 cm Not fixed	Size > 5 cm May/may not be attached	Any size Fixation to chest wall or skin ulceration
Lymph node status (N) Description of nodes	N. 0 Axillary nodes not palpable	N. 1a Axillary nodes palpable No tumour	N. 1b Axillary nodes palpable Tumour	N. 2 Nodes: > 2 cm May/may not be fixed	N. 3 Enlargment of supra-clavicular or infra-clavicular nodes
Distant metatasis (M) Description of metastasis	M. 0 Not clinically obvious	M. 1 Obvious			

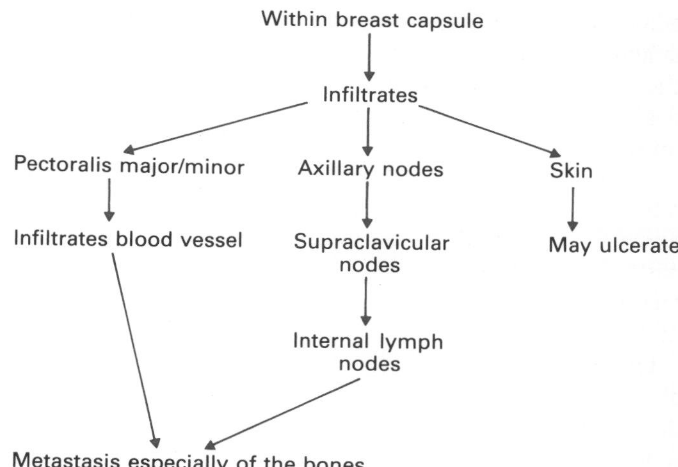

Fig. 44.2 Simplified staging of a tumour.

taken for biopsy. The nipple and areolar tissue are removed, which will leave a transverse suture line with wound drainage.

A *modified mastectomy* includes the removal of the pectoralis minor muscle, axillary lymph nodes and axillary tract in addition to the breast tissue. The incision line will extend from the epigastrium to the shoulder with drainage from the axillary bed.

A *radical mastectomy* includes the removal of both the pectoralis major and minor muscles with a complete axillary clearance as well as all the breast tissue. The incision line will be extensive from the epigastrium to the arm of the affected side coupled with axillary drainage.

Chemotherapy

Chemotherapy is reserved for advanced cases of breast cancer and the course of drugs is prescribed over a period of 3–6 months, a popular combination therapy being vincristine, adriamycin, 5-fluorouracil, and cyclophosphamide.

Hormone Therapy

Hormone therapy combined with bilateral oöphorectomy may be attempted on patients who are premenopausal or within 5 years of the menopause. If the breast cancer shows a response with this initial regimen, the clinicians may decide to then proceed to ablation of the endocrine glands, i.e., the pituitary and adrenals, to contain the levels of circulating oestrogen, progesterone and testosterone.

Radiotherapy

Radiotherapy alone or in combination with surgery is usually employed for stages 2 and 3. The breast area, axilla, supraclavicular and internal mammary lymph nodes are irradiated with 6000–9000 rad over a period of 3–6 weeks.

PREOPERATIVE CARE

Advising the Patient

As the operative procedure will not be decided upon until after a frozen section biopsy is completed, the nurse should prepare the patient as though for a radical mastectomy. The patient should have the benefit of receiving this advice and information from an experienced nurse. The nurse will make the judgement as to whether the patient would be receptive.

This counselling may take the form of the patient having a **woman to woman chat** with a sympathetic ex-patient who is a member of the local Mastectomy Association, or with a mastectomy nurse. This person will be able to advise on the postoperative problems of adaptations to underclothing, i.e., bras, social difficulties which have to be overcome, and the type of exercises which may be needed to deal with any persistent swelling of the arm on the affected side.

The **programme of events** from the evening prior to surgery until recovery from the anaesthesia should be discussed with the patient, her partner or family who will be giving the emotional support so vitally needed at this time.

Literature and pamphlets are usually available from both local and national organisations. In addition there are several well-written layman's texts on breast cancer which should be offered to the patients to read if in the nurse's judgement they could cope with this and their emotional distress.

The **temporary or permanent breast prosthesis** which the patient may have to wear should be discussed if not actually demonstrated. Certainly the lightweight breast form temporary prosthesis which the patient will wear on discharge should be available. The NHS and private firms issue permanent prosthesis after precise measurements are taken following recovery from the operation.

Trusting the medical and nursing staff is vital. Should the nurse detect any doubts or concerns the patient may have, these should be brought to the surgeon's attention so that further explanations can be offered. Positive attitudes lead to a more rapid recovery and encourage the patient to adapt more quickly to the changing circumstances in her family and social circle.

Preparing the Patient

The specific nursing preparation includes shaving both axilla and if necessary the epigastric area. One thigh should also be shaved in case the patient will require a radical mastectomy when a skin graft may be needed. The physiotherapist or nurse should demonstrate then supervise the patient in performing certain exercises for the arm of the affected side. These include flexion and extension from the elbow, abduction and adduction of the whole arm, and circumduction through the shoulder joint. The evening prior to surgery the patient will normally be prescribed potent sedation to reduce anxiety and fear and to ensure a restful sleep.

POSTOPERATIVE CARE

The specific postoperative care following recovery from the anaesthetic is to check the wound site for drains and to ensure they are secure and patent. The breast area may be secured by a compression crêpe bandage if a graft has been transferred from the thigh to the chest wall and this will require frequent checking for stains from any wound exudate.

The arm of the affected side should be slightly elevated on several pillows and note made of any obvious or increasing swelling. A nurse **must** be at the bedside when a mastectomy patient regains full consciousness, either to reassure her that all is well and a complete mastectomy was not required or to calm the emotionally distressed patient when the reality of a radical mastectomy having been performed finally dawns. Such distress combined with the pain of the wound site, shoulder girdle, and arm warrants the use of powerful analgesics every 4–6 hours for the next 24 hours.

If the affected arm is on the dominant side and the alternate arm has intravenous therapy in place, the nurse will obviously include in the care plan such assistance as is needed with toileting, dressing, feeding, cosmetic appearance and hair care. At the same time the patient must be encouraged to do the arm exercises demonstrated in the preoperative preparation period.

The first dressing is the second emotionally critical phase. This is the first time the patient may or may not take the opportunity to look at the amputation of the breast. The nursing skill of rapport and judging the right moment to ask the patient if she wishes to look at the wound is a most testing time. A refusal should be accepted quietly and the dressing completed competently. If the patient has the courage to wish to look, she will require a mirror to view the wound completely. In the majority of cases a mild sedative drug should be administered 1 hour before the first dressing is taken down and, if possible, the surgeon should be available to inspect the healing of the tissue.

Should the arm remain swollen it may be because of the complete axillary clearance decreasing the normal venous return and lymphatic drainage of the arm. In addition to the exercises a limb compression bandage may be applied to promote venous blood flow.

Fitting of a Prosthesis

When the wound is ready to receive its first temporary prosthesis, usually the Spenfil type, the patient is shown how it is fitted into a false pocket sewn into the cup of the brassière. At the same time accurate measurements are taken for the size of the permanent prosthesis. There is now a wide range of these prostheses, some of the more commonly known ones being:

Spenfil is made of silicone and is usually of a temporary nature
Trulife is a fluid filled type
Confidante is filled with fluid and air
Malpro is a granule filled model
Poisette is made of silicone and gel and has to be obtained from private sources

Normally the patient will require 3 prostheses for laundering and changing purposes and most models are designed to take into account the every day problems of odour and staining from perspiration.

Possible Complications

During the early postoperative phase the nurse should observe for and report on any complications. There may be *haemotoma* of the incision line, or at the axilla. Either will have to be released, for it is not only painful and a serious focus for infection but it will damage the chances of good cosmetic wound healing.

Pneumothorax may occur if both the pectoralis major and minor muscles have been removed during a radical mastectomy. The risk of the pleura or lung being punctured is increased and normally a chest X-ray will be routinely requested to detect this risk, in the first postoperative day. If, however, the patient is becoming increasingly breathless which is accompanied by peripheral cyanosis the nurse should request a surgical opinion immediately.

Surgical emphysema or 'air' in the superficial tissues near to the incision line may occur if a graft has been taken from the thigh to the chest wall to compensate for lack of tissue. The tissue tends to crackle and be very painful requiring more than the usual amounts of analgesia. This complication is usually left to resolve spontaneously.

DISCHARGE FROM HOSPITAL

As the patient regains independence of her arm and the wound begins to heal plans will be made for hospital discharge unless a course of teletherapy or chemotherapy is being planned. A rest interval between surgery and any adjuvant therapy is normally taken until complete wound healing has taken place.

A prolonged convalescent period well beyond the normal healing time is strongly recommended for the mastectomy patient not only to regain complete use of the affected arm but also to regain correct posture from the excised muscles. In this convalescence a great deal of psychological adjustment must also be made to realign the altered body image and the normal fears associated with the loss of femininity. Adjustments related to the problems of clothing and dressing style have also to be carefully thought through. A mastectomy nurse is the best possible contact to have for she with her experience will have the insight to help the patient make the necessary adjustments in both her close relationships and in her social life. A useful address to give the patient before she finally leaves the ward is:

Mastectomy Association of Great Britain
1 Colworth Road
Croydon
London CRO 7AD

Chapter 45
Cerebral Tumours

Primary tumours of the nervous system arise within the tissues which contribute to its structures, while *secondary* tumours are metatastic from another primary site. Depending on its location, a primary or secondary tumour is further classified as being either *intrinsic*, i.e., from nervous tissue, or *extrinsic*, being of the system but not arising from the nervous tissue.

Tumours of the cell of a neurone are very rare. Growths whether benign or malignant are more likely to arise from the tissues which support the nerve cells: the meninges, blood vessels within the brain, nerve sheaths, the pituitary gland, and the ventricles of the brain (Fig. 45.1).

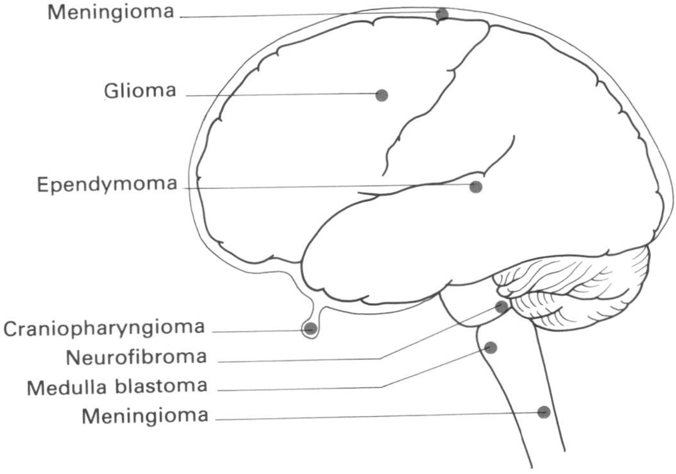

Fig. 45.1 Cerebral tumour sites.

Gliomata

Glia is the supporting connective tissue of the brain. The 2 main cell types from which it is derived are the astrocyte and oligodendrocyte cells. Tumours or *gliomata* constitute by far the largest group of intracranial tumours. They are intrinsic, arising from the cells as:

Glioblastomata developing from immature glial cells

Astrocytomata developing from the astrocyte cells

Oligodendrocytomata developing from the oligodendrocyte cells

Such tumours are closely invested into healthy brain tissue, their rate of growth is unpredictable, as is their likely location. If surgery is undertaken to remove this type of tumour a certain amount of healthy brain tissue has also to be removed with unpredictable postoperative prognosis. Even after surgery the tendency for the tumour to recur after 1–2 years remains a possibility.

Meningiomata

Extrinsic tumours arising mainly from the subarachnoid coat, *meningiomata*, develop to press upwards against the outer meningeal coat, the dura mater. As such they are outside the brain substance and can easily be surgically removed. Invariably they are benign. Spinal meningiomata are more frequently seen in newborn infants, and tend to block the flow of cerebrospinal fluid creating hydrocephalus (*see Nursing 1*).

Ependymomata

Tumours arising from the ependymal cells lining the ventricles of the brain are known as *ependymomata*, and like meningiomata can obstruct the flow of cerebrospinal fluid. Another type of tumour developing from the ventricles of the brain is a medulloblastoma, which grows and presses downwards upon the medulla oblongata increasingly embarrassing the functions of the base of the brain.

Neurofibromata

Tumours arising from the sheaths of nerve fibres, *neurofibromata*, affect the cranial or spinal nerves as they enter or leave the brain and spinal cord. Although invariably benign, the symptoms they cause are the result of pressure on closely related structures. An acoustic neurofibroma is a good example of this. The eighth cranial nerve (acoustic) is closely related to the fifth and seventh cranial nerves. Pressure exerted on any of these can cause a variety of symptoms such as deafness, vertigo, imbalance, facial palsy, and speech impediment.

Craniopharyngiomata

Craniopharyngiomata refers to tumours specifically within or pressing into the pituitary fossa, and affecting the functions of the pituitary gland and detailed discussion of this is outlined in chapter 36.

Haemangioblastoma

Haemangioblastoma are tumours, usually of a benign type, arising from immature blood vessels within the brain. They tend to be cystic encapsulating an arteriovenous junction and may remain asymptomatic for many years until they suddenly rupture causing a severe cerebral haemorrhage.

There is a wide disparity in the age group affected by these tumours. There is a tendency for tumours of this nature to have a peak incidence either in early childhood and after the age of 40 with an preponderance of male victims.

EARLY FEATURES

The early features arising from a cerebral tumour are due to 3 main alterations within the cerebral structure. There is *increased pressure* within the enclosed structure of the skull, which is referred to as increased intracranial pressure. There is *compression* of structures within the brain near to the site of the tumour. If the ventricles of the brain are affected there

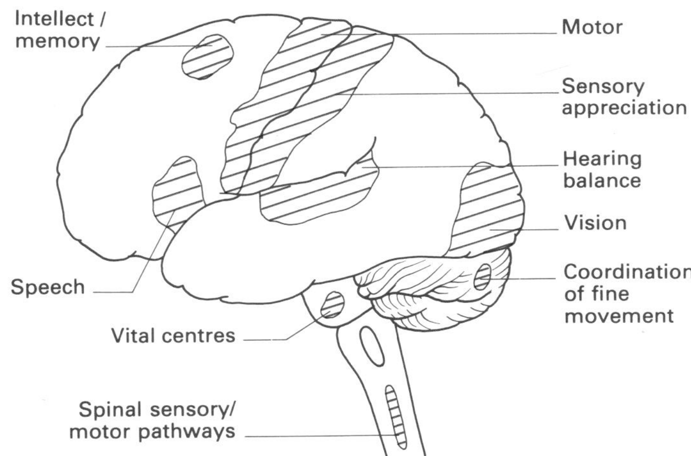

Fig. 45.2 Functional areas affected by tumours.

is also usually an effect on the flow of cerebrospinal fluid into the subarachnoid space. If the pituitary gland is compressed a wide variety of symptoms, both cerebral and endocrine, can result. There is *destruction* of healthy brain tissue either from the invasiveness of a malignant intrinsic tumour or if a benign tumour is progressively enlarging depriving nerve cells of an adequate blood and oxygen supply.

The particular problems from which the patient may suffer will depend on the location of the tumour or on its overlap effect of nearby structures (Fig. 45.2). The earliest signs and symptoms are vague and misleading. Headaches, for example, although persistent tend at first to be generalised. It is not until the intracranial pressure increases from an oedema that the headache will cause the patient to seek medical advice.

Personality changes are also subtle, and it is usually a long lost friend or someone from the patient's past who is the first to remark on any significant personality change. Intellectual ability may be only marginally affected. A poor memory for recent events is a useful indicator, but more helpful are the emotional changes. Abrupt changes of mood, unexplained anger, disinterest but not depression, any loss of personal esteem and self-regard, unaccountable restlessness and agitation are all noteworthy. The neurosurgeon will be interested in learning of these changes during the clinical assessment.

A single event convulsion without a previous history of epilepsy is most relevant. If the nurse should observe one of these epileptiform fits, it should be noted if the convulsion is of a focal type (Jacksonian) or a true psychomotor fit. The former may implicate the motor area of the frontal lobe, and the latter the temporal lobe. Sensory appreciation may also be in default and a significant finding is that of paraesthesia or weakness to one side of the body which suggests a tumour in the sensory area of the parietal lobe.

Expressive aphasia and general difficulties with speech may suggest that the speech area of the patient's dominant side in the temporal lobe is affected.

An important early finding is alteration to the vision; bilateral hemianopia, papilloedema, and diplopia which do not resolve or cannot be explained suggest further investigations for a tumour within the brain. The combination of severe headache, nausea and vomiting, and visual loss all suggest an increased intracranial pressure, and in the absence of other causes suggest an intracranial tumour.

Apart from an exhaustive and detailed medical and social history the patient may be required to go through a series of very demanding investigations. Some of the tests outlined are as major as the treatment, and the nurse in preparing and explaining the reasons and purposes of the tests must also ensure that the arrangements are secure so that repetition of the tests can be avoided.

INVESTIGATIONS

The simplest investigation is the request for an X-ray of the skull. The film is examined to note if there are any calcification areas, erosion of bone, and obvious shift in the midline, and if the skull contour is proportionate to the skull size.

A complete neurological examination, if completed correctly, takes a considerable length of time and requires the assistance of the nurse.

Intellectual Orientation

The patient is asked questions related to time, places, dates, and events. Confused answers are the cue to simplifying the questions even more to ensure that any disorientation of the patient is genuine and not due to misunderstanding. During this orientation testing the patient's speech should be noted for its quality of articulation, lucidity, and pronunciation. Any local dialect or idioms are ignored.

Co-ordination Tests

Tests of coordination examine the complex neurological arrangement which controls both fine motor and sensory appreciation.

Romberg's Sign

The patient is asked to stand upright in the anatomical position with the eyes open. The ability to maintain this posture without wavering is noted, and then compared with the ability to maintain the posture with the eyes closed. During this the patient may be gently nudged forward and backwards or side to side to see if he or she can adjust positions quickly and correctly. Any loss of postural coordination suggests disease of the cerebellum.

Point-to-Point Testing

The patient is asked to touch the tip of the nose with the finger. If the finger wavers as it approaches the target with either the eyes open or closed it would also suggest a loss of the sense of position related to the surrounding environment, i.e., imbalance due to cerebellar disease.

Alternate Rhythmic Movement Test

Tasks of a moderate complexity such as tapping the back of the left hand with the right hand and then alternating the task cannot be sustained for too long by patients with cerebellar disease.

Sensory tests

The sensory receptors of taste, smell, tactile appreciation, and colour vision and hearing are tested, usually to detect any change in common every day experiences. The 4 tastes of sour, sweet, salt and bitter if depreciated may suggest compression of a part of the sensory area in the parietal lobe. Any depreciation in noting the aroma of distinctive odours such as the oil of cloves may implicate the olfactory bulb. Hearing tests such as Weber's, Rhine's, and the labyrinth test establish if hearing or balance are normal. If they are not the temporal lobe may be affected by a tumour.

Extensive testing of the visual fields is carried out by perimetry; distant and near vision is clarified by the acuity tests. Ophthalmoscopic examination of the optic disc for oedema or vascular changes is strongly diagnostic of increased intracranial pressure.

The nurse should note any default in sensory depreciation which may give rise to problems of coping with simple tasks. Pain appreciation if diminished may lead to minor burns going unnoticed. Imbalance and poor posture may cause patients to fall and hurt themselves. Extrapolation of the doctor's assessment may be of great value to the nursing plan of care in addition to the nurse's own assessment.

Further investigations requested from other hospital departments will require the nurse to be conversant with local hospital procedures as they relate to X-ray, physics, and pathology departments.

Lumbar Puncture

When measured by manometer the cerebrospinal fluid pressure is excessive. If above 150 mlH_2O it is suggestive of a raised intracranial pressure due to a blocked third ventricle. The Queckenstedt's test is done to exclude the possibility of a spinal lesion confusing a brain lesion. A cerebral tumour may utilise glycoproteins for its metabolism thereby increasing the cerebrospinal protein level above 200–400 mg/l.

24-Hour Urine Save

A neuroblastoma increases the level of vanillylmandelic acid (VMA) which is a waste product of noradrenaline. If the renal and endocrine functions are normal yet the VMA level is raised, it may suggest further investigations are necessary for the cerebral tumour.

Computer Assisted Tomography

Computer assisted tomography (CAT or EMI Scan) involves an X-ray machine synchronised to a computer and has replaced the majority of previously used investigations. Serialised sections of the brain are displayed on the computer screen and gradually built up to show a clear image of the brain's anatomy. Practically all areas of the brain can be studied over a period of 20–40 minutes. The patient lies perfectly still while the X-ray machine moves over the patient's head through a 180° circle. If the patient is restless, or confused, the doctor should be requested to prescribe a sedation for administration 30 minutes before the procedure is due to take place.

Electroencephalography

The electrical activity of the brain using electroencephalography (EEG) can be shown on a trace as the activity is transmitted via electrodes connected to the patient's skull. The electrical activity over a tumour area shows a slow electrical discharge rate despite having the machine at a high amplitude.

Echo Encephalography

Using the ultrasonic sound wavelength of an echo encephalography (echo EEG) the resulting trace of the brain shape may show deviation of the cerebral longitudinal fissure, i.e., the midline, possibly caused by a meningioma.

Pneumoencephalography

Small amounts of air up to a maximum of 25 ml are injected into the subarachnoid space via a lumbar puncture after a small amount of cerebrospinal fluid has been removed. The patient's position is altered to encourage the air to flow towards the ventricles of the brain and the subarachnoid spaces. Ependymal tumours or meningiomata are accurately detected by the method of pneumoencephalography (PEG).

Gamma Encephalography

With gamma encephalography a radioactive isotope, usually technetium, is injected either via a ventricular needle (isotopic ventriculography), or via a lumbar puncture. After a few minutes the brain is scanned to note those areas of the brain which have a heavy concentration of the isotope, this is known as a 'hot area'. Tumours attract the isotope because of their increased temperature. There is a 95% detection rate if the tumour is 2 cm in size or over.

Cerebral Angiography

A contrast medium is injected into the femoral, carotid or vertebral arteries which will enable the cerebral circulation to be outlined. The contrast medium may highlight arteriovenous angiomata, the vascularity of a tumour, or will indicate the size of a laterally placed tumour. Following a cerebral angiography the nurse should expect the patient to have a severe headache. The site of the arterial injection must be monitored for the risk of haemorrhage.

TREATMENT

Following these exhaustive and disturbing series of investigations which should confirm the presence, size and location of the tumour, the nursing plan is altered to accommodate the proposed treatment. Several therapeutic measures are possible. *Deep X-ray therapy* can be performed directed at the tumour. Alternatively, deep X-ray therapy following surgical removal of the tumour bulk will effectively decompress the surrounding brain tissues. This form of therapy is usually of temporary benefit especially so if the tumour is extensive and malignant.

Combination chemotherapy using several cytotoxic agents, e.g., vincristine, methramycin and methotrexate may be used. This therapy is increasingly effective in dealing with gliomata which are intrinsic and invasive to healthy brain tissue.

Intracranial surgery is the most prevalent form of treatment and in reality is the only therapy which will finally confirm if the tumour is actually benign or malignant. Apart from taking a biopsy, surgery can be used to decompress the tumour or to remove it by total excision. Total excision is certainly recommended if the tumour arises from the meninges, blood vessels, bone, or the pituitary gland.

Intracranial Surgery

Preoperative Care Plan

There are preparations which must be included as part of the specific nursing care plan preoperatively.

The patient's hair is shampooed the day prior to surgery. The shaving of the skull is usually done when the patient is under the general anesthetic. Useful advice is to ask the patient to provide either a silk headscarf (female) or any type of hairpiece (male) which will disguise this baldness until the hair grows again.

The crevices and external meatus of both ears should be thoroughly cleansed and the auditory canal checked for the presence of wax, and if present, removed by ear syringing.

The mucosa of the mouth and pharynx should be inspected and swabs taken of the throat to exclude the possibility of infections. Scrupulous oral hygiene is vital to minimise ascending infection via the nasal and paranasal sinuses.

A small enema is administered the evening prior to surgery and again the following morning to ensure the lower colon is clear of faeces to reduce the need for toileting for at least 48 hours postoperatively.

In the majority of cases both intravenous therapy and bladder catheterisation are established on the morning of surgery, as both will be required postoperatively.

A great deal of time should be devoted to patient counselling, both advising the patient on what is the likely course of events and answering any questions simply and directly which arise following the surgeon's explanation. Wherever possible these counselling periods should also involve the family to reduce anxieties at every level. Those patients who are properly advised make a better and more rapid recovery. The areas of patient–nurse concern which may require detailed explanation tend to be: fear of loss of intellectual ability and memory, the timetable of events, postoperative difficulties and a variety of social factors.

It is now unusual for patients to suffer from any impairment of either intellect or memory following brain surgery, and this knowledge is most reassuring as it is one of the greatest areas of anxiety.

Brain surgery usually lasts for 3–6 hours and this information is needed by the relatives so they can timetable their telephone enquiries and visits. They often need the verbal reassurance that free visiting is possible in the immediate postoperative period when their anxieties will be at the highest level.

Postoperative difficulties for the patient will include coping with the tubes, wound drain, bladder catheter, intensive repetition of nursing observations, remaining flat for 1 or 2 days, and being nursed in the intensive care unit. If carefully taken through these points, the personal coping skills, following surgery, will be such that a more rapid recovery can be anticipated, simply because the patient will know what to expect. If possible the nurse-patient allocation system should also be explained to the patient. A one-to-one nurse-patient relationship is desirable if for no other reason than that the crucial observations are on a continuum and adverse problems will be spotted and resolved more quickly.

Social factors which the patient may consider problematical can be discussed with the medical social worker, or indeed the spiritual adviser.

Postoperative Care Plan

Following surgery the anaesthetist may bring the patient to a rapid conscious level. This reduces the need for prolonged endotracheal intubation, but it is vital for the nurse to appreciate that a relapse into coma may be due to anaesthesia rather than postoperative complications. A bed and suitably equipped area are prepared for the patient and on the patient's arrival the nurse should make immediate checks. The type and location of the craniotomy flap (curved suture line) should be assessed and whether it has a drain. A ventricular drain may be connected to a tap system which must be in the off position whenever the patient is moved. Alternatively the drain may be attached to a suction bottle. The drain will limit the patient's choice of position until it is removed some 24–36 hours later. If the skull is bandaged the location of the sutures must be known so that the actual wound site can be checked for exudate. A 'wet' bandage must not be removed but covered with further sterile dressings held in position by a Netalast head cap dressing.

The patient is usually nursed in the prone position with the bedhead tilted to a 20° or 30° elevation to counteract the risk of increased intracranial pressure due to oedema. This position is maintained until the drains have been removed. It is a wise precaution to have the bed fitted with cotsides during the early phase of recovery.

Observations

Observations must be carried out every 30 minutes until the surgeon instructs otherwise after he or she has examined the patient.

Airway patency at all times until the patient has both a swallow and cough reflex.

Blood pressure to note either hypotensive or hypertensive changes.

Pulse for a reduction in rate and volume, i.e., bradycardia. A raised blood pressure and a slow pulse imply increasing intracranial pressure, and **must** be reported immediately.

Respiratory rate for obvious altered rate and depth, combined with any cyanosis of the skin.

Rectal temperature to denote the risk of hypothermia or hyperthermia, a function controlled by the hypothalamus and a major risk following brain surgery.

Pupil reaction to light, noting if the pupils are equal in size, equally dilate and constrict reflexly when light is directed into the eye.

Limb movement and **reflex responses** to touch when repositioned or when turned during nursing procedures. Flaccid or spastic reactions **must** be reported immediately.

Response to quiet sound, i.e., simply phrased questions.

Restlessness of any degree.

Focal or psychomotor **convulsions.**

Note Any of the above observations, when erratic, must be reported to the surgeon because of the real danger of increased intracranial pressure and subsequent poor muscle coordination. It is possible that diuretic drugs, e.g., mannitol, may be prescribed to reduces these dangers.

The blood pressure, pulse, and respiratory rate are functions controlled by the medulla oblongata. If they are all erratic, the pressure being exerted on this area of the brain is increasing which is extremely dangerous.

Analgesia

In the immediate postoperative phase, analgesia if used tends to be of the milder type since powerful analgesia may disguise important neurological assessment and observation. Intravenous mannitol, a sugar-based diuretic, can be of temporary benefit in those patients suffering from raised intracranial pressure due to oedema. In practice it would not be used for more than 10 hours. More usual is the administration of dexamethasone (fluorinated corticosteroid) on a reducing sliding scale which effectively prevents cerebral oedema. Antiemetics are vitally important, and prochlorperazine (Stemetil) 12.5 mg is normally prescribed every 6 hours for a period of 24 hours.

Site of Incision

Specific problems with brain surgery relate to the point of incision. Craniotomy incision, if approached from the front, creates problems of periorbital and periocular oedema and bruising. It will be 4 or 5 days before the discolouration and swelling recede which may be serious enough to hinder observation of the pupil size and reaction. Until the bruising recedes, frequent eye toilet with 0.9% normal saline will reduce the risk of corneal ulceration. Diplopia and photophobia are another two problems related to vision. These may be partially overcome if the patient can have a pair of photochromic spectacles to wear, e.g., Foster Grants.

Fluid Needs

The immediate fluid needs of the patient are initially met by the administration of intravenous fluids. Once the swallow and cough reflex are present, and with the surgeon's permission, oral fluids are commenced. If vomiting is occurring despite antiemetics, it suggests increased intracranial pressure and fluids should be discontinued until the surgeon gives instructions to the contrary.

Nasogastric feeding may be used to ensure that calorific requirements are being met in those patients who are making slow progress to recovery. When able to eat patients will usually prefer very small amounts of easily digested food, nevertheless they should have the full choice of the menu, and in time their normal appetite will return.

Speech Defect

If problems arise from speech defect, the probable cause may be due to damage to the glossopharyngeal or vagus nerve. If the patient displays any laxity of facial muscles on one side, then the facial nerves may be involved. After reporting the observation, the nurse must then consider which form of communication would best meet the needs of the patient, e.g., bell system, pad and pencil, hand signalling, or picture cards.

Excretion

Excretion of urine will be by continuous drainage via the bladder catheter connected to a drainage bag, and will remain so until any danger of increased cerebral pressure has passed.

Several days prior to its removal it is a useful precaution to clamp off the tubing for periods of 4 hours so that the bladder can once again tone up with residual volumes of urine. After its removal the patient should not expect to automatically return to normal micturition, but should be warned to expect for several days, until the urethral sphincters are toned up once more, a little problem with accidental incontinence. On the third postoperative day if required the patient should be offered some assistance to evacuate the lower colon either by use of suppositories or a very small enema.

Mobility

Mobility of the patient cannot begin until after the wound drains have been removed. A slow programme towards ambulation is commenced over a period of 5 days. With the advice of the physiotherapist the first day should be no more than the patient sitting by the bedside for 10 minutes with a few leg and arm exercises later in the day. Sitting out of bed is progressively increased over the next 4 days when the patient may then be allowed to take a very short walk. During this period the nurse should note the motor and sensory responses and report on any obvious difficulties.

Complications

The complications of intracranial surgery are for the most part evident within 24 hours of the operation. Changes in the vital signs, using skilled observation and interpretation, if reported **immediately** will enable action to be taken to forestall any further deterioration.

1. There may be increased intracranial pressure from cerebral haemorrhage, cerebral oedema or extradural haematoma. This complication is noted by restlessness, meningitis, vomiting, headache, a slow pulse, and increased blood pressure.
2. Abnormal body temperature may be either hypothermia or hyperpyrexia. This complication involves the hypothalamus and for accuracy only a rectal thermometer reading should be used. Since it is not due to infection, nursing measures could include cooling measures, e.g., tepid sponging or use of a fan, or alternatively keeping the patient warm by raising the room temperature and giving additional clothing. A close watch must be kept on the fluid balance of the patient in either case of abnormal temperature.
3. Dysphagia or difficulty in swallowing should be reported immediately as it may be due to damage of the glossopharyngeal or vagus nerves.
4. Cerebellar herniation of the medulla through the foramen magnum of the occiput may occur as a result of compression due to increased intracranial pressure. The vital signs are extremely erratic and surgical intervention is critical if the pressure is to be relieved.
5. Convulsions may occur if the surgery was near to the motor cortex. The convulsion if it does occur is most likely to be of the psychomotor type, i.e., grand mal. To prevent this happening many surgeons prescribe drugs preoperatively and continue them in the postoperative period with, e.g., Epanutin and phenobarbitone.
6. Personality changes are not immediately obvious but may arise when the surgery involves the frontal lobes. Poor memory recall, deterioration of the intellect, decreased spans of concentration, emotional distress, and total apathy are a few examples of those factors which may contribute to overall personality changes. This assessment, however, is usually reserved until several weeks after surgery and is completed by a psychologist.

Chapter 46
Pancreatic Tumours

Benign or malignant tumours may arise within the pancreatic tissues. Although tumours may occur in the head, body or tail of the pancreas they are more commonly located in the head of the organ. Occasionally the tumour may affect the insulin-secreting cells within the islets of Langerhans causing a hypersecretion of insulin (hyperinsulinism) which leads to episodes of hypoglycaemia.

EARLY SYMPTOMS

The early symptoms of a pancreatic tumour tend to be vague and ill-defined; as a consequence the patient may not seek medical advice for some time. It may be over 4 months before investigations are instigated by which time the patient is usually extremely ill. The worsening symptoms centre on 3 major discomforts. These are a profound and progressive loss of weight, pain centred in the mid-abdominal region and radiating to the mid-back, and a worsening jaundice; this last symptom being quickly obvious if the tumour is located near the ampulla where the pancreas meets the duodenum causing an obstruction to the flow of bile.

To cope with these symptoms the patient makes several adaptations which are often noted on assessment. To relieve the pain they prefer to sit upright when at rest or sleeping, if walking they adopt a stoop which relieves the constant ache of the abdomen and back. Those who drink alcoholic beverages tend to give them up, as alcohol worsens their symptoms. Indeed, alcohol may be the initial cause of the tumour.

ASSOCIATED DISCOMFORTS

Associated with the 3 cardinal symptoms of pancreatic tumour are other discomforts: feverish attacks alternating with severe chilling is quite common. If jaundice is present then there is the associated constipation with a pale stool, dark concentrated urine, and **pruritis** (or itching). Should the insulin-secreting cells be affected there may well be a glycosuria. Accompanying all these problems is the persistent occurrence of many abdominal discomforts such as nausea, vomiting, abdominal distension and heartburn. The typical patient tends to be male, rather thin, between 55 and 70 years of age with a history of heavy alcohol consumption.

TESTS

While the symptoms suggest a pancreatic tumour the series of tests required would identify the exact location of the tumour, whether it is malignant or benign, its size, and if it involves related structures or has metastasised.

The nurse should expect to prepare the patient for the following investigations:

Barium meal to exclude involvement of the stomach, especially the pyloric region.

Abdominal X-ray to outline any mass distorting neighbouring organs.

Endoscopic retrograde cholecystopancreatography (ERCP) which is a fibreoptic examination of the biliary and pancreatic ducts and may require a general anaesthetic.

Cholangiography, i.e., an opaque X-ray of the gallbladder to exclude the presence of gallstones which may be a cause of jaundice.

Computerised axial tomography (CAT scan) to detect the presence of any abnormal mass within the abdomen. A tumour as small as 0.5 cm can be detected by this X-ray technique.

Isotopic or **ultrasonography** of the pancreas.

Glucose tolerance test will be performed if the patient has a glycosuria not related to a diabetes. It may suggest that the tumour is affecting insulin-secreting cells.

Blood level estimations for:

Serum bilirubin if there is biliary obstruction

Alkaline phosphatase to assess liver function

SGOT to assess both liver and cardiac function

Prothrombin time if jaundice is present

Skeletal scan to detect if there is secondary spread to the bones.

TREATMENT

Once the diagnosis has been accurately made the doctor may suggest several courses of action. Treatment may be conducted along conservative lines, i.e., the control of symptoms, or alternatively surgery. The type of operation offered can vary from a laparotomy, a pancreatectomy or pancreatic bypass, but the most common elective procedure is Whipple's operation (Fig. 46.1). This last procedure is the surgical resection of the head of the pancreas (pancreo-duodenectomy) providing that related structures and neighbouring organs have not been invaded by the cyst or tumour. All patients for pancreatic surgery require extremely detailed preoperative care if they are to overcome the multiple hazards associated with this operation. If the patient has a malignant tumour of the head of the pancreas the chances of success are currently 25% with 5 year survival.

Preoperative Care

In the preoperative phase the challenge to the nursing skill is to prepare the patient for extreme surgery. This must take into account the condition of the patient who will be severely undernourished and quite ill. Initially the plan will be to prepare the patient as if for any major abdominal operation with concentration being given to:

Ensuring a daily calorific value intake of at least 8400 kJ (2000 cal). This is achieved by giving a diet of high protein foods, some carbohydrate and avoiding fatty foods. The diet decided upon may be complemented by adding pancreatic enzymes to aid digestion

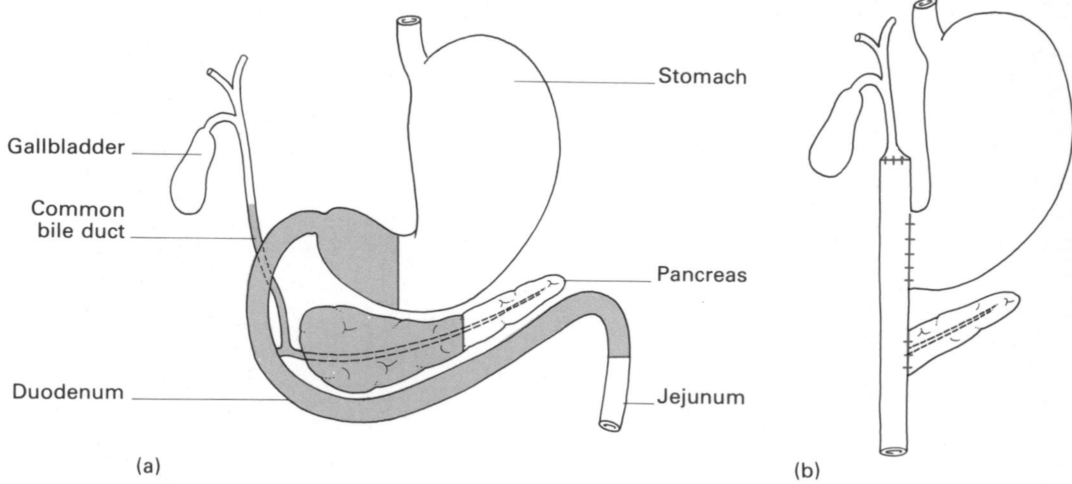

Fig. 46.1 Whipple's operation: resection and excision (a); anastomosis (b).

Daily injection of vitamin K to counteract the risk of postoperative haemorrhage due to jaundice and surgery

Correction of anaemia usually by blood transfusion

An absolute ban on any type of alcoholic beverage

Administering prescribed anticholinergic drugs to relieve the many abdominal discomforts

Postoperative Care

The operation itself usually takes some hours and arrangements are made for the patient to be nursed in the intensive care unit for the first 48 hours after recovery from anaesthesia. These arrangements should be explained to the relatives and the patient to allay undue anxiety at a very emotional and critical time.

On the return from theatre explicit arrangements are detailed to control hypoglycaemia or hyperglycaemia usually by measuring the blood glucose at hourly intervals and administering soluble insulin on a sliding scale. The wound usually has a pump drain to allow pancreatic, biliary or intestinal juices to escape. These digestive juices are extremely excoriating to the skin which is usually protected by a seal dressing. Wound drains may remain in position for quite a few days until the underlying structures heal at their anastomotic junctions. The patient also has to cope with a plethora of tubes, such as:

a nasogastric aspiration every 2 hours

urinary bladder drainage to permit for 2-hourly urinalysis for glycosuria

an intravenous infusion to maintain hydration for so long as the patient is restricted from having oral fluids.

The basic nursing care is also quite intensive as the patient is totally dependent on the nurse for all physical needs and the promotion of comfort. As the days go by there should be a gradual relief of any jaundice. Abdominal pain recedes along with the discomforts, and the appetite returns. When diet commences the patient may require to take supplementary pancreatin to ensure correct digestion and absorption of foods in the intestine.

Part 6
Care of the Traumatised Patient

Chapter 47
The Role of the Nurse

Regardless of the size of the department, whether it is a major accident centre with a wide catchment area, or a minor unit in a small town, the role of the nurse follows a similar parallel. The nurse's main role is to:

Receive, recognise, and determine the priority of care required by the injured patient

Guide and warn medical staff of untoward and sudden changes in the patient's condition

Make both subjective and objective observations continuously, before, during and after treatment

Assist medical staff with resuscitation techniques

Complete minor treatments in a competent and safe manner

Act as an intermediary between the patient and his or her relatives, the medical staff and other hospital personnel

These 6 aspects are an integral part of the main aim of the department which is to determine the type of injury sustained, severity of any illness, and then to confirm its degree and initiate treatment. An understanding of these roles does make a positive contribution to the team approach required within the department, among medical staff, nurses and the other specialists working within the periphery of the unit, i.e., X-ray staff, theatre staff, ambulance crews, and outpatient staff.

Nurse learners will usually be allocated specific areas of work during their period of experience in the department and the emphasis of roles will vary in each area. The nurse may

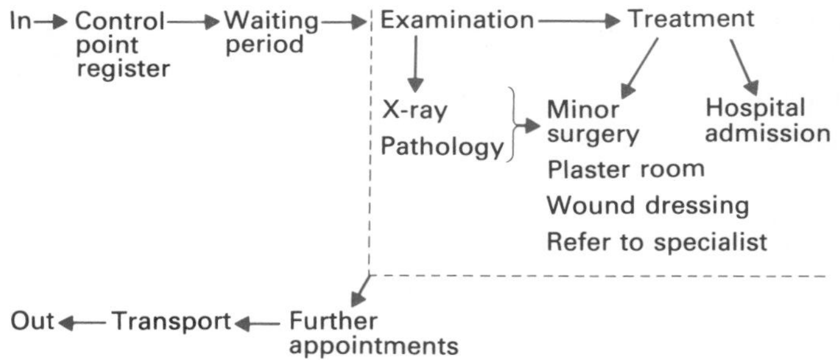

Fig. 47.1 Flow plan for moderately ill or injured patient.

be assigned to the control point, the resuscitation area, the examination and minor treatments area, the observation and waiting areas, the admission ward (24 hours) or the minor theatre, e.g., fracture clinic, or plaster room.

DEPARTMENTAL LAYOUT

The design of a modern accident and emergency department centre allows for a *flow method* when dealing with an injured patient (Fig. 47.1). Indeed the importance of space and the vital need to be in constant readiness will soon become evident to the nurse if the flow method is to work efficiently.

The Control Point

The first point of contact between an injured person and the hospital is the control point. This area of the department is the communications centre and it is here that many admissions are notified before their arrival. Advance warnings by either telephone or radio link are only of value if the communication can give the priority of care the patient will need.

Priority of Care

The term *priority* can be used in several contexts. From the point of view of receiving patients, the nurse will need to know:

Is resuscitation required, e.g., respiratory or cardiac arrest?

Is the patient in shock requiring emergency therapy?

Does the patient require examination and non-urgent treatment?

A diagnosis does not clarify whether the patient is stretcher-dependent, wheelchair-bound, or a walking injured victim. Both the police and ambulance crews are trained to advise the department of the priority needs of the patient. Advance warnings are extremely valuable as they advise the staff of what to prepare. This state of readiness increases the patient's confidence in both the staff and the treatment to be received and psychologically helps to reduce the element of shock which accompanies all injuries.

Minor Injuries

The majority of patients, however, have minor injuries, though they are not minor to the patient. This type of patient will have to report to the control point. Here personal details are recorded on a treatment/admission card before the patient is seen by the casualty officer. More seriously injured patients usually bypass the control point, though are still received by nursing staff, so they can receive immediate care and treatment; their details being noted at a later time. The minor injury may have to wait and if so the nurse must once again decide on priority. Where there are no separate reception areas, stretcher patients should not have to wait in the main waiting area but should be escorted to a treatment cubicle as soon as possible.

Nurses should as part of their role regularly check on the patients waiting in the main reception area at, say, half-hourly intervals. Often, patients with minor injuries suffer from delayed shock from which fainting attacks, vomiting, frequency of micturition, aggression, or overt anxiety may develop, even from what at first glance may seem a trivial injury. Reassurance as to how long they may have to wait for their turn to be seen by the casualty officer and the provision of a reasonably comfortable waiting area will do much to avert these responses to delayed shock.

Nursing Action

If a patient who is seriously ill is admitted to the examination cubicle, the nurse must stay with the patient until after the casualty officer has completed the initial assessment and indicated that he or she will be safe if left alone. Often, there are secondary injuries disguised or hidden by clothing and it is normal practice to assist the patient to undress to the underclothing. Then, cover the patient with a warm blanket. Clothing may already have been removed by the ambulance crew at the scene of the accident and the nurse should check that such clothing has been retrieved. When circumstances require assistance by the nurse the conscious patient's permission should always be sought before the nurse removes any clothing. Privacy and discretion are absolutely essential as sometimes patients soil themselves at the time of an accident, as one response to being very frightened.

When undressing the injured person the nurse is advised always to commence with the clothing on the uninjured side and manoeuvre the clothing over the injured limbs, with the limb being kept still. Otherwise unnecessary pain will be caused. If the injury makes it impossible to undress the patient then, with permission obtained when feasible, heavy duty scissors should be used to cut along the seams of the clothing, and the material drawn back to expose the injured site but left underneath the patient. Lifting or rolling a patient is inadvisable until after the casualty officer's first examination, especially so for fractures. Emergency splints or dressings that have been applied at the site of injury should not be removed until the doctor advises that he or she is ready to begin the examination.

If the patient is unconscious a second nurse is required as a witness to any search of the clothing to establish the patient's identity. When necessary, pockets, handbags and wallets should be searched not only for identity but also to check whether the patient is having any medication for a current illness. During the procedure of undressing a patient the nurse should visually assess if the patient has any obscure cuts, bruises, laceration, or grazes, and direct the doctor's attention to their presence as they may indicate the presence of underlying secondary injury. Equally important is to alert the doctor to the presence of any medi-alert emblem or card the patient may possess.

Observations

As a matter of routine the following observations are taken and recorded prior to the doctor's examination:

Blood pressure—often low due to shock
Pulse—usually rapid because of shock
Temperature—invariably low
Respiratory rate—tends to be shallow and rapid

The level of consciousness will be assessed in all head injury cases and in those with a history of unconsciousness. If possible, a urinalysis may be of value to exclude glycosuria, in suspect diabetes.

The location of pain should already be established, but its persistence despite any analgesia given must be reported. A history of entonox gas if used by the ambulance crew should also be noted. The frequency of recording the vital signs is usually every 15 minutes unless advised otherwise, especially in all cases of shock and unconsciousness. The observations should be available to the casualty officer for appraisal prior to the initial physical examination. In the majority of instances the doctor will physically examine the patient in a logical pattern from head to foot, despite the injury sustained. This is a useful pointer for the nurse if she or he wishes to be helpful to both patient and doctor during the actual examination.

MEDICOLEGAL ASPECTS

Some of the medicolegal implications of accident and emergency nursing which affect the learners most frequently must be considered to avoid the unnecessary embarrassment of future litigation against the employing hospital authority.

Personal Possessions

One of the most frequent complaints against the hospital authorities refers to the loss of property, i.e., personal possessions, on arrival at, or within, the accident and emergency department. For this reason the management policy of the department should clearly identify that 2 nurses *must* check the personal possessions of a patient, especially if the patient is unconscious. If a relative accompanies the patient then, with the patient's permission if possible, they should be asked to take charge of any valuables which the patient is carrying.

When admitting the patient to a ward from the department the escorting nurse should draw the attention of the ward nurse to the admission slip which normally indicates those possessions which the patient has. It is common practice for the ward nurse to take charge of valuables such as money which will be secured in a locked safe for which the patient will receive a receipt.

Incorrect Treatment

If treatment is incorrect it could be that the nurse has misinterpreted the doctor's written instructions. Treatment cards should be double-checked by 2 nurses, especially so in the case of drug administration. If in doubt a confirmation **must** be sought from the prescribing doctor.

The correct treatment can be given, but the doctor or nurse may not have screened the patient for any allergic reactions to the prescribed drugs, i.e., antibiotics. Failure to check with the patient is a serious omission of care, and to reduce this hazard the case notes should carry the information on known allergies as a matter of routine.

Correct identification of the site of injury is equally important when a patient is to be admitted directly to surgery.

Consent to Treatment

For minor treatments in adults it is accepted practice to seek verbal consent, which implies the patient understands the purpose of the treatment and will co-operate once an explanation has been given by a casualty officer. In the case of children and minors, the consent of the parent or guardian is necessary before treatment is given. If general anaesthesia is to precede treatment, a written consent must be obtained by the casualty officer after an explanation has been given to the patient. When dealing with unconscious patients, the consent of the immediate next-of-kin is always obtained wherever possible. On those occasions when relatives are unavailable, the senior surgeon on duty usually acts *in loco parentis*.

Refusal of Treatment

Though uncommon, it is occasionally found that once the patient understands the implications of the treatment being offered he or she may for some reason refuse to accept, even though the patient initially sought treatment. A prescribed treatment **cannot** be forced on anyone, and in this instance the nurse should refer the patient back to the casualty officer who must give a second explanation. This is particularly important when on grounds of religion, parents or guardians may refuse treatment for their child.

If the patient persists in his or her refusal then the patient must sign a refusal form which releases the departmental staff of any responsibility for any consequences arising from the untreated unjury. It is usual, however, for the staff to treat the patient if he or she returns at a later time having decided that the doctor was correct in the initial prescription.

Co-operation with the Police

The most frequent enquiries come from the traffic police and while medical and nursing staff, including students, may co-operate with the police they may do so only with the patient's permission. Requests by the police to remain with a patient are decided by the casualty officer. If the patient agrees to be questioned by the police it is done in privacy. In the larger accident units, there is usually a small room for such purposes. The police do not have access to a patient's notes. Although referred to as the patient's notes they do in fact belong to the doctor as they are his or her notes about a patient.

Complaints Procedure

If a patient wishes to lodge a complaint about the department, the patient should be advised to write giving explicit details, including time and date, to the hospital administrator who will investigate the complaint. Complete and accurate documentation is essential for all nursing and medical records. The accident and emergency nurse sees and treats many patients in a day, and unless treatment is clearly documented it is increasingly difficult to remember a situation which occurred several years ago and is now the subject of a legal action.

However, many complaints can be dealt with within the department and possibly avoided with some tact and reassurance, e.g., an explanation concerning the reason for long waiting periods.

Violence Towards Staff

Unfortunately there have been increased reports of violence towards medical and nursing staff. Often it is unintentional, especially so from drunken patients, drug addicts or hysterics. Where aggressive patients display a tendency towards violence, 2 or more nurses should be present during any treatment. The presence of a male porter or male nurse may be enough to discourage any tendency on the part of a patient to be violent.

Deliberate violence cannot be condoned in a hospital department and the staff should have no hesitation in contacting the police for assistance. It is at the discretion of individuals if they wish to bring an assault charge against a patient who indulged in deliberate violence.

Chapter 48
Emergency Resuscitation

To feel and be competent in such a situation as cardiac arrest takes time. The nurse learner must take every opportunity to become acquainted with the resuscitation room and the equipment provided (Fig. 48.1). The more modern suite will resemble a small operating theatre with a complexity of resuscitation machinery which is an extension of the more simple cardiac arrest trollies held on most acute wards. From previous experience on the acute wards the nurse learner should already know the basic procedures and also know how to recognise either a cardiac or respiratory arrest (see *Nursing I*).

A nurse learner should be able to carry out a number of procedures making a positive contribution in an emergency situation.

1. Correctly position the patient's body

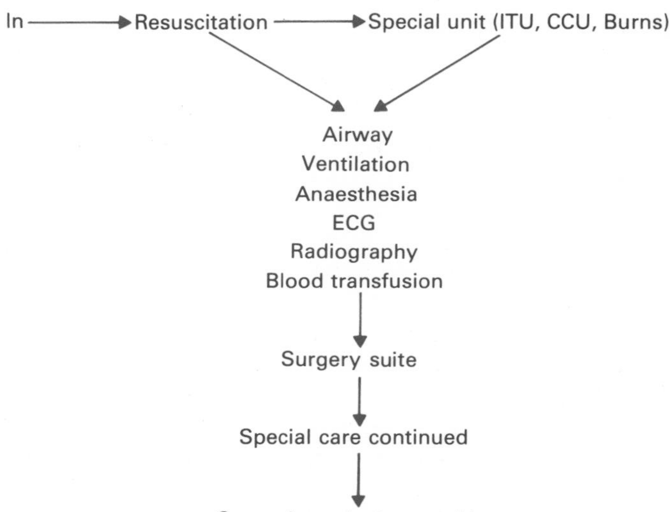

Fig. 48.1 Flow system for seriously ill or injured patient.

on a firm surface, adjust the head to ensure a patent airway, and quickly remove any clothing covering the patient's neck and thorax.

2. Using the index and middle fingers of one hand, clear debris from the mouth and, where applicable, remove any dentures. If necessary the nasal chambers should also be cleansed. Occasionally suction may be required.

3. Locate the carotid pulse. If it is absent, immediately commence external cardiac decompression.

4. Insert either a Guedel or Brook's airway. The Guedel airway is inserted upside down until the distal end reaches the back of the mouth when it is turned into the correct position. A Brook's airway contains a one-way valve system which is valuable for giving mouth-to-mouth resuscitation, and is inserted in the same way as a Guedel airway.

5. Alternate cardiac decompression with mouth-to-mouth or mouth-to-nose artificial respiration. Working alone, the ratio is 5 cardiac decompressions to 1 respiratory cycle. Working with a colleague, 15 cardiac decompressions to 2 respiratory cycles.

When working with a medical team the nurse will usually continue to administer cardiac decompression and a colleague will:

1. Administer the oxygen from the available source, i.e., cylinder or wall-mounted point.

2. Pass both a laryngoscope and an endotracheal tube to the anaesthetist who will establish a patent airway. The Ambu bag will be connected to the endotracheal tube, this then being connected to the oxygen tubing. The Ambu bag will inflate the lungs rhythmically, alternating with the nurse or doctor carrying out the cardiac decompression.

3. Draw up drugs on the verbal request of the doctors, in readiness for emergency administration.

4. Prepare an intravenous-giving set by running through the tubing the most likely solution to be used, which is sodium bicarbonate 8.4%.

5. Locate and unwrap intravenous needles or cannula for the doctor's use.

6. Apply the electrodes of the cardiac monitor either directly to the chest wall or alternatively to the wrists and ankles, depending on which type of monitor is available.

7. Connect the electrical cables and plugs to the mains socket of both the cardiac monitor and the defibrillator.

If there are secondary or tertiary injuries the preceding suggested outline would be adapted, but it should be noted that cardiac and respiratory function precede in priority over any other injury.

RESUSCITATION TROLLEY

Within the resuscitation room, the equipment on the trolley and in the immediate vicinity should allow the medical staff, with the assistance of the nurses, to:

1. Establish a patent airway and provide oxygen

2. Gain access to a vein either by direct venepuncture or cut down. In some instances access to an artery may prove necessary for blood gas analysis

3. Commence external cardiac massage, monitor the conduction of the heart rate and rhythm, and apply defibrillation to correct cardiac arrhythmias

4. Supply a selection of drugs and intravenous solutions to meet the variety of causes of cardiac or respiratory arrest

Drugs Available

Standard drugs normally within the resuscitation trolley are available for cardiac and respiratory emergencies, head injuries, poisoning and anaphylactic reactions.

For cardiac/respiratory emergency
Aminophylline 250 mg in 5 ml
Adrenaline 1/10000 in 10 ml
Adrenaline 1/1000 in 1 ml
Atropine Sulphate 60 mcg in 1 ml
Calcium Chloride inj. 13.4% in 1 ml
Calcium Gluconate inj. 10% in 10 ml

Disopyramide 10 mg in 1 ml
Isoprenaline 2 mg in 2 ml
Lanoxin 0.5 mg in 2 ml (Digoxin)
Lasix 20 mg in 2 ml (Frusemide)
Lignocaine Hydrochloride 5% in 10 ml
Mephentermine 15 mg in 1 ml
Sodium Bicarbonate 8.4% w/v 200 ml
Sodium Chloride inj. 0.9% in 10 ml
Water for inj. 10 ml ampoules

For head injuries
Diazepam inj. 10 mg in 2 ml
Diazepam inj. 20 mg in 5 ml
Dexamethasone 4 mg in 2 ml
Methylprednisolone 40 mg in 1 ml
Methylprednisolone 500 mg in 7.5 ml

Common Poison Antidotes
Naloxone 0.4 mg in 1 ml
Doxopram 100 mg in 5 ml
Amylnitrate

Anaphylactic Reactions
Adrenaline as above
Hydrocortisone Sodium Succinate 100 mg
Dep-Medrone 4 mg in 2 ml

NB It is the duty of the nursing staff to check the drug and equipment stock *at least* once daily. Following each use drug replacement must be ensured and it must be checked that the drugs are within their expiry date.

BASIC MANAGEMENT PLAN

Resuscitation in the event of cardiac arrest, coma, chest injuries or collapse:

1. Airway	Obstructed or threatened following oropharyngeal clearance	Guedel airway Intubation Intermittent positive pressure ventilation
2. Heart	Absent carotid and femoral pulse	External cardiac massage Defibrillation Intravenous lignocaine
3. Blood pressure	Below 90/50 mmHg	Intravenous line established to infuse large molecular fluids
4. Diagnosis of cause	Precise history required Complete physical examination Blood biochemical analysis X-rays or CAT scan Specialist opinion	Treat primary cause
5. Admission to specialist unit	Intensive care unit Coronary care unit Emergency theatre	Stability of vital functions; admit to general ward

Chapter 49
Surgical Toilet for Minor Wounds

The guidelines for the treatment of minor wounds is firstly to establish:

The type of wound

The extent, depth and length of wound

Whether the wound is contaminated by soil or other debris

If deeper internal structures or organs are involved

As the doctor examines the wound he or she will carefully record and assess the history often to find out if other injuries are likely to be present and to see if the history of the accident actually matches the visual evidence of the wound. Other factors which will determine the treatment of the wound are the presence of haemorrhage, the risk of infection, and the possibility of residual deformity.

TYPES OF WOUND

The more common types of wound can be described as incised, contused, blunt and burst, puncture, lacerated, gunshot and blast injuries (Fig. 49.1).

Incised

An incised wound is a clean cut with the edges well approximated usually caused by a razor, sharp glass or the sharp edges of metal. The wound may be superficial or deep but tends to heal with minimal scarring once the bleeding has been arrested by pressure bandage or suture.

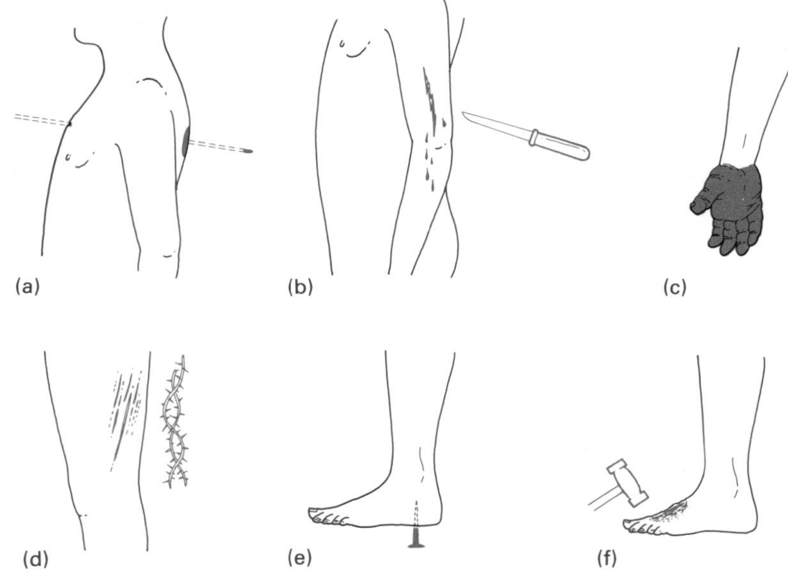

Fig. 49.1 Types of soft tissue wound: gunshot (a); incised (b); burns (c); laceration (d); penetrating (e); contused (f).

Contused

The skin is broken in a contused wound with some bruising around the site of injury due to damage to the superficial blood vessels. The cause of this type of wound arises from pressure or a crushing effect upon the skin.

Blunt and Burst

The skin may be split in a blunt and burst wound with severe bruising around the edges of the wound. This may have been caused by a blunt object, e.g., a cosh, boot kick, fist punch, or a fall from a height. The underlying blood supply is affected, often being inadequate for oxygenation of the wound area, in which case necrosis might occur. If the skin edges are necrosed they will require excision under local anaesthetic and approximating for suturing. In more serious instances skin grafting may be required.

Puncture

A puncture wound has a small entry and may be caused by a stab wound from a knife. The depth of such a wound is important and may require probing to identify if underlying structures have been affected. Observations for internal haemorrhage, i.e., taking the blood pressure and pulse, and close scrutiny for undue restlessness, thirst and pallor are required at 15-minute intervals. The wound may require exploration under general anaesthetic if there is any suspicion of foreign bodies retained within the wound.

Puncture wounds are also caused by nails, part of which may remain in the wound necessitating an X-ray.

Lacerated

The edges of a lacerated wound are extremely jagged and are often a feature of injuries from 'flying' glass. This type of wound requires full surgical toilet and removal of debris. The wound edges need to be excised, and underlying damaged tissue removed along with any residual debris.

Gunshot

A bullet entering the body at high velocity does so by creating a small entry puncture wound and on exit from the body causes a large burst and lacerated wound. Where it enters a bone cavity, e.g., the skull or pelvis, the bullet may come to lodge in the bone. After X-ray such a wound will require full exploration under general anaesthetic not only to remove the bullet, if still within the tissues, but to repair the damaged soft tissues.

Blast Injuries

Whether from a bomb blast or explosion, flying debris will cause multiple lacerated wounds requiring extensive surgical wound toilet and then plastic surgery after the initial recovery period is over.

SURGICAL TOILET

There are 2 types of surgical toilet: primary suture and debridement.

Primary Suture

The nurse must arrest the haemorrhage by applying steady pressure over the wound using a sterile pad. If glass is present in the wound, the patient's limbs should be elevated and indirect pressure applied. While this is being done the casualty officer will complete his or her examination searching for second obscure injuries. The wound area is cleansed carefully of any blood and other obvious contamination, e.g., dirt, dust, grease and perspiration by the nurse. A small amount of local anaesthetic is injected into the surrounding area and after a few minutes a simple suture technique is employed to bring the edges of the wound together by the doctor, or trained nurse. The tension of the suture should not be too tight, otherwise scarring may form as the wound heals by primary suture.

Treatment

In some cases, antibiotics are given as a prophylactic measure to control any tendency to infection. Invariably one of the broad spectrum antibiotics are prescribed, usually a large single intramuscular injection of penicillin, tetracycline or one of the sulphonamides.

For support of the sutured wound a firm but simple dressing should be applied over the wound. It should not be forgotten that however minor the wound appears, a degree of shock, usually neurogenic, always accompanies a wound and a sympathetic and reassuring confident manner will do much to reduce 'shock reaction'.

On completion of the wound suturing, an appointment is arranged for the patient to have the sutures removed in 5–7 days' time. Facial and scalp wounds requiring primary suture usually have a great deal of blood loss which can be extremely alarming for everyone concerned, and its control requires firm pressure for a longer than usual period of time, i.e., about 20 minutes.

Incisional wounds of the face may not in fact be sutured, but the edges of the wound approximated by a Butterfly tape and Steristrips. For such a dressing to be successful the skin must be absolutely dry when the Butterfly tape is applied.

Patient Counselling

The healing time for facial wounds is usually very short, about 3 days. The patient requires advice on keeping the wound dressing dry and intact and if concerned about any reactions of persistent pain, swelling or obvious infection he or she should be told to return to the department without delay.

Debridement

Surgical toilet usually applied to burst, punctured, or lacerated wounds is *debridement*. The first step in surgical toilet would be to give an analgesic by injection, to deal with any pain, to calm the patient and to gain maximum cooperation while the patient is still in a state of shock. The wound is cleansed superficially and covered aseptically while preparations are made for a general anaesthetic. In theatre, the wound may be dealt with in several ways.

Management

Dead tissue may be excised, the wound edges approximated and secured by sutures, or the wound may be probed to remove any foreign material. Alternatively the wound may be thoroughly cleansed by skin antiseptic lotion and prepared for a skin graft, or a drain sutured into the wound and then covered with a dressing, or thoroughly cleansed and left open.

Wounds which have to be probed or drained may then be sutured several days later if healing is taking place from the base upwards, i.e., by granulation. If this is done it is referred to as either a *delayed primary* suture or *secondary* suture.

In all cases antibiotics will be prescribed and administered, and the possibility of tetanus and gas gangrene is always considered. The organisms which cause these conditions are spore-bearing and anaerobic, which means they can survive and thrive without air or oxygen. If they gain access to dead or damaged tissue their toxins are lethal. To combat this serious infection risk one of three things can be done:

1. If the patient is not immunised against tetanus he or she is given a dose of tetanus toxoid immediately and again in 6 weeks' time. This is combined with a 2-week course of antibiotics, with a third dose given 12 months later.
2. If the patient has been immunised within the last 12 months, a booster dose of tetanus toxoid is given combined with a 2-week course of antibiotics.
3. If the case is an extremely high risk, e.g., a wound injury over 6 hours old and contaminated with soil, severe burns, or a wound with an extremely poor blood supply, then antitetanus (Humatet) serum is used. A test dose of 0.05 ml is given subcutaneously and after a period of 30 minutes. If there is no reaction, a further dose of 1500 units of antitetanus serum is given regardless of the age of the patient.

During the waiting interval of 30 minutes, the nurse must observe for the slightest reaction to the serum. The most severe reaction that can occur is anaphylactic shock or serum sickness, which requires that both adrenaline and hydrocortisone be on hand. These reactions include respiratory failure, hyperpyrexia, nausea and vomiting with a severe fall in blood pressure. Antitetanus serum is never given to those patients with a history of any allergy.

Follow-up Nursing Care

When seeing the patient at a follow-up appointment the nurse should check the following factors before removing sutures: if there is continuous pain at the wound site; if the pulse is rapid; if the patient has been persistently feverish; if there is a distinctive unpleasant odour from the wound; if the wound edges appear tense, red or inflamed. If any of these are present the patient must be seen by the casualty officer since the wound may be infected. It should be noted that deep wounds are not always visually or superficially infected, the infection being in the deeper tissue layers.

Chapter 50
Acute Poisoning by Common Drugs

IN ADULTS

In adults the majority of cases of acute poisoning are deliberate acts of attempted suicide. About 10% of a total of some 300 000 attempted suicides succeed, that is, the victim dies as a result of taking an overdose of a common drug. The actual statistics reveal an incidence of some 100 000 cases per annum, but the true figure is more likely to be in the region of 300 000.

In seeking for a motive for self-poisoning, psychiatric analysis suggests that many suicide attempts are *impulsive* acts during a bout of reactive depression. In some cases the victim is *experimenting* with drugs, particularly the young adult, while a third group use the threat of attempted suicide as a form of *manipulative* behaviour. The impulsive and the manipulative act of attempted suicide suggests that the victim is unable to communicate his or her stress verbally. In itself, this is one of the most limiting factors to a nurse-patient relationship after the patient has recovered.

The ratio for attempted suicide is approximately 3 females to 1 male, mostly between the ages of 16 and 25 years. Peak admission rates to the department are during the summer months, mainly at weekends, and during the night. When the victim is a male, there is an increased chance that the 'poison' has been combined with alcohol. The impulsive type of victim often takes a mixture of drugs with an unpredictable effect on the body systems.

Immediate First Aid

The first aid for a victim with acute poisoning revolves around the principles of maintaining a patent airway. This involves correct lateral positioning of the victim with his or her head tilted forward and upward to keep the mouth and oropharynx clear of obstruction, especially so if there is vomiting. The patient needs to be kept warm and any restrictive clothing around the neck and waist loosened.

Advance warning to the department will help them to prepare the necessary equipment and if the drug(s) are known to the first aider this will indicate if an available antidote is required. Both the pulse and respiratory rate should be monitored to indicate if the vital cardiac and respiratory functions are threatened.

The drug containers and their contents should be brought to the department along with any other relevant material such as a 'suicide note'. Certainly the containers will help with a quick identification of the drugs taken. In those circumstances when the first aider knows the name of the drug, it is suggested that he or she tickles the victim's oropharynx which will cause reflex vomiting. This should be done **only** with a conscious patient and **never** when the patient has taken corrosives or if the poisoning is by volatile hydrocarbons. In these instances the first aider would encourage the conscious patient to drink a buffer solution, e.g., water.

Nursing Priorities

On receiving the patient into the department the nursing staff will pursue the principles of first aid which have been established at the scene of the incident.

1. Establish and maintain the airway by correct positioning of the head and, if necessary, passing a Guedel-type airway until the casualty officer can introduce an endotracheal tube. If the coma is very deep than the patient may require intermittent positive pressure ventilation by means of an artificial respirator to ensure continuous oxygenation of the tissues.

2. Maintain the circulatory level by elevating the lower limbs, keeping the patient warm, and preparing to establish an intravenous infusion which will be sited by the casualty officer. Both the pulse and blood pressure will be recorded every 15 minutes until the neurological signs indicate that the patient is over the phase of 'unconsciousness' and 'hypovolaemic shock'. If the cardiac rhythm is erratic an ECG may be requested.

3. Administer the prescribed antidote if the poison is known.

4. Employ techniques to help eliminate the poison from the body via the renal system, i.e., administer prescribed diuretics, if a massive diuresis is the treatment of choice. A gastric lavage may be administered to remove the poison from the stomach if the time interval between the poison being taken and arrival at the department is of a short duration.

Identification of Poisons

The importance of knowing the poison taken **before** the treatment of choice begins cannot be overemphasised. Every effort should be made to achieve accurate identification.

Reference Books

To help in identification of poisons the department should have basic references available for guidance within their toxicology file:

Martindale: The Extra Pharmacopoeia
Data Sheet Compendium
Approved Products for Farmers and Growers
Clinical Toxicology of Commercial Products

Poison Centres

In addition to references, the telephone numbers of Poison Centres in the UK and Ireland should be displayed.

London 01 407 7600
Cardiff 0222 569200

Edinburgh 031 229 2477 Ext 2233
Belfast 0232 240503 Ext 2140
Dublin 0001 723355
Leeds 0532 432799

Antidotes

It is useful to have the listed antidotes to the more common forms of acute poisoning by drugs. Some of these are:

Naloxone 0.4 mg intravenously every 10 minutes which is effective against opiates, narcotics, and alcohol

Benztropine (Cogentin) 1 mg per ml which is effective against Maxolon and Stemetil

Co EDTA (cobalt edetate) and **Kelocyanor** 500 mg intravenously immediately and then 200 mg 1 minute later to counteract cyanide poisoning

Physostigmine salicylate 1–3 mg intravenously which is effective against the tricyclic antidepressants

Methionine 2.5 g orally or via a nasogastric tube every 4 hours up to a dose of 10 g. Alternatively N-acetylcysteine 150 mg/kg body weight intravenously in 15 minutes pursued by an intravenous infusion of Dextrose 5% if severely poisoned with paracetamol (within 10 hours of ingestion)

On Admission

In most cases of self-poisoning, the patients are admitted for a 24-hour period to ensure physical recovery and for psychiatric observation. Before being discharged it is the normal policy for this type of patient to have an interview with a psychiatrist, who will decide if the patient requires psychiatric therapy as a day patient or if he or she should be admitted to a psychiatric institute by means of Section Order.

CHILDREN

Accidental poisoning in children has an incidence of some 700 cases per annum in children from 1–4 years of age, and about 300 cases involving children aged 5–14 years old. Various studies show that the access to poisons occurs mainly in the kitchen, living room and dining room of the child's home when the poison has been left on a low level surface. The substances most frequently cited are:

Medications, e.g., aspirin, iron tablets, barbiturates, laxatives

Cleaning products, e.g., disinfectants, washing soda, bleach

Flammable corrosives, e.g., spirits, petrol, oil

Other poisons include: poisonous berries and seeds, e.g., laburnum; alcohol in the form of whiskey, brandy, gin; and the contraceptive pill.

Immediate First Aid

The first aid rendered **immediately** to a poisoned child is the same as that for an adult. It must be appreciated that many children will vomit profusely after taking an inordinate amount of any of the mentioned poisons, though this is not necessarily the case when corrosive poison is taken.

In the absence of vomiting the first indications of poisoning are increased *drowsiness* and *abdominal pain*. The urgency of departmental treatment cannot be overemphasised and the child should be brought to the department by the quickest means possible. The substance should also be brought to the hospital for rapid identification of the poison.

Nursing Priorities

The immediate priority is to maintain the airway, especially if the child is semicomatose and vomiting. The conscious level is rapidly determined by a swift neurological examination, and the effect of the poison on cardiac function is estimated by pulse and blood pressure recordings. If the observations are within acceptable, normal limits for the age of the child and the vital functions are not threatened, then one of several treatments is commenced to rid the body of nonabsorbed poison still within the gastrointestinal system.

Gastric Lavage

A restraining blanket is wrapped around the child to secure both the arms and legs. With the child's head tilted slightly forwards a wide-bore gastric lavage tube is passed into the stomach via the mouth and oesophagus. The mere act of passing the tube irritates the epiglottis and may be sufficient to induce vomiting. If this happens the nurse should check with the casualty officer before proceeding further, especially if the vomitus contains undigested tablets.

Once the tube is securely situated in the stomach, a small volume of tepid water (**not** normal saline or salt water) is passed into the stomach and then siphoned off via a funnel into a bucket. The resulting vomitus should be retained for examination by the casualty officer and then despatched to the pathology department if the poisonous substance has not been identified. Gastric lavage may be continued until the contents of the stomach show a clear return on repeated siphonage. This is a most unpleasant treatment for everyone concerned, not least of all the child but also the parents or guardian. If they show an aversion to the treatment they should be escorted to a quiet waiting area in the department.

Inducing Vomiting

Oral paediatric ipecacuanha 10–30 ml, mixed with water or orange juice, is administered to the child and within a short interval the child will vomit, reflexly emptying the stomach of the poisonous substance. Once again the vomitus should be retained for inspection and pathology examination if the substance is not identified. This is an effective and more gentle treatment, requiring fewer restraining methods, but is only relevant if the time interval between ingestion and treatment is of a short duration.

Observations and Nursing Action

Observations accompanying treatment include recording the body temperature to note if there is a tendency to hypothermia or pyrexia, and the respiratory rate and depth are continuously monitored as they may indicate increasing hyperventilation in the case of respiratory acidosis and alkalosis.

If possible a specimen of urine should be tested to note the pH of the sample. This may indicate if the poison has reached the kidneys. Specimens of blood are required for certain poisonings such as with aspirin and iron tablets, when it is possible to determine the blood level.

A child should never be separated from his or her parent or guardian, even during treatment. This is essential if the nurse wishes to observe the child-parent/guardian interactions. The expected behavioural reaction of the parent or guardian is one of guilt combined with anxiety, tinged with anger and possibly fear for the child's safety. A parent who shows indifference, accuses the child of being naughty, or makes too many excuses may cause the nurse to wonder if the child is 'at risk'. Any suspicion of this should be discussed with the casualty officer, who has the authority to pursue the matter with the help of a health visitor or social worker's report on the home conditions.

Specific Poisons

Barbiturates

With barbiturate poisoning, the nurse should expect the child to be in or to develop a coma. The primary care is that for the unconscious patient, with special care given to protect the patency of the airway. If the child is unconscious, then an endotracheal tube must be *in situ* before gastric lavage. A gastric lavage is routinely a part of the treatment before the child is admitted to the ward.

There are 4 recognised problems with barbiturate poisoning in children:

1. The complications of a prolonged coma.

2. Pneumonia which may develop as a result of aspiration of vomitus or from respiratory failure. Antibiotics are prophylactically prescribed to try to prevent this serious complication.

3. Respiratory failure if the blood level of the barbiturates is affecting the respiratory centre. It may prove necessary to commence positive pressure ventilation on the child by means of a respirator. The child will be admitted to the intensive care therapy unit, after an endotracheal tube has been inserted to maintain the airway.

4. Urinary retention is unusual but possible, with excessive barbiturate poisoning and may necessitate the insertion of a urinary catheter to ensure continuous bladder drainage until the child has recovered completely.

Aspirin

Ingestion of aspirin (acetylsalicylic acid) and its absorption alters the blood pH from its neutral level of 7.4 downwards, which means that the blood becomes more acid. As a consequence of this chemical change the child will begin to hyperventilate. Hyperventilation will usually return the blood back to its normal pH. Concurring with this blood change, the child may suffer from vomiting, perspiration, and a haematemesis. Other side effects of aspirin include *tinnitus* (ringing in the ears) and a possible deafness.

On admission the child may appear to be severely dehydrated and have an extremely low blood pressure. Blood tests will show an electrolyte imbalance. The initial treatment of choice is to empty the stomach either by gastric lavage or by giving oral ipecacuanha. An intravenous regimen of sodium bicarbonate 2.4% is rapidly infused to cause a diuresis, i.e., a rapid increase in the volume of excreted urine. When the blood pH and electrolyte levels have returned to within normal limits, the intravenous regimen is altered to dextrose saline with added potassium and this is infused until the urinary pH is 7.5 and above, i.e, an alkaline urine. If forced, diuresis therapy is unsuccessful and the child may then have to be treated with either peritoneal or haemodialysis until the blood salicylate levels are cleared. This estimation is made every 3 hours until the blood picture is normal. Only then is the treatment discontinued.

Iron Tablets

Iron is absorbed in the upper small intestine and any overload of iron leads to a haemosiderosis if doses as low as 2 gm are taken at once. If left untreated the symptoms of iron poisoning develop within 30–60 minutes when the child develops abdominal pain, diarrhoea and vomiting severe enough to cause the child to physically collapse. Within 4–6 hours the child may succumb into a coma and in about 20% of cases this leads to death. If the child does not develop a coma, there may be recovery after a period of vomiting only to be followed by a relapse within 8–16 hours of taking the iron tablets. Even those who escape, within a month the more serious symptoms of intestinal obstruction from scarring of the small intestine may develop.

The specific treatment involves giving a gastric lavage, using a solution of sodium bicarbonate. Once the stomach is cleansed of any residual iron the circulating iron is neutralised by the administration of the antidote, desferrioxamine, via a nasogastric tube (often put down the stomach tube after gastric lavage) or intravenously. This antidote will *chelate* (bond in a ring or rings) the iron, which allows it to be excreted harmlessly. Should haemosiderosis be evident from the examination of a blood specimen an exchange blood transfusion may be considered as essential. With the increased blood viscosity due to the iron the blood pressure will rise (hypertension) and renal function is threatened. Both complications cause a coma, requiring treatment of the child in the intensive care unit.

The child is always admitted for 24-hour observation following iron poison.

PREVENTION

The prevention of accidental poisoning in children is of major concern and has received wide publicity over the years. In an attempt to reduce the incidence of poisoning, the pharmaceutical companies have designed and issued child-proof drug containers. The individual packaging of drugs in a plain container has done much to reduce the visual attraction, and the labelling on containers does carry warnings to parents on the dangers of leaving drugs within easy access of children.

Children do have a natural curiosity and tend to imitate parental behaviours, i.e., taking tablets, if it is a regular feature of domestic life. Securing drugs in a child-proof domestic drug cabinet, fixed to a wall well above adult head height, has proved the most effective way to reduce accidental poisoning of children within the home.

Compounding the problem of acute poisoning in the adult is the ready availability of drugs 'over the counter'. There is an increased tendency in the adult population to self-prescribe for minor ailments. Often the drugs bought are kept within the home and, if left lying around, may act as an easy source for the 'impulsive act' of self-poisoning.

To counteract abuse of some drugs, e.g., barbiturates, paracetamol, distalgesics and benzodiazepines, many have now been taken off the commercial market and are only available on prescription. As a general rule prescribed drugs are issued on a weekly or fortnightly prescription which helps to reduce the chance of an accidental overdose becoming an acute poisoning. Nursing staff do have a responsibility for advising their patients on the correct storage and, when necessary, disposal of unused drugs.

Chapter 51
Initial Care and Management of Injuries

BURN INJURIES

Causes

The wounds resulting from burns may be classified by cause:

Dry heat from flames, molten metals or friction

Wet heat from boiling water (scalds), boiling or hot fat or steam

Chemical burns from acids or alkalis

Electrical burns and shock

Sunburn

NB Ice, paradoxically, can also cause a burn of the skin.

The majority of victims suffering from burns are children under the age of 6 years. They are admitted to the department with scalds usually as a consequence of a domestic accident. Actual deaths related to fire are in the main due to housefires. The cause may be smoking in bed, a faulty electrical appliance, or electrical wiring which has been overloaded with appliances.

Physical Reaction

The body's reaction to a burn, when taken to its logical conclusion without any intervention, would follow a certain sequence of pathophysiology. There would be:

1. Extreme pain and neurogenic shock
2. Superficial tissue destruction
3. Oedema and blistering of skin thickness
4. Tissue necrosis

5. Fluid loss from tissues and circulation, i.e., plasma, leading to oligaemic shock

6. Retained heat which continues the tissue destruction

7. Haemoconcentration, i.e., blood viscosity, increases due to fluid loss. Renal secretion is decreased combined with adrenal insufficiency which increases both oligaemic and neurogenic shock

8. Exposed necrotic tissue with the risk of infection. This would not occur with superficial burns but is likely with severe burns, from whatever the cause. It gives a useful background against which to place the most effective method of first aid treatment.

Immediate First Aid

As with other emergency measures, the efficacy of immediate help relies heavily on the first aider remaining absolutely calm and acting swiftly.

1. If possible isolate the cause of the burn without putting the rescuer at risk, e.g., insulate against electric current, switch off gas, isolate the flames. If the cause is not evident, the casualty must be moved quickly to hospital.

2. If the cause of the fire is associated with smoke, the victim's airway takes priority over the burn. The inhalation of smoke damages the lining membrane and surfactant of the lungs, leading to a pulmonary oedema and suffocation. The patient must be removed from the scene of the fire as soon as possible and kept as near to the ground while doing so, and artificial respiration commenced immediately it is safe to do so.

3. Should the victim's clothing be on fire, roll the person in a blanket, a coat or a rug, if available, on the ground to extinguish the flames. There is a tendency for the victim to run, pulling at the burning clothing. It may be necessary to trip the person over *deliberately* so that the flames can be extinguished.

4. A high voltage causing an electrical burn will 'shock' the vital centres of respiration and cardiac function into arrest. Artificial respiration with external cardiac massage may be necessary once the victim and rescuer are insulated against the electricity.

Having established that both the airway and cardiac function are satisfactory the next step is to:

1. Remove any articles near the burnt area (e.g., jewellery, belts, loose garments, pocket contents) which are likely to retain any heat.

2. Irrigate or immerse the affected burned area with cool water for at least 10 minutes. This will cause vasoconstriction of the local blood vessels and limit further damage to deeper tissues from the heat. For deep burns, cool packs (not ice) are helpful in reducing the local heat.

3. Check for singed hair in the nasal mucosa, which will indicate if smoke has been inhaled.

If time permits, when sending for an ambulance, it is helpful if the crew can be informed of the depth of the burn and the area. This information will in turn be relayed to the hospital, and the departmental staff will prepare the necessary equipment.

Depth of a Burn

The depth of a burn is an unpopular method of assessing its severity. It does, however, help the rescuer to assess immediately the possible degree of shock and how the patient can be handled.

Physical Appearance

The depth of a burn can be assessed by its physical appearance.

Erythema. If the skin is red and inflamed, only the upper layer of the skin is damaged. This superficial burn, however, can be extremely painful even if the burn is only slight in area. The immediate care would be to immerse the part or irrigate the area with cool water for several minutes until the pain recedes. This will limit not only the extent of further damage but also the effect of blistering.

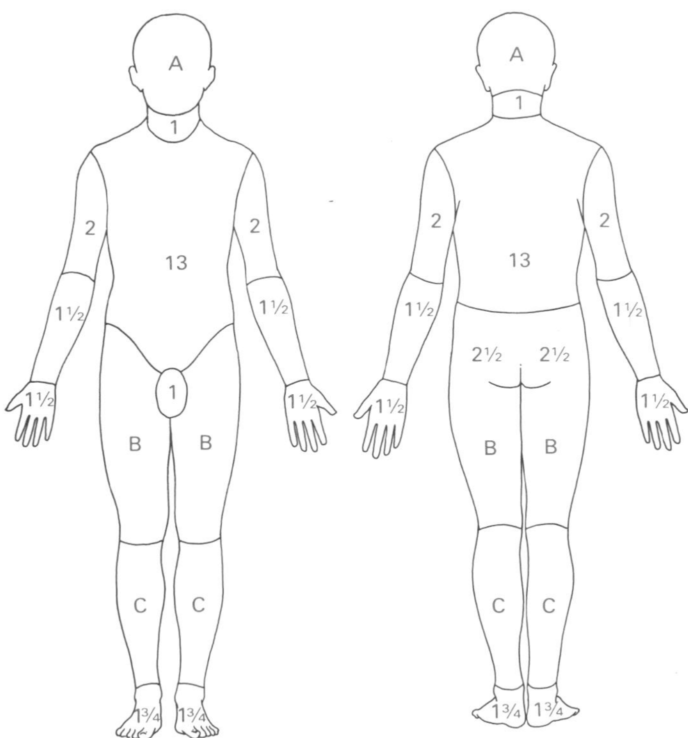

Relative percentage of areas affected by growth

Area	Age in years					
	0	1	5	10	15	Adult
A – ½ of head	9½	8½	6½	5½	4½	3½
B – ½ of 1 thigh	2¾	3¼	4	4¼	4½	4¾
C – ½ of 1 leg	2½	2½	2¾	3	3¼	3½

Fig. 51.1 Estimation of area burnt using Wallace Rule of Nine.

Blistering. If the skin blisters, the burn has involved a partial thickness of skin and the first aid is similar to that for erythema. Blisters should **not** be burst as a part of first aid, but left to the hospital staff. The blistered skin acts as a temporary aseptic barrier, preventing infection risk.

Whole thickness. The full thickness of the skin is lost and the burn may extend downwards to the subcutaneous fat, muscle or even bone. In appearance the flesh will be black and charred and have an offensive odour. It will do no harm to immerse the burnt part in cool water or, if this proves impossible, to apply cool packs to reduce further damage from retained heat. Clothing should **not** be removed from burns as it will pull away with it any viable tissue and cause further severe pain. Whole thickness burns are said to be 'analgesic', i.e., without pain, since the nerve endings have been destroyed.

Area of the Burn

The area of the burn can be roughly assessed using the Wallace Rule of Nine (Fig. 51.1). In principle, each area of 9% represents a fluid loss of about 1000 ml depending on the age and weight of the victim. This is valuable information as it gives the medical staff an immediate calculation of the amount of fluids which will require replacing. From a treatment point of view in dealing with shock, the area of a burn is far more relevant than the depth.

In first aid, oral fluids should **not** be given to the patient. If the person is within one hour of hospital treatment then it is recommended he or she be given hot sweet tea.

Admission to Hospital

A person will be admitted to hospital if the burns are exceeding:

10% in a child
15% in an adult

If the burns exceed 35%, there is a high risk of renal failure because of haemoconcentration and the victim will need catheterisation. Circumferential burns, i.e., all around a limb or body, will require the person's admission because of loss of function and immobility. The greater the area of the burn is, the more likely will be the incidence of hypothermia and, therefore, the need to keep the patient warm in a room with a temperature of 22–28 °C.

Nursing Care

After making these assessments and giving the initial care, the nurse should ensure that the victim is cared for in the dorsal position, with the burns covered with clean material. Keep the patient warm but do **not** overheat him or her with excess use of blankets or coats.

It is a false assumption to apply creams, lotions, grease, butter or other such 'soothing' agents to a burn. If the patient requires debridement of the burn it should be remembered that such applications will have to be *scrubbed off* (literal meaning) while the patient is under anaesthetic. Creams are usually required *once* the burn has healed. The new skin, being thin and friable, will need to be moisturised to prevent it breaking down.

Assessment and Intervention

On admission to the department the admitting nurse's first assessment should follow a set pattern.

Assess the airway. Check for scorch marks at the nostrils and look for burns to the lips. Listen carefully for any distressed respiratory effort such as dyspnoea, wheezing, or coughing. This will indicate if the lungs have been damaged by inhaled smoke and heat. Oxygen therapy administered via an *MC* or similar oxygen mask should be commenced immediately.

If the throat tissues are oedematous this will soon lead to respiratory obstruction, and intubation by an anaesthetist will be done urgently. A tracheostomy is not performed until a few days later when the patient's condition is more stable and the procedure can be conducted electively. Severe damage to the lungs invariably means that the patient will require intermittent positive pressure ventilation on an artificial respirator, for several days.

Record the pulse. The pulse will usually be rapid and weak. If the burn is over 10%, the tachycardia will be due to both neurogenic and oligaemic shock. The fluid being lost from the body is plasma, and this must be replaced by the intravenous route as soon as possible. If the peripheral vessels have collapsed, or are not available due to the burn, the casualty officer may have to perform a cut down to reach a suitable vessel. The rate of flow of the plasma infusion is important.

Fluid replacement. The fluid replacement required must take into account that haemoconcentration threatens renal function. To counter the risk of renal failure the fluid replacement is measured over a 36-hour period. This calculation is based on one of several formulae.

The Muir and Barclay formula (see Table 51.1) states that the percentage area of a burn times the patient's weight in kg divided by 2 equals the volume of plasma required in each 6-hour period for 36 hours. If, for example, a patient weighing 70 kg had a 20% burn area, then

$$\frac{20\% \times 70\ \text{kg}}{2} = 700\ \text{ml}$$

plasma will be needed in each 6-hour period for 36 hours.

The importance of initiating a fluid balance record at the very outset of therapy and of

Table 51.1. Muir and Barclay formula applied

Period	Hours	Accumulative intake (ml)
1	0–4	700
2	4–8	1400
3	8–12	2100
4	12–18	2800
5	18–24	3500
6	24–36	4200

ensuring that the handover to ward staff is absolutely clear cannot be overemphasised. It is essential if this twofold therapy, i.e., the treatment of oligaemic shock and the prevention of renal failure, is to be successful.

Pain relief. Morphine (Diamorphine 10 mg) or pethidine 75–100 mg is usually required and for a more rapid effect is normally administered intravenously. With the rapid relief of pain the consequences of further shock are diminished.

Control of shock. Once the patient has been transferred to a Dean's trolley, to control shock the patient should be positioned head down to promote blood flow to the brain. Without causing further loss of body heat, the nurse must ensure that the patient is kept reasonably warm.

Secondary Assessment

The burn should not be regarded as an isolated wound, secondary injuries may be present, especially if the history indicates that a blast or explosion occurred at the same time as a fire. Fractures, ruptured organs, head injuries and other flesh wounds require the second examination to be as thorough as possible. Loose clothing is carefully cut away and left lying beneath the patient rather than unnecessarily moving the patient too much. A careful examination should be made for obscure burns, e.g., behind the ears and knees, and the perineum.

In conjunction with the second assessment, the casualty officer would normally request grouping and cross-matching of several units of blood, an assessment of the patient's haemoglobin level and the haematocrit.

An initial large dose of broad spectrum antibiotics and tetanus toxoid are administered as a prophylactic precaution whether or not the patient is to be admitted. If the burns exceed 35% in area the patient will undoubtedly be admitted directly to a Burns Unit Hospital, or transferred there when stable, but a urinary catheter may be passed into the bladder before this happens.

Burns patients who require admission are normally seen by a plastic surgeon in the accident and emergency department before their admission to the ward. After an examination, the surgeon will decide on precise treatment to be pursued for the next 36 hours. In some instances, the patient may go straight to theatre.

Treatment of Minor Burns

Prior to dressing a minor burn the nurse should ensure that the patient has been given the prescribed analgesia necessary to minimise the distress of having the burned area handled. It is preferable to have the patient positioned lying down flat with the head supported by one pillow and looking away from the burn. The surrounding area is cleansed of any debris or grease using a weak solution of cetrimide (Savlon).

Burn Dressing

The burned area itself must be dressed according to strict aseptic techniques. Using gentle wiping strokes from the centre of the burn outwards, the nurse cleanses the area of superficial debris with swabs soaked in cetrimide. Necrosed tissue requires to be cut away, blisters incised, their fluid expressed and the blister skin replaced onto the burned part. Nonadhesive dressings are then applied to the area. Three common dressings are tulle with gauze, tulle with a dry, nonadherent absorbent dressing (e.g., Melolin), and Melolin alone. Superimposed onto this basic dressing is placed a thick layer of gamgee secured firmly in position with a crepe bandage. The crepe bandage **must** be firm as any looseness will cause rubbing on the burned area. This first dressing is normally left in place for at least 48 hours, and the patient must be warned to expect the outer layer of the dressing to stain with exudate but not to be alarmed as this is quite normal.

Before a patient is sent home he or she will require enough analgesic to ensure a pain-free 48 hours, and they should be questioned on how they will cope with everyday activities of living. If the arms or hands are dressed the patient will need more than the usual help for things such as cooking, undressing and washing.

Subsequent Dressings

In subsequent dressings the nurse must be very careful to remove the dressings layer by layer, soaking each layer with copious amounts of cetrimide, as the exudate tends to harden the dressing. If bleeding occurs, over the healing burn, then the nurse is being far too rough and this will lead to delayed healing and unnecessary pain which is unforgivable. Sloughing of the tissue as the burn heals can be expected and this will be removed carefully. When the healthy skin begins to appear the covering or occlusive dressings are discontinued and ointments are introduced, e.g., silver sulphadiazine, smeared into a layer of Melolin and then lightly secured to the burned area. As healing progresses, a continual assessment should be made of functional ability. If needed, the patient can be advised on mild exercises to tone up the muscles, especially of the limbs and digits.

For very minor burns, the treatment consists of antibiotic sprays and the exposure technique, i.e. no occlusive dressing.

CHEMICAL BURNS

Immediate First Aid

The immediate first aid in dealing with chemical splashes to the skin is to irrigate the tissues with water for a minimum of 10 minutes regardless of whether it is an alkali or acid. Water is the most readily available neutralising agent. In industrial processes using specific chemicals, the precise antidote is usually on site and can be applied immediately. Many chemical burns, however, occur in the home or in schools. Clothing which has been splashed should be removed immediately to avoid any further burn to the underlying skin.

Common Chemicals

Specific common chemical burns are caused by hydrofluoric acid, bitumen, phosphorus, phenol and chromic acid.

Hydrofluoric Acid. Calcium gluconate gel 2.5% is applied to the area burned by hydrofluoric acid as a first aid measure. On arrival at hospital, if the area is a full thickness burn, it may require excising and irrigation with cetrimide solution. If it is a splash burn to the eye, sterile water is used to irrigate the sclera, cornea and conjunctiva followed by instillation of calcium gluconate 10% eyedrops.

Bitumen. The bitumen should not be forcibly removed, but will require to be softened and then removed by a slow infusion of liquid paraffin.

Phosphorus. Particles of phosphorus remaining on the tissues after irrigation with water must be removed as soon as possible. Use any implement to hand, e.g., a spoon if forceps are not available. Do **not** use the unprotected fingers. Once the phosphorus has been removed, a dry clean dressing should be applied until the burn is examined in hospital.

Phenol. The area affected by phenol (carbolic acid) should be thoroughly washed using copious amounts of water. Then, a wet compress is applied, and the patient must be seen by the casualty officer in the department.

Chromic Acid. Immediate irrigation with water will reduce the incidence of ulceration from a chromic acid burn. A second danger is damage to the respiratory passages from the fumes, and the patient must be taken into the fresh air as soon as possible. After the skin has been covered with a clean dry dressing, the patient must be examined to exclude further damage to the respiratory passages.

PREVENTION

Since 75–80% of burns accidents occur in the home, it is always useful to explore those measures which can be taken to prevent their incidence. The Royal Society for the Prevention of Accidents (ROSPA) places particular emphasis on the safety of children under the age of 6 years. Fireguards should always be placed in front of open fires and secured to the wall. Matches should not be left lying around. The kitchen should be a restricted area unless the child is closely supervised. Children's nightwear should be made from noninflammable material.

Some regard should be given to home furnishings for their fire resistance, notably upholstered armchairs and settees. This type of furniture should carry a warning label if it is not fireproof and, even more importantly, if it gives off dangerous fumes when ignited. Flammable solutions such as petrol, kerosene, paint, oil, or grease should not be stored in the house but preferably in a shed or self-contained unit away from any main dwelling area. Houses should have their electrical wiring checked at least every 20 years and frayed insulation should be a warning sign that a fire from an appliance is a high risk. Equally, the overloading of any electrical socket with the incorrect ampage is a serious hazard.

Dwellings with many rooms and, certainly, multistoreyed dwellings should have a smoke detector installed to raise the alarm when the residents may well be some distance from the source of the fire. For larger institutions such as hospitals the fire risks are too numerous to mention. The most serious hazard is permitting patients to smoke cigarettes in bed. To counter the hazards of fire in large buildings, legislation does require: frequent inspections by the local appointed fire officer, staff to have frequent fire drills, and fire notices to be displayed in every unit and subunit occupied by either employee or patient. Additionally, heat and smoke detectors should be installed.

LOCOMOTOR INJURIES

A vast number of the patients admitted to the accident and emergency department arrive as the result of locomotor injuries. These may be due to muscular strain, ligamentous sprains, fractures, fracture plus dislocation, or dislocations.

Immediate First Aid

At the scene of the accident, it is often impossible to say if the injury is a simple strain or a fracture unless the skin is obviously broken by a wound. Only an X-ray can actually confirm the suspicion of a fracture. It is, therefore, better to treat all locomotor injuries as fractures until diagnosis in the department states otherwise.

Signs and Symptoms

Classically, a fracture will present with certain features:

1. Intense localised **pain** at the site of injury which contributes to the state of shock. If touched the patient will complain of tenderness over the affected area. This reaction in itself is enough to advise the first aider to be careful and gentle when moving the injured person.
2. Inability to move the injured part (**immobility**).
3. **Deformity** of the injured part, e.g., the limb may appear or actually be shorter than the healthy limb, or if it is the lower limb it will adopt a position of internal rotation with the ankle and toes pointing into the midline of the body.
4. **Swelling** of the injured site, if it occurs rapidly, implies bleeding into the tissues.

Improvising Splints

Having first ensured the safety of the area where the accident victim is lying and enlisted assistance to contact emergency services, the first aider sees to the comfort of the victim. It is now recognised that applying improvised splints does increase the handling of the injured site.

Immobilising the injured part should be done using the simplest forms of improvisation, e.g., secure the injured leg to the other with a scarf or tie, bearing in mind circulation, and pad the spaces between the natural limb contours with any form of material. An arm can be secured to the torso by the jacket or cardigan the patient may be wearing.

With serious limb injuries, the patient should be lying down and must be kept warm. With chest injuries, the patient is nursed in a sitting position. Reassure the patient that aid, i.e., the ambulance, has been or is being sought and is 'on the way', and keep to a minimum the amount of movement required to ensure the safety of the patient.

Bleeding

If there is any bleeding over the injured site apply firm but consistent direct pressure using either the fingers or a clean piece of material. On arrival the ambulance crew will immobilise the part, if this is required, before the patient is correctly lifted onto the ambulance stretcher. A history of how the accident occurred is invaluable to help the casualty officer in the assessment of the injury.

Initial Assessment

On arrival at the department the receiving nurse should make an initial assessment for all locomotor injuries:

1. The degree of shock must be measured by recording the pulse and blood pressure. If there is hypotension and tachycardia accompanied by pain then the shock will increase and medical intervention with analgesia becomes the first priority. If the casualty officer would like X-rays before giving analgesia, the patient needs reassurance that the pain will be relieved after the diagnosis is confirmed.

2. The circulation of the limbs is assessed by: feeling for the distal pulses, e.g., the dorsalis pedis in the foot; noting the colour of the skin; observing the injured part for bruising or haematoma; and checking that any temporary splint is not too tight. When exposed the toe nails or finger nails can be sharply depressed to see if the normal pink colour beneath the nails blanches to white and then returns to pink. If not, the venous blood return may be impeded.

3. Sensory responses of touch, texture and temperature along with pain should all be present. If there is paraesthesia or absent feeling then a nerve has been injured and a paralysis would be possible. It is usually obvious by the laxity of the limb.

4. The posture or adopted position taken up by the patient is often a clue not only to where the injury is but what the type of injury is, e.g., supporting the arm against the body may imply a fractured wrist.

5. Visually assess the degree of any swelling by comparing the injured limb with its opposite. Note also that muscles around a fracture site may be in spasm especially those of the femur.

6. If the skin is broken, i.e., a wound, then the handling and moving of the patient must obviously be completed with gentleness, though of course this must be done with any suspected fracture. Equally important is the presence of any debris in the wound, which will be an infection risk.

7. Temporarily applied splints are normally left intact until the casualty officer is ready to complete the initial assessment, but if they are obviously too tight, or inappropriate, they require to be removed. These splints are often replaced so the patient can be undressed.

FRACTURES (Fig. 51.2)

The Skull

Direct or indirect violence to the skull may cause a simple linear fracture to the bones of the cranium or be associated with a wound. Wounds to the skull, even minor ones, tend to bleed profusely and can be alarming to everyone concerned. Superficial bleeding will be easily controlled by digital pressure over the laceration, until such time as it can be cleansed and dressed in the department.

If the injury to the skull is accompanied by a history of unconsciousness, however brief, a neurological assessment is commenced

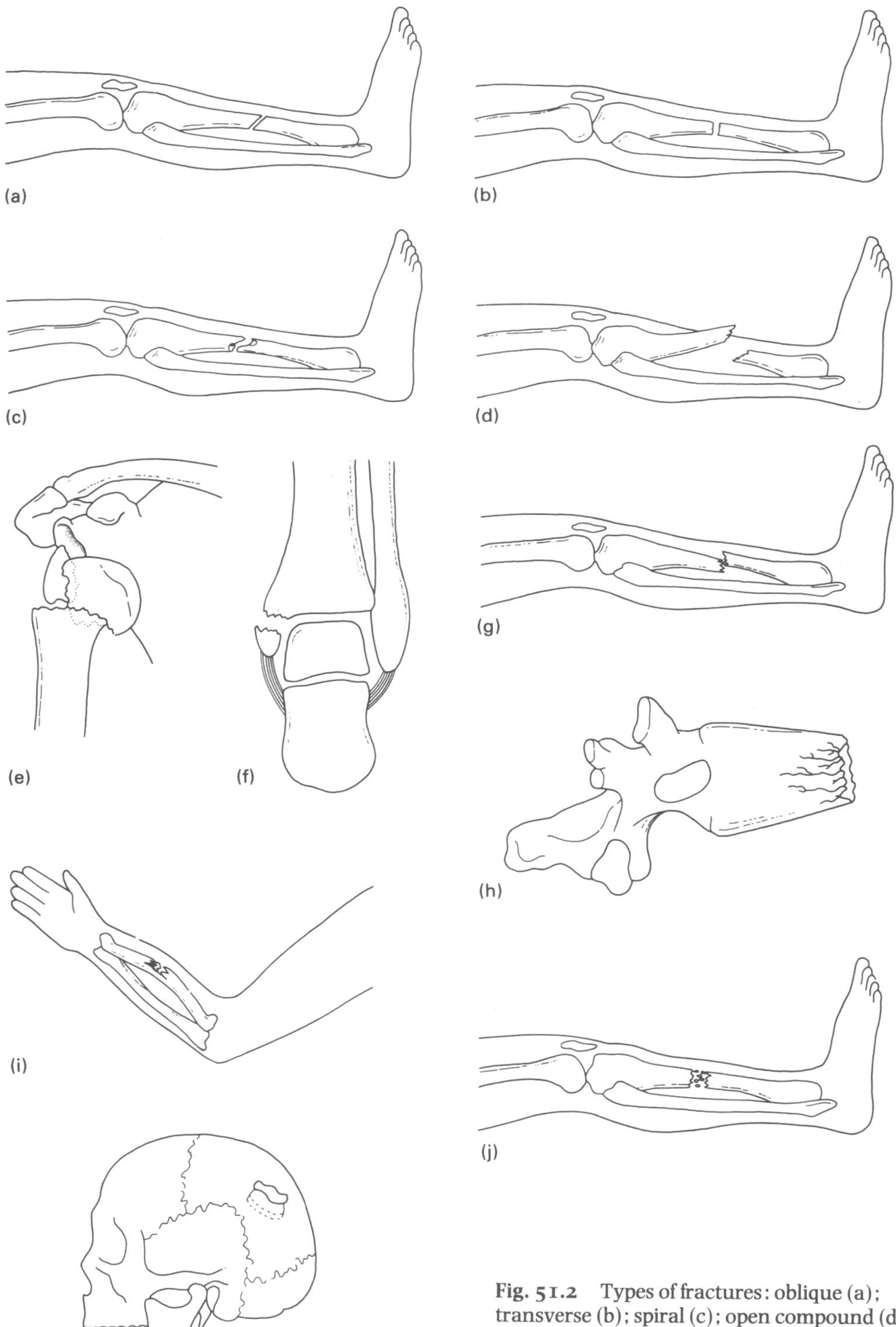

Fig. 51.2 Types of fractures: oblique (a); transverse (b); spiral (c); open compound (d); fracture dislocation (e); avulsion (f); impacted (g); crush (h); greenstick (i); comminuted (j); depressed, where broken skull bone is driven inwards (k).

immediately and may be continued over a period of 24 hours. This ensures that the complications of increased intracranial pressure from any cause, i.e., *subdural haematoma, cerebral haemorrhage* and *cerebral contusion,* can be detected at the earliest opportunity and surgical intervention can be implemented quickly. All skull injuries should be X-rayed to eliminate the possibility of hidden fractures. In some instances, and if available, a CAT scan may be employed to detect if there is any unusual object within the skull as the result of the injury.

Conscious Patient

The patient may be admitted to the observation ward in the department. The nurse will be required to make frequent checks on the pulse, blood pressure, temperature, pupil reaction, and level of consciousness.

Observations

If the pulse becomes reduced in rate or if the blood pressure rises over a period of time increased intracranial pressure may be indicated. The temperature may rise or fall. In either case, it indicates cerebral irritation. The pupils' reaction to light, and their size if altered, i.e., pinpoint or dilated, implies there is increased pressure on that side of the brain. The level of consciousness is determined by asking simple questions to denote if the patient is orientated to time, place and event.

Distressed or laboured respiration, vomiting, or restless and confused behaviour are noted. If any of the above observations are causing the nurse concern because they are not within normal limits, even if the patient is conscious, they **must** be reported to a senior colleague without delay. In addition, any discharge from either the nose or ears must be reported immediately as this is a sign of cerebral damage which requires surgical opinion. If, however, the observations remain normal for a defined period of 24 hours the chances of cerebral damage are greatly reduced.

Discharge from Hospital

If the injury sustained to the skull occurred without any loss of consciousness, the casualty officer may discharge the patient home after treatment. In this case the patient should be issued with a card advising a return to the department if headaches, vomiting, pyrexia, or a feeling of being unwell develops. Before discharge the patient should be assessed by X-ray for hidden fractures particularly of the zygomatic arch, nasal septum, and malar bones. These particular fractures require specialist treatment from senior surgical staff, e.g., an orthodontic surgeon and ENT surgeon.

Unconscious Patient

Unconscious head-injury patients are admitted immediately into the resuscitation room to establish a patent airway and for a full neurological assessment before further treatment is decided upon. In carrying out the observations already outlined, the nurse should particularly **note** and **report** immediately any discharge from either the nose or ears. If it is a clear fluid, it may be cerebrospinal fluid. This is a sign of *cerebral damage* which requires **immediate** surgical opinion.

The Spine

Fractures to the cervical spine are described as being *unstable,* particularly if they are of the atlas and axis vertebrae. It is vital that the patient, if moved, **must** be lifted by 3 nurses and not rolled. Under no circumstances should the injured patient's spine be flexed in case further damage is done to the spinal cord. The head must be held in a firm position by applying either a soft cervical collar or placing sandbags, one each side of the skull. If the patient appears to have a neurological paralysis, this may be caused by *spinal shock* as opposed to spinal injury.

Fractures of the thoracic and lumbar spine must be treated with the same principle, and if proven by X-ray will require the patient to be admitted for bedrest and orthopaedic opinion as to whether conservative or surgical treatment is required.

The Ribs

A simple fracture of a rib is quite painful initially, and affects the respiration depth. By and large the ribs heal quite quickly if left alone, and for a temporary period it may be sufficient if the patient has the arm on the affected side in a full sling.

Adhesive strapping strips if applied over the fracture site do not promote healing but can be comforting and reassuring. If the pain persists after several days the doctor may infiltrate the local costal nerve with a small volume of local anaesthetic, which is very effective.

The far more serious injuries affecting the thoracic cavity include: a depressed sternum, a flail chest, and a stove-in chest. All require intensive resuscitation.

The pain of a **depressed sternum** is excruciating requiring either morphine or pethidine administered intravenously immediately. A **flail chest** injury implies that there are multiple broken ribs, the breaks being segmented with loose flails. After endotracheal intubation and positive pressure ventilation have been established it is vital that the fractured segments are fixed by surgical means as rapidly as possible. A **stove-in chest** injury requires the same approach of immediate resuscitation and intensive therapy nursing.

The Pelvis

In the young adult, fractures of the pelvis are caused mainly by car or horse accidents, while in the elderly they are the result mostly of falls. In the elderly, it is important to distinguish between a fracture of the femur and of the pelvis and both possibilities should be assessed. At the time of the injury there is severe pain which becomes quiescent if the patient is placed in the dorsal position with feet secured together.

In the department, the patient must be undressed without rolling, i.e., if necessary, the clothes must be cut along their seams.

Observations

Observations include examination of the external urethra for blood. Haemorrhage from the urethra indicates either contusion of the bladder or a ruptured urethra. In either case, the patient will be unable to pass urine. A catheter must **not** be passed without the express permission of the surgeon, in case the tip of the catheter is inadvertently placed into a rupture of the urethra.

A second major consequence of pelvic fractures is haemorrhage into the pelvic cavity from any of the major blood vessels traversing this region, e.g., the internal iliac artery. The lower abdominal cavity can easily hold 2–3 litres of blood which will be noted only by the increasing severity of shock, i.e., low blood pressure and increasing pulse. Emergency grouping and cross-matching of blood is completed while Group O blood is transfused in preparation for emergency abdominal surgery to ligate the torn blood vessels.

Depending on how the injury was sustained, the upper abdominal organs may also be involved, again noted only by the degree of shock. In an uncomplicated case, the patient will still require admission to hospital for pelvic traction to correct any malalignment of the pelvic girdle.

The Upper Limbs

The Radius

Colle's fracture is an extremely common fracture of the lower end of the radius with an upward (*posterior*) displacement of the bone fragment along with a degree of impaction. The radius may also be displaced towards the thumb side of the affected arm.

Under the effects of an anaesthetic the surgeon applies traction using the *Charnley method*. While this traction is being applied, the nurse applies a plaster of Paris backslab which will secure the forearm in pronation and hold the hand in moderate flexion. The ulnar side may be secured in slight deviation to prevent future displacement.

Simple precautions such as removing rings and thoroughly cleansing the arm before plaster of Paris is applied will avoid the discomforts of swelling and itching. The plaster of Paris remains in position for several weeks when the fracture will be reviewed.

A juvenile Colles's fracture affects children under the age of 15 when the epiphysis of the radius becomes displaced posteriorly. A cylindrical below-elbow plaster of Paris is applied immediately following manipulation under general anaesthetic.

Smith's fracture is the opposite of a Colles's fracture, and usually occurs when the patient falls onto the back of the wrist. In this fracture, the lower end of the radius is broken but with an *anterior* displacement. The treatment following confirmation by X-ray is as for a Colles's fracture.

Barton's fracture is similar to a Smith's fracture, but tends to be more unstable and affects the anterior base only of the radius. The treatment is manipulation followed by application of an above-elbow plaster of Paris with the hand and wrist secured in full supination and extension.

Related Fractures

Fractures of the shaft of the radius and the ulna once diagnosed by X-ray, and ensuring the blood supply, sensory and motor nerves are intact are manipulated under the effects of a general anaesthetic followed by the application of plaster of Paris from axilla to metacarpals.

Bennett's fracture is a combined fracture dislocation of the bones and joints within the thumb. After reduction by manipulation the injured part usually will require internal fixation with K wire or an orthopaedic screw and then be held in a temporary external splintage for several weeks.

The Scaphoid

A scaphoid fracture is a common injury and carries a risk of avascular necrosis. Once manipulated, a plaster of Paris is applied which holds the thumb of the affected hand in opposition to the middle finger. This position has to be held for 3 weeks when the fracture will be X-rayed again and further treatment reviewed. Injuries to the other carpal bones are less common but they too would require to be held in a plaster of Paris cast for 3–4 weeks.

The Metacarpals

Individual metacarpal fractures are normally splinted by 'ring strapping' which holds the affected finger in extension until the fracture heals. For several days it is wise to support the hand and wrist in a sling until all signs of swelling have gone.

Multiple metacarpal fractures of one hand require detailed assessment to ensure that the nerve and blood supply to the hand are unaffected. Therefore, the hand is encased in a plaster cast with the hand positioned in optimum function.

Amputation Injuries

Amputation and crush injuries of the hand require emergency surgery as an inpatient to save the maximal function, normally using microsurgical techniques to re-establish both the blood and nerve supply. Such operations may be successful only if the amputated parts have been recovered and are brought to the department with surgery beginning within the shortest period possible.

The Phalanges

A *mallet finger* refers to a fracture at the base of the terminal phalanx. If a plaster cast is applied to the individual finger with the distal joint flexed and the middle joint extended, there is a 50% chance that the fracture will heal within 4 weeks.

Hand injuries are a highly specialised field of casualty work, not only from a surgical point of view but in the adroit application of plaster of Paris. Keen observation of the blood supply is needed for noting undue blanching, peripheral temperature and sensory responses of pain, temperature and texture. Pain in such cases is very severe, often leading to fainting, if not nausea and deepening shock. The use of analgesia is of paramount importance, and as a temporary measure the availability of Entonox is invaluable.

The Elbow

Elbow fractures are rare. When they do occur, there is an immediate threat to the nerve distribution of the lower arm and its blood supply. Because of these two major problems, it is usual to refer the patient for immediate orthopaedic specialist opinion after an X-ray has confirmed the fracture.

After specialist manipulation the joint is maintained in a sling support for some time and analgesia has to be prescribed at regular intervals for a temporary period. Children with elbow fractures are usually admitted to hospital for observation.

The Humerus

Humeral fractures, especially to the shaft, are encased in a plaster of Paris cast with the elbow in a flexed position at a right angle. Once the cast is dry, the arm is supported by a full length sling. At a later time, when the swelling has reduced and the plaster of Paris has been replaced, a simple collar and cuff support is all that is required to keep the limb stable until it is healed.

The Clavicle

Clavicular fractures are a consequence of falling on the outstretched hand. This small *S*-shaped bone can be held in position only by applying a bandage over both shoulders.

It is applied with the patient in a sitting position and undressed to the waist. The bandage (wide-width) is anchored to the chest wall by 2 circular movements and then, usually in a figure-of-eight movement, is taken under the padded axilla and across the back to go over and under the opposite axilla. This is repeated several times until both shoulders have been pulled backwards into alignment with each other.

It is possible to apply this using a triangular bandage. The knots should finish in the natural depression at the nape of the neck so that they do not create an uncomfortable pressure. The arm of the affected side is then supported by a full arm sling. At the conclusion of this, the nurse should check that the radial pulses and sensory responses are normal before allowing the patient to go home.

The Scapula

Scapula injuries are invariably the result of direct violence and require the support of a full arm sling.

Injuries of the upper limb all benefit from elevation, using either a pillow or a cushion, when the patient is at rest. The nurse should advise the patient that if the limb is elevated at frequent intervals any tingling sensations or constant aching that he or she may be experiencing will gradually recede. Tingling sensations may indicate the presence of a nerve injury and **must**, therefore, be reported.

The Lower Limbs

The first aid for any fracture to the bones of the lower limbs is essentially to bring both limbs together and secure them with temporary splintage. This action alone should reduce the severity of the acute pain. More sophisticated splints are made, such as the air inflatable type. This type of splint has a full length zip and is made of 'see-through' material. They are popular with ambulance crews, not only to splint the fracture but to observe any wounds sustained at the time of injury.

The Femur

Fractures of the femur whether of the trochanter, neck, or shaft of the femur invariably require the patient to be admitted to hospital. The full facilities of a theatre may be required to fix the fracture internally, or to apply skin traction for a prolonged period of time, i.e., a Thomas Splint (see *Nursing 1*).

The muscles surrounding the broken femur go into a rigorous spasm, which accounts for a great deal of the associated pain. In addition, the amount of blood which can be lost into these large muscles is quite considerable and would account for the degree of some of the extensive swelling at the site of the fracture. Should the broken ends of the bone prove to be impacted into each other and combined with severe muscular spasm, continuous traction should be applied as soon as possible to relieve the pain.

The Tibia and Fibula

When possible it is better to rest the injured lower limb in a foam-type splintage rather than the air inflatable splint. The blood loss may be as great as 0.5–1 litre into the surrounding tissues, requiring the patient to be hospitalised not only for correction and reduction of the fracture but to receive blood transfusions.

A simple fracture may be manipulated in the department while the patient is under a general anaesthetic. The affected limb is flexed over the end of the operating table. Once manipulated into correct alignment a plaster of Paris cast is applied in 3 parts:

Between the heel and knee with the leg held in extension

From the heel to the toe

From the knee to midthigh

The Ankle

Pott's fracture involves the lower end of the fibula and tibia where it articulates with the malleolus, the break either being associated with an inverted or everted injury which also affects ligaments and tendons around the joint. From this primary point the injury will be diagnosed by degree; some surgeons will consider doing an internal fixation of the broken bone, while others may request for only a plaster cast to be applied.

Nursing Action

In either instance considerable thought has to be given to the removal of footwear before examination and for X-ray purposes. Prior to removal of tightly fitting footwear an analgesic should be prescribed and administered. It may prove necessary to cut downwards towards the sole of the footwear on either side of the shoe before it can be removed. A great deal of the pain arises from the swelling around the injury which will increase once the footwear has been removed. Equally gentle techniques must also be used when removing socks or stockings. To reduce handling of the injury it is always better to request the patient's permission to cut the sock before removing it from the foot.

If the malleoli are affected, the fracture is regarded as being *unstable* requiring internal fixation and the ligaments connecting the fibula to the malleoli may also require operative repair.

The Foot

A fracture of the main tarsal bone, the calcaneum, usually occurs with a forceful landing directly onto the heel. It is an extremely painful injury requiring pethidine to reduce the extreme discomfort. This type of injury is also indicative of possible fractures higher up on the skeleton, e.g., tibia, spine and base of skull.

The local treatment is to support the heel with a layer of Tubigrip covered by a layer of wool and secured by a figure-of-eight crepe bandage to the whole foot. The patient will be unable to weight-bear and will need to be issued with a pair of crutches and taught how to use them correctly before being discharged home.

Injuries to other tarsal bones are rare unless it is a crush injury to the foot and in every case they require to be assessed by a senior orthopaedic surgeon before treatment can be prescribed. Such injuries would normally require the patient to be admitted to hospital.

If the small metatarsal bones are not displaced, even when fractured, they require firm support which holds the contours of the sole of the foot and toes in natural alignment. A prolonged period of rest is necessary to avoid any weight-bearing. When fractures are complicated, they require specialist orthopaedic opinion before treatment can be prescribed.

Individual fractures of the phalanges of the foot heal well when they are 'ring strapped'. Advice must be given on the wearing of correct shoewear, i.e., low heels and preferably leather to give reasonable support and protection to the injured toe.

Dislocations

The Mandible

When the mandible is dislocated from the temporomandibular joint, the lower jaw bone comes forward (anterior). This is normally a spontaneous dislocation as the result of laughter or yawning. Speech is of course impossible and swallowing is difficult, with an excess of saliva, and there may be an accompanying blood loss due to broken teeth or a gum injury.

To correct the injury it is usual to give an injection of valium intravenously to relax the tense and frightened victim. The surgeon stands in front of the seated patient and places the thumbs on each side of the posterior mandible and presses downwards while at the same time pressing the angle of the jaw upwards and forwards, which should reduce the dislocation. To prevent an immediate redislocation, the lower mandible is supported by a firm bandage which lifts the mandible upwards. The patient should remain in the department for several hours after this treatment to ensure that redislocation does not occur and because the effects of the valium may make the patient feel very drowsy.

The Shoulder

When the head of the humerus dislocates from its scapular socket, usually from the impact of a direct fall onto the shoulder joint, it tends to come forwards (anterior) into the musculature of the upper arm. The preferred position for the patient is to be rested lying down in the prone position with the arm hanging over the edge of the stretcher. This position of itself will sometimes bring about a spontaneous reduction.

One of two methods may be employed to reduce the dislocation following the administration of an analgesic:

Kocher's method, which is the simpler, is in 4 stages. The surgeon will:

Flex the arm at the elbow and apply traction for several minutes

Rotate the flexed arm externally

Carry the arm into the centre of the body (adduction)

Rotate the arm internally

Hippocratic method. The operator's foot (without shoes) is placed in the patient's axilla and the affected arm is extended. Traction is then applied by gently pulling the arm over the foot which is being used as a fulcrum.

After either treatment the shoulder requires to be X-rayed again to confirm that the dislocation is completely reduced. If it is not, the patient will require an anaesthetic for a more forceful reduction to be attempted. When a shoulder dislocation is accompanied by a fracture, then it requires open surgery through the humeral neck for which the patient must be admitted to hospital.

The Hip

When the femoral head dislocates from the acetabular socket, it is usually as a result of the femur being forcefully pushed towards the pelvic girdle. This might occur if the knees were forced against the dashboard of a car involved in a collision. The pain of this dislocation is so severe that it overrides any other associated injury, e.g., to the abdominal organs.

Vomiting, extreme nausea and deepening shock need to be countered by the use of Entonox in the first instance and followed by a significant dose of pethidine. Providing that second injuries do not preclude reduction, the patient is taken immediately to theatre to have the dislocation reduced. Following a general anaesthetic, the patient is normally placed on the floor while the surgeon manipulates the affected leg with the knee at a 90° flexion and applies prolonged upward traction with adduction and flexion of the hip. The patient is then admitted to hospital for a period of rest and further observation, especially because of the intense degree of shock which has been sustained.

The Knee

A knee dislocation is rare and unusual. It is dangerous, however, because it threatens the integrity of the blood vessels and nerves located behind the knee in the popliteal space; both must be intact before the dislocation is reduced under the effects of general anaesthesia.

The Patella

When dislocated, the patella usually shifts from its normal anterior position to the lateral or outer aspect of the knee. After dealing with the shock, the leg is extended and the patella is manipulated manually into place and then usually supported by a Robert Jones bandage. This bandage consists firstly of a layer of wool extending from midthigh to midcalf secured by a firm crepe bandage. A second layer of wool is then applied with a second crepe bandage. This is a very firm support allowing a few degrees of movement. The Robert Jones bandage is also used for other injuries of the knee such as effusions or haemarthrosis.

Before being sent home, the patient should be issued with a walking stick to give support when walking; the patient will only require this aid for several days.

SENSORY STRUCTURE INJURIES

A person with injuries to the eye, ear, nose, throat or mouth is for the most part always referred to a specialist after the initial first aid has been given. In each case it is important for the nurse to take an accurate history of the accident: how, when, where and what the circumstances were. The history should also take note of the first aid actually given at the time of the injury.

The Eye

Regardless of the type or degree of injury, any trauma to the eye generates extreme anxiety and restlessness in the victim. A main skill of the nurse will be to calm the patient enough to gain his or her cooperation. This calming effect is often obtained by taking the history, showing interest and concern.

Examination

The eye will obviously have to be uncovered of any first aid dressing, to permit a preliminary examination. When making the patient comfortable, he or she should be so positioned that the nurse or doctor can work from behind and from the affected injured side of the patient. A good light which casts no shadows is vital to detect the most minor of abrasions. A Cobalt lamp is excellent for this purpose.

Equipment

The basic equipment which will be required for an examination of the eye includes:

- Ophthalmoscope to examine the posterior chamber of the eye
- Topical anaesthetic eyedrops, e.g., Amethocaine 1%
- Schiotz tonometer to measure intraocular pressure
- Magnification eye glass
- Fluorescein staining eyedrops or reagent strips
- Visual acuity test chart, e.g., Schellen Chart
- Mydriatic eyedrops, antibiotic ointments, steroid ointments
- Sterile swabs and cotton wool buds
- Antitetanus serum or toxoid if wound contaminated by soil

Foreign bodies

The Conjunctiva

Small particles, e.g., dust, grit, or a broken eyelash, can easily become lodged and fixed to the mucosa, usually of the upper eyelid. Persistent rubbing, while increasing the tear flow, can irritate the cornea even further and cause an abrasion.

By **everting the upper eyelid** the offending particle can sometimes be easily removed either with a wisp of damp cotton wool or a piece of damp tissue. If the particle proves stubborn, repeated **irrigation** with normal saline may prove effective. As a last resort the ophthalmologist may insert a few drops of local anaesthetic, waiting 2 or 3 minutes, before needling the object free from the conjunctiva. This needling procedure should **not** be done by nurses in training unless supervised by an expert.

To establish whether the cornea has been damaged, a few drops of the fluorescein stain are instilled into the lower conjunctiva. If there is an abrasion the colours of yellow and green remain within the abrasion surface after the stain has been washed away. For corneal abrasions antibiotic ointment is applied and the affected eye covered by an eye pad.

Intraocular Injuries

A small particle travelling at high velocity can penetrate the outer coat of the eye and embed itself within the interior of the eye, often leaving an imperceptible entry point. Particles of metal, stone or glass are often quoted and found to be the causative agent of the injury.

In the early stages the victim of this type of injury may have minimal symptoms apart from a localised pain. If the history suggests metal, glass or stone fragments the patient must be referred to the ophthalmologist without delay as this is an emergency. The particle will invariably have to be removed at surgery requiring a general anaesthetic.

Early **complications** of intraocular foreign bodies include haemorrhage into the anterior chamber of the eye (hyphaemia), retinal detachment and loss of vision.

Trauma

Trauma to the eye should be considered in association with head injury or other secondary injuries. Likewise, all head injury patients should have trauma to the eyes considered as part of their examination.

As a first aid measure, both eyes should be covered to reduce muscular movements. If the patient is unconscious the upper eyelid should be temporarily taped to the lower lid after an examination to remove any contact lenses. The majority of trauma injuries to the eye result from not wearing protective goggles in dangerous industrial processes. For this reason it is vital to know and obtain a most accurate history of how the injury occurred.

The Eyelid

Cuts and wounds require to be **cleansed** and **irrigated** to remove dried blood and contaminating debris. Pressure to the eyelid will be necessary to arrest the expected profuse haemorrhage. The edges of the wound are approximated and held secure by a butterfly suture. If any eyelid tissue is missing the patient will require referral to a plastic surgeon to reconstruct the eyelid to prevent scar tissue healing with ultimate deformity of the lid.

Orbital Injuries

Injuries accompanied by blunt or penetrating force invariably cause a periorbital ecchymosis (black eye). Initially this type of injury will require a straightforward X-ray to exclude fractures of the bone orbit surrounding the eye. The examination includes checks for types of visual disturbance and if there is any clear fluid escaping from the nose, i.e., cerebrospinal fluid, or rhinorrhoea. If bruising is the only problem, an icepack over the eye will contain further swelling to the eye orbit.

Orbital blowout describes an injury in which the pressure within the orbit is so great as to cause a fracture of the thin bony orbital framework. Usually it is associated with a maxillofacial impact injury. Between the space created by the fracture, the inferior rectus muscle may become trapped thus limiting the movement of the eyeball. Haemorrhage into the anterior chamber occurs quickly and both these consequences of injury require emergency referral to an ophthalmologist. Usually the patient will require to be heavily sedated, and the eyes covered with eye pads before he or she is admitted to hospital for bedrest and further treatment.

Burns to the Eye

Chemical

It is possible to classify the burn if the type of chemical is known.

Acid burns actually destroy tissue on contact and are therefore *nonprogressive*, i.e., tissue destruction is limited.

Alkali burns continue to destroy tissue after contact and are therefore *progressive* after the initial contact with tissue.

Gases and **fumes** cause excess tearflow at first and then leave the membranes *dry* and *irritated*.

In all cases copious irrigation with tap water at the time of injury is the standard first-aid therapy. If available the precise antidotes to burns of the eye are:

Sodium bicarbonate 2% solution for acid burns

Citric acid for alkali burns

Ammonium tartrate 5% for irritant gases and fumes

Irrigation with normal saline would be continued in the department until the pH of the eye returns to its normal reaction (pH 7, i.e., neutral). To deal with pain and for purposes of examination a few drops of local anaesthetic are used. If further damage is precluded, a course of topical antibiotics or steroids are prescribed for 4–5 days. Apart from teaching the patient how to instill the prescribed ointments correctly, he or she should be advised to rest quietly away from glaring light, and discouraged from watching television or from reading.

Thermal

Singe burns to the eyelashes or eyelids may accompany facial burns, in which case the risk of eyelid contracture may be a major complication. Initially, the patient will require to be heavily sedated with systemic analgesia and the eyes irrigated with normal saline. Antibiotic ointment is applied to both lower conjunctiva prior to bilaterally blindfolding the patient with eye patches. This will keep both eyelids at complete rest and closed until healing takes place within the next few days.

Radiation

Either ultraviolet or infra-red light can cause radiation burns. The sources of ultraviolet light are from sunlamps, snow/ice glare, welders' arc flame, and reading in direct sunlight; these can lead to conjunctivitis or keratitis within 3–6 hours. More serious is infra-red light which can lead to cataracts and the source may be either X-rays or intense heat. In either case, systemic analgesia and topical antibiotics will reduce the worst effects of inflammation. Bilateral blindfolding with eyepatches for several hours to rest the eyes will ensure an improvement within 24 hours.

Nursing Action

Minor treatments for the eye which a nurse should be able to carry out include: eye irrigation, staining of the cornea, eversion of the upper eyelid, and instillation of ointments.

Eye Irrigation

The suggested method for eye irrigation involves:

1. Cleansing the orbital margins and skin around the eye.

2. Preparing a sufficient amount of normal saline solution at tepid temperature, at least 500 ml to 1 litre. If the irrigation is to be continuous it may be best to arrange

the solution to be delivered via an infusion set.

3. Placing the patient in either a dorsal or semirecumbent position. Turn the patient's head to the affected side, so that the injured eye is immediately above the receiver which is positioned to collect the used irrigation solution.

4. Pulling the lower eyelid downwards, maintain this gentle pressure, and ask the patient to look upwards to keep the upper eyelid open.

5. Directing the flow of irrigation fluid over the eyeball working from the nasal side of the eye to its outer aspect. Between each irrigation ask the patient to blink repeatedly.

6. Frequently test the conjunctival pH with litmus paper and continue the irrigation until the pH is neutral (when dealing with chemical burns).

Staining the Cornea

The cornea is stained by:

1. Moistening the reagent end of the chemical strip with normal saline.
2. Pulling the lower eyelid downwards and maintaining this pressure.
3. Touching the exposed conjunctival mucosa with the reagent strip and asking the patient to blink several times to disperse the stain effect over the cornea.
4. Examining the cornea with a cobalt lamp looking at the eye in every direction for an obvious abrasion or injury.
5. Irrigating the eye to remove the stain.
6. Repeating the eye examination to note any retained stain, usually either green or yellow, over the cornea.

Eversion of the Upper Eyelid

The eversion of the upper eyelid can be achieved thus:

1. Standing behind and to one side of the patient with the fingertips grasping the eyelashes, ask the patient to look downwards.
2. With the index finger of the free hand, press downwards on the eyelid and at the same time pull the eyelashes upwards and backwards.

The everted eyelid should now remain steady for further examination and staining.

Instillation of Ointments

Ointments can be instilled by:

1. Cleansing the lower eyelid and conjunctiva with moist wool swabs.
2. Depressing the lower eyelid and asking the patient to look upwards.
3. Instilling the ointment from the nasal side to the outer aspect of the conjunctiva, but ensuring the applicator does not touch the eye.
4. Asking the patient to close the eyes but not to squeeze them tight.
5. Gently massaging the closed lower eyelid and removing any excess ointment from between the eyelashes.

The Ear

Foreign Bodies

Foreign bodies impacted into the auditory canal, if not removed within a short time, can lead to a painful oedema, infections, extreme tenderness, and a loss of hearing. Since this type of emergency is mainly confined to children, any prescribed treatment should, if at all possible, be carried out with the parent or guardian holding the child.

Treatment

Treatment should be carried out as soon as is possible after arrival at the department when the child is less likely to be bored and fidgety from waiting and in a more cooperative frame of mind.

Small objects can sometimes by floated out after instilling some warm oil drops. They may become sufficiently loose for their easy removal by angled forceps. If this is not successful, it is no use struggling with an uncooperative child. It is better if the child is mildly sedated so that a more extensive examination can be carried out **especially** if there is an otitis externa which can be extremely painful. Once the object has been removed the child should be referred to an ENT specialist for any further investigations or treatment in case of damage to the auditory canal or tympanic membrane.

The Nose

Foreign Bodies

Foreign bodies impacted within a nasal chamber may be dislodged by occluding the free nostril and asking the patient to *blow down* the obstructed chamber. This simple technique, however, does not work in children, and children are the main victims of this type of accident. An object may be trapped within the nasal chamber for some time, only becoming obvious when the child develops an offensive nasal discharge indicating an infection.

Treatment

After a few drops of nasal topical anaesthesia have been instilled, it may be possible to apply suction to dislodge the object. If this fails, nasal instrumentation will be required which gets behind the obstruction so that it can be pulled forwards. Since most victims are children it is strongly suggested that nasal instrumentation is only used when the child is under the effects of a general anaesthetic.

Epistaxis: Minor and Persistent

A small and brief nosebleed should respond to first aid measures; whereas persistent epistaxis, which occurs more readily in the elderly with hypertension, requires more involved treatment and usually admission to hospital.

Treatment: Minor

The patient is sat forward with the head placed in a downwards position, the clothing around the neck should be loosened, and the nasal chambers cleansed of any blood clots with nasal buds. The patient is asked to pinch the nostrils together just below the bridge of the nose for about 10 minutes. While doing this the patient should breathe through the mouth, and not speak or swallow. Any dribbles of blood are mopped away and the patient's shoulders are supported during the period.

The amount of blood lost appears to be quite copious but in reality is very small. The pulse and blood pressure should be checked for tachycardia or hypotension since the degree of shock can be considerable. The patient should be allowed to rest for an hour.

Treatment: Persistent

Persistent epistaxis will not usually respond to the preceding treatment, so nasal packing will be completed before admitting the patient to hospital. In most cases the blood is escaping from vessels located in the anterior septal mucosa known as *Little's* area or *Kiesselbach's* triangle.

Initially, the patient will have to be sedated. This is ideally done with an injection of morphia, a most useful drug in cases of haemorrhage since it reduces blood pressure combined with sedatory effects. Both nasal chambers are cleansed of any blood clots, if need be with suction apparatus. A nasal decongestant and anaesthetic, such as cocaine 5% or tetracaine 1%, are instilled into the nasal chamber using gauze wicks or cotton wool pledgets packed into either chamber. The nostrils are then pinched together for about 10 minutes to achieve a vasoconstrictor effect.

If the nasal packs are then removed, the ruptured blood vessel may be identified and subsequently cauterised to stop further bleeding. If this is not possible, a nasal balloon (*nasostat*) is packed into the affected nasal chamber and inflated to compress the ruptured blood vessel. Following this treatment, the oropharynx must be checked to ensure that fresh blood is not trickling down into the oesophagus. Invariably, the patient has to be admitted under sedation for several days before the nasal balloon is removed.

Fractures

A blunt assault to the front or side of the nose will cause depression, swelling, deformity and crepitus of the nasal septal bone and cartilage. A plain frontal X-ray is taken to determine the extent of the fracture and the presence of any other injuries to the skull. The internal mucosal membranes of the mouth and pharynx are checked with a good torch light to exclude damage to these structures.

Treatment

Fractures of the nose are always treated as open fractures, implying that tetanus and a single dose antibiotic injection are prescribed and administered. A serious **complication** of nasal fractures to look for is a *septal haematoma*. This is caused by the separation of bone and cartilage allowing blood to accumulate within the fracture space. Untreated it will split the tissues permanently causing a deformed nasal structure.

A cold pack is applied to the bridge of the nose and a temporary splint arranged until the ENT surgeon can administer regional anaesthesia to the nasal area. If there is minimal swelling, the nasal septum and cartilage are manipulated into correct alignment and then secured by nasal packing either side of the manipulated septum. An external splint usually made from plaster of Paris may be made to cover the nose. Both internal and external splinting is left in place for 2 weeks in which time the nasal septum should have started to heal.

The Mouth

Dental Injuries

Dental pain has a multiplicity of causes such as oral ulceration, fractures, gum disease, sinusitis, haematomas and tooth decay. Any of these is sufficient to cause the patient to seek urgent treatment in the absence of a dentist.

Toothache can be temporarily relieved by applying the tincture of oil of cloves and a systemic analgesic, and then referring the patient to a dentist.

Chipped teeth are quite common injuries in contact sports and children are especially vulnerable. The 4 front teeth of the upper mandible are usually affected, and the nurse should always consider the possibility of head injury. A careful history of how the accident happened and to exclude any period of brief unconsciousness is necessary.

The oral cavity and pharynx should be checked for any damage to the soft tissues and impacted tooth chippings. Once it is established that there is no other injury and that any haemorrhage has stopped, the patient is referred to a dentist for further treatment.

Avulsed teeth are in fact torn from their gum sockets by facial trauma. It is violently painful and copious bleeding should be expected, both contributing to a deepening shock.

Treatment

When the patient has been cleansed, and the extent of injury assessed and treated, the upper and lower mandible are secured together. The patient's head is directed forwards while the body is maintained in either a semirecumbent or lateral position. If possible, the avulsed teeth should be taken to the hospital department. Ideally, the principle will be to replace any recovered teeth back into their own sockets and to secure their position by dental wiring. Within several days the dental pulp will regenerate once the blood supply is re-established.

On arrival at the department, a strong analgesic is required before examining the mouth. Haemorrhage and obvious bleeding is cleared away by suction to detect the actual bleeding point. Digital pressure on a bleeding gum is far better than indirect methods. Once the basic condition is stable the patient will be admitted to hospital for further orthodontic treatment.

Dental abscesses are extremely painful, requiring analgesia in the first instance. If possible, the abscess should be drained via an incision as soon as possible. Applying hot packs to the local site is quite effective in reducing the discomforts, and combined with an antiseptic mouthwash will rid the mouth of any offensive taste. Since the abscess is usually accompanied by pyrexia, an anti-pyretic such as Aspirin is helpful. The patient will require further dental treatment, and a course of antibiotics is usually prescribed to help contain secondary infections.

Chapter 52
Aspects of Unusual Situations

There are instances in an accident and emergency department which may be referred to as unusual and require action on the part of the nurse additional to standard nursing care. For example, the change of season may bring to the department patients suffering from acute systemic reaction. Other examples would include special action required for patients whose injuries would not indicate admission but who would be unable to cope without assistance by a community service; the suspicion of nonaccidental injury; the patient brought in dead on arrival; the victims of a major disaster.

ALLERGIC REACTIONS

Allergic reactions can be briefly summarised as an acute systemic reaction which is usually induced by the release of chemical mediators after an antigen–antibody reaction occurs at cellular level. Hay fever is the more common example of allergic reactions. In this the grass pollen (protein antigen) stimulates an antibody response which releases toxic amines from damaged cells. The toxic amines (chemical mediators) cause the obvious symptoms of rhinitis, wheezing respirations and anxiety. This would suggest that the individual possesses an inadequate defence mechanism from the immunoglobulins which normally protect the individual's tissues.

Anaphylactic Shock

The more severe allergy reactions which the accident and emergency nurse may have to deal with include anaphylactic shock. This severe reaction can be induced by factors such as injections of horse serum or antibiotics, and insect venom.

Horse Serum

Antitetanus injections contain horse serum (Humatet). If this substance is prescribed the nurse would safeguard against a reaction by firstly giving a small test dose by subcutaneous injection waiting for an interval of 30 minutes before proceeding to give the prescribed dose. This precaution is recommended even if the patient has no history of previous or other allergies.

Antibiotics

Antibiotics often cause a mild reaction and in the case of penicillin in particular, hypersensitivity is an increasing phenomenon. Therefore both the prescriber and the nurse must double-check with the patient on his or her previous history. Any suggestion of allergies would normally preclude the use of penicillin and another group of antibiotics would then be considered for the treatment plan. The patient's treatment card should be marked clearly in red **Allergic to Penicillin** if there is a known allergy to the drug.

Insect Venom

Insect venom can come from the stings of bees, wasps and the hornet. The **immediate local reaction** to insect venom is a very localised pain, a rash and a persistent itching.

Treatment

If the sting is located in a vulnerable area, e.g., within the oral cavity, then emergency treatment may be required to protect the airway in case of severe tissue oedema. Otherwise a cold compress applied over the sting will counter the pain, and an attempt to remove the sting by firmly scraping the skin with a dull edge implement will if successful give immediate relief.

The sting should **not** be pulled out as this will only release more venom into the tissues. Soothing lotions such as calamine may help contain the itching. If the rash persists, as it may well do for several days, then antihistamine drugs such as chlorpheniramine (Piriton) may be prescribed.

Delayed local reactions include oedema, erythema and the development of small nodules at the site. These delayed discomforts may persist for several days. Rest, a very mild sedation to promote sleep, and continued topical applications such as an antihistamine cream may control the more severe of these reactions until they finally resolve. In the hypersensitive individual the local reactions may persist for several weeks or months.

Immediate generalised reactions may vary from that of a vasovagal attack (fainting) to the more severe anaphylactic reaction. In the hypersensitive individual, the amount of insect venom in a sting is about 60 μg of foreign protein. This exceeds the foreign proteins in the air during the grass pollen season. With such a high volume therefore the chances of a severe reaction are multiplied many times over. A generalised response can occur 10–20 minutes after the initial sting and when it occurs it is important to distinguish between vasovagal attack and anaphylaxis.

Vasovagal attack

Pallor
Perspiration
Rapid respiration
Bradycardia
Fainting

Anaphylaxis

Anxiety and restlessness
Flushing of the skin
Intense itching of hands and feet
Violent headache
Urticarial rash
Coughing, wheezing and stridorous breathing
Husky and stammered speech
Rhinitis
Dysphagia from laryngeal oedema
Urinary and/or bowel incontinence

Tachycardia with extrasystoles
Dramatic hypotension

If both anaphylaxis and vasovagal attack are combined the symptoms together will produce visual disturbances, chest pain, unconsciousness and an imperceptible blood pressure. It is important to remind the reader that this reaction may follow if the patient is hypersensitive to horse serum or penicillin.

Treatment

Emergency treatment for anaphylactic reaction has of necessity to be swift and it may be that a senior nurse will have to act on her or his own initiative to commence the standard treatment:

Place patient on trolley
Summon doctor
Prepare equipment

Adrenaline 0.5 ml of 1/1000 solution is injected intramuscularly or subcutaneously and a second injection given after 5–10 minutes; this is to increase the blood pressure. Hydrocortisone 100 mg intravenously injected over a 2-minute interval to counter the allergic reaction, i.e., inflammatory response at cellular level.

Maintain the airway if necessary by proceeding to intubation if laryngeal oedema occurs. Constantly monitor the heart rate and rhythm in case of arrest from the very low blood pressure or the arrhythmias. Admit the patient to hospital for a minimum of 24 hours for continued observations and further therapy.

For the **milder** hypersensitivity reactions and vasovagal attacks, it is advised to rest the patient in the head down position for at least 2 hours and to be vigilant in observing for the possibility of an anaphylactic reaction occurring. On recovery this type of patient requires advice from a dermatologist on his or her hypersensitivity, and may have to be offered a series of desensitisation injections against a particular foreign protein once it can be identified.

Since many 'stings' occur in the countryside, the patient may well arrive in the department having overcome the worst of the symptoms. However, the patient would still require a complete examination and possibly be prescribed antihistamine therapy to minimise the risk of a delayed general reaction. Such a reaction may not occur for 12–24 hours later and will usually take the form of a vasovagal attack. Apart from giving the appropriate advice on how to deal with the fainting episode such patients should always be referred to their general practitioner for further advice and follow-up.

LIAISON WITH THE COMMUNITY SERVICES

The accident and emergency nurse is the one person who must exercise personal discretion when deciding if it is necessary to call upon any of the agencies in the community services. There are many groups of patients who while suffering a handicapping injury, are not seriously ill enough to warrant admission to hospital.

Incapacitated Patients

Injuries to the hands or feet will reduce the individual's ability to meet their own physical needs and the normal activities of daily living. An elderly person living on his or her own, suffering from such an injury, is the prime example of when the nurse should go beyond thinking about the injury itself but consider how well the individual will be able to cope.

In the first instance, the nurse would contact a relative or friend to ensure that the patient is escorted home and can be cared for in the interim. Unfortunately, many people, the elderly in particular, live alone and have no relatives. The next action would be to call upon the district nursing services to arrange that the patient will be visited at regular intervals and that the district nurse will arrange a schedule to meet the patient's physical needs. This liaison is normally conducted via the nursing officer in charge of the health centre nearest to the patient's home. Additional to this, it may prove necessary to inform the hospital's medical social worker so that services, e.g., Meals-on-Wheels, can be provided.

Future visits to the hospital for further treatment would necessitate liaison with the ambulance service to arrange dates and times of future visits, so that an ambulance can be provided.

Non-accidental Injury

Non-accidental injury will always require liaison with a multiplicity of professional colleagues. For children at risk, large accident units may well have a paediatric liaison officer on call, alternatively a medical social worker may have to be sent for to deal with the administrative aspects of the custody order required to admit the child into hospital for a prescribed period. Liaison with the police and a paediatric consultant will also be required.

The *battered* or *bashed* patient is not always a child; the common factor is the victim's inability to defend himself or herself against physical violence. There is usually an established policy for the nurses to follow if such a patient is admitted into the department.

Self-inflicted Harm

In every case of drug overdose or self-inflicted poisoning or injury, the nurse has to liaise with the psychiatrist on call to the hospital to arrange for an examination and interview to take place before the patient is allowed to go home. Usually, such patients would be admitted for at least 24 hours, but this may be into the 24-hour observation ward of the department and not into a main hospital ward.

Vagrants

Homeless and elderly vagrants often seek refuge in the accident department, and while sympathetic to their basic needs, the hospital is limited in what it can actually offer by way of comforts. Often, if the department liaises with a voluntary group in the community, e.g., Shelter, such a group may be able to offer temporary warm accommodation, especially during the winter months.

Injured Employees

Employers of injured victims are often grateful if the accident department liaises with them about any admissions or accidents in which their employees have been involved. The degree of anxiety from which many patients suffer is often reduced if the nurse is able to inform their employer of where they are and what has happened to them.

Follow-up Letters

Liaison with general practitioners is usually completed by a letter which is normally written by the casualty officer. Such letters are considered confidential and if given to the patient to take to his or her doctor should always be put in a sealed envelope. The information in the letter would refer to diagnosis and treatment given with some reference to future intention if the patient has to return for further hospital treatment.

DEAD ON ARRIVAL (BROUGHT IN DEAD: BID)

The policy for dealing with a victim dead on arrival at the hospital varies from area to area. If the ambulance crew suspect that their patient is dead, they would advise the senior nurse in charge, who along with the casualty officer would examine the victim while still in the ambulance. Only a medical officer may legally confirm the diagnosis of death by examining the corpse and checking for:

Complete absence of spontaneous respiratory effort

Absence of the heart beat and carotid pulse

Fixed and dilated pupils in both eyes

Complete absence of reflexes

NB Brain death requires the testing of cerebral reflexes by 2 doctors on 2 occasions spaced over an interval of 24 hours if the victim has been supported by intubation and intermittent positive pressure ventilation, i.e., a life-support system.

Procedure

Once the death has been confirmed, a senior member of nursing staff with a colleague will ensure absolute privacy for the deceased while they:

1. **Identify** the corpse by accurately written labels which are secured to the clothing.
2. **Tidy** the body only, which requires the limbs and skull to be placed in correct alignment, clearing away any blood or other debris, and adjusting the clothing.
3. **Check** the property of the corpse, not only clothing but any articles found within the pockets, and jewellery attached to the victim. In the absence of relatives the property is listed and valuables (not clothing) are then secured within an envelope and, with a copy of the list, handed over to the hospital administrator for safe keeping until collected by the next-of-kin.

If there is a *police interest*, they would normally direct their enquiries to the casualty officer who has confirmed the diagnosis of death.

The deceased is then conveyed to the city mortuary for temporary internment until arrangements are made by the next-of-kin, unless a postmortem has been requested in those cases where suspicious circumstances surround the cause of death.

Informing Next-of-kin

If the death occurs within the department, it usually falls to a senior nurse to advise the next-of-kin or relative. If they are actually present in the department the relative should be taken to a quiet area, preferably a private room, and offered a warm drink.

Prior to imparting such sad news the nurse should have as many details as possible of not only the cause of death but the circumstances leading to the death and the treatment given. When imparting the knowledge it is best to be seated with eye-to-eye contact with the relative. Speaking quietly and using the simplest terms and without any evasiveness the news should be given.

The reaction of relatives is so varied that no one can give practical advice on what emotional response the nurse will have to deal with. By far the best thing to do is wait for a few minutes and listen respectfully for the first verbal response which may cue the nurse as to the best way to proceed. Many relatives do not demonstrate any shocked response, the very fact that they are in a hospital has implications of the worst of possible connotations for most people.

It is a matter of personal and professional judgement as to when to ask for the telephone numbers of other relatives or friends who would be most supportive at such an emotional time. Certainly, no relative should be allowed to leave the department on his or her own to go home to an empty house, if at all tearful or emotionally distressed.

Counselling

The relative will need advice on the following points before leaving the department:

1. From whom to collect the signed death certificate. Usually this is ready the following morning and is collected from the administrator's office.
2. The method by which the deceased will be released from the mortuary to a resting chapel. This is often organised by the relatives responsible for nominating an undertaker.
3. Whether the medical officer signing the death certificate requires a postmortem.

As a final gesture the relative should be escorted to waiting transport and not left to find his or her own way from the department.

MAJOR DISASTER

The larger accident and emergency unit will have written policy and definite procedure which will anticipate the needs of a major disaster. Such calamities as motorway pile-ups, air crashes, mining accidents, terrorist activities or serious fire usually include multiple victims with an undetermined degree of single or multiple injuries.

The 'Flying Squad'

The initial hospital reaction will be to despatch a team of doctors and nurses to the site of the disaster to render immediate first aid treatment, i.e., the Flying Squad. Normally only fully qualified nurses would be part of this team. From their reports, usually by radio link, the department will organise itself to receive the injured victims. Where multiple victims are involved the co-ordination between the police, ambulance services, and fire brigade and the hospital is a vital component of quick and effective evacuation from the scene of disaster to hospital.

Priorities

A first priority is that the accident and emergency unit be cleared of all non-urgent patients who are either rerouted to other outpatient departments or to a designated area or ward within the hospital, if not actually sent home or referred to their own general practitioner.

Every square metre of **space** will be needed and this may necessitate all corridors, annexes and cubicles being cleared to give enough floor space for several teams of doctors to work and deal with the critically injured.

Resuscitation **equipment**, drug stocks, intravenous therapy, blood transfusion (Group O) and immobilisation splinting will all be required. Someone should be nominated for the task of preparing to increase these stocks and check that they are available and to hand.

From a **standby list**, the staff in the department is immediately increased by the telephonist who will call on duty senior nurses, doctors, anaesthetists, surgeons, pathology department and X-ray technicians. Often the appeal is made to hospital personnel to come on duty over the local radio as well as by personal contact.

Designated Areas and Teams

An area of the department is nominated to receive shocked patients while other areas are earmarked for the various categories of injuries. These are usually classified as being:

- Shocked only
- Injured but walking
- Injured but stretcher-dependent
- Critically wounded (multiple injury)
- Dead

Each area of the department has its own team of doctors and nurses to deal with the specific category of patient. Further teams within the hospital will have received advance warning of a major disaster and these should include:

- Emergency operating department
- Intensive care unit
- Emergency admission ward
- Blood transfusion service
- Pharmacy
- X-ray department
- Designated ward area for admissions

The hospital administrator would, if the need were there, establish an **incidents room** to collate the names and locations of the injured as they are admitted to the various units in the hospital after treatment. The value of such a room is that relatives can be kept constantly aware of information as it becomes available. This leaves the other telephone lines of the hospital free to conduct its normal communication system. The same room can also be used to collate information from the site of the accident and to advise the senior medical staff of what exactly is to be expected. The best that one can plan in fact is to give a staged response as the disaster unfolds itself.

At the Disaster Site

Rescue teams going to the site of a disaster will have the basic equipment to sustain life until the victim reaches more advanced medical aid. The **5 golden rules** which will act as the guiding principles for treating the injured at the site are:

1. Regardless of the injury sustained, maintain and protect a patent airway.
2. Control obvious haemorrhage.
3. Minimise shock reaction by dealing with pain and establishing intravenous therapy.

4. Transport the most critically ill first from the scene.

5. Conserve ambulance transport for those who really need it, and use other transport for the shocked victims.

These same principles will guide any nurse at the site of even a minor accident, and if working alone or on escort duties when transferring a critically injured patient to another hospital.

Chapter 53
Code of Conduct in Theatre Practice

On commencing a secondment to the operating department for the relevant period of training the learner nurse may be issued with a pamphlet outlining local policy and expressing a code of conduct which will help the nurse to meet the aims and objectives of the department. Regardless of whether the experience gained is in a large general hospital with every surgical speciality or within the theatre unit of a small hospital, certain fundamental principles remain similar. The nurse will have to respect the team approach dealing with those aspects of care revolving around medicolegal requirements; theatre dress, and hazards such as those from static electricity, radioactive materials, anaesthetic gases, drugs, infected materials, and sharp objects. Depending on the type of surgery (see Table 53.1), local policy may adapt slightly from theatre to theatre requiring a flexible approach, however the principles outlined here apply to all general surgery.

MEDICOLEGAL ASPECTS

The law demands that professional standards are equitable with professional qualifications. Possessing or pursuing a professional qualification implies a *responsibility* and a *conduct* which precludes negligence, and effectively ensures the highest possible integrity and standard of care towards patients admitted to theatre for a surgical procedure requiring a general anaesthetic. Any policy or procedure should therefore be followed to safeguard the patient's safety, and learners in particular

Table 53.1. Common operations

Operation	Procedure
General surgery	
Abdominal perineal resection	Excision of the rectum via both the abdomen and perineum
Appendicectomy	Excision of the appendix
Cholecystectomy	Excision of the gall bladder
Choledochotomy	Opening into the common bile duct
Cholejejunostomy	Anastomosis of the gall bladder to the jejunum
Gastrectomy	Partial or total removal of the stomach
Gastroenterostomy	Anastomosis between the stomach and small intestine
Herniorrhaphy	Repair of a hernia
Laparotomy	Opening into and exploration of the abdomen
Ramstedt's operation	Opening of and dilation of the pylorus
Splenectomy	Removal of the spleen
Thyroidectomy	Total or partial removal of the thyroid gland
Vagotomy and pyloroplasty	Dissecting the gastric branch of the vagus nerve and reconstruction of the pylorus
Orthopaedic surgery	
Arthrodesis	Fusion of structure within a joint
Arthroplasty	Repair or reconstruction of a joint
Arthrotomy	Opening into a joint
Laminectomy	Excising the process/lamina off the vertebral column
Meniscectomy	Excision of cartilage from the knee joint
Open reduction	Realignment of fractured bone ends after surgical exposure
Osteotomy	Division of bone to correct a deformity
Tendon repair	Suturing a ruptured tendon
Gynaecological surgery	
Caesarian section	Removal of the fetus from the uterus via an abdominal incision
Colporrhaphy	Constructive surgery to repair the anterior or posterior vaginal wall following a rectocele or cystocele
Dilation and Curettage	Dilation of and scraping of the inner wall of the uterus
Hysterectomy	Partial, total, or radical excision of the female internal reproductive organs
Laparoscopy	Endoscopic examination of the uterine (Fallopian) tubes
Oophorectomy	Excision of one or both ovaries
Salpingectomy	Excision of one or both uterine tubes
Vulvectomy	Excision of the vaginal vulva
Vascular surgery	
Embolectomy	Removal of an embolus from a vein or artery, (Trendelenburg's operation)
Endarterectomy	Excision of atheroma plaque from the arterial intima
Resection of aneurysm	Excision of the bulging portion of the aneurysm and its replacement with a graft
Ligation of varicosities	Tying off the veins affected by, e.g., haemorrhoids or varicose veins
Valvotomy	Opening of a valve, as in mitral stenosis
Neurosurgery	
Chordotomy	Division of anterolateral nerve columns within the spinal cord
Craniotomy	Opening of the skull to reach the brain tissue
Leucotomy	Division of the white fibres in the frontal lobe of the brain
Rhizotomy	Division of a nerve root
Sympathectomy	Excision of a part of the nerve chain parallel to the vertebral column

Table 53.1 (*continued*)

Operation	Procedure
Trephining	Excision of a disc of bone from the skull to reach the brain tissue
Ophthalmic surgery	
Cataract operation	Excision of the lens of an eye
Corneal grafting	Transplanting of a donor cornea
Enucleation	Removal of an eye
Iridectomy	Removal of a section of the iris preliminary to a cataract operation
Tarsorrhaphy	Suturing the eyelids together to protect the eye, e.g., in fifth cranial nerve damage
Urological surgery	
Circumcision	Excision of excess foreskin
Cystectomy	Excision of the urinary bladder
Cystoscopy	Endoscopic examination of the urinary bladder
Cystostomy	Creating an opening into the urinary bladder
Epididymidectomy	Excision of the epididymis
Nephrectomy	Partial or total removal of the kidney
Orchidectomy	Excision of one or both testes
Prostatectomy	Excision of the prostate gland
Urethrotomy	Opening of the ureter to remove a renal stone
Ear, nose and throat surgery	
Adenoidectomy	Curetting and removing the adenoids
Antrostomy	An opening into the maxillary sinus, usually through the upper palate, e.g. Caldwell Luc's operation
Laryngoscopy	Endoscopic examination of the larynx
Laryngectomy	Excision of the larynx; includes the vocal cords
Mastoidectomy	Excision of diseased bone above and behind the ear
Myringotomy	Incision into the tympanic membrane to drain the middle ear
Polypectomy	Excision of benign small tumours from the nasal cavity
Stapedectomy	Excision of the stapes bone from the middle ear
Submucous resection	Excision of bone which is causing nasal septal deflection
Tracheostomy	Creating an opening into the trachea
Tonsillectomy	Excision of the tonsil structures
Thoracic surgery	
Bronchoscopy and oesophagoscopy	Endoscopic examination of the bronchus and oesophagus
Lobectomy	Excision of one lobe of a lung
Pneumonectomy	Excision of a lung
Thoracotomy	Incision into the chest wall to create an opening
Plastic surgery	
Skin graft	Split, whole, or pedicle grafts taken from a donor site to an injured skin area
Cleft lip and palate	Closure of an opening of either the lip or upper palate, usually combined with reconstructive surgery
Rhinoplasty	Reconstruction of the nasal septum

should *ask* if they are in any doubt about their responsibility.

Written Consent

Written consent, as opposed to verbal or implied consent, for elective surgery is obtained by the surgeon only:

after the operation has been explained to the patient by the surgeon

before any premedication has been administered

after ensuring there are no extraneous influences, such as drugs or alcohol, which would impair the patient's understanding

after ensuring no duress had been exerted by hospital staff to have the operation

that psychiatric illness had been excluded from influencing the patient's consent

Should a theatre nurse knowingly allow anaesthesia to be given, or surgery to commence, when the consent form has **not** been signed by the patient, she or he is guilty of professional misconduct, in the legal sense of the term 'misconduct'. The only exception to this would be in the event of emergency surgery when the patient cannot give his or her consent, or when the immediate next of kin are not available. The chief surgeon would then act as 'locus parentis'.

Identification

Patient on Leaving the Ward

For identification purposes, on leaving the ward the patient's wristband, case notes and X-rays are checked. They are checked again on the patient's reception in theatre before anaesthesia is administered and immediately before surgery begins.

Operation Site

Only the surgeon may mark the skin of the operation site with indelible ink or pencil, and the proposed operation should be written in full in the case notes and on the consent form. Abbreviations are **not** acceptable. For example, the words *left* and *right* should be used **not** L or R.

The fingers for surgery should be clearly identified indicating if it is the thumb, index, middle, ring, or little, finger. Surgery of the toes uses the number system: big, second, third, fourth and small. The written statements on the consent form and case notes should agree with the typed operation list. If not, it must be questioned with the surgeon before surgery begins.

Operation Lists

Two statements from the Joint Memorandum of the Medical Defence Union and the Royal College of Nurses (1978) underpin the importance of following the procedure of identification.

1. Mistakes may occur when changes are made in theatre lists after the start of the operating session, particularly if such changes have not been notified to all concerned immediately they have been made. Operation lists should be altered as little as possible and never by telephone.

2. The operation list should be typed and photocopied and should show the nature of the operation, the patient's full name and hospital number. A copy of the operating list should be displayed in the anaesthetic room, the operating theatre, and postoperative recovery room. The list should also be sent to all wards in which patients are awaiting operation and displayed in all places where the patient is to undergo operation.

Operation Register

An operation register is maintained and contains the full details of each operation, indicating the full names of the patient, the operation, the time of surgery, the names of the surgeon and his or her team, the anaesthetist and the scrub nurse. The register is retained for several years in the department, not only for statistical purposes but also if there is litigation at any future date by a claimant.

Theatre Dress

A light cotton dress or trouser suit with very short sleeves and preferably without pockets, freshly laundered and comfortably fitting at the waist without the need for belts is recommended for theatre nurses. It is preferred if the hair is kept short, because theatre can become very hot during an operation. Certainly for hygienic reasons during surgery the hair must be completely sealed beneath the theatre cap.

Court shoes with leather or rubber heels and soles have antistatic properties and are essential for theatre. Manmade shoe fabrics should not be worn in theatre, or, if they are, should be covered by cotton overshoes. During surgery it may be recommended that the nurse change footwear to antistatic rubber boots, or clogs; this will depend on local policy.

Jewellery is **not** to be worn in theatre. This is partly for the patient's safety; he or she should not come into contact with any type of metal and this includes all forms of jewellery. Jewellery also carries a proven infection risk.

Cosmetics can be worn in moderation but, bearing in mind the humidity of an operating theatre, it is preferable to keep them to the minimum. Nail varnish, however, should **not** be worn. The fingernails should be trimmed quite short and to the shape of the finger tip.

Static Electricity

Everyone builds up some degree of static electricity in clothing and the hair, the best example of this being the friction of wool and cotton being rubbed over each other. If there is a great deal of static electricity it may disperse as a spark. In areas such as an operating theatre where there are flammable anaesthetic gases and other agents it is obvious that there is a **risk** of explosion and fire. This potential hazard is almost excluded if the following antistatic measures are observed:

1. Apparatus such as trollies and theatre tables are earthed; this is done by attaching a wire from the apparatus which trails to the floor.
2. Antistatic shoes are worn at all times in the theatre.
3. Trolley wheels, operating table mattresses and anaesthetic tubing are composed of conductive rubber and are coded in black and yellow colours to identify that they are antistatic.
4. Antistatic rubber flooring, wherever possible.
5. Overgarments, theatre dress, etc., are made of cotton; woollen blankets should **not** be used in theatre.
6. The humidity of the theatre during surgery should be between 50 and 60%.
7. Alcohol or spirit lotions should be stored in a separate area away from the main operation area, **not** in the operating theatre suite.
8. Aerosol sprays should **not** be used or stored in theatre.
9. All electrical appliances within the theatre should be regularly tested so that they comply with the safety regulations.
10. Electrical apparatus should be positioned at least 137 cm above floor level, and switches should be explosive proof.

Radioactive Materials

The rules relating to the handling of radioactive materials in the theatre are very strict. Radioactive materials such as caesium, radium needles, and radon seeds are delivered to the operating department in sealed lead containers. Both the radioactive material and the containers should be manipulated with rubber protected handles of extra long forceps. The lead containers are placed on a special trolley which can be shielded by a portable lead screen, being positioned to protect the person manipulating the radioactive material. The exposure time and the proximity to the radioactive materials should be as short as possible.

A qualified nurse should carry out the checks required on the containers, the number of needles used, the number of threads attached, or the type of applicator used to contain the caesium. These details are entered on the radiotherapy treatment chart together with the time of insertion and the time due for removal before the card is returned to the patient's ward. As soon as possible the lead containers should be returned to the radioactive safe, normally located in the medical physics laboratory.

Anaesthetic Gases and Drugs

The storage, supply, prescription and administration of drugs in the theatre and anaesthetic room are subject to the Control of Drugs Act, and the Poison's and Schedules Act. A major difference between these two Acts is that the prescription is usually written on the patient's anaesthetic sheet rather than on the drug chart.

Hazards

The major hazard relating to anaesthetic gases is that many of them are either combustible or flammable, and antistatic measures in the anaesthetic room need to be just as vigorous as in the operating theatre.

A second hazard is that the connections between the anaesthetic cylinders and the delivery masks require to be double-checked every day. However, this is the responsibility of the anaesthetist and this duty should not be delegated to anyone else.

Spirit-based lotions and other alcohol solutions should not be stored in the anaesthetic room.

Nurses who are in the early stages of pregnancy, i.e., up to 12 weeks, should inform their theatre sister, nursing officer or clinical teacher so that they may be advised on the risks to the fetus from anaesthetic gases. Where there is a *scavenging* system to collect anaesthetic gases from the atmosphere in the theatre there is little risk to the fetus, however not all theatres have this system installed.

In addition to knowing the precise location of drug and lotion cupboards within the theatre precinct, the nurse should also learn the international colour coding for medical gases.

Specimens and Infected Materials

Tissue specimens are usually passed to the circulating nurse for immediately **sealing** into a specimen jar containing either formalin or alcohol. Once sealed the jar requires to be correctly **labelled** with the name of the patient and the date and be accompanied by a *pathology request form* stating the medical details and the requested pathology examination.

Following surgery both the specimen and request forms are despatched to the pathology department. Frozen section biopsy is normally done in a small sideroom, within the theatre, equipped for this purpose and the circulating nurse acts as the courier between the theatre and the pathologist.

Infected tissues or amputated tissues are sealed in waterproof nonopaque plastic wrapping and despatched for incineration by a separate route to that normally used for rubbish.

Sharp Objects

Sharp objects including needles, scissors, blades and broken ampoule glass (usually simply called *sharps*), all represent hazards not only to those in the theatre but also to hospital personnel who have to handle the postoperative debris. These will include porters removing rubbish, and the laundry workers. It is imperative that items which can lacerate, cut, or which in any way represent a hazard, are disposed of correctly. A Sharps disposal bin is located in both the anaesthetic room and the disposal room for this purpose, and the scrub nurse has a special responsibility to ensure that the correct counting and disposal procedure is pursued.

Many of the foregoing principles come within the remit of the Health and Safety at Work Act 1974, and it is to meet this requirement that operating departments have and adhere to strict and formalised procedures to ensure the safety of both the patient and theatre personnel.

Chapter 54
Assisting the Anaesthetist

Prior to the operating list commencing, the nurse ensures that the anaesthetic room has been damp-dusted. The equipment and working surfaces should be wiped clean with a damp disposable duster that has been soaked in an approved disinfectant, e.g., 1 % phenolic solution (i.e., Stericol).

EQUIPMENT

The standard equipment used for general anaesthesia is prepared and checked. If any item is faulty, this fact **must** be reported to a senior colleague so that it can be replaced immediately or, if necessary, inspected and repaired before the first patient arrives.

Basic Equipment

Basic equipment for general anaesthesia usually includes:

1. Tourniquets for temporarily obliterating the venous arm flow before venepuncture.
2. Laryngoscope, with the bulb checked. This is used to guide the endotracheal tube through the vocal cords into the trachea.
3. A variety of different sized endotracheal tubes with operational and correct connections. Following intubation, this tube will be connected to the anaesthetic machine.
4. The suction machine, connecting tubing and suction catheters are checked. If the suction is fitted to the wall, this is also checked and the suction jars should be

partially filled with an approved antiseptic solution, e.g., Phenol.

5. Intravenous needles, syringes, wool swabs or sterets should be arranged in size order on a clean working surface. A Sharps disposable container should be close to hand and available for wasted needles.

6. A variety of airways and anaesthetic/oxygen face masks should be neatly arranged on a tray and positioned near to the anaesthetic machine.

7. The gauges of each cylinder on the anaesthetic machine should be checked for the residual volume of gas remaining in each cylinder, and each connection checked that it is freely moveable.

The ultimate responsibility for the anaesthetic machine and wall mounted anaesthetic gases is that of the anaesthetist and before commencing the anaesthesia for each patient he or she is responsible for checking the machine.

Specialist Equipment

Specialist equipment, if required, will depend on the operation list and the experienced nurse will know that specialist surgery requires specialist anaesthetic techniques. A copy of the operation list **must** be posted on the anaesthetic room for the checking of the patient's identity.

Drugs

The anaesthetist uses a wide variety of muscle relaxant drugs and these would be available but **not drawn up** except in the presence of the anaesthetist who is responsible for checking the drug prescribed before it is actually administered. The keys to the controlled drugs and scheduled drugs cupboard and the drug refrigerator are held by the registered nurse in charge of the theatre for the operating session.

PATIENT CARE

When receiving a patient into the anaesthetic room the nurse must remember that this may be a new experience for the patient and therefore very frightening. The two important forms of reassurance that will ease the patient's anxiety are firstly to greet the patient by his or her name, and secondly to give an assurance that until recovery from the anaesthetic he or she **will not be left alone at any time.**

The majority of patients are quiet and may seem unresponsive, but this is due to the effects of premedication which disguises the true feelings of fear that the patient is actually experiencing. A calm friendly manner and holding the patient by the hand will do much to diminish anxiety, and make the individual feel safe.

Preanaesthetic Check

The anaesthetist and nurse will conduct a series of checks **before** the administration of anaesthesia:

1. If possible obtain a verbal response from the patient to reconfirm his or her personal identity. For this reason, hearing aids are often left in until either the transfer area or anaesthetic room.

2. Check the name written on the wrist identity band and confirm that the name stated correlates with that on the operation list, the case notes and the verbal response.

3. Check that the consent form to surgery has been signed by the patient and witnessed by a doctor.

4. Check that the operation site, if marked with indelible skin pencil, corresponds to the operation listed and that indicated on the consent form.

5. Jewellery, except for a wedding ring (which must be taped over), must not be worn by the patient. Facial make-up, if worn, must be cleansed off and a last check made to ensure that dentures or dental plates have been removed.

6. Note is made of any known allergies and current medications such as insulin, steroids, or monamine oxidase inhibitors are brought to the attention of the anaesthetist.

7. If blood has been ordered, the form

denoting the group and cross-matching should be with the case notes and such blood should be available for collection from the blood bank.

8. If requested to do so, the pulse and blood pressure are taken and charted. This reading may be used as a base line and to guide the further readings given during surgery.

Procedure

The anaesthetic machine and venepuncture equipment should not be in the direct visual line of the patient so that the anaesthetist's preparations of the drugs and masks do not add any further anxiety to the patient.

When the tourniquet is applied to the upper arm and tightened, the needling of a prominent vein normally selected from the dorsal surface of the hand is usually quick and uneventful. The nurse times the release of the tourniquet with the commencement of the drug being injected. Usually the patient is asked to count from 1 to 20 and as the drug takes its effect of quickly relaxing the voluntary muscles and inducing the first stage of anaesthesia, the nurse should retain a hold on the patient's hand.

During this procedure, a quiet calm atmosphere is essential; hearing is acute and is one of the last senses to recede under the effect of anaesthesia, therefore loud speech or noise will only cause the patient to resist the anaesthesia and make them restless. It is usual for the intravenous needle to be secured to the vein site for further use during the time of anaesthesia.

Once the patient is in a fully relaxed state the anaesthetist will work quickly to establish control over the patient's airway by passing an endotracheal tube into the trachea. This tube is held in place once the cuff balloon is inflated. The connection piece of the tube is then attached and taped to the anaesthetic machine. The appropriate anaesthetic gases, which will maintain respiration and anaesthesia, are controlled by the anaesthetist.

A diathermy plate is now secured to the patient's thigh, this apparatus being the ineffective electrode to the diathermy machine used to seal off small haemorrhaging blood vessels during surgery. When transferring the patient from the anaesthetic room to the operating room, several people are required to guide not only the patient's trolley but also the anaesthetic machine and any other item of equipment attached to the patient.

A 4-person lift is used generally to transfer the patient from anaesthetic trolley to the theatre table if stretcher poles are not used. The nurse assigned to the anaesthetist should remain with him or her and follow any instructions given during the anaesthetic period. On the conclusion of surgery the anaesthetic nurse will help transfer the patient to the care of the recovery nurse.

Chapter 55
Theatre Nurses

THE CIRCULATING NURSE

The circulating nurse is directly responsible to the scrub nurse during the course of an operation. The main defined area of activity is concerned with what can only be described as the *unsterile circuit*, because it is outside the sterile circuit.

Duties

Prior to surgery the circulating nurse will check both the suction and diathermy machines, and ensure that they are pre-tested by having plugged them into the electric mains socket. To be an effective team member the circulating nurse should know the principles of diathermy.

Diathermy

Diathermy is a means of sealing blood vessels with a low frequency electrical discharge, but can also be used for cutting (*cauterising*) tissue if a high frequency electrical discharge is used. The electrical circuit is obtained by an *active* electrode which the surgeon uses within the operating site, and an *indifferent* electrode which is an aluminium foil plate, also known as the diathermy pad. This pad would normally be applied to the patient's thigh following anaesthesia either in the anaesthesia room or in the operating theatre.

Both electrodes are plugged into the diathermy machine which regulates the desired frequency. In turn this machine is plugged into the electrical mains. The surgeon controls

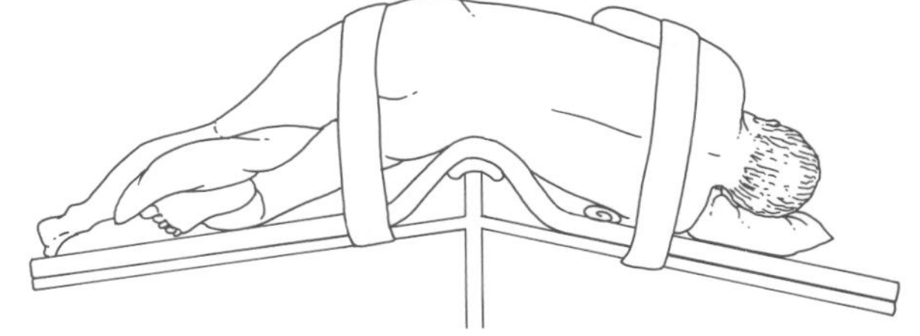

Fig. 55.1 Kidney operation position.

the active electrode by means of a foot pedal located at his or her feet. The leads from both electrodes and the foot pedal should be of sufficient length so that no pull or strain will threaten any of the connections.

The coagulation point and cutting dials are presterilised and attached to the active electrode by the scrub nurse immediately before surgery. If metal is touching the patient at any point on the body surface, the electrical current will bypass the diathermy machine and travel a direct course to the earth via the operating table. In doing so the point of contact between metal and body surface will be burned. Hence, the patient's position on the operating table **must** be safe not only from pressure on blood vessels and nerves but also from contact with a metal surface.

Positioning the Patient

The main positions into which the patient can be placed for particular general operations are outlined in Figures 55.1 and 55.2. While the nurse is not responsible for the ultimate position requested by the surgeon, it may be required of the circulating nurse to adjust the position of the operating table during the course of surgery. A sound knowledge of the mechanisms of the operating table is required of everyone in the team, but since it is a duty in the unsterile circuit the circulating nurse usually performs this task.

The Operating Table

The operating table can be adjusted in both height and length. It is divided into 3 sections: the *head* and *lower* sections can be either tilted upwards and downwards or if necessary removed; the *middle* section can be raised to elevate the lumbar spine. Many attachments can be added to the table's main framework and these include head and arm extensions, chest or hip supports, lithotomy poles, X-ray plates and cine camera, anaesthetic screen and a sectioned mattress.

The main position of the table is secured by a locking device, which on release allows for easy moving of the table for floor-cleaning purposes. It is strongly recommended that the nurse should practise putting these attachments in place, and develop a thorough grounding in the location of the tilt mechanisms, releasing pins and other fine adjustments so that there is no hesitation in helping during the operation. Again, this is regarded as an unsterile circuit duty.

Lighting

The nurse should also be familiar with the overhead lighting and whether it has satellite attachments. The tilt and angle of these lights give a most accurate focus onto the operating site, which may change as the operation proceeds when quick and fine movements are necessary to comply with the immediate request for a better focus.

Gowning

Apart from assisting the scrub nurse to gown, all other sterile personnel will require this assistance after they have scrubbed up. This help usually involves opening the outer wrapping of the sterile gown and glove packs. In handling the tapes only, the circulating nurse can help the sterile personnel manoeuvre their arms and body into the

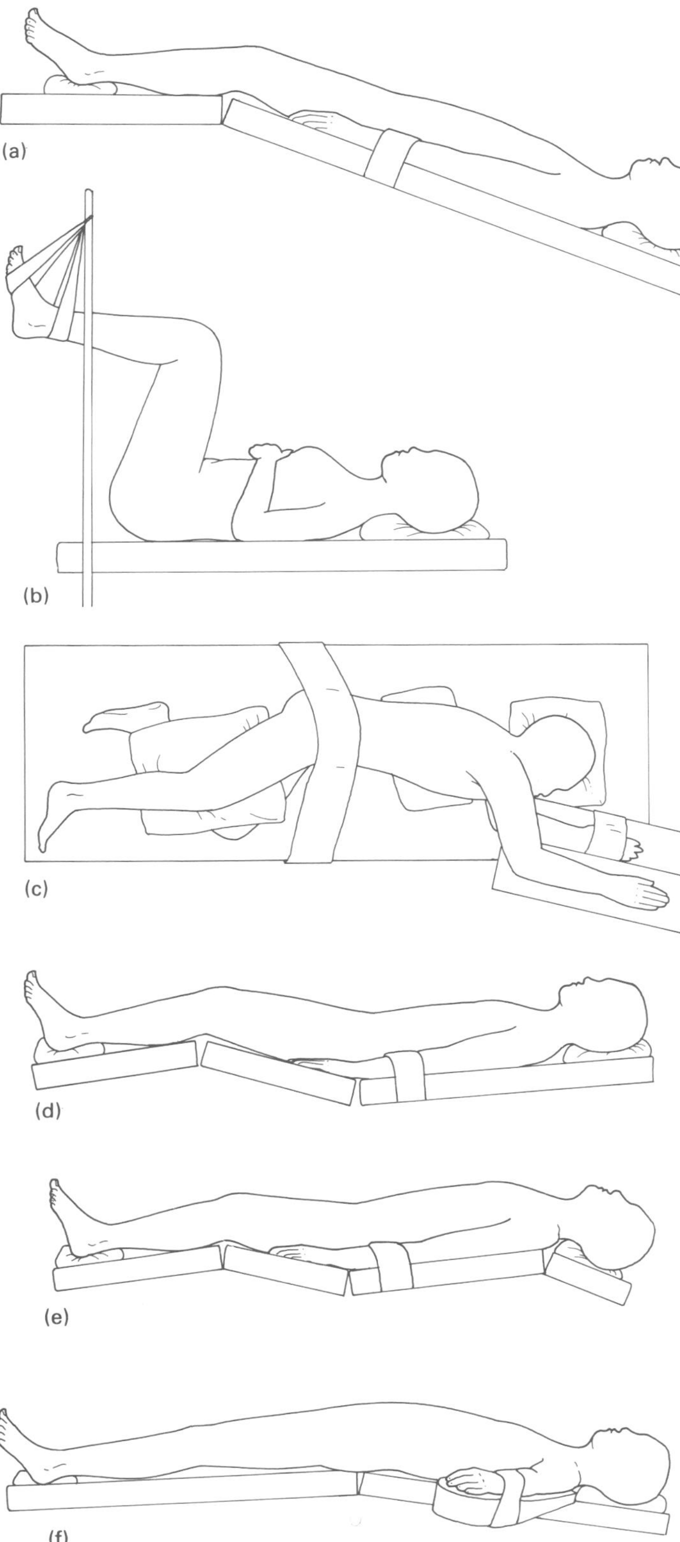

Fig. 55.2 Positions for general surgery: Trendelenburg position for pelvic surgery (a); lithotomy position for gynaecological and rectal surgery (b); lateral position for thoracic surgery (c); supine position for cholecystectomy (d); supine position with neck extension for thyroidectomy (e); supine position for laparotomy/abdominal surgery (f).

gown and, without touching the outer surface of the gown, tie the tapes at the back and those around the waist.

Equipment

When the scrub nurse is preparing the trolley and Mayo table, the circulating nurse should be available to open all the outer wrappings of the presterilised surgical packs. Once the preparations are complete, both the scrub and circulating nurse check together the following items:

Instrument count, usually in set numbers

Swabs, normally in packs of 5 with each swab having a radiopaque band, are counted. The ties holding the swabs together are also retained

Abdominal packs are counted

Needles are counted

In some theatres it is routine practice to chalk up these 'counts' on a board or swab rack so that the final tally at the end of the operation can be counterchecked.

Other Tasks

During surgery the circulating nurse will have many small but important tasks to carry out to help in the smooth running of the operation. These tasks should be performed quietly and without ever contaminating the *sterile circuit*. Such tasks include acting as messenger for the scrub nurse, e.g., fetching additional packs, correct positioning of the diathermy foot pedal, attaching the diathermy leads, adjusting the overhead lights at frequent intervals, mopping the surgeon's forehead to clean away perspiration, if necessary cleaning the spectacles of any team member who is sterile, and labelling specimen jars ready for despatch to pathology.

At the conclusion of surgery, the surgeon will pause when the scrub and circulating nurses make a final check on the number of used and unused swabs, packs, instruments and needles. It is the duty of the scrub nurse to insist on a double-check if the numbers do not tally, and the duty of the surgeon to make the final decision on whether to close the wound. On the completion of surgery, and discontinuation of anaesthesia, the nurse will then make final adjustments to the patient's position and clothing in preparation for a 4-person lift from the operating table to the recovery trolley, and then escorting the patient to the care of the recovery nurse.

The theatre will then have to be cleared and cleansed in preparation for the next operation. Many of these duties are the remit of the circulating nurse.

THE SCRUB NURSE

The scrub nurse is directly responsible to the surgeon during the course of an operation and for the discipline of personnel in the theatre other than the surgeon's team.

Duties

The conduct of procedures which maintain sterility at the operating table is the main duty of the scrub nurse, in addition to anticipating the particular requirements of a specific surgeon. Working repeatedly with the pre-set sterile trays and trollies is the only method of mastering the unique skill of knowing the names and purpose of each type of surgical instrument.

Theatre Layout

Prior to surgery the nurse should check the layout of the theatre (Table 55.1), ensuring that the equipment within the operating room is minimal and what is there is actually needed

Table 55.1. Basic theatre layout

Adjustable operating table
Adjustable overhead light with satellite attachments
Mayo table, instrument tray set for surgeon's use
Basin stand containing sterile water for used instruments
Diathermy machine
Suction machine
X-ray viewing screen
Swab rack
Adjustable stool for anaesthetist

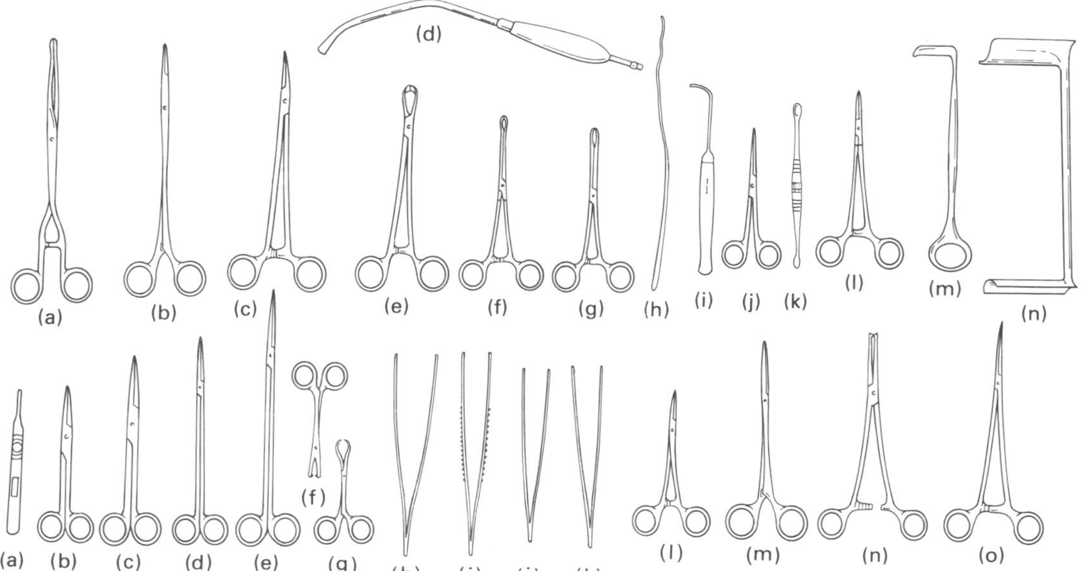

Fig. 55.3 'Major General Set'

Top

(a) Sponge holder
(b) Roberts artery forceps
(c) Moynighan artery forceps
(d) Lanes tissue forceps
(e) Babcock tissue forceps
(f) Allis tissue forceps
(g) Probe
(h) Aneurysm needle
(i) Sims forceps
(j) Volkmans spoon
(k) Mayo's needle holder
(l) Langenbeck retractor
(m) Morris retractor (double ended)
(n) Pharyngeal sucker

(a) Bard Parker handle
(b) Mayo's curved scissors
(c) Mayo's straight scissors
(d) McIndoes dissecting scissors
(e) Nelsons dissecting scissors
(f) Towel clips
(g) Towel clips
(h) Toothed dissecting forceps
(i) Non-toothed dissecting forceps
(j) Gillies dissecting forceps
(k) McIndoes dissecting forceps
(l) Dunhill artery forceps
(m) Spencer Wells artery forceps
(n) Oschner artery forceps
(o) Lehey artery forceps

for the particular operation. Unnecessary equipment is undesirable. The temperature of the operating room should be between 20° and 22 °C, while the humidity should register between 50 and 60%. Most theatres have an air extraction system and an anaesthetic scavenging air system which should both be functioning during the course of an operation. The cleanliness of the theatre should be checked at the beginning of each operation session, the ledges and fittings being damp-dusted to remove all dust.

Instruments

Many operating departments have operation cards which identify the required instruments for any type of operation (Fig. 55.3). These cards also have the surgeon's specific needs listed for the guidance of the scrub nurse (Table 55.2). They are very useful in that they will help the scrub nurse plan the layout of the instrument trolley and forewarn the nurse of any special points to anticipate at certain times in an operation. It is useful to know before planning the layout of instrument trolley and Mayo table if the surgeon is

Table 55.2.

Amputation	Partial gastrectomy	Colectomy
General set and amputation pack, i.e., Medium bone cutter Medium bone nibbler Sequestrum forceps Rasp Amputation saw Amputation knife Blake's amputation guard	General set plus 5 Spencer Well's artery forceps 5 Oschner artery forceps Retractor pack Intestinal pack Pozzi's retractor	General set plus Retractor pack Intestinal pack 2 Einsell Foss Clam Appendicectomy General set plus Dennis Browne dissecting forceps
Repair of Hernia	Abdominal perineal resection	
General set required for Epigastric hernia Inguinal hernia Femoral hernia Incisional Umbilical Hiatus hernia Additional instruments are toothed and nontoothed long dissecting forceps, or a thoractomy pack	General set plus St Marks retractor Retractor pack Intestinal pack Balfour self retaining retractor Naunton Morgan needle holder Toothed and nontoothed long dissecting forceps	

lefthanded or righthanded, as this will alter the ultimate position of the trollies and the theatre team working around the operating table.

Scrubbing

The term *scrub* describes the preparation to assist the surgeon: the nurse has to scrub the arms from the finger tips to the elbows with a sterile nail brush using an approved soap solution for a period of between 3 and 5 minutes, under continuously running water. The tap controlling the water flow must be operated by either the foot or the elbow to avoid contaminating the hands after they are scrubbed. After this scrubbing, especially between the fingers and the finger nails, the arms and hands are rinsed and then carefully dried on a sterile towel (this may be disposable). An alternative is to rinse the hands first and the arms second and then apply an approved antiseptic soap solution which is carefully rinsed off. Then very thoroughly dry first the hands and then the arms.

Donning Theatre Apparel

With the assistance of the circulating nurse, who opens the outer wrapping of the *gown* pack, and by handling the gown only by its inner surface, the scrub nurse is aided to manoeuvre her or his arms into the sleeves of the gown. The circulating nurse will then tie the tapes at the back of the gown.

After the *glove* pack has been opened by the circulating nurse, the scrub nurse will disperse the provided sterile powder either over the hands or into each glove, or both, depending on personal preference. The first glove is pulled on touching the inner surface only. This technique prevents the nurse touching, with a socially clean hand, a sterile surface. Scrubbing the hands and arms renders them as clean as possible, but does not make them sterile.

The gown sleeves are secured under the cuff of each glove, and after this the circulating nurse may then tie the gown tapes at waist level.

Masks may either be made of cotton, or disposable; in either case they should be

Table 55.3. Suture materials

Absorbable	Nonabsorbable
a Catgut. Plain, absorbed after 10–14 days Chromic, which is catgut treated with chromic salt solution, absorbed after 14–21 days b Polyglycolic acid. A liquidised polyester stretched and braided to form a suture. Like cutgut it is absorbable within the body and can also be used to suture skin incisions	a Silk. Silicone-treated protein fibre which has been spun by the silkworm b Cotton. Made from the vegetable material of plant seeds c Linen. Made from flax fibres which have been twisted d Human hair. Occasionally used for nerve repair e Nylon. Synthetic fibre f Dacron, terylene, polythene, polyprolene. All synthetic fibres g Stainless steel wire. For dental and orthopaedic surgery h Silver wire. Used to repair rectal prolapse i Metal clips. E.g., Michel clips to close wounds

handled by the tapes only, and when applied to the face should cover both nose and mouth. When they are removed it should be by the tapes only.

The hair is completely secured beneath the theatre *cap*. Once the scrub nurse is gowned for surgery, her or his hands should be brought forwards and clasped together at waist level, or alternatively clasped over the chest with the elbows at waist level, to avoid touching any unsterile article and also to indicate to others that sterility must now be observed.

Positioning Equipment

Instructions from the scrub nurse to the circulating nurse must be quite clear and specific as to where to position the instrument trolley, Mayo table and portable washbasins. These positions are related to the operating table and are opposite the surgeon. All outer wrapping of any theatre pack, and this includes the additional packs, suture containers and blade pack, **must** be completed by the circulating nurse.

The scrub nurse will indicate the order of opening of the packs and, as the instrument trolley and Mayo table are prepared, both nurses double-check the swab packs, abdominal packs, instruments, needles and suture materials; the total number of each is recorded either on a chalkboard or on the swab rack.

During the course of the operation, the scrub nurse should have the skill of being able to locate at any given time the whereabouts of all instruments, plus keeping a constant check on the swab numbers and abdominal packs.

The **drapes** which will surround the operation site are prepared on the instrument trolley and handed to the surgeon in the order that they should be placed over the unconscious patient, the drapes being maintained in position by towel clips.

Blades are mounted on their scalpel handles by using clip forceps. Several scalpel handles are prepared, since the first incision blade is normally discarded. With careful and concentrated observation of the progress of the operation the scrub nurse can anticipate the surgeon's requirements. Some surgeons have a preferred method of being handed the surgical instruments, e.g., curved forceps being handed curve downwards. Whichever preference is used must be respected. The nurse must, however, place each instrument, handle firmly end down, in the palm of the surgeon's hand.

Table 55.4. Suture methods

1. Anchor method. Drains and tubes leading from a cavity to the outside of the body are anchored in place by a single suture
2. Continuous suture. This is a running stitch to approximate the wound edges, with only the first and last suture being tied
3. Interrupted suture. Each stitch is tied separately and is independent
4. Ligature. A suture is used to encircle and close off a blood vessel when it is tied
5. Mounted suture. The suture is threaded into the serrated jaws of a pair of artery forceps which are beneath a blood vessel. As the forcep is withdrawn it pulls the suture through and under the vessel
6. Purse string. A continuous suture sewn around a circular opening. When both ends of the suture are pulled together it closes the opening
7. Stay suture. A pair of sutures are threaded through a structure, the ends are then pulled tautly to raise the structure so that it may be incised
8. Traction suture. The suture is inserted into a structure then pulled so that it retracts the tissue for surgery, e.g. the tongue
9. Transfixion. A suture is fixed crosswise over a vessel to prevent a ligature from falling off a tied vessel
10. Tension sutures. A strong suture material encased in either plastic or rubber sheathing which is used to close the wounds of obese patients, or those wounds liable to infection, risking burst abdomen

Suture materials should not be released from their container until actually required (Table 55.3). The coil of the material is taken around the finger, the free end is grasped with the opposite hand and held securely, while the coil of suture material is allowed to unravel of its own volition. The other free end is then taken up and either end pulled straight to release any kinks. Suitable lengths are then cut and, when handed to the surgeon, both ends are held tautly. Some surgeons prefer to thread their own needles; atraumatic sutures have the needle already attached (Table 55.4).

Conclusion and Completion Procedures

At the end of surgery, but before the wound is closed, the following checks must be made to everyone's satisfaction:

- Swab count
- Abdominal pack count
- Instrument count
- Blade count
- Needle count

The instrument trolley, Mayo table and washbasins are taken to the disposal room and the scrub nurse is usually responsible for separating the instrumentation from the linen. Blades are released from their scalpel handles by using the clip forceps in a downward releasing action but away from the body and, with nobody in the immediate vicinity, blades are disposed of in the Sharps bin.

Instruments are either cleaned by hand or placed in an especially designed washing machine and immediately after this cleaning they should be checked for any defects. Scissors may require sharpening, joints on the larger instruments may require lubrication. This should be done before they are despatched for resterilising in the theatre sterile supply unit or in the central sterile supply department.

NB The careless disposal of instruments means that some may end up in the laundry, with serious consequences to the laundry workers and often damage to the laundry machines.

THE RECOVERY NURSE

Prior to receiving patients from the operating room, the recovery nurse should check that the following equipment is available and functional:

1. Piped oxygen points, connection tubing and oxygen masks. The flowmeter of

the oxygen point should be turned on to check it is functioning properly.

2. Portable oxygen cylinders with an adequate supply of masks. The volume gauge should be checked to note the residual volume of oxygen in the cylinder. The main valve should be in the open position, but the flowmeter valve in the off position, ready for immediate use.

3. A variety of anaesthetic masks suitable for children and adults should be arranged on a tray and sited in a central area of the recovery room.

4. Suction points (wall-mounted) or a suction machine should be tested to see if it can achieve minimal and maximal pressure. The connection tubing and suction catheters should be attached and ready for immediate use. The jar which receives any material sucked from the oropharynx and mouth should have a small amount of approved antiseptic added to it.

5. A tray or trolley containing an adequate supply of intravenous cannula, giving sets and a variety of intravenous solutions should be in constant readiness. When used, the equipment should be immediately replaced, the trolley cleaned and checked each day and particularly, the expiry dates of the solutions checked daily.

6. A pre-tested laryngoscope, bronchoscope set, endotracheal tubes and a tracheostomy set are additional to the cardiac arrest trolley. All this equipment should be available, positioned centrally and clearly labelled. The drugs within the cardiac arrest trolley require immediate replacement when used, and checking daily for their expiry date.

7. The emergency bell located at each trolley bay should be tested for both sound and flash light daily, these will normally be heard and seen in various strategic areas throughout the theatre suite, especially in the anaesthetic room and in the anaesthetist's rest room.

Duties

Following surgery, the patient is transferred from the operating table to a narrow tilt-type recovery trolley. In routine cases, the patient will be positioned either on the back with the head turned to one side or semi-prone, and the airway kept patent by an artificial airway, usually of the Guedel type. **The primary duty of the recovery nurse is to maintain the patient's airway.** The recovery nurse is responsible to the anaesthetist until he or she gives permission for the patient to return to the ward.

The lumen of the airway should not be occluded with garments, linen, towels, or the pillow edging. On gradual recovery, the patient will eject the airway, but this does not mean that the patient has gained complete control of the swallowing and cough reflex. To counter the risk of the tongue falling backwards and occluding the pharynx and the lower jaw becoming slack, a gentle upward pressure of the rear portion of the lower mandible is exerted until the patient demonstrates he or she has regained reflex control. If the patient has excess saliva, or vomits and is without a reflex, the material may be inhaled into the lung and can be regarded as an airway obstruction. The immediate response to this is to:

Clear the mouth of any material

Tilt the trolley into the head down position

Insert a suction catheter into the mouth so the tip reaches the pharynx and apply suction

Press the emergency bell

Turn the patient, with the help of colleagues, onto the side, *operation permitting*

Observations

Four essential observations should be taken and recorded every 15 minutes. Any sudden or dramatic changes should be reported immediately to the anaesthetist if:

1. The respiratory rate falls below 12, or exceeds 30 per minute, and there is obvious embarrassment of the rib cage movements.

2. The pulse rate is below 50 or exceeds 90 beats per minute. If the pulse is irregular in rhythm, or has a weak

Table 55.5. Interpretation of surgical terminology

		Prefix		*Suffix*	
A or an	without or not	intra	within	desis	fusion
ante	before	poat	after	ectomy	excision
anti	against	pre	before	lysis	freeing of
dys	difficult	retro	behind	orrhaphy	repair of
ecto	outer			oscopy	examination of
endo	inner			ostomy	create an opening
hyper	above			otomy	cut into
hypo	below			plasty	restore or reconstruct
inter	between			pexy	fix into position
			Roots, or derivations		
adeno	gland	gastro	stomach	os	opening or bone
arthro	joint	haema	blood	ot	ear
blepharo	eyelid	hepato	liver	pharyng	throat
cardi	heart	hystero	uterus	phleb	vein
chole	gall	jejun	jejunum	pneumo	lung
cholecyst	gallbladder	lamin	vertebral arch	procto	rectum
col	colon	mast	breast	pyelo	pelvis of kidney
colpo	vagina	myo	muscle	rhino	nose
cranio	skull	nephro	kidney	salping	fallopian tube
cysto	urinary bladder	neuro	nerve	sphlancho	viscera (organs)
dent	tooth	oophor	ovary	teno	tendon
derma	skin	ophthalm	eye	trachel	neck of uterus
entero	intestine	orchio	testes	vas	vessel or duct

Common surgical procedures during operations	
Anastomosis	joining of two structures, e.g. gastroenterostomy
Biopsy	removal of tissue for microscopic examination
Curettage	removal of excess tissue by currette or spoon, e.g., of the uterus
Cauterization	use of electrical current to destroy or remove tissue
Diathermy	sealing of blood vessels or cutting tissues with electrical current
Dissection	separation or division of tissues and their removal
Excision	removal of an organ or of tissues
Ligation	tying off a blood vessel or a structure

pulsatile strength, either observation may indicate shock or haemorrhage.

3. Cyanotic changes of the skin, face, lips, nose or the periphery which may indicate haemorrhage in the absence of respiratory obstruction.

4. A systolic blood pressure below 90 and a diastolic pressure below 50 may imply shock.

The slightest suspicion of deterioration requires the nurse to press the emergency bell without hesitation. It is better to summon help in error and feel some temporary embarrassment, than to dither in uncertainty in the vain hope that your observation is perhaps a mistaken judgement.

Other observations for which the recovery nurse is responsible, include reporting any restless or agitated behaviour during recovery from anaesthesia. This may be due to pain which, for obvious reasons, the patient cannot verbally express. Many anaesthetists routinely prescribe analgesia to be given during the recovery period. The safety of the patient is paramount while he or she is unconscious. The limbs and body should be aligned so that no pressure is exerted on any vulnerable area, e.g., blood vessels and nerves.

Intravenous infusions are quite common following surgery and apart from securing the needling site with a short splint and bandage, the flow rate of the infusion should be monitored and controlled by the gate clip to conform with the prescribed flow rate. When blood transfusion is in progress the nurse should make observations for any allergy or reactions to a potentially mismatched blood transfusion. Wound drainage tubes, vacuum drains, wound packing and suture lines should be checked for oozing or excessive fluid loss and, if required, adjustments made for the comfort of the patient.

Urinary catheters are usually open for free continuous drainage of the bladder and the principle of closed circuit to prevent infection should be observed. The connection between catheter and tubing should be intact. The drainage tubing should be secured to the outer thigh and the collecting urine bag positioned below the level of the patient's pelvis to prevent reflux.

Returning the Patient to the Ward

After the anaesthetist has given permission for the patient to return to the ward, the recovery nurse in handing over the patient to the ward nurse, should ensure that the ward nurse understands:

The surgeon's written instructions on the care of the patient

The anaesthetist's written instructions regarding postoperative medications, e.g., analgesia and antiemetics, and the prescribed rota for intravenous therapy

The recorded observations made during the recovery period and any treatment given

Case notes, X-rays, and pathology forms should be available for return to the ward with the escorting nurse. The ward nurse should be of sufficient seniority and training to ensure that if an emergency arises during the return journey to the ward she or he would respond in a competent manner to the emergencies of respiratory obstruction, cardiac arrest and internal haemorrhage.

Chapter 56
Burns and Plastic Surgery

Apart from dealing with burns, the specialist branch of plastic surgery deals with reconstruction and remodelling of tissues damaged by trauma other than burns, i.e., congenital abnormality, disfiguring lesions and with benign or malignant tumours. Only a few topics have been selected here for the study of plastic surgery, i.e., those which lend themselves to an understanding of the underlying principles used in plastic surgery. The congenital deformity of cleft lip and palate is dealt with in some depth in the paediatric section of *Nursing 1*.

The principles of care advocated in the specialist burns units can be extrapolated and used as a guide for those occasions when a burned patient is being cared for in an acute ward of a main hospital. A major consideration is the therapeutic regimen prescribed by the surgeon and in the majority of cases this will be to nurse the patient with their burn injury *exposed*, though usually a plastic bag is used to cover the hands when burnt. A second important principle is the measures necessary to contain the risk of infection, which is always very high whenever the integrity of the skin has been breached. For the purposes of study, the care of a burned patient may be looked at in 3 distinct phases:

1. The first 36 hours for the **immediate care**.
2. The second to seventh day for **continuing care**.
3. Final stage of healing for **grafting procedures**.

PHASE ONE: IMMEDIATE CARE

Fluid Replacement

The most critical phase of therapy is the first 36 hours during which the major concern will be to replace lost body fluids. This replacement will be by intravenous therapy and should have already been commenced in the accident and emergency department, with the rota clearly stated. The rota should be written to cover either 6 or 8 defined periods of time during the first 36 hours.

The solutions prescribed can be variable, from plasma to normal saline, and the nurse must constantly check the drip counter to ensure that the prescribed rota is infusing to the prescribed time. The most minor problem arising from the infusion **must** be reported immediately to senior staff so that corrective measures can be taken immediately.

The principal reason for such a strict fluid balance monitoring is that with an excessive fluid loss from the body the viscosity of blood will increase, leading to a concentration of erythrocytes (*haemoconcentration*). As this 'thickened' blood attempts to pass through the kidney, the concentration of red cells is likely to block the renal tubules with a risk of acute renal failure. Fluid therapy, therefore, is not only replacing lost fluid on a given time basis but also trying to prevent haemoconcentration.

Assessments

During the infusion programme, the following assessments are carried out at the discretion of medical staff:

Haemoglobin level. This can be expected to fall 24 hours after the burn injury giving rise to an anaemia. It may necessitate the giving of whole blood.

Haematocrit, or packed cell volume (PCV), refers to the ratio of plasma to the erythrocytes, normally being 55% plasma and 45% red cells. With a fluid loss the plasma ratio will be reduced while the cell ratio is increased. As the infusion programme progresses this tendency should be corrected back to normal levels.

Blood urea levels. If renal function is inadequate, blood urea levels will persistently rise if the renal tubules are becoming blocked by the concentrated blood cells.

Potassium and sodium levels are bound to be imbalanced if there is a fluid loss. The blood levels of these electrolytes will guide the medical staff on the additives required for the infusion regimen to correct any imbalance.

Nursing observations

The nursing observations made during this 36-hour period are also crucial to the success of fluid therapy. These would include:

Fluid balance charts are checked each hour during the critical 36 hours.

An **output** showing at least 30 ml of urine each hour indicates that the kidney is at a basic healthy excretion rate; below this indicates renal failure. If an indwelling urinary catheter is in position, then samples can be tested every hour for:

Specific gravity, if above 1030, implies a concentrated urine with a possible danger of renal failure.

Sugar, protein and blood, which can be expected in the first few samples of urine, but if their presence persists it should be drawn to the attention of medical staff, especially a persistent haematuria.

If at all possible during this 36-hour period the patient should be encouraged to take small amounts of clear oral fluids. The surgeon will include this in the total fluid requirement. When there is difficulty, part of the therapy may be for a nasogastric tube to be passed and prescribed volumes of milk to be given every few hours.

Vital signs of blood pressure, pulse, respiration and oral temperature should be taken on a time-graduated basis; every hour for the first 6 hours then spaced at increasing intervals as they become stable. Each observation needs to be assessed on its own merits. For example, a low blood pressure accompanied by a tachycardia would indicate shock, while a pyrexia may indicate infection.

Burns to the mouth, throat, neck or face are likely to give rise to an oedema which, if near the airway, may cause an obstruction to respiration. Apart from correct positioning of the patient and a medical appreciation that this is a potential risk, the nurse should have both suction and oxygen available for use when required. Elective tracheostomy may be performed for severe burns to the face and neck.

Response to analgesia is a vital observation and the patient should be questioned as to the degree of discomfort arising out of pain. Even if the burn is deep enough to be 'anaesthetic', the surrounding tissues will be contracted into the burned area. Pethidine, while a potent analgesic, is not necessarily effective in every patient and an alternative such as morphine may prove necessary. Analgesia combined with sedation is the normal practice to control the restlessness this type of patient is likely to suffer.

Complications

The complications which should be observed for and for which investigations may be aimed at detecting during this initial period are:

Massive blood cell destruction, i.e., *haemoconcentration*, which is indicated by continuing shock despite intense treatment and an obvious haematuria

Acute renal failure usually due to necrosed distal tubules within the kidney as a result of obstruction from haemoconcentration. The blood urea level if persistently rising over a period of 24 hours is an early warning sign, indicating that peritoneal dialysis may be required

More rarely, the massive blood cell destruction may contribute to a *necrosis* of the liver, pancreas, or the gall bladder

Other Nursing Actions

For other patients admitted from the accident and emergency department with a burn injury exceeding 20% of the body surface, it is recommended they be nursed in a Clinitron-type bed. This bed consists of a 30 mm depth tank which contains silicone-type chips through which a regulated volume of air is constantly distributed. The chips are restrained in their tank by sterile sheeting on which the patient will rest.

The immediate advantage to the patient is that the constant air flow beneath the patient will speed up the drying process of the burned tissue, thus reducing loss of body fluid from the wound exudate. With the constant, but imperceptible movement of a chip mattress, the risk of pressure ulcers is also greatly reduced. For burns below 20% and not located on the back or buttocks a standard hospital bed is used.

Exposure

Exposure of the burn to the air will also speed up the drying process. Occlusive dressings are rarely used today, even when the burn is circumferential. If the burned surface becomes infected then it may prove necessary to cover the burn with an occlusive dressing, but this will be to promote sloughing of the wound. Burns near to the genitalia or buttocks will be masked for modesty reasons by sterile sheeting held away from the wound by the adroit positioning of bedcradles.

Advantages

The acknowledged advantages of the exposure method include:

It *limits* the *variability of abnormal body temperature*. Occlusive dressings, for example, would increase body temperature and may cause pyrexia. Related to this aspect of care is the need to nurse the patient in a warm dry atmosphere which is thermostatically controlled between 24° and 27 °C, and apart from aiding the drying process of the wound reduces protein catabolism with less loss of nitrogen.

Rapid drying of the burn *limits* the ultimate degree of *scar tissue* formation.

Tissue regeneration will commence from the base of the burn wound more quickly and the decision as to when to graft can be taken that much earlier, usually some time between the second and seventh day of therapy.

The crusts of dried tissue which form over the tissue are known as *eschar*. Eschar separation, i.e., the dead epithelium separates from the underlying regenerating tissue, will occur more readily if the wound is dry. The deeper the burn is, the more important it becomes to aid eschar separation since grafting will be a very necessary part of therapy. Occasionally, the eschar will have to be split by longitudinal incisions (*escharotomy*) if it is limiting respiratory movement of the rib cage due to burns of the thorax.

Risk of infection is *reduced* if the wound surface is dry, and if this principle is combined with that of reverse barrier nursing techniques, the infection risk is even further reduced.

Handling, moving, turning, or lifting the patient can be somewhat *reduced* when the wound is exposed. This is important in the early stages of care; the more handling of the patient there is, the greater the degree of shock and the more prolonged the shock remains.

Nursing observations of the wound itself are easier. Infection can be detected at an earlier stage, allowing the nurse to advise medical colleagues, and to initiate positive steps to prevent the infection from becoming worse.

Disadvantages

A major disadvantage of the exposure method is that the patient is constantly visually reminded of his or her disfigurement. It is likely that the patient's concept of his or her body image will be adversely affected, giving rise to a wide variety of emotional responses such as fear, anxiety or depression.

If the burn wound becomes infected, an occlusive dressing using eusol-soaked gauze swabs and paraffin gauze (tulle gras) is placed over the affected area and secured by a layer of gamgee and crepe bandage. This type of dressing will promote desloughing and cleanse the infected area, thus speeding up the healing from the base of the wound so that a decision about grafting can be taken.

Burns confined to the hands are another example of when the burn is not exposed. In this instance, the hands are encased in plastic gloves after the burn has been treated by an antibiotic cream, e.g., Flamazine. The plastic gloves are sealed at the wrists. Exudate and serum escaping from the wound provides a volume of trapped fluid which in fact condenses inside the bag and promotes the absorption of the applied antibiotic creams. At the same time, this gloving technique allows for some degree of movement of all the digits, an important principle for any injury to the hands.

Reverse Barrier Nursing

Any type of wound which breaches the integrity of the skin poses a major threat of infection. The reverse barrier nursing technique is employed to reduce the risk of infection from any outside source. Ideally, the isolation area or cubicle should be equipped with all the therapeutic and domestic resources to sustain the patient during the period of risk, and have the minimum of contact with other people.

Infection Risks

The risk of infection from *nursing uniforms* is considerably reduced if a plastic apron, as opposed to a cotton gown, is worn over the uniform. Cotton apparel does in fact have a permeable surface through which contamination is possible. A second major source of infection is the *nurse's hands*, which must be scrupulously washed and dried before and after each nursing procedure, and also on entering and leaving the cubicle.

A warning notice that reverse barrier nursing is being carried out should be displayed at the entrance to the cubicle and give clear instructions to all *visitors* on the precautions required before entry. In the early stages of care it is recommended that visitors to the patient be limited to the minimum. This includes relatives and medical staff. Presterilised *linen* is normally supplied either from a central supply department, if not actually sterilised within the burns unit. The disposal of used linen is via the normal laundry service.

The bacterial air count in the cubicle can be considerably reduced if it has a laminar *air flow*. Rather than circulating, the air travels in straight lines, implying that the air is changed within a 2-minute period as opposed to the normal circulating air time of 20 minutes. This difference of air time means that bacteria have less time in which to settle on to an exposed wound.

Prophylactic antibiotics, normally administered via an intravenous route, will contain some of the infection risk from within the patient as the body's natural defence mechanisms act against infection, and immunity will be low.

Wound debridement (the removal of separating eschar) is also an infection risk if the nurse does not perform this type of dressing in the strictest manner when employing the aseptic technique. Removing dead epithelium is a slow process involving the cutting away of very small pieces of tissue at a time, using a non-touch technique with fine instruments.

PHASE TWO: CONTINUING CARE

From the second to the seventh day of care the critical period should become more stable and permit the nursing staff to plan further care on a day-to-day assessment of the patient's needs.

Nutrition

From a major burn, it can be expected that there will be considerable weight loss. The nutritional requirements to promote healing and restore this weight loss are in the order of between 150% to 300% above normal values. A quick formula for estimating is the patient's weight times 25, plus the area of burn, times 40, equals the patient's daily calorific requirements. For example, if the patient weighed 65 kg and had a 25% burn, the formula would read

$$65\text{ kg} \times 25 + 25\% \times 40$$

$= 2625$ calories (11 025 joules) per day.

To calculate the amount of protein from this calorific assessment, the second formula is the patient's weight, plus 3 times the area of burn, equals the daily protein requirement in grams. From the preceding example, this would be:

$65\text{ kg} + 3 \times 25\% = 4875$ g protein per day.

If each gram of protein yields 4.1 calories, then

$$4875\text{ g} = 1190\text{ cal}$$

made up of protein.

Planning Meals

It is important to supplement the calories and protein requirements with vitamins C (ascorbic acid), B complex and A, because all are required for the regeneration and continued integrity of the epithelial cells and membranes. Apart from being high in protein with supplementary vitamins and a high fluid intake, the diet should also be of low fibre in the first few days. This low fibre is suggested because of the loss of appetite and feelings of anorexia and nausea. Small-sized meals presented 6 times a day are more beneficial than the 3-times-a-day average-sized meals.

The manipulative skills of the patient in handling crockery and cutlery should be taken into account. In the early phases of therapy, nursing assistance should be offered to the patient; his or her ultimate independence in self-care should also be promoted.

If the burn affects the lips or mucous membranes of the mouth, table salt or spices should not be added to the patient's food. If the burns are located in those areas where it is impossible for the patient to lift or turn the head, then alternative means of maintaining nutrition must be explored. This is usually that a nasogastric tube will be passed and the same calorific values are given as in a liquidised diet.

Personal Comfort

Before giving attention to any of the patient's very personal needs, the nurse assesses whether the patient can co-operate without suffering any undue pain or discomfort. Many surgeons do prescribe analgesics or sedation on an As Required basis. Such drugs should be used half an hour prior to extensive and prolonged procedures which cause either pain or exhaustion.

Adaptations to the standard procedures of bedbathing, oral toilet, hair care and pressure area care, all require reappraisal to meet the particular needs of the individual patient. Singed hair is normally cut away and long hair should be braided so that it is well out of reach of any burned skin.

Cleansing of the skin is limited to healthy skin, bearing in mind that the skin creases such as the groin, perineum and axilla are very moist and merit extra attention. Once the burn area is dry the surgeon may consent to the patient having saline baths daily. Such baths do promote eschar separation and, in addition, allow the patient to move the burn area in water without undue pain.

Mobility

In principle active movement is desirable as early as possible. To assess and plan when this can be implemented, the advice of a physiotherapist should be sought. The risks of contractures to all joints are assessed, and it may be that soft splinting rather than active physiotherapy will be recommended.

The surgeon's opinion as to the type of grafting planned also needs to be known so that particular joint movements and muscle tone exercises can be implemented. Any active physiotherapy should be considered only if the patient is pain free.

If the patient cannot sit out of bed, then the risks of pressure ulcers to prone areas of the body may be relieved by utilising the many aids which are now available. Chest infection is a high risk in the immobile burnt patient, and careful consideration should be given to the most comfortable position which will promote deep breathing and the expectoration of sputum.

Social Factors

Even in the very early stages of hospital care, some consideration should be given to the effects that the injury will have on the patient's future. Immediate thought should be given to the type of work/occupation of the patient.

Informing and Reassuring

Initially, the patient and family will need to know a rough estimate of how long the patient is likely to be in hospital. A second consideration in the mind of the patient will be that of possible permanent disability. This particular anxiety is often relieved if someone in the nursing team explains the total aims of the therapeutic regimen and that the main aim is to prevent any disability and to correct a possible disfigurement. Patients do not readily appreciate that isolated incidents or procedures are in fact part of the total aims of care and explanations should be given with this total concept in mind.

The emotional responses of both the patient and his or her family vary from extremes of anger and fear to those of grief. It is usually necessary to try to dispel these more extreme emotions by giving a careful and repeated explanation of the intent of treatment and assuaging some of the guilt feelings by positively reminding both patient and relatives of how well they are coping with a difficult situation. Discussion with relatives should take place **only** after the surgeon has had a preliminary interview with the immediate next-of-kin.

Second-stage Complications

During the second stage of healing, the nursing assessments and care combined should have as one of its aims the early detection of possible complications.

Wound surface infections should be relatively straightforward in the exposure technique, but will be more difficult if occlusive dressings are used. Swabs despatched to the pathology department for culture and sensitivity tests are usually required every second day.

Septicaemia or bloodborne infection may be noted by a persistent pyrexia, extreme restlessness, rigors and an extremely shocked patient. Specimens of blood for cultures may reveal the causative pathogen and powerful antibiotics may be prescribed to deal with what is a fulminating condition.

Urinary tract infection is an increased risk when a catheter has been inserted into the bladder, and also when there is a decrease in renal flow. Regular samples of urine should be despatched for culture and sensitivity tests every second day.

Oral infections, Candidiasis (Thrush) are more likely to occur when the patient's defence mechanisms are reduced or, in a very dependent patient, because of inadequate oral hygiene.

Gastrointestinal upsets are quite common after burns, but when they persist into the second stage of therapy a review of the possible causes should be made. Gastric motility is reduced after burns for some days and it may be that the patient's diet is too bulky. Alternatively, the antibiotics prescribed may have reduced the intestinal bacterial flora causing a diarrhoea. In children ulceration of the stomach and duodenum may occur (Curling's Ulcer).

Respiratory tract infections are quite common and may be due to the very poor circulation of air within the cubicle rather than any limitation placed on the ability to breathe correctly from the burns. Sputum specimens are collected in the early morning and despatched for culture and sensitivity testing which may identify the causative pathogen.

Electrolyte imbalance. Persistent electrolyte imbalance, despite intensive intravenous therapy and daily electrolyte monitoring, may imply that the adrenal glands have not yet recovered from the 'shock' of the burn injury. This complication will cause a wide range of symptoms varying from complete lethargy to irregular cardiac rhythm. It implies that the electrolyte balance will have to be measured at least twice daily and the fluid balance rota reviewed every 12 hours.

Anaemia. From 24–48 hours following a major burn injury, iron deficiency can be expected and corrected by whole blood transfusion. A persistent anaemia implies, however, that renal function in the production of the hormone erythropoietin is failing.

Pulmonary embolism and deep vein thrombosis are both potential risks if a haemoconcentration occurred in the early stages of treatment. This is especially so in an immobile patient.

Reduced liver metabolism may occur for several days following a major burn, which has implications for any drugs administered. Many such drugs, e.g., antibiotics, have to be removed from the body by conjugation with bile in the liver. Therefore, blood levels of certain drugs may remain high for a rather longer period than usual.

Joint contractures are generally preventable providing that correct positioning and support of the affected joint with soft splinting is implemented as soon as is feasible and that the principle of active movement is implemented as soon as possible.

PHASE THREE: GRAFTING

Between the second and tenth day of treatment, the surgeon will make a decision as to if and when the burn will require a graft to promote the final stage of healing. Alternatively, the decision may refer to the correction of a deformity arising from the burn or to correct a post-burn contracture. There are many forms of grafts used in post-thermal injuries.

Autograft

Basically, an *autograft* is the transfer of a piece of tissue from a donor site to the injured site and can be done by one of the following methods:

1. Free graft
2. Fixed graft
3. Other tissue grafts

Free Graft

A piece of skin of variable depth is transferred from a donor site to the injured site and can be either a split skin graft, full thickness graft, or pinch graft (Fig. 56.1). Free skin grafts are also used to promote healing in varicose and decubitus ulcers.

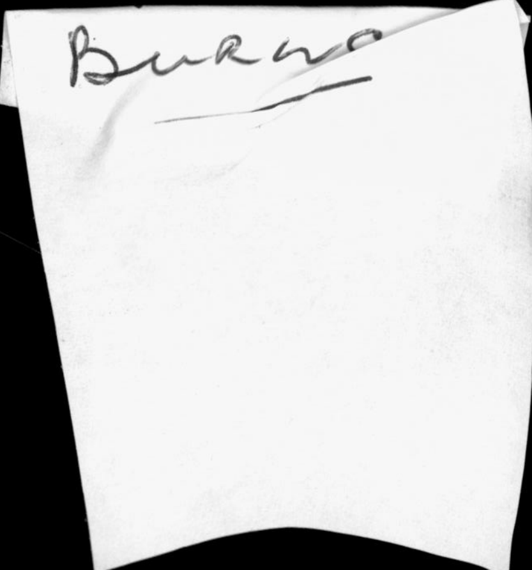
Burns

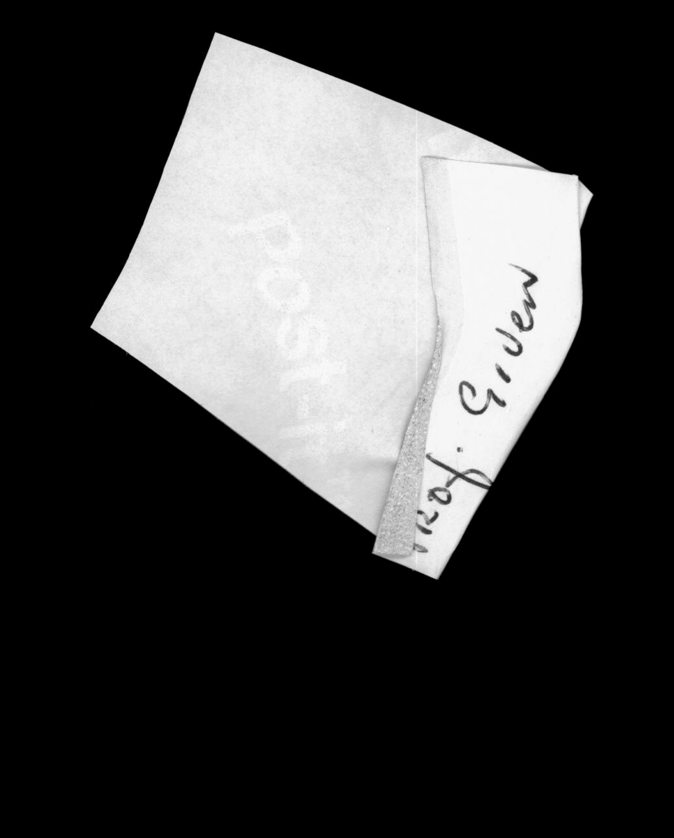

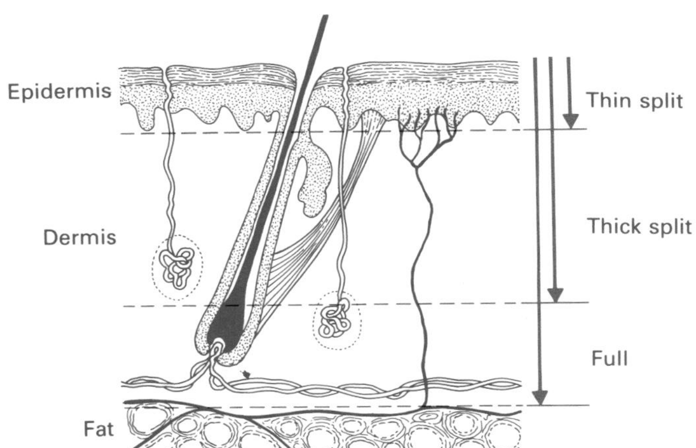

Fig. 56.1 Depth of split and full thickness skin grafts.

Split skin graft (Ollier-Tiersch graft), when applied, overlaps the boundaries of the injured site.

Full thickness skin graft (Wolfe Kraus graft) implies that the donor skin is the full thickness and taken from just above the subcutaneous fat layer. When applied to the donor site it is usually sutured into place within the boundaries of the injured site. Full thickness grafts are normally taken for burn injuries of the face where facial reconstruction is required. Benign or malignant tumour removal may also require full reconstruction to the lesion site and a full thickness graft may also be needed to correct a post-burn contracture.

Pinch grafts are tiny pieces of split skin taken from the donor site by raising the skin with a fine needle and cutting away a diameter of skin (about 1 cm) which is then placed on a partially healed recipient area.

Composite grafts are precisely cut grafts which must fit into the lesion site exactly. This type of graft is often planned to meet the needs of the cosmetic finish of a graft to the face or hands.

Fixed grafts

More commonly known as *skin flaps*, a fixed graft involves the fixing of a flap of skin to a neighbouring injured site. Such grafts can be local or distal skin flaps.

Local skin flaps, when fixed to a neighbouring site, are transposed directly or are rotated. Either method ensures that the recipient site is completely covered and that the flap has a good blood supply. A local skin flap is more commonly used in reconstruction surgery for facial lesions, e.g., from the nasal alae to the upper lip, or from the neck to the lower jaw.

Distal skin flaps are used to cover large recipient areas and the flap may be created from skin of the hand and fixed to a lesion on the neck, or abdomen. With injuries of the lower limb the flap may be a connection between the healthy and affected leg.

Once created, however, a distal skin flap must contain within itself an independent blood supply to keep it alive while it regenerates the recipient area (Fig. 56.2). The size of the skin flap may be either large or small. A great deal depends on the size of the recipient area. Pedicle and tube pedicle grafts are extensions of a distal flap constructed to form a tube of tissue which has an independent arterial and venous blood flow.

Other Tissue Grafts

Apart from the dermis, cartilage, bone and synthetic substances are used primarily to reconstruct appendages such as the nose and ears, as well as to correct deformities of contour. Synthetic materials do not pose the same problems of rejection as those of live tissue. Silastic is a most popular substance as

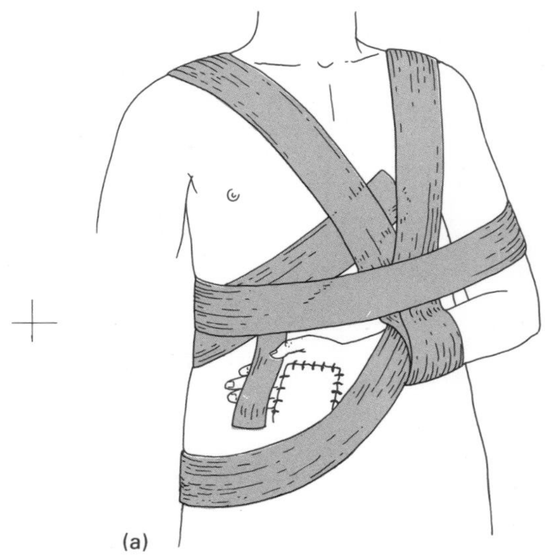

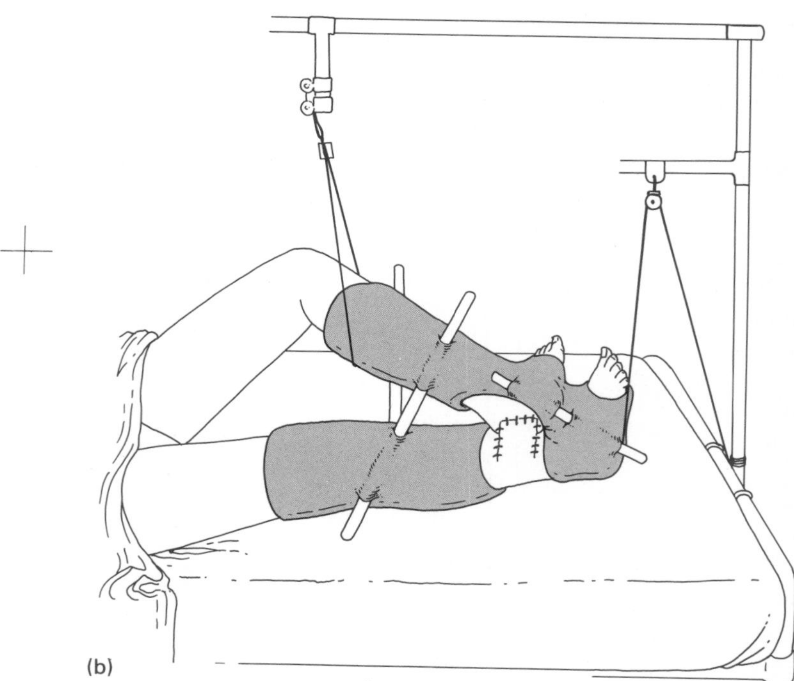

Fig. 56.2 Examples of immobilisation of flaps.

it can be shaped to fit the exact requirements of the reconstruction of an individual's nose, chin, breast, or be used as finger and joint implants. In the lower jaw, metal or chrome cobalt is often used to fill the space created between excised bone ends.

An external prosthesis usually composed from acrylic or silicone can be made to replace an excised nose, ear or eyelid. A major advantage to the external prosthesis is that it can be incorporated into the spectacle framework and can temporarily disguise any cosmetic disfigurement of the face until surgery can take place at a later date.

Choice of donor site

The choice of donor site, in decreasing order of frequency and if available to the surgeon, is:

Outer aspect of either thigh

Outer aspect of either lower and upper arms

Outer aspect of lower leg

Abdomen, buttocks and back are usually selected if the area to be grafted is very large. Whenever possible the donor skin would be taken from the 'bikini area' to reduce the embarrassment of residual scarring.

Removal of Donor Skin

Donor skin is removed from the patient under the effects of general anaesthesia and the method of removing the skin depends on the depth of graft required. Instruments such as the Humby knife are used for fairly deep grafts, while an air electrical dermatome is used for thin split grafting.

Once the skin is removed it is placed outer surface downwards on a piece of sterile tulle gras, after being stretched. Until the recipient site is ready, the donor graft is stored in a container of sterile normal saline. If the graft is to be applied at a much later date, i.e., delayed grafting, the stretched skin is stored for up to 3 weeks in a refrigerator at a controlled temperature of 4 °C.

The donor area is covered with a sterile piece of crease-free tulle gras over which crease-free layers of gauze swabs are placed and then secured with a firm crepe bandage (Fig. 56.2). Some bleeding can be expected from the donor site, but the original dressing is not normally disturbed until 7–10 days later. When due for removal the adhered gauze should be soaked liberally with a mild antiseptic to disengage the hardened blood.

Patients complain more about the pain from the donor site than that of the recipient site and for this reason mild analgesia given 30 minutes before the dressing is due for removal would be a useful measure.

Risk Factors from Grafts

The planning of any type of graft takes into account several common risk factors of which the nurse must be aware so that the care plan is adjusted to meet the needs of the individual patient.

The donor site from which the skin is taken usually is one which:

Is non-weight-bearing

Has a good blood supply

Is free from infection, especially of *Staphylococcus aureus* which can cause graft rejection

Is a non-friction area, i.e. not an obvious skin crease

Has a low microbial count at the time of graft taking. The donor site is usually prepared by cleansing with a skin antiseptic 3 or 4 times daily for 2 days prior to surgery. Shaving of the donor site is at the discretion of the surgeon, who will often not want to risk accidental nicking of the donor skin with a razor blade.

The recipient site of a skin graft should be pink, vascular, and moist. When the surgeon considers there will be a risk of *sheering*, or tearing, strain on or around the recipient site, a form of splinting the area will have to be planned before the operation. It is usual practice to take a swab of the recipient area for culture and sensitivity to any pathogens the day before operation so as to eliminate the risk of infection being present.

Prevention of Haematoma

At the time of surgery the recipient area would have any necrosed tissue excised, excess granulation tissue may also be excised if it threatens the ultimate cosmetic finish of the graft. Haematoma is one of the greatest risks to the graft and to prevent it occurring any superficial vessels will be either ligated or coagulated by diathermy. Any threat of bleeding which risks a haematoma will spoil the chances of the graft taking successfully.

The donor skin will be placed to overlap the recipient area, secured by suture within the boundaries of the lesion, or cut as a composite to fit exactly into the lesion area. After careful suturing, the graft may be compressed onto the area by either flavine-soaked cotton wool swabs or with a polyurethane foam pledgelet which is tied over the graft area by one long suture thread. The whole area is then covered by further pressure and the dressings held secure by a firm crepe bandage.

Grafted areas would in the normal course of events be left alone for between 7 and 10 days and the first redressing performed by the surgeon who carried out the operation. During this waiting period the area may have to be immobilised if the graft is subject to any shearing or pulling forces which would threaten the graft.

Chapter 57
Surgical Reconstruction Techniques

From the wide variety of repair and reconstructive surgery undertaken in the field of plastic surgery, it is proposed to highlight only a few of the conditions which a general learner nurse may meet during a period of training. From the few examples given, the main principles underlying the care of patients with repair of tissues due to congenital defect or trauma can be extrapolated and used as a general basis before going on into specialised care, after becoming qualified.

THE HAND

Deformity arising from congenital abnormality, traumatic injury or burns can include one or several of the following deformities to the anatomy of the hand:

Hyperextension of the metacarpal and phalangeal joints

Flexion of the phalangeal joints

Contracture of the thenar web space (between thumb and first finger)

Flexion of the carpal joints

These deformities carry a high risk of failure to heal if at the time of the injury or during the course of therapy any of the following factors are present:

Oedema can only be prevented by continual elevation of the whole arm, promoting early activity of each individual finger and the palmar surface of the hand. Promoting self-care such as independence in eating and encouraging movements of the shoulder and elbow joint will promote venous return from the affected arm and limit the amount of oedema.

Infection will delay healing and the period of rest required until the localised infection has resolved will increase the risks of flexion and extension deformity.

Incorrect positioning of the injured part of the hand, especially if the hand has been splinted, e.g., with plaster of Paris. If the splint was incorrectly applied in the first instance, there is an increased risk of contractures. With the hand in the elevated position, attention should be given to the correct positioning of each finger, as well as the wrist and elbow joint, to reduce any risk of flexion contracture.

Prolonged immobilisation in any form of splinting will cause those tissues in flexion to contract. If a hand is splinted in extension, this may lead to a hyperextension deformity, especially of the metacarpal and phalangeal joints.

Delayed grafting, in the case of burns, may lead to the risk of tendonitis which is increased the longer the wound is left.

Reconstructive Surgery

One of 4 criteria is used when reconstructive surgery is being planned, and it will be to

1. Skin graft to restore lost tissue
2. Restore bone architecture
3. Repair a severed nerve
4. Restore motor function by tendon graft, tendon repair or transfer

Procedure

The actual surgery may be undertaken by regional anaesthesia using Lignocaine 0.5% infiltrated into the tissues of the hand via a butterfly needle. Where the patient may be overly upset by the procedure, a general anaesthesia is used. The surgeon should, with an indelible skin pencil, clearly identify the part of the hand which is to be the site of surgery, even if the hand is obviously deformed.

Immediately before surgery, the blood flow through the arm is firstly occluded by applying the inflated cuff of a sphygmomanometer, followed by the application of Esmarch's bandage, or tourniquet, from the wrist upwards (to exclude the venous blood). Elective surgery of the hand should, therefore, be completed more quickly if the actual site is a bloodless field.

After the corrective surgery is completed the surgeon will usually advise the application of one type or form of temporary immobilisation to prevent contractures or extension deformity until the healing is completed. This will usually mean that the hand and arm should be nursed in the elevated position to reduce the tendency to oedema. This position should be maintained for at least 24 hours, if not longer (Figs. 57.1–2).

Aftercare

The first dressing following the surgery is generally done by the surgeon who performed the operation. Until this time, the nurse will implement a care plan which meets the specific needs of the patient. If the operation is performed on the dominant hand then obviously the patient will be more dependent on nursing assistance to cope with the normal activities of daily living.

The hand is a notoriously painful area when subject to any kind of trauma, including surgery, and a strong analgesia should be available to the patient on an As Required basis for the first 48 hours following operation.

Microsurgery

Severed Nerves

Surgery to repair a severed nerve would normally be completed using microsurgical techniques to establish sensory and motor response via one of the following:

The **radial nerve,** which permits normal extensor movements of the fingers

The **median nerve,** which permits normal flexor movements of the fingers and hand

The **ulnar nerve,** which permits normal intrinsic hand movements

The **digital nerves** within each finger

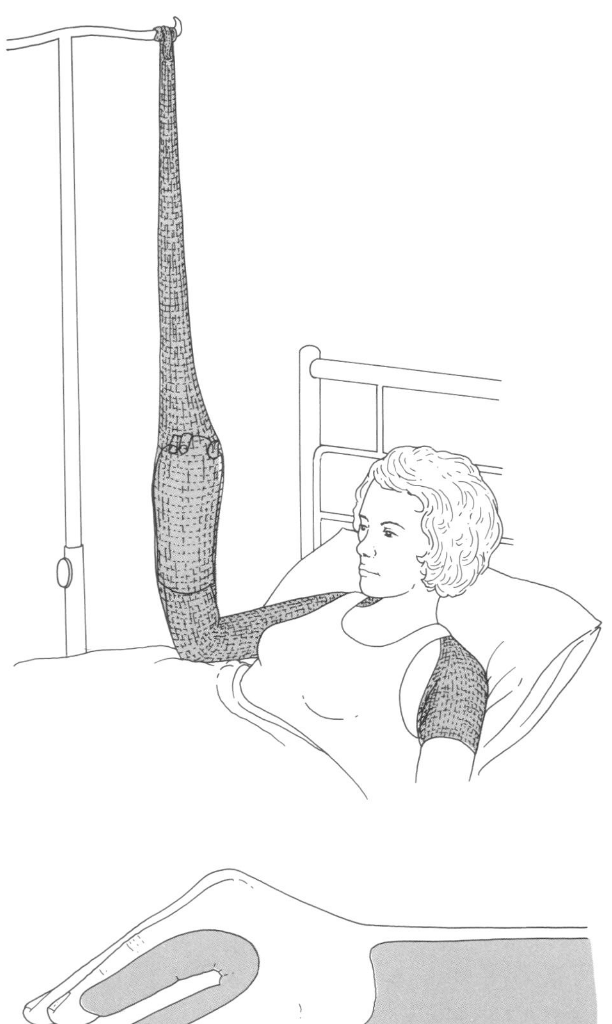

Fig. 57.1 Upper limb elevation following hand burns, injury or surgery.

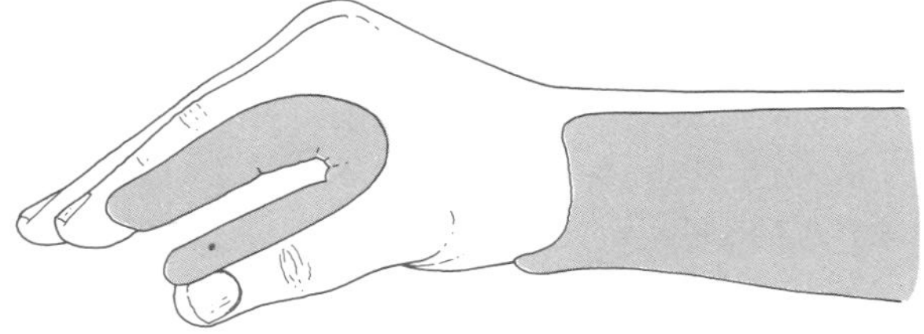

Fig. 57.2 Ideal position for prolonged immobilisation of a hand in burns, trauma or after surgery.

which are the terminations of the median and ulnar nerve

Blood vessels which may give rise to problems in the course of surgery are the branches arising from the radial and ulnar arteries which supply the deep palmar arch with further sub-branches to the digital arteries.

Guillotine Injuries

Microsurgery is more appropriate for guillotine injuries either of the digits or at the wrist. Avulsion or crush injuries are not amenable to microsurgery. Reimplantation of an individual digit, or indeed the whole hand, is possible providing the amputated part is retained at the time of injury and the time of operation is between 4 and 6 hours after the injury.

If the retained amputated part is stored in a sterile container, which is kept cool, surgery can take place up to 24 hours later. The main principle employed is that if at least 1 artery and 2 veins can be resutured together, combined with digital nerve repair, then correct realignment of bone architecture and a reasonable amount of skin flap can connect the severed parts at the amputation site.

The diameter of the vessels is so small that a microscope is employed to visually enlarge their diameter. Very fine instruments are employed to anastomose and approximate their edges, with the use of extremely fine soluble suture material.

Aftercare

The same principles of nursing care for reconstructive surgery are adopted. An additional observation required is that the amputated part has a healthy re-established blood flow and, consequently, is as warm as the opposite healthy hand. Again, the first dressing should be done by the surgeon who performed the operation. Microscopic surgery of the hand takes a considerable amount of time. With the associated risks this has of prolonged anaesthesia, the nurse may have to consider this potential **risk** in the first 24 hours of care.

Surgical Excision

Dupuytren's Contracture

Dupuytren's Contracture is a condition in which bands of fibrous tissue lying underneath the skin of the palm and fingers may develop. Their presence causes a static or progressive flexion contracture of the fingers. It may at first appear as a nodular thickening along the palm of the hand in line with the ring finger. As it increases in thickness it pulls on both the metacarpophalangeal and interdigital joints which in turn pull the fingers into the palmar surface (*contractures*).

The contractures are released by surgical excision of the fibrous tissue from the palmar fascia. The sutured wound is covered by a nonadhesive dressing which is then covered by a layer of supportive cotton wool over which a plaster cast is applied. The plaster remains in position for one week, after which it can be removed. Active exercises of the digits are encouraged for a given period, each hour, every day for a further week before sutures are finally removed.

Carpal Tunnel Syndrome

The carpal tunnel syndrome refers to a compression of the median nerve within the carpal tunnel at the wrist, which is located at the palmar surface of the wrist. The compression causes localised pain and a parasthesia of the thumb and index finger which were innervated by the median nerve.

Gradually, the whole hand feels weak and the fingers cannot grip objects firmly. With an increasing lack of use the thenar muscle begins to waste and hypertrophy. The various causes of median nerve compression may be due to a fracture of a carpal bone, rheumatoid arthritis of the wrist joint, or a synovitis. It may affect one or both wrists.

A surgical removal of part of the transverse carpal ligament may relieve the median nerve compression. Following the operation, there will be some local oedema for several days, but after this the patient should find it possible to begin graduated exercises of the digits, palmar surface and the wrist without too much discomfort. The sutures can be removed after 5 days.

THE NOSE

Rhinoplasty

Disfigurement to the nose may be congenital, may be consequent to trauma, or result from tumours. In all cases there is a strong underlying psychological stress due to the disfigurement, and the optimism with which many patients enter the proposal of surgery is infectious. Professionally, the nurse should try not to be carried away with the patient's enthusiasm in case the results are not all the patient has been led to expect.

When surgery is being planned, careful measurements are made of the facial contours to determine the correct proportions. Frontal and lateral skull X-rays are usually taken to check on the underlying bone structure. The patient **must** be free of any upper respiratory tract infection prior to the proposed time and date of surgery.

Procedure

The underlying structures are the tissues which will be reshaped, and access to these is made through incisions made into the mucosa of the nasal chamber, implying that there will be no visible scars after the operation. Several examples of reshaping the nose include the surgeon removing excess septal bone for a pronounced nasal bridge, removal of excess soft tissue (i.e., alar cartilage) for very broad nostrils, and the reconstruction of nasal tip.

Aftercare

After surgery the nasal chambers are packed with a nasal splint either side of the septum to support the reconstruction. There is usually a great deal of nasal secretion during the next 2 or 3 days. This is collected into a nasal gauze sling which is fixed under the nostril apertures, and the sling obviously requires frequent replacement with regular nasal toilet until the splint packs are removed by the surgeon.

Oral breathing will lead to some discomfort for the patient and adequate oral hygiene will have to be offered at very frequent intervals. Sleep is usually impossible, unless some sedation is offered each evening until the packs are removed. If surgery is near to the bridge of the nose, then *periorbital ecchymosis* (black eyes) can be expected for 3 or 4 days after surgery.

It is quite usual for this type of surgery to be accompanied by a submucous resection to correct any septal deflection. One of the benefits of this should be an improved tonal quality to speech, since the malar sinuses should have an improved ability to contain uninfected air in addition to better airflow over the turbinate bones.

THE MALE URETHRA

Urethroplasty

Hypospadias is a congenital defect in which the urinary meatus is located on the underside of the penile shaft instead of at the penile tip. A second deformity accompanying hypo-

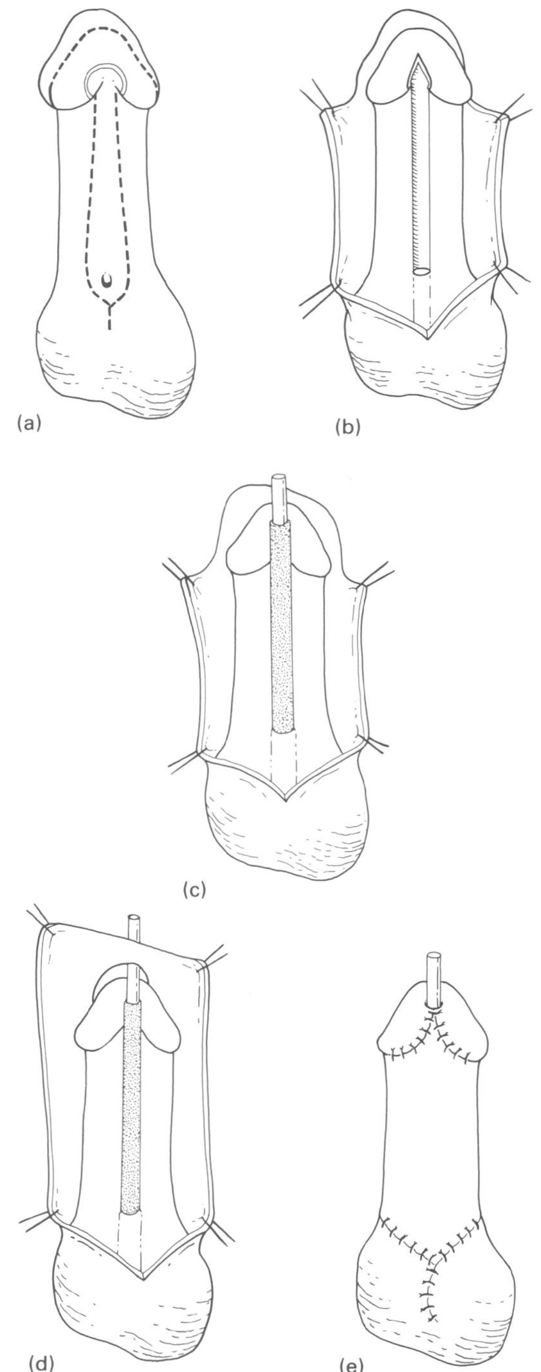

Fig. 57.3 Surgical correction of hypospadias: release of chordee (a); urethral gutter established (b); skin positioned around urethra (c); prepuce readied to cover raw area (d); wound edges sutured (e).

spadias may also be the malformation of chordee. In this, fibrous bands along the penile shaft keep the penis in a permanent downward bowing position. The aim of plastic surgery would be to correct the positioning of the urinary meatus and, if necessary, to straighten the penile shaft (Fig. 57.3).

Procedure

Urethroplasty is a two-stage operation with an interval of time between each operation.

The *first stage* usually, is to correct the chordee, by the surgeon making a circular incision or a dorsal slit into the penile shaft to enable the fibrous bands to be excised via the anterior surface of the penis. This may correct the abnormal curvature of the penis. At the same time, a buttonhole incision is made to bring through the glans penis to the urethral tip.

The *second stage* is the reconstruction of the urethra itself. This is completed using a variety of techniques such as burying a skin tube graft along the urethral track, doing a free skin graft, or a buried skin flap. The implied surgery is quite extensive and to restrain the new urethral tract a restraining urinary catheter with continuous bladder drainage is maintained for several days while the graft takes.

Similar operations are carried out for the reverse condition known as *epispadias*, when the urethral meatus is located on the anterior surface of the penis and may be combined with the congenital absence of the external sphincter.

Both preceding defects may occur in the female urethra. In hypospadias, the urethra opens into the vagina; in epispadias, the fissure would be above the clitoris. Incidence of either, however, is very rare.

THE JAW

Hemimandibulectomy

Surgery to excise and resect part of the jaw (lower mandible) is usually reserved for those patients with proven cancer of the mouth. Preoperatively there are major problems to be overcome, which include dysphagia, speech difficulties, oral hygiene, excess salivation and pain control. Significantly, these same problems will have to be dealt with postoperatively.

Patient Care

Dysphagia

Dysphagia will usually require the patient to have a soft or liquid diet, if they can in fact swallow. If the patient cannot swallow, then the alternative method of nasogastric feeding would be necessary. Straws may be a useful alternative after trying very small spoons, if the patient is able to swallow anything at all. This effort is aimed at correcting any dietary deficiences before undergoing a major operation.

One form of communication will have to be agreed upon between the nurse and patient. This may be by sign language, picture cards, or the written word. Whichever method is decided upon should also be appropriate for postoperative care. Many investigations will be completed to exclude the possibilities of secondary deposits of cancer cells (see also Part 5, Oncology).

The suture line will be within the oral cavity, and the resected bone may have been filled with cobalt chrome prosthesis. In addition, the upper and lower jaw may be temporarily fixed together by wire suture. In extreme cases the surgeon may have performed a tracheostomy to bypass temporarily the problems of respiration until the incision lines within the mouth are completely healed. The major problems for the patient will be the inability to swallow with any degree of comfort. Therefore feeding may be continued for some time via a nasogastric tube.

Oral Toilet

Oral toilet may only be possible via an irrigation syringe, using a solution of dilute hydrogen peroxide and sodium bicarbonate. In this technique, the head of the patient must be brought forward to allow the irrigation fluid to escape from the aperture between the wired teeth.

Emotional Reactions

The emotional responses of the patient are somewhat muted without their ability to express themselves verbally. It should be appreciated that the patient's feelings require to be vented somehow. Emotions such as fear, anger, and those of grief because of altered body image may have to be diminished by the use of sedation for several days following surgery.

Postoperative Outcomes

The response to this type of reconstructive surgery is not very good, especially if it is accompanied by a tracheostomy and for this reason, is not frequently seen. Another limiting factor to the possibility of surgery is the high incidence of secondary cancer.

Successful operations, however, do occur and when the reconstruction is complete, and the healing of tissues is satisfactory, the patient can then be encouraged in more positive self-care techniques as the various catheters and tubes are removed. Once the problems of dysphagia are overcome it may be necessary to introduce speech therapy in the early part of convalescence.

THE BREAST

Reduction Mammoplasty

In those female patients with excessive and gross breast tissue, it may be appropriate for the patient's doctor to offer an operation (Fig. 57.4) which will reduce the size of the breasts and, at the same time, shape the breast contour so that they are symmetrical with the patient's body weight and build.

The bulk and weight of excessive breast tissue would cause respiratory difficulties and backache. The breast tissue is rather tender to the touch and the patient may complain of diffuse pain throughout the breast tissue.

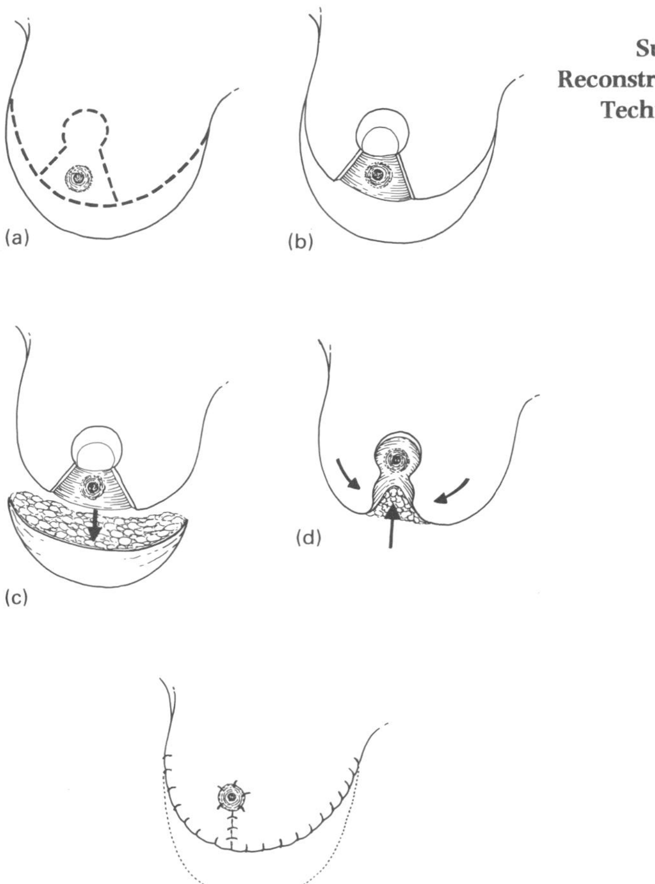

Fig. 57.4 Reduction mammoplasty: incisions (a); upper resection and de-epithelialisation of dermal bridges (b); lower resection (c); positioning of nipple (d); completed (e).

This, combined with fatigue, may be sufficient grounds to offer the operation. The symptoms are more pronounced at menstruation. The social difficulties and embarrassments the patient may have to cope with should never be underestimated, often being so humiliating that the patient becomes a recluse.

Careful planning is completed prior to a reduction mammoplasty so that the problems resulting from enlarged breasts are dealt with effectively, e.g., obesity, risk of chest infections and backache problems. The timing of the operation may be arranged after or before the menstrual period.

Procedure

While under the effects of a general anaesthetic the surgeon carefully marks out the area of where the normal nipple position should be, i.e., in alignment with the fourth intercostal space. The next lines drawn will be along those creases where the incisions will be made, through which the excess tissue will be dissected.

The first stage of surgery is to remove the nipple areolar complex. This is retained in a solution of normal saline and will be grafted back onto the reconstructed breast. The redundant tissue is then excised. The incision lines are then closed by sutures from the subcutaneous layer upwards and a drain is secured into the wound and held by a suture. The nipple areolar complex is then grafted onto the correct breast position and secured by sutures.

One suture will be rather long and is used to hold in position over the graft a pressure gauze dressing. The wound dressing applied must both cover and support the reconstructed breast while allowing the drain to rid the wound site of any exudate.

Aftercare

Postoperatively, the patient is best nursed in the recumbent position to allow for wound drainage. The drain should be removed 24-48 hours after surgery to allow the incision line to heal without any obvious scarring. After a few days, when the pressure dressing over the nipple area is removed, there is likely to be a blackened scab over the nipple. This falls away once the underlying tissue has regenerated, and the patient should be reassured that this is quite normal. The younger female patient should be told that a reduction mammoplasty may produce a non-lactating breast.

Breast Augmentation

Breast augmentation, or enlargement, is an operation which may be offered to the female patient who suffers from hypoplasia of the breasts, has tissue involution, as a compensating technique following mastectomy, or if either breast is asymmetrical. A psychological assessment of the patient is absolutely vital, not only for the surgery itself but for the postoperative period when the patient must cope with the problems of an altered body image.

The enlargement of the breast is created by implanting an inert prosthetic device. This may be composed of silastic gel semi-inflatable material, or inflatable material, e.g., Jenny Prosthesis.

Procedure

Surgically, a pocket is created by separating the breast tissue and the subcutaneous fat from the underlying pectoral fascia via an incision made at the undermargin, or base crease, of the breast. Both bleeding and risk of infection may cause a rejection of the prosthesis. Therefore, the most minor of bleeding points are sealed with diathermy and strict asepsis is essential. After the implant has been inserted the incision line and wound are rechecked for bleeding.

The closure of the wound is equally carefully done with soluble fine suture material from the base upwards. The incision line is then covered by a gauze dressing secured to the skin by an elastic tape dressing which creates pressure on the wound to press the suture line towards the chest wall.

Aftercare

During the postoperative period the patient should wear a supportive bra which allows the nipple area to be exposed. The nursing plan of care should highlight the importance of reducing the risk of wound infection.

The sutures are usually removed 5–7 days after surgery. The risk of rejection or infection remains a hazard for several months after the implant, and to detect either the surgeon will arrange to see the patient at frequent intervals for the 6 months following the operation.

Part 7
The Special Senses

Chapter 58
The Eye: Structure and Clinical Examination

STRUCTURE

Extrinsic

The structures external to the eyeball are mainly protective and include the bony orbital cavity, the eyelids, eyelashes and the eyebrows.

Many of the facial bones combine to form the orbit within which the eyeball rests, its walls aligned at an angle of 45°. The bones contributing to this framework are the orbital margin of the frontal bone, the nasal bones, maxilla, zygoma, ethmoid and lacrimal bones. Within this bony orbit there are 3 main apertures which allow vessels to enter and leave: the principal foramen being on the posterior wall allowing the optic nerve to leave the eyeball and travel on to the occipital lobe and lobes of the brain. The lacrimal gland, orbital arteries and veins, and several cranial nerves gain access to the eyeball via the other 2 apertures. Growing from the skin covering the orbital margin are the eyebrows, their only function being slightly protective in that they can trap any sweat from the forehead and if thick enough can limit the amount of light from above the eyebrow reaching the eyeball.

Eyelids

The upper and lower eyelids are formed from folds of skin extending and being continuous with the facial skin. Within each eyelid there is some muscle tissue, i.e., *orbicularis oculi*, which lends not only movement to the eyelid but gives the upper eyelid in particular more rigidity. A further form of strengthening comes from a plate of fibrous tissue in each eyelid, its increased weight giving the eyelid more shape.

On the inner surface of each eyelid lies a serous membrane, the *conjunctiva*. Being a serous membrane it has two layers: the outer and inner layer. The *outer* layer reflects over the eyeball and is known as the **bulbar** conjunctiva. The *inner* layer facing into the eyelid is called the **tarsal**, or **palpebral**, conjunctiva. The potential space between these two layers is the *conjunctival sac*. At the point where the upper and lower eyelid meet and recess, lies the inferior and superior fornices.

Both the conjunctiva and the eyelid are liberally supplied with blood vessels, goblet cells secreting mucus, and serous Meibomian glands which secrete a lubricating sebaceous fluid. A protective blink reflex ensures that the eyelids can quickly open and close whenever the cornea is threatened by dust or other irritations. This rapid reflex movement is innervated by the third cranial nerve.

Eyelashes

Growing from the anterior edge of each eyelid are the eyelashes, these being more profuse and longer on the upper eyelid. If the eyelashes are cut they will grow again to their former length within 6 to 8 weeks. As with other body hair each eyelash has its own hair root and glands. On blinking, the eyelashes help to prevent particles of dust from reaching the conjunctiva and cornea.

The Lacrimal Apparatus

The conjunctiva are kept moist by a constant flow of tears from the lacrimal glands, located at the upper outer corner of each orbital cavity and are not palpable (Fig. 58.1). Tears are composed of water, sodium chloride and a mildly antibacterial enzyme, **lysozyme**. The constant secretion of tears across the conjunctiva keeps the membrane moist and also washes the cornea.

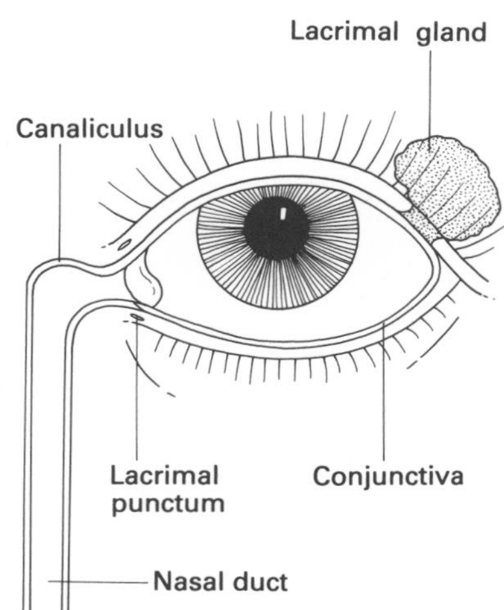

Fig. 58.1 Lacrimal apparatus.

Secreted from the lacrimal gland, tears enter each eye via the superior fornix, wash across the eye and are drained into the common canaliculus via a tiny aperture, the **punctum**. The tears then drain downwards into the inferior meatus of the nose via the nasolacrimal duct.

Ocular Movement

Six extrinsic muscles enable the eyeball to move in every direction. Four of these muscles lie in straight alignment between the sclera, running backwards to be inserted into the wall of the orbital cavity. The other two muscles are placed at an oblique angle on the superior and inferior poles of the eyeball. Innervation to these extrinsic muscles is derived from the fourth and sixth cranial nerves.

Intrinsic

The eyeball measures 2.5 cm in diameter and depth, has a spherical shape, and rests on a pad of fat lining the orbital cavity (Fig. 58.2). It has 3 distinct layers, or coats:

Sclera, or outer layer
Choroid, or middle layer
Retina, or inner layer

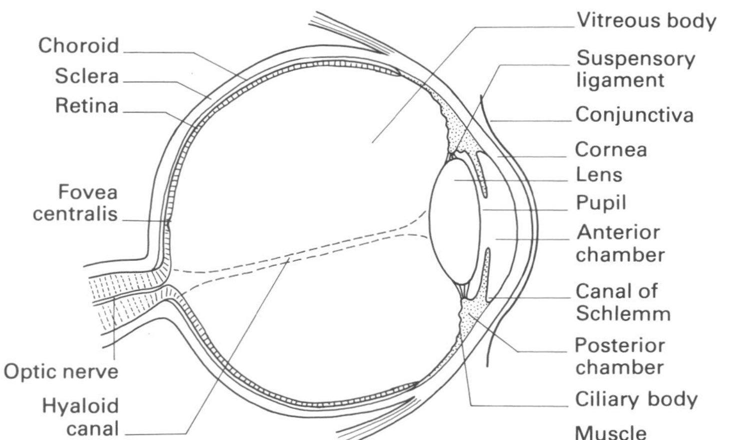

Fig. 58.2 Intrinsic structures of the eye.

The Sclera

Composed of a tough fibrous tissue, the sclera is white in colour and completely surrounds the eye except on the anterior surface of the eyeball where it is interrupted by a transparent area, the **cornea**. The cornea is arranged in layers of highly specialised tissue of which the main feature is its transparency through which light rays can enter the pupil of the eye. The main layers are:

Non-keratinised epithelium, which prevents the tears entering the cornea and is dependent on its function of a free access to atmospheric air.

Bowman's capsule is a resistant tissue. If perforated by injury, it cannot regenerate. Its presence assists with the curvature of the cornea.

The **stroma** layer is a precise arrangement of collagen fibres permitting light rays to enter the eye to reach the lens. A disturbance of this layer scatters light rays, instead of refracting them so that they can reach the lens immediately behind the cornea.

An **inner endothelial** layer is continuous with the iris (coloured area) which also lies behind the cornea. This layer prevents aqueous humour in the anterior chamber from coming forward into the cornea.

The cornea is an avascular structure and the corneal sensitivity is dependant on perfect transparency through its layers and the normal curvature of its surface.

Choroid coat

The middle coat is also known as the **pigmented** layer because of the blood vessels which traverse through to reach the retina. On its anterior surface it is interrupted by 3 important structures: the iris, pupil and ciliary body, all of which lie immediately behind the cornea.

The **iris**, or coloured disc, surrounding the pupil of the eye, is composed of two involuntary muscles, *radiating* and *circular*. Radiating muscle fibres dilate the size of the pupil, while the circular muscle fibres constrict its diameter.

The size of **pupil** is reflexly controlled, constricting in diameter for near vision and bright light and dilating for distant vision and dim light. This reflex movement is controlled by the third cranial nerve. The pupil is literally a black circular hole within the centre of the iris, and it is through this hole that light must pass to reach the lens and retina.

At the point where the iris meets the choroid layer lies the **ciliary** body. This structure has a dual function, *muscular* and *glandular*:

1. The ciliary muscle fibres are attached to the lens and by its muscular action can alter the shape of the lens. As light passes

through the lens it can be refracted according to the lens shape. This ability to accommodate light rays refers also to the ciliary body being known as the *muscle of accommodation*.

2. The glandular tissue of the ciliary body secretes intraocular fluid for the nourishment of both the anterior and posterior chambers of the eye.

In the anterior chamber the intraocular fluid is called *aqueous humour* and in composition it is slightly dense containing some protein and sodium chloride. Excess aqueous humour is drained from the anterior chamber via the filtration angle situated immediately below the iris and leaves the eye via the canal of Schlemm to reach the veins situated above and behind the eye.

In the posterior chamber, however, the intraocular fluid known as *vitreous humour* is far more dense, being of a jelly-like consistency containing much more protein and hyaluronic acid. Both fluids contribute to the rigidity and spherical contour of the eyeball, creating an intraocular pressure of between 18 and 25 mmHg. Since they are both transparent media, light rays can pass through to reach the retina.

The *lens* is a biconcave crystalline disc surrounded by a transparent capsule held in position by suspensory ligaments attached to the ciliary body. Because it is very elastic its curvature can be altered to focus on distant or near objects by the contraction or relaxation of the ciliary muscle pulling on the suspensory ligaments. In the lens, light can be refracted, i.e., light rays can be bent, and this refraction can also occur in the aqueous and vitreous humours. However, the lens is the only structure which can refract light by *accommodation*, i.e., changing its shape.

The Retina

The inner coat of the eye is the area containing the specialised nerve cells known as the **rods** and **cones**. The rods respond to dim light and are placed forwards on the retina, while the cones respond to bright light and colour and lie behind the rods. Where the cones are gathered most profusely at the back of the eye, this area is known by several names: *yellow spot*, *macula lutea*, or *fovea centralis* and is the area of perfect vision in the healthy eye.

The rods contain a pigment known as visual purple. This pigment alters chemically in its reaction with light and is essential in altering the light ray via a chemical reaction into a nerve impulse. In reacting chemically the visual purple loses its pigmentation, becoming bleached. It has to be reformed from dietary vitamin A and protein, otherwise night blindness may result. The rods and cones deepen into a complex layer which ultimately ends up with optical neurones and optic nerves. These travel towards the optic disc (or optic head) and leave the orbit as the optic nerve to travel along the visual pathway to reach the occipital lobe. The retinal artery enters the eye at the optic disc.

The Visual Pathway

Impulses travelling from the retinal nerve fibres leave the eyeball via the optic disc and travel along the optic nerves until they reach the optic chiasma (Fig. 58.3). On reaching the chiasma, however, the nasal portions of the retinal impulses come together.

Normal Vision

In normal vision, light rays passing through the air and then through the different densities of the optical transparent structures, are refracted. This refraction is essential since light rays travel in parallel lines and, therefore, must be refracted to reach the retina. The power of the eye to refract light depends on 3 important points:

1. The convex surface of the cornea causes parallel light rays to converge.
2. The lens then reduces the convergence of light rays to the centre of the lens by altering its shape.
3. The axial length of the eye should then permit the convergent light rays to reach the retina from any distance.

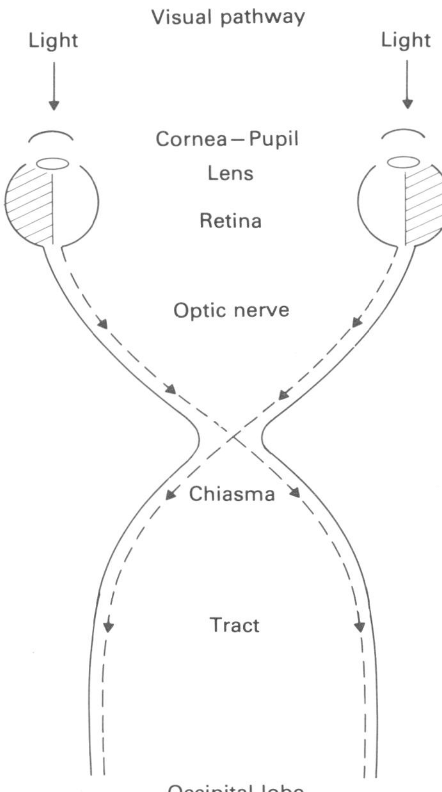

Fig. 58.3 Visual pathways.

Disorders of Refraction

If the refraction of light is normal (**emmetropia**) the individual can be said to have perfect vision.

With natural ageing the lens loses its ability to alter shape with an increasing tendency towards errors of refraction and near objects tend to appear blurred. Any of these refractive errors can be corrected by prescribed lens or contact lens.

Disorders of refraction are quite common, the main errors being hypermetropia, myopia and astigmatism.

Hypermetropia is also referred to as the *long-sighted* eye because the light rays focus on a point behind the retina. This can be due to either poor lens refraction or a short axial eye length. If the refractive error is ignored it can lead to severe eyestrain.

Myopia is also known as *short-sightedness*. The light rays tend to focus in front of the retina, which implies that the axial eye length is greater than normal and the curve of the lens is more convex than usual. Myopic eyes tend to be rather large with some atrophy at the optic disc.

Astigmatism occurs where the light rays are not focusing on any given point because the shape of the eye prevents correct refraction in the lens. The eye tends to be oval-shaped instead of spherical. Astigmatism may also be combined with hypermetropia or myopia.

CLINICAL EXAMINATION

Important to the ophthalmic examination is a detailed history, noting not only the individual's personal health but any familial disease pattern such as diabetes, hypertension or renal disease. Any of these has an adverse effect on the retina of the eye. The subjective examination of the eye includes noting any of the following:

- Redness of the conjunctiva or sclera
- Obvious infected discharge
- Lacrimation or excess tear flow
- Squint
- Prominence of the eyeball
- Distortion of the eye or the eyelids
- Movement of the eyeball
- Conjunctival oedema or injection (redness)
- Conjunctival mucosa

Any abnormal sign from the preceding list should be related to the very common symptoms of ocular pain, visual disturbance and double vision (*diplopia*).

The Cornea

When inspecting the cornea the physician may instil a few drops of dye, e.g., fluorescin 2% or Bengal Rose 1%, which is washed out after a few moments. Any stain remaining on the cornea would indicate an abrasion or perforation of the cornea. The cornea may appear opaque. A slight opacity is called *nebula*, but if there is a marked density the term *leucoma* is used. It is important not to confuse this condition with a cararact. A wisp of sterile cotton wool can be used to stroke the cornea to test its sensitivity, i.e., the blink reflex should occur immediately.

The Anterior Chamber

The anterior chamber which contains aqueous humour is inspected for both depth and clarity. If the aqueous humour is hazy, it is called *hypopyon*, whereas if there is blood present in the anterior chamber it is known as *hyphaemia*. Cells deposited immediately behind the cornea are known as *keratic precipitation*, suggesting an abnormality of the non-keratinised corneal layer coming backwards into the anterior chamber.

The Iris

In disease the normally well-defined shape and contour of the iris may alter. If it has an ill-defined shape and there is new vessel formation within the iris it suggests a disorder known as *rubeosis* of the iris. The iris can adhere either to the cornea at the front or to the lens behind, i.e., anterior or posterior synechia respectively.

The lens would normally support the position of the iris, but should there be a displacement of the lens the iris will become tremulous, i.e., oscillate rapidly (more correctly termed *iridodonesis*).

The pupil of the eye can be quickly assessed for its size, shape and position, as well as its reaction and accommodation to light.

Testing

Ophthalmoscopy is used to test the lens, the vitreous humour of the posterior chamber and the retina. A poor opacity of the lens suggests the development of a cataract. A close examination of the retina includes an assessment of the retinal blood vessels at the optic disc to check if they are dilated or have, in fact, haemorrhaged. This may also show if the retina is becoming detached, or separated, from the middle coat.

Tonometry will measure the intraocular pressure of the eye (18 to 25 mmHg). Usually amethocaine 2% eyedrops are instilled to anaesthetise the eye. While the eyelids are held widely apart, the tonometer is then placed on the cornea. The needle deflects across a translatable scale giving the exact intraocular pressure. The condition of glaucoma will raise the pressure to above 25 mmHg.

Testing of one or both eyes may continue with an assessment of:

- Visual acuity and form sense
- Field of vision
- Colour vision
- Light sense, or adaptation

Visual Acuity

Visual acuity is the ability of the eye to perceive the shape of a given object, or letter, at near or distant vision. It can be assessed by the use of a Snellen's chart, Landolt's rings or the E-test for those who cannot read. Distant vision implies that the eye can refract light from an object 6 m distant (20 ft), while near vision, which requires increased refraction, enables the patient to be able to read standard print size at a distance of 33 cm (13 in).

When tested the focusing power of the lens may be recorded as 6/6 m or 20/20 ft. The upper figure represents the actual distance, while the lower figure represents the distance at which the eye should be able to focus. Therefore, 6/6 m means perfect vision. Perception of objects may also be tested by asking the patient to finger count the doctor's upheld hand or by indicating if he or she can follow hand movements.

Field of Vision

The field of vision test can describe the ability of each eye to appreciate visually objects around the central field of vision, i.e., at the extreme of the temporal field. When drawn graphically, the actual field of vision of a normal eye somewhat resembles a pear lying on its side with the narrow end pointing towards the nose. The loss of peripheral vision is subtle and often the patient does not notice how much loss there can be in a short period of time. Many patients mistakenly blame their advancing years as the cause, while it may be due to a disease of the retina.

Perimetry is used to test the actual perception of peripheral vision. There is little by way of actual preparation except to advise the patient that it is a painless procedure which lasts for a short period of time and involves mapping out on a graph what he or she can actually see through a perimeter.

Colour Sense

The colour sense test would discriminate whether the cones of the retina can distinguish the spectrum of wave lengths in white light. The spectrum in normal light consists of the colours red, orange, yellow, green, blue green, blue, and violet. The Young–Helmholtz theory suggests that the cones appreciate three distinct colours (red, blue and green) and the appreciation of all other spectral colours is based on the intermingling of these three dominant colours. A common and simple test for colour vision is either by asking the patient to examine Ishihara colour plates or by completing the Eldridge–Green test. These tests are so constructed that if the patient is colour blind he or she will be unable to assess what is being examined. Congenital colour deficiency usually involves red and green appreciation. Red and green are vital colours for drivers, pilots etc.

Light Sense

Adaptation to light or dark is measured by photometry and may indicate if the patient is suffering from vitamin A deficiency, or if retinal degeneration is interfering with the rhodopsin cycle which produces visual purple, the pigment needed for the chemical reaction to convert a light ray into a nerve impulse.

Chapter 59 Ophthalmic Nursing Procedures and Surgical Guidelines

PROCEDURES

Bacterial Eye Swab

A swab from the lower conjunctiva is routinely taken prior to ophthalmic surgery and before commencing antibiotic therapy. The patient is advised to look upwards and, while the lower eyelid is pressed downwards, a sterile wool swab is gently taken across the exposed conjunctiva from the nasal side of the eye to the outer aspect. The swab is immediately sealed in its container and correctly labelled with the patient's name. The container and the pathology form should both clearly state if the swab was taken from the left or right eye. Results of the culture and sensitivity tests on the swab are not usually available for over 24 hours. It is normal practice for the physician immediately to commence treatment pending the results.

Instillation of Eyedrops

As with any drug (Table 59.1), two nurses are required to check the drug container and the prescription chart before the drug is actually given to the patient. The nurse's hands must be thoroughly washed and dried before handling the drug container or touching the eye.

The patient's head, resting comfortably, is titled slightly backwards. If the patient is in a recumbent position, the chin should be tilted upwards. A sterile swab is placed and held against the lower eyelid margin and a slight downward pressure exerted to reveal the conjunctiva. With the pipette or drug container

Table 59.1. Commonly used drugs in ophthalmology

Group	Purpose	Name
Antibiotics	Infection	Chloromyecetin (chloramphenicol) drops 0.5% ointment 1% Genticin (gentamycin) drops 0.3% Soframycin (framyecetin sulphate) drops or ointment 0.5%
Local anaesthetics	To paralyse the local parasympathetic system	Cocaine hydrochloride drops 2 or 4% Benoxinate oxybuprocaine hydrochloride 0.4% Amethocaine hydrochloride 0.5 or 1%
Stains	To examine the cornea for abrasion	Fluorescein sodium 2% Bengal Rose 1%
Mydriatics	To dilate the pupil for examination of the retina and for surgery	Atropine sulphate 1 or 2% Homatropine hydrobromide 1 or 2% Mydrilate (cyclopentolate hydrochloride) 0.5 or 1% Phenylephrine hydrochloride 10% Topicamide (mydriacyl) 0.5–1%
Miotics	To constrict the iris and the diameter of the pupil, and also aid the drainage of aqueous humour	Eserine (physostigmine) 0.25 or 1% Pilocarpine nitrate 1–4% DFP (di-isopropylfluorophosphate) 0.01–0.05% Phospholine iodide 0.06 or 0.12%
Steroids	Anti-inflammatory agents	Predsol (prednisoline sodium phosphate 0.5%) Betnesol (betamethasone sodium phosphate 0.1%) Neo Cortef (hydrocortisone plus neomycin)
Diuretics	To reduce aqueous humour production and relieve high intraocular pressure	Diamox (acetozolamide)

held about 2.5 cm from the eyeball, release the drops into the middle of the conjunctival membrane as the patient looks upwards. Immediately following the instillation of the eyedrops, the patient should keep the eyelids closed for several minutes, and any excess tearflow is absorbed by the swab resting below the eyelid. Rubbing the eyelid is inadvisable as it will force the drug out of the eye.

Absorption of drugs via the conjunctiva is an unreliable method of giving drugs and repeated instillation every few hours is necessary if the drug is to be effective. Eyedrop containers are **not** interchangeable between patients, each eye having its own individual prescription supplied by hospital pharmacy. Also, eyedrops are **not** warmed before they are administered. The number of drops per instillation should be indicated on the prescribed container. On average, 6 drops per instillation are prescribed.

Application of Eye Ointment

It is usual to take a swab first for bacteriology sensitivity tests before commencing on a course of antibiotic ointment. The prescription chart should clearly indicate if the ointment is to be applied to the skin around the eye, to the eyelid margin, or to the conjunctiva.

Skin Application

For skin application the ointment should be squeezed from its tube onto a sterile gauze swab, which is then gently massaged onto the affected area. If this is to be combined with eyedrop instillation, the eyedrops should be instilled before the ointment is applied.

Eyelid Margin

Before the ointment is applied, the eyelid margin should first be bathed with normal saline to cleanse away any crusted material. Ointment is then massaged into the eyelid margin with the patient keeping the eyelids closed during the treatment.

Conjunctiva

Ointment to the conjunctiva is applied from a single dose container. The nozzle of the tube **must not** be touched when the tube is released from its outer package, and the nozzle should **not** touch the eyelashes during the application. While holding the lower eyelid downwards with a sterile swab, direct the ointment onto the exposed conjunctiva from the nasal side to the temporal side of the eye. The patient should then close the eyelids and excess ointment be removed with the swab. If both eyes are being treated, the ointment should be applied from different dispensers to reduce the risk of cross-infection.

Hot Spoon Bathing

The aim of hot spoon bathing is to steam the affected eye without applying direct heat. It is a comforting measure to the painful eye, which increases blood flow and hastens the absorption of drugs from the conjunctiva. Prior to hot spoon bathing, any drugs such as eyedrops or ointment should be administered.

A wooden spoon is padded with any absorbent type of material and then soaked in a jug containing 1 litre of boiling water. The patient should preferably be sitting at a table. If the patient is in bed, however, then the recumbent position is used with the patient leaning forwards over a bedtable which is firmly anchored or braked to the floor. Before commencing the treatment, ensure that the patient has a protective waterproof cape placed across the shoulders and thorax.

The padded spoon is held close to **but not** touching the closed eye so that the patient actually feels the heat. At the same time, the patient's head is brought forwards so that the eye feels the steam rising from the jug. This treatment should be continued for about 5 minutes and repeated for as long as it brings the patient relief from his or her pain. The eyelids and surrounding skin require to be dried with wool swabs after each treatment. Since boiling water is being used, the nurse **must** stay with the patient throughout the entire treatment.

Eyebathing

Eyebathing is a comforting procedure. It should always be done **prior** to the instillation of eyedrops or the application of eye ointment. The equipment used is sterile and the technique itself should be an aseptic procedure. Before proceeding with the treatment, the eye should be inspected for:

- Bruising or oedema of the eyelids
- Redness of the lower conjunctiva, i.e., infected conjunctiva
- Hazy or oedematous cornea
- Hyphaema or hypopyon of the anterior chamber
- Size and shape of the pupil
- Colour and shape of the iris
- Progress of any surgical incision or wound

The patient should be made comfortable in a recumbent position with the head resting on one pillow and be able to look upwards and downwards on request. The nurse, after carefully washing and drying the hands, wipes the sachet of normal saline clean with a steret before opening it and pouring the contents into a sterile gallipot. A sterile wool swab is moistened with the normal saline and the lower lid is swabbed in a single stroke from nasal side outwards. One swab is used for each stroke until all crusted debris has been removed. The same procedure is used for the upper eyelid. Both lids are then carefully dried with sterile wool swabs.

A major hazard is cross-infection between the eyes. Apart from always swabbing from the nasal side outwards, it is suggested that separate equipment be used for each eye and, in addition, the nurse **must** wash her or his hands thoroughly before proceeding to the next patient.

Trimming the Eyelashes

The advice of the surgeon should always be sought before cutting a patient's eyelashes. However, this procedure does reduce cross-infection hazards in ophthalmic surgery and makes subsequent eye-dressings easier. If cut, the eyelashes will grow again within 6 to 8 weeks, and the patient should be advised of this fact before they are trimmed.

An extremely good light-source is required to enable the nurse to see the eyelashes. With the patient in a recumbent position and his or her head resting on one pillow, the nurse should reassure the patient that what seems to be a cruel and possibly painful procedure is, in fact, quite painless and very swift, providing the instructions are followed as they are given, i.e., looking downwards with eyelids open for upper lashes, and upwards for the lower lashes.

A pair of blunt-ended but sharp-bladed scissors (ophthalmic type) are used and each blade is smeared with paraffin gel. This traps the hairs as they are cut.

As the patient looks downwards with the eyelids open the upper lashes are trimmed towards the nose. For trimming the lower eyelashes, the patient is asked to look upwards. It is unnecessary to cut the eyelashes immediately against the eyelid margin. Trimming eyelashes is never done on a conscious child and, if necessary, is done after the general anaesthetic has been given. This same option could be offered to very nervous or frightened patients. After each use the blades of the scissors should be wiped clean with sterile wool swabs to remove the paraffin gel.

Eye Dressings

Unlike other surgical dressings, ophthalmic wounds have to be dressed using the hands and fingers. It is essential that the nurse has an excellent handwashing technique, ensuring that the fingernails are absolutely clean and trim, so that there is never any risk of scratching the eyelids or cornea.

A basic sterile pack, along with sterile eyepads, blunt-ended sterile ophthalmic scissors and Moorfield's forceps, are prepared on a trolley or tray. With the patient in a recumbent position and the head resting on two pillows, the nurse must decide the most appropriate position from which to dress the eye. Some nurses prefer to stand behind the patient's head while others can manipulate the dressing more effectively when working from the side. In either position a good light-source is essential.

The eyedressing to be removed is usually retained by either a Cartella shield or an elasticated eyepad. These coverings should be removed without undue or unexpected movement of the patient's head. If the eyelids are sutured together (*tarsorrhaphy*), the single suture is removed using the ophthalmic scissors and Moorfield's forceps. Eyebathing may then be essential to encourage the eyelids to open without too much discomfort. Before proceeding with the dressing the nurse should inspect the eyeball and report upon:

Conjunctival infection
Hyphaema or hypopyon of the anterior chamber
Scleral wound edge approximation

A bacteriological conjunctival swab is then taken as a matter of routine for culture and sensitivity. Scleral or conjunctival sutures are only removed by a trained member of the nursing staff and the normal policy is that the first dressing following surgery is always done by a nursed trained in opthalmology.

After any sutures are removed, the whole eye and its external structures are bathed with normal saline before any further treatment is given, e.g., antibiotic ointments or eyedrops. A sterile eyepad is replaced over the affected eye and retained by either a Cartella shield or an elasticated eyepad.

NURSING GUIDELINES FOR INTRAOCULAR SURGERY

Increasingly, with the sophistication of intraocular surgical techniques, a patient's stay in hospital is likely to be very short, making 'day-patient' surgery common. However, the basic principles of care remain unaltered if the surgery is to be completed in safety, and the nurse makes a considerable contribution to the eventual outcome.

Hospital Admission

On admission to an eye ward the nurse should expect that the anxiety levels of a partially blinded or totally blinded patient will be higher than those of the sighted person. To reduce these levels of anxiety the nurse should use both the voice and physical contact to reassure and orientate the patient to his or her environment. This means walking with the patient, linking the arms. At the bedside, it is necessary to persuade the patient to touch and feel the bedside furniture and fittings so that he or she knows their precise location. This early orientation is essential for postoperative care when all required items not only should be within easy reach but also remain in the same place at all times.

Procedures

The usual pattern for obtaining written consent for intraocular surgery is observed but some emphasis should be given to the correct identification of whether it is the right or left eye which is for surgery. To avoid errors, abbreviations should not be used on any of the patient's documentation.

Conjunctival eye swabs are taken routinely for culture and sensitivity to any bacterial infection. If any are obviously present, an infection would delay the time of surgery. Infections of the upper respiratory tract or the lungs would likewise delay surgery, as would any coughing or sneezing which will raise intraocular pressure and disturb any incision made into the eyeball.

The lower colon should be empty or, if necessary, evacuated with the aid of 2 glycerine suppositories. The desire to defaecate may have to be suppressed for 2 to 3 days postoperatively because following major surgery, the act of defaecation also increases intraocular pressure. If necessary the eyebrows and eyelashes are trimmed (see p. 459). A broad spectrum antibiotic, e.g., chloramphenicol 5% eyedrops, may be instilled into the lower conjunctiva the day prior to surgery as a prophylactic measure.

Reducing the patient's anxiety

For many patients the anxiety level is reduced if the following details are discussed with them during the preoperative phase of care:

1. If one or both eyes are to be padded the patient will be nursed in full view of the nursing station so that any needs can be anticipated promptly and dealt with quickly. It should be stressed to the patient that any dressing covering the eye should not be touched by the patient and if it is causing discomfort the nurse should be asked to check the dressing.
2. If the eyes are double-padded the nurse will use the same technique each time she or he approaches the bed, that is, approach quietly and simultaneously address the patient by name and touch the hand or shoulder to indicate on which side of the bedside she or he is standing. Every procedure, however minor, will be preceded by a detailed explanation so that the patient will know how to cooperate.
3. If required to remain on bedrest for several days, the patient should be advised that unexpected movements of the head or other activities such as sneezing, coughing, blowing the nose or vigorous chewing will increase intraocular pressure. Smoking is obviously dangerous if the eyes are double-padded, but is normally banned anyway since the acrid smoke will irritate the conjunctiva. These activities all threaten the success of the operation and a detailed discussion may reveal that medical intervention may be needed to suppress them, e.g., a linctus to suppress coughing.
4. In general, the patient should be given a menu choice for all meals, but advised to select the softer foods for the first few postoperative days, unless prescribed a specific diet. A decision has to be made about the wearing of dentures; they are either to be retained or completely left out for several days postoperatively. If the eyes

are double-padded the nurse must feed the patient until visual independence is regained.

5. Relatives should be included in the preoperative counselling sessions so that they have been given exactly the same information. They may need to be guided on what gifts to avoid bringing into the patient who is double-padded, i.e., puzzles, books, magazines, newspapers or games. The radio may be a main diversion. Foods which require vigorous chewing should also be avoided and generally relatives should be persuaded to bring fruit in preference to bringing sweets.

Given this programme of advice, most patients relax since they have the knowledge with which to face what for many is an emotionally harrowing time, the underlying fear being the permanent loss of vision. However, in addition to counselling, a mild hypnotic given the evening prior to surgery to ensure a restful sleep is recommended.

Preoperative Care

In the immediate preoperative period the nursing plan should be flexible enough to ensure a fasting period of 4–6 hours before surgery is scheduled. After the general bath the hair should be arranged so that it is clear from the forehead and face. This should also be considered if the patient is to be double padded for several days. Facial cosmetics cannot be allowed and all jewellery must be removed. Premedication may take one of two forms or be combined:

Intramuscular injection of omnopon or pethidine.

Local anaesthetic eyedrops, e.g., cocaine 2 to 4%.

Mydriatics (to dilate the pupil), e.g., haematropine 1 or 2%

tropicamide 1%

mydrilate 0.5 or 1%.

usually instilled into the affected eye every 5 minutes until the pupil is widely dilated, which may take about 30 minutes.

Following the patient's physical preparation for surgery the nurse should then complete a check on the patient's documentation. This includes noting if the identity wristband matches the details on the documents, that the eye to be operated on is correctly identified not only on the patient's notes and consent form but also on the theatre operating list. The ophthalmic prescription sheets, observations charts and any pathology reports should all be assembled and taken to the theatre along with the patient.

Postoperative Care

Postoperatively, the patient remains in the recovery area until both the swallow and cough reflexes are regained. Once returned to the ward, the patient is gently lifted into a prepared bed, being careful to keep the head as still as possible. Quiet reassurance that the operation is over often settles the patient and prolongs sleep for a further few hours. During this period it is preferred that the patient be nursed in the semirecumbent position with the head and neck well cushioned by pillows. Any further lifting, moving or turning must be cautiously undertaken to avoid sudden or unexpected movement to the head.

Analgesia, anti-emetics, or sedation are invariably prescribed to ensure a restful first 24-hour period of recovery, and a quiet pleasant ward atmosphere is also essential to promote a calm and uneventful recovery. If the eyes are padded, it does not mean that the eyeball movement is restricted. The eyeball will turn reflexly towards the direction of any sudden noise. To reduce eyeball movement in the early phase of recovery, the nurse ensures that the environment is quiet.

The nursing plan of care following recovery will very much depend on how much independence of action the patient has, if double-padded it implies total dependence on nursing skills for the interim, while a partially blinded patient should be encouraged to do as much for himself or herself as possible. In any event, the needs of the individual such as personal hygiene, toileting, pressure area care, feeding or diet, oral toilet and hair care can be planned to fit in with the patient's day so long as he or she is confined to bed. When permitted to get up from bed the advice to keep the head still and avoid sudden movements must be repeated and on no account must the patient be allowed to stoop or bend. Otherwise, the intraocular pressure will rise and cause unnecessary eye pain. Straining at stool should also be avoided with the use of mild aperients, if required.

Dressings covering the eye will not be touched until indicated by the surgeon and the first dressing should always be done by a trained member of staff. If the eyelids are sutured together (*tarsorrhaphy*), the removal of the suture is usually painless but nevertheless still requires a skilled manipulative action for its removal. Thereafter, eye dressings, ointments and eyedrops may be done twice a day until the surgeon indicates the patient is fit for discharge from hospital.

Counselling for Discharge

Prior to being sent home the patient should have further counselling. If dark glasses are prescribed to be worn it is usually for 4–6 weeks. Thereafter, the patient will be tested again for lens prescription. Dark glasses reduce the glare of sunlight or bright artificial light and will aid the healing process within the eyeball. To this end, the patient should also be advised not to indulge in strenuous activity either at work or in sports.

The nurse should assess whether the individual who lives alone could possibly benefit from any of the community services, such as a home help, district nurse, or meals on wheels. This would only be for a temporary period until vision is fully restored. If drugs are prescribed, the patient will not be able to read any of the instructions on the container labels. The nurse will have to instruct verbally on what to do and show how to instil eyedrops or apply ointments, if these have been prescribed. Until instructed otherwise, the patient should avoid social events where bright lights are in use. Television may also present problems, as would the cinema or reading.

The complete healing process for intraocular surgery may take as long as 6 weeks and for this period the patient may have to live a quiet and undemanding life. The general practitioner should also be advised by letter of the type of surgery the patient has received and any further drugs required, since he or she will have to prescribe these. In every case of intraocular surgery, an outpatients' appointment is made. The nurse should consider whether transport is available to the patient so that he or she can keep this important follow-up appointment. If not, then an ambulance should be ordered to ensure that the patient keeps the appointments.

Chapter 60 Common External Disorders of the Eye

The proximity and direct connection of the orbital cavity with the nasal sinus and upper teeth make the eye socket a prime target for ascending infection and inflammation. If there is a craniofacial defect, either from a congenital cause or arising from a traumatic injury, this too makes the orbit more than usually prone to infection. An inflammation localised to the orbit is referred to as *orbital cellulitis* and, apart from pain and infection, it also induces a systemic pyrexia resulting in a very ill patient.

If the orbital space is reduced by any factor, it will force the eyeball forwards against the nonresistant eyelids, i.e., **proptosis**. The principal causes of a proptosis are tumours that may not always be amenable to surgery, located as they are in the orbit behind the eye. Examples of such tumours are sarcomas, melanoma, glioma, angioma and rhabdomyosarcoma. This last tumour, although rare, is seen in children.

The pressure exerted on the eyeball causes it eventually to become immobile, oedematous and infected eyelids develop, these factors contributing to a gradual loss of vision in the affected eye. A pseudotumour often confuses the diagnostic testing, but its presence would still cause the same symptoms. If the tumour proves to be cancerous, both surgical removal and a course of radiotherapy are attempted in an overall aim to save the vision. If the cancer is invasive to the actual orbital bone, the eye is *exenterated*, i.e., totally removed along with the connective tissues holding the eye in place within the orbit.

A second example of proptosis is when the

eye bulges forwards and is very prominently advanced against the eyelids, either as a result of thyrotoxicosis or as a consequence of treatment using thyroid stimulating drugs in myxoedema. This *exophthalmus* threatens to cause 3 problems; lid lag, conjunctival oedema and a paresis or weakness of the superior rectus muscle. Apart from medication or surgery to control the thyrotoxic state, the ophthalmic surgeon may recommend a tarsorrhaphy (suturing the eyelids together) to protect the cornea and eyelids from further damage, which may lead to problems with vision.

DISORDERS OF THE EYELIDS

There are many minor disorders of the eyelids that are usually dealt with in the outpatients departments. Occasionally, however, they are also seen in the acute wards of large hospitals, where the nurse may have to deal with them. These disorders are discussed below.

Blepharitis

Blepharitis is an infective inflammation of the sebaceous glands which line the eyelid margin, the principal pathogen being the *Staphylococci*. Predisposing conditions to a blepharitis are allergic conditions, adverse reactions to vaccinations, infectious childhood diseases and seborrhoeic dermatitis of the scalp. The eyelid margin appears very red, is obviously swollen and, if the area is ulcerated, threatens the integrity of the cornea. To soothe and cleanse the obvious irritation, frequent eyebathing with a solution of normal saline should be completed several times daily. An antibiotic ointment such as chloramphenicol 1% will in most cases control and defeat the infective organism.

Stye (Hordeolum)

A stye is a boil of the hair follicle (eyelash) as it stems from the eyelid margin. There will be extreme enlargement of the eyelid tissue since the lymphatic drainage of the tissue is blocked. To release the infective material, hot spoon bathing should be applied several times daily. This will bring a great deal of relief, though it may prove necessary to remove the eyelash to allow the infective material to escape, i.e. depilation.

Chalazia (Cysts)

The tissue within the Meibomian gland may granulate to form a cyst, usually on the tarsal surface of the conjunctiva. There is a noticeable swelling and the eyelid may be inflamed. If the cyst liquefies, the cyst content may discharge into the conjunctival sac and create an infection. If the cyst is relatively small, antibiotics may resolve the granulation. If the cyst is large, surgical excision may have to be done, which is followed by a course of antibiotic therapy.

Rodent Ulcer

A rodent ulcer is a basal cell carcinoma which may appear as a solid lump or more likely be seen as an ulcerated area which is extending from the eyelid towards the face. Surgical excision followed by a brief course of radiotherapy is the standard treatment once the biopsy proves positive.

Xanthelasma

Xanthelasma are patches of lipid material deposited on the submucosal layer of the eyelids, occurring mostly in the elderly, and may be indicative of either an undiagnosed diabetes or hyperlipidaemia. Such lipid patches are painless, but if the patient is very conscious of a cosmetic disfigurement, they can be removed surgically.

Trichiasis

Trichiasis refers to an eyelash which is growing inwards and into the conjunctiva and may be the cause of a great deal of discomfort as well as risking conjunctivitis. Surgery is required to remove the eyelash and the eyelid may have to be reconstructed, i.e., plastic surgery. This operation may be accompanied by electrolysis.

Entropion and Ectropion

Entropion is the term used when the eyelid turns inward, and when the eyelid turns outwards it is termed *ectropion*. It may be due to old age, a facial palsy, or fibrosis of healing tissue, i.e. scars or laceration. In all cases the normal tear flow is disturbed. In the case of entropion, the tear flow is prevented from crossing the cornea, and in ectropion the tear flow escapes over the conjunctiva in a constant spillage. The conjunctiva becomes thickened and the cornea may be damaged if the eyelid is turned inwards. The threat to both the lacrimal apparatus and the cornea may warrant a surgical reconstruction of the eyelid to ensure correct lacrimal drainage.

DISORDERS OF THE LACRIMAL APPARATUS

Obstruction either at the conjunctival sac, punctum, canaliculus or nasolacrimal duct can be simply proven by attempting to syringe the system. Often, syringing will release the obstruction. If it remains blocked there is excess tear flow escaping over the conjunctival rim onto the face, i.e. *epiphora*, and the ophthalmologist may attempt to probe the duct system while the patient is under general anaesthetic. If probing fails then an operation to construct a new opening between the duct and the nasal cavity, i.e., dacryocystorhinostomy, may be attempted. If the apparatus is inflamed, i.e., acute dacrocystitis, then it is usual for another condition such as conjunctivitis or keratitis to be present, which, when treated, allows the inflammation or infection of the lacrimal system to resolve.

CONJUNCTIVITIS

Inflammation of the conjunctival membranes may be attributed to one of the following causes:

- Bacterial infection
- Viral infection
- Allergic reaction
- Atopic conditions
- Chronic inflammation

The inflammatory process may be graded or classified as being either acute, subacute, or chronic. Whatever the cause of the conjunctivitis, the subsequent irritation produces a consistent series of symptoms. The conjunctival blood vessels become *injected* with blood, producing a hyperaemia, and there is an increased redness and a swelling of the membranes. This is accompanied by an increase in tear flow, although the eye feels dry and very gritty and is accompanied by a feeling of tightness in the eyeball within the orbit. The eyelids are swollen and it is only with difficulty and some pain that the patient can keep them open. The corneal endothelium is also irritated, causing the patient intense discomfort when in bright light, i.e., photophobia. If the cause is bacterial or viral, the conjunctiva may discharge a watery, serous, mucopurulent, or frankly purulent material. This would indicate the severity of the infection, as opposed to the inflammation. The infective type of conjunctivitis is highly contagious in overcrowded and unsanitary conditions, being transmitted by dirty towels or other articles. The causative organism is exogenous to the body, but present in the environment. Those who smoke a great deal, drink alcohol indiscriminately, or live or work in poorly ventilated rooms are more than usually prone to conjunctivitis.

Bacterial Conjunctivitis

The most frequently quoted pathogens which are causative of infective conjunctivitis are one of the following:

- Staphylococci species
- *Haemophillus influenzae*
- Pneumococci
- *Pseudomonas pyocyanea*
- *Neisseria gonococcus* (gonorrhoea)

The treatment of bacterial conjunctivitis follows two principles:

1. Frequent eyebathing with sterile normal saline at 4-hourly intervals during the day reduces many of the discomforts

caused by the symptoms and will keep the conjunctiva moist. The wearing of dark glasses may reduce the discomfort from the glare of sunlight or other bright lights. Despite temptation, the eyes *should not* be covered. This is important in the unconscious patient who may develop a conjunctivitis, from dust particles or pressure from pillows or bedsheets.

2. Chemotherapy following the identification of the causative organism after taking a conjunctival eye swab for culture and sensitivity. The following antibiotics may be prescribed:

Chloramphenicol eyedrops $\frac{1}{2}$% or ointment 1%

Systemic penicillin by intramuscular injection for *Neisseria gonococcus*

Systemic polymixin for *Pseudomonas pyocyanea*

Neomycin and bactricin are broad spectrum antibiotics for other pathogens

Viral Conjunctivitis

Although this is an infective conjunctivitis, the causative virus may not respond to antibiotics, which may still be prescribed to act as a prophylactic measure. Comforting measures, such as instilling artificial tears, often soothe the irritated conjunctiva. An untreated viral conjunctivitis may lead to the development of small patches of lymphoid tissue on the conjunctival membranes. These are referred to as *follicles*, hence the term *follicular conjunctivitis*. This latter condition may be transmitted in the water of public swimming pools and is one of the reasons why the water is heavily chlorinated. Another two types of viral conjunctivitis which the nurse may meet in the course of his or her work are inclusion body conjunctivitis and trachoma.

Inclusion Body Conjunctivitis

Inclusion body conjunctivitis is caused by the TRIC virus *Chlamydia oculogenitalis*. This virus is found in the genitalia tissues and when transmitted to the eye by touch will cause an inflammation of the conjunctiva after a short period of incubation, about 5–8 days later. The symptoms are usually well controlled with antibiotic therapy and the viral infection runs a very short course.

Trachoma

Trachoma is also a viral conjunctivitis caused by *Chlamydia trachomatis*, another TRIC virus. This form of conjunctivitis is highly contagious in Third World countries, being a major cause of blindness. The word *trachoma* is derived from the Greek meaning 'roughness', which partly describes the inflammatory process, the development of follicles and eventual keratitis (inflammation of the cornea). On healing, a considerable amount of scar tissue develops on the conjunctival membranes which causes aberrant eyelashes and corneal infection which will eventually limit vision and, if untreated, lead to blindness. The treatment plan offers a wide choice of options and may not always be feasible in Third World countries:

1. Prevention is the best avenue and can be achieved by public education, improved social and hygienic conditions and mass screening of a susceptible population in the endemic areas of the Third World countries.
2. Antibiotic therapy over a 2-month period will limit the active infection, e.g., topical application of chloramphenicol, albucid or tetracycline are the most frequently used.
3. Removal of the follicles from the conjunctival membranes by 1% silver nitrate.
4. Surgical correction of distorted and aberrant eyelashes and reconstruction of the conjunctival sac.
5. Corneal grafting, if there is a corneal opacity.
6. Instillation of artificial tears to maintain the moisture of the conjunctival membranes.

Chronic Conjunctivitis

Prolonged inflammation of the conjunctiva may be caused by repeated attacks of the acute type or by the repeated use of topical drugs, e.g., steroids. Mechanical disorders which may cause a chronic inflammation include;

1. Exophthalmos, or the forward bulging of the eyeball, which is sometimes seen in thyrotoxicosis.
2. Proptosis is very similar to exophthalmos, but in this case the bony orbit is gradually becoming too small for the size of the eyeball.
3. Facial paralysis, e.g., Bell's palsy, may cause the conjunctiva to droop and be constantly exposed to irritation.

Often the primary condition is amenable to treatment, in which event the chronic conjunctivitis will usually resolve. However, a chronic inflammation does lead to scar formation which may require surgical removal and perhaps some reconstruction of the eyelid to preserve the cornea from further irritation.

Allergic Conjunctivitis

The inflammatory response is most often seen during the late spring and summer months, when the pollen count is high. It is seen most frequently in children who tend to suffer from eczema, asthma, or hay fever (Spring catarrh). The conjunctiva is threatened by the development of *papillae*, which can be compared to conjunctival thickening. This can cause intense itching during an active inflammation. In addition the conjunctival thickening threatens the corneal surface, i.e., keratitis. Treatment is limited to the extremely cautious use of steroids, e.g., prednisolone eyedrops, which although anti-inflammatory do carry major side effects of both glaucoma and cataract in susceptible patients.

Atopic Conjunctivitis

Certain skin diseases may involve the conjunctiva as part of their pathology, i.e., acne rosacea, pemphigus and erythema multiforma. Often the inflammation is accompanied by an exudate, keratitis, fibrosis of the cornea, obstruction of the lacrimal ducts, and scarring of the conjunctival membranes. The symptoms of the skin disease may in fact disguise the threat to the conjunctiva, unless the physician takes time to scrutinise carefully the health of the external structure of the eyes. If the skin condition is successfully treated, then the threat of conjunctivitis retreats. However, an examination of the eyes remains of paramount importance in future therapy.

Chapter 61
Internal Disorders of the Eye

DISORDERS OF COATS OF THE EYE

Episcleritis or Inflammation of the Sclera

Episcleritis is often associated with rheumatoid arthritis or one of the collagen diseases. The sclera may heal spontaneously after either a deep or superficial inflammatory attack, but in so doing may cause the scleral coat to bulge and atrophy disturbing the mechanics and intraocular pressure of the eye. To prevent this the eye is treated during an acute attack with atropine eyedrops and steroids. Hot spoon bathing during an acute attack is very comforting to relieve the pain of increased pressure. Systemic phenylbutazone may be prescribed to deal with the associated collagen disease.

Corneal Grafting

The cornea of a cadaver donor, if removed and transplanted within 24 hours into a living eye, is very successful in dealing with the problems of a scarred cornea. The scarring may be the result of corneal ulceration, trauma or mechanical distortion. Corneal transplant is rarely if ever done during the active phase of a corneal disease. The grafted cornea is held in place by very fine suture material, i.e., 10/0 nylon, which is left alone for 12 months or more until the graft is secure. All transplants are subject to the risk of rejection by the host's immunological system, which considers the graft as a foreign tissue. Rejection risk is usually suppressed by the use of steroids given systemically for a period of time. The nursing care is very similar to that for any ophthalmic surgery.

DISORDER OF THE CHOROID (UVEAL TRACT)

The middle layer of the eye comprises the iris, ciliary body and, extending backwards to encircle the globe, the heavily pigmented choroid coat carrying the optical arteries and veins onwards to the retina. Inflammation of the iris and ciliary body (iridocyclitis) is known as *anterior uveitis*, while inflammation of the choroid coat (choroiditis) is a *posterior* inflammation. If the whole layer is affected the term *panuveitis* is used.

Anterior Uveitis (Iritis, Cyclitis, or Iridocyclitis)

Inflammation of the iris or the ciliary body may be either acute or chronic, being caused by a wide variety of primary diseases. The acute form can be caused by syphilis, ankylosing spondylitis, Reiter's disease and the allergies. Chronic uveitis is more likely to be due to tuberculosis, sarcoidosis, brucellosis, toxoplasmosis viral infections, or the cause may remain unknown, despite extensive investigation. The changes in the eye somewhat resemble glaucoma, but the pressure remains normal and vision remains good. The ciliary body becomes enlarged, being swollen with blood, the iris appears a muddy colour, the pupils are small and of an irregular shape, and the cornea may develop a thickening due to keratitis. In the chronic form there is a definite keratatic precipitation, and opacities can be seen in the vitreous body via ophthalmoscopy. If the uveitis causes a secondary glaucoma the patient will also suffer from orbital pain, photophobia, lacrimation and corneal oedema, all combining in a restless, anxious and very ill patient. Uveitis also predisposes to cataract and if the patient suffers repeated acute attacks the iris becomes atrophied. The most common symptom of uveitis is a blurring of vision and a gradual loss of peripheral vision.

As there is usually a primary disease, this will be receiving treatment systemically, but the local eye treatment usually involves the following:

1. Mydriatic eyedrops combined with hot spoon bathing to enhance their effect, e.g., atropine 1%, hyoscine 0.25%, cyclopentolate 1%, and phenylephrine 10%.
2. Topical steroids, e.g., Predsol eyedrops every 2 hours for acute uveitis.
3. Systemic steroids, e.g., Prednisolone 15 mg daily for posterior uveitis.
4. Systemic analgesia to control and relieve orbital and eye pain.
5. Topical antibiotics for proven infection.

COMMON DISORDERS OF THE RETINA

Macular Degeneration

The macula is the avascular point on the back of the retina which is most sensitive to light rays because of the vast number of rods and cones located in this area. Its degeneration occurs mostly in the older eye, but can be found in children, juveniles, adolescents, and in middle age. Its main symptom is the reduced appreciation of central vision. On examination the macula appears pale, there may be some pigment deposit and small haemorrhages. Sometimes a cyst develops, carrying with it the risk of a tear or hole in the macula itself. The physician may investigate to exclude or confirm the presence of hyperlipidaemia, which would cause lipids to be deposited in the macula. Central vision can be improved by prescribing telescopic lenses to enhance reading ability and near vision, and a second pair of spectacles for distant vision.

Retinal Detachment

The retina may detach itself from the choroid layer when there is a break or tear in the retinal layer, which allows vitreous fluid to escape into the subretinal space forcing the two layers apart. This break or hole in the retina may be due to primary or secondary causes. A primary cause is degeneration of the retina (occurring in old age), injury to the eye, or to vascular changes. Secondary causes include toxaemia of pregnancy, malignant melanoma of the retina, or vitreous haemorrhage. The eye is often myopic and on ophthalmoscopy the vitreous body may appear scarred as a consequence of any inflammation. The retinal folds press forwards against the vitreous body and alter vision. Perimetry can often determine the exact loss of vision from the peripheral field. Prior to any surgical treatment to re-attach the retina, a period of rest is recommended both for the body and eye itself. This may involve the instillation of a variety of eyedrops and the routine preparation for operation. The surgeon may employ one of the following methods to re-attach the retina:

1. Indirect diathermy or cryosurgery applied to the sclera immediately overlying the tear or hole in the retina will encourage union between the separated layers.
2. Photocoagulation will enhance the union between the two layers if the separation between them is minimal.
3. Drainage of the subretinal fluid via a small incision into the overlying sclera will allow the two layers to come together spontaneously.
4. Scleral resection shortens the eyeball and may be done if there is extreme loss of vitreous fluids.

Peripheral Retinal Degeneration (Retinitis Pigmentosa)

Peripheral retinal degeneration is mainly an inherited disease affecting both eyes, although the symptom of night blindness may not be complained of until the patient reaches adolescence. The deposit of pigment in mainly the peripheral retina increasingly migrates and branches to cover the whole retina. Thinning or 'attentuation' of the retinal arteries and optic disc atrophy contribute to a gradual loss of both central and peripheral vision, which may lead to complete blindness by middle life. Unfortunately there is no known cure at this time.

Retinal Vascular Disease

The retinal arteries frequently reflect the state of health of the systemic arteries and are often examined in great clinical detail to give some measure of the degree of both local and systemic illness. Retinal arteriosclerosis causes the vessels to become thickened and also narrow, making them easily become occluded. These changes can lead to retinal haemorrhage and thrombosis. The loss of vision may be either central or peripheral, or a combination of both depending on which part of the retina is affected. Systemic anticoagulent therapy often limits the degree of retinal damage and deeper investigations are pursued to establish whether the systemic blood vessels are healthy (especially the internal carotid artery and its branches). If the patient suffers from hypertension the retinal vessels may haemorrhage and the optic disc becomes oedamatous. Diabetic retinopathy often causes retinal venous dilation, haemorrhages, small aneurysms and retinal exudates. In addition, the diabetes may cause retinal haemorrhage into the vitreous body, i.e., retinitis proliferans, which is soon followed by the formation of fibrous tissue in the vitreous body. Occasionally the anaemias, e.g., pernicious anaemia, contribute to retinal haemorrhage and a retinal neuritis. Renal failure is often accompanied by hypertension and the raised blood pressure causes retinal oedema. The nurse must therefore also assess the visual problems the patient may be experiencing in all these primary diseases.

Cataract (See also *Nursing 1*)

By definition cataract is an opacity of the lens. Since the lens permits light rays to fall onto the retina any opacity will block the light ray leading to a gradual but increasingly severe blurring of vision within the affected eye. The protein, electrolyte and water content of the lens increases in density if the lens becomes dehydrated. This is a naturally occurring degenerative change in the ageing process, being the most common cause of cataract. However there are many other causes of lens opacity:

1. Congenital cataract. German measles in the first trimester of pregnancy can damage the developing lens of the fetus.

2. Hereditary cataract. In some families there may be a tendency for cataract to pass from one generation to the next, occurring in early adulthood.

3. Traumatic Cataract. Rupture of the lens capsule from a penetrating injury causes a dense opacity of the lens. Surgical procedures of the eye can also be regarded as traumatic insults leading in some instances to a cataract.

4. Inflammation. Chronic iritis will eventually cause a cataract tending to be an opacity of the aqueous around the lens, rather than within the lens itself.

5. Neoplasms. Tumours adjacent to the lens, e.g., the ciliary body, have an adverse effect on the lens capsule disturbing the lens contents.

6. Metabolic (Endocrine). A persistently raised blood sugar level does not reach the intraocular fluids, but indirectly induces an increased cataract at an early stage of untreated diabetes.

7. Ionising Radiation. Prolonged exposure to infrared light on the unprotected eye will lead to a classical cataract.

8. Toxic causes. Drugs, such as steroids, if used over a prolonged period of time induce degenerative changes within the lens.

An opacity can vary a great deal in its shape, size and position within the lens. The time taken to cause symptoms is also very variable, the earliest symptom being an awareness of some loss of central vision which is worse when in bright sunlight. On such occasions the pupil becomes very constricted. False haloes, i.e., orange rings around a light, can easily be confused with the haloes suffered by those with a glaucoma. If the opacity is placed centrally within the lens, the light rays are split equally and can cause double vision or diplopia. Diagnosis is relatively straightforward. Ophthalmoscopy through a dilated pupil will reveal the opacity as a silhouette against a red background. Visual acuity testing may be used to identify the best time when surgery can be offered, i.e., lens extraction. If the lens is soft, ripe and swollen it may rupture at any time, and surgery become more urgent.

Cataract patients are usually well screened in the out-patients department to exclude those diseases which would threaten the successes of the operation, e.g., upper and lower respiratory tract infections, or diabetes. Lacrimal syringing may be requested in addition to the normal preoperative care for eye surgery. Since the patient will be on bedrest for several days the nurse should ensure that they can cope with such things as bedpans, or urinals, can handle a feeding cup if they are singly or doubly eye-padded, and are advised on the limitations they will have for several days.

Prior to surgery, several conservative measures may be attempted; atropine eyedrops instilled 3 times weekly would be sufficient to keep the pupils permanently dilated to improve central vision. If the lens of spectacles is tinted with sodium yellow, it reduces the glare of bright sunlight preventing the pupil from constricting. However these are delaying tactics until the appropriate time for surgery. Several techniques may be employed to remove the lens: e.g., needling and aspiration of the nucleus of the lens, surgical evacuation and ultrasonic probe lens extraction.

Needling and Aspiration of the Nucleus of the Lens

A wide bore needle is directed through the corneal scleral junction to the pupil during a general anaesthetic. The lens nucleus is aspirated and this is immediately followed by replacing the extracted material with a salt solution to maintain the optical balance. The aspiration is possible because the lens material remains soft until about the age of 30, the operation can therefore be done on children and young adults, whatever the cause of their cataract.

Surgical Evacuation of the Lens

Surgical evacuation of the lens is completed by an incision around the corneal scleral junction. The lens is extracted via this incision by either forceps or a freeze probe. When the lens has been dislocated from its suspensory ligament, and both lens and lens capsule are removed, this is referred to as an extracapsular lens extraction. If however the lens cannot be dislocated, and this is increasingly difficult in the older eye, the lens capsule is referred to as an intracapsular lens extraction. The corneal scleral junction is then sutured and the eye covered. It takes between 4 and 5 days for the wound to heal completely.

Ultrasonic Probe Lens Extraction

Ultrasonic probe lens extraction is completed by directing sound waves via a small incision into the corneal scleral junction at the lens, giving an easy lens evacuation. However this procedure carries some risk of damage to the corneal endothelium, and is reserved for a few selected patients, with cataract.

Postoperative Care

Postoperative recovery is planned on a firm programme. The first dressing is always completed by the senior nurse on the first postoperative day. This may be no more than eyebathing, instilling prescribed atropine eye-drops, and checking the anterior chamber for hyphaema or hypopyon. If there is a risk of surgical iritis, then cortisone eye drops may also be prescribed at each daily dressing. Between the fourth and fifth day the corneal scleral sutures are carefully removed after a local anaesthetic has been instilled into the eye. Between these times the nursing plan should attain the goal of keeping the patient at rest, in the greatest degree of comfort, and without any vigorous movement of the head.

When plans are being made to send the patient home, a pair of dark glasses are normally prescribed to wear for a period of between 4 and 6 weeks. This will reduce the discomforts of bright glaring light. If the social assessment indicates the need for the primary health care team or social services, the nurse should implement these requests as soon as possible. After 6 weeks the patient is seen again in the out-patients department to be fitted with a powerful lens for both near and distant vision. A selected few may be fitted with contact lenses, but this depends to a great extent on the patient's tolerance and manipulative skill with such a small article.

GLAUCOMA

This term *glaucoma* describes a raised intra-ocular pressure, i.e., above 25 mmHg. The increased pressure is caused by either the glandular tissue of the ciliary body increasing its secretion of aqueous humour, or a failure within the filtration angle to drain away the aqueous humour into Schlemm's canal. A raised pressure of this magnitude is sufficient to cause optic nerve damage and dramatically reduce peripheral vision. One of several factors may cause this increased pressure:

1. The glandular tissue of the ciliary body is overproducing aqueous humour.
2. The filtration angle is partially or totally occluded, preventing excess humour draining from the anterior chamber via the filtration angle into Schlemm's canal.
3. There is an obstruction to aqueous humour flow within the Schlemm's canal or in the trabeculated veins.
4. There is damage to the vitreous humour behind the lens.

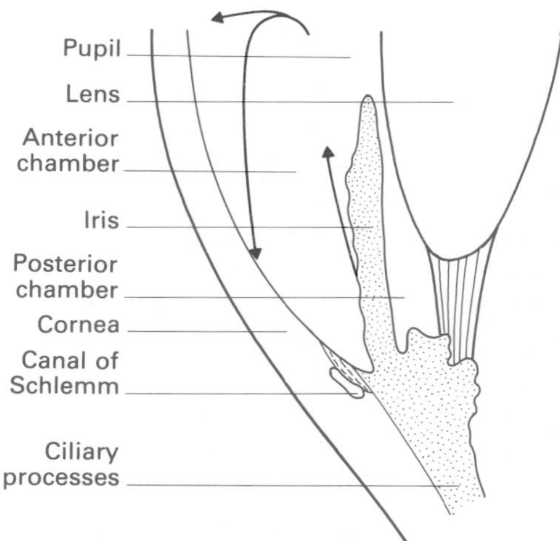

Fig. 61.1 Production, flow and adsorption of aqueous humour.

The condition may occur either as a congenital defect, or be acute, chronic or secondary to a primary disease. It may affect one eye or occur bilaterally. In each condition the physician would have to assess if the filtration angle is open or closed, and these latter terms may indicate if the obstruction is localised or at another point in the drainage system.

Congenital Glaucoma (Infantile) (Buphthalmos)

If the embryonic tissue within the anterior chamber fails to disappear it obstructs the filtration angle with a consequent increase in the intraocular pressure. To compensate for the increased pressure the sclera stretches, causing the eye to increase its tear flow. The Scleral stretching also causes photophobia. In appearance the cornea is hazy and if the condition is neglected the optic disc becomes damaged leading to blindness of the affected eye. Once diagnosed the treatment is by *goniotomy*. This is a simple needling procedure to clear away the embryonic tissue from the filtration angle. After recovering from the surgery, normal drainage and vision should then develop.

Chronic Glaucoma

Chronic glaucoma is a painless, symptom-free condition often confused by the patient with another eye condition, i.e., cataract. No symptoms are reported by the patient until they are aware of a loss of peripheral vision. The basic underlying mechanism is the disturbed balance which occurs between the pressure of the eye itself and the pressure of blood in the vessels supplying the optic disc. When the optical blood pressure is higher than the intraocular pressure, it prevents the drainage of aqueous humour. Often no cause can be found for the disturbance between the two pressures. Any signs are to be seen within the eye itself with coalescing patches from the blind spot to the macula. On testing with perimetry there is a marked loss of peripheral field vision.

Prevention of chronic glaucoma is possible if those who wear prescribed lens have their eyes tested at least every 2 years. Treatment for chronic glaucoma aims at either increasing aqueous drainage or decreasing aqueous production. This may be achieved by instilling eyedrops which will constrict the ciliary muscle, open the trabecular veins and pull the iris away from the filtration angle. For example

Parasympathetic drugs. Pilocarpine eyedrops, encourage aqueous drainage

Anticholinesterase. Eserine (neostigmine) constricts the pupil pulling the iris away from the filtration angle

Sympathetic drugs. Adrenaline, plus guanethidine, reduces the ciliary blood supply decreasing aqueous production

Carbonic Anhydrase Inhibitors. Acetozolamide (Diamox) is given systemically and reduces aqueous production

Diuretic drugs. Mannitol, urea, sorbital. Any of these may be given intravenously if the ocular pressure is excessively high

One or several of these drugs may be prescribed and, if successful, the treatment is for life. However the drugs are not often well tolerated and their side effects may be worse than the glaucoma. If the patient does suffer severe side effects, and tonometry proves a consistent high pressure and perimetry shows increasing visual field loss, then one of several surgical procedures may be offered to improve the aqueous drainage.

Trabeculectomy or Schere's Operation

This creates a fistula at the corneal scleral junction to create a new channel through which the aqueous humour can drain into the conjunctiva and then be absorbed into the conjunctival vessels.

Cyclodialysis

A cleft is created at the root of the iris between the ciliary body and the sclera to reduce aqueous humour secretion.

Cryotherapy

Freezing or applying diathermy to the ciliary body through an intact sclera may reduce aqueous humour secretion.

Secondary Glaucoma

As the term 'secondary' implies, a glaucoma may follow upon a primary disease in another part of the eye, or from a systemic illness. Iritis, cataract and dislocation of the lens all tend to block the blood flow through the trabecular veins, with a consequent increase in the intraocular pressure. An untreated diabetes, usually of mature onset type, also contributes to an increase in intraocular pressure. The primary disease must of course be treated first as a matter of urgency before the glaucoma reduces and destroys peripheral vision. Once the primary condition is stable, the glaucoma is treated as for chronic glaucoma.

Acute Glaucoma (Closed Filtration Angle Glaucoma)

A sudden increase in intraocular pressure is seen mostly in people with a long sighted eye, which has a shallow anterior chamber. Because it is shallow the anterior chamber hinders the pupil in its dilation and pushes the iris against the filtration angle obstructing aqueous flow. The eye is very painful and appears very red and angry-looking. In addition, vomiting, nausea and anorexic feelings can be quite pronounced and in severe cases of tunnel vision are accompanied by a blurring of vision.

Acute glaucoma represents an ophthalmic emergency, especially if the iris appears muddy coloured with corneal oedema. One of the effects of an oedematous cornea is to refract light into the rainbow spectrum, producing a rainbow circle which matches the size and shape of the cornea. These rainbow circles (which the patient can see) are 'haloes'. If these are complained of, a detailed ophthalmic examination should differentiate between glaucoma haloes and cataract rings.

The patient is obviously terrified by the severity and suddeness of their symptoms, being agitated and restless. Psychologically they have difficulty in comprehending the threat of sudden blindness. The prognosis, even with immediate surgery, is most uncertain and nurses should be cautious in their use of terms and reassurances should be phrased to avoid over-optimism.

Prior to surgery the patient may receive acetozolamide (Diamox) 500 mg intravenously to reduce the secretions from the ciliary body. Atropine or pilocarpine eyedrops are liberally instilled to try and open the filtration angle. The unaffected eye may also require some protection and pilocarpine or eserine eyedrops may be instilled. An emergency peripheral iridectomy (Trephining) is usually performed and this involves an incision into the iris to create a hole from which the aqueous humour can drain freely from the ciliary body to the filtration angle. After surgery the eye is kept covered and the patient advised to remain on bedrest for several days. When there is no apparent hyphaemia or hypopyon the patient can then be more independent. If the tension in the eyeball remains high, gentle massage over the closed upper eyelid may promote drainage as will hot spoon bathing. Any sutures are removed on the third postoperative day. A detailed assessment is made of the second eye to establish if this too requires a peripheral iridectomy in the next few days.

STRABISMUS (SQUINT)

The word *strabismus* means 'to turn' and refers to the inability of both eyes to fix simultaneously on an object and relay the image to the retina using binocular vision. If one eye cannot synchronise its movement to the other, it is impossible to have a single image, regardless of the angle or distance of the object in focus. The causes of poor binocular vision focusing ability are manifold and are shown in Table 61.1.

Diplopia or double vision can be suppressed by the squinting eye and results in the eye not being used at all (*amblyopia*). In this event the

Table 61.1. Causes of poor binocular focusing

Sensory input defects	Motor impulse defects
Poor illumination	Central vision defect
Incorrect lens prescription	Emotional distress
Ptosis	Teething
Cataract	Inability to learn
Penetrating injury	Orbital defects
Inflammation	Extrinsic muscle defect
Optic nerve lesion	Extraocular tumour
Poor proprioception	

eye will have very poor visual acuity and if the squint is left untreated there could be a complete loss of vision in the affected eye. For this reason diagnosis and treatment should be made as early as possible. Strabismus is most frequently seen in children, mainly because the optical reflexes are not fully developed until a child is about 5 years old. If there are any deep emotional problems children may experience difficulty in learning how to use their eyes. This can lead to what is commonly known as the *lazy* eye. The squint can take many forms, being either convergent, i.e., towards the centre, or divergent, away from the centre. The more serious forms of squint are when there is a paralysis due to a defect in the optical nerve pathway, or a paralysis of one of the extrinsic eye muscles responsible for moving the eyeball. A latent squint is in fact a symptom of an underlying disease, or defect in the structure of the eyeball, e.g., there is usually a refractive error of the lens, i.e., hypermetropia, astigmatism or presbyopia. There may be a chronic conjunctivitis, uveitis, glaucoma or keratitis. If the latent squint is accompanied by severe headache, there may be a need for deeper investigations to exclude retinal artery damage, sinusitis, or temporal arteritis.

The terms used to describe a squint include

Esophoria. Divergent and vertical squint combined

Esotropia. Convergent squint

Exotropia. Divergent squint

Hypertropia. Vertical squint

Phoria. Latent squint

Tropia. Manifest squint.

The tests used to confirm the degree of the squint include visual acuity of both eyes, the cover–uncover test, using a prism to assess the angle of deviation and ocular movement tests. Additionally, the Hess screen test can plot the amount of eye movement possible.

Treatment for Strabismus

Once the squint is proven, a series of treatments are possible to correct the deviation:

1. **Optical lens prescription** to improve the focusing ability and correct any refractive errors within the lens is the primary form of treatment.
2. **Occlusion therapy** involves covering the unaffected eye to force the 'lazy' eye to work by focusing, which therefore corrects the deviation. This treatment is reserved for children under the age of 8 years old. It both restores normal vision and reduces diplopia.
3. **Drugs** such as miotics would dilate the pupil and so help to correct a convergent squint if they are combined with orthoptic exercises over a period of 6 months.
4. **Orthoptic therapy** attempts to obtain and preserve normal central and binocular vision. The therapy consists of a series of exercises to improve extrinsic eye movement to correct the diplopia. As a bonus it also improves the cosmetic appearance, once the deviation is corrected, by placing the cornea in its central position.
5. **Surgery** is reserved for those occasions when it is necessary to either strengthen or release an extrinsic eye muscle. If an extrinsic eye muscle is 'recessed' it is released from its original point of insertion

and placed further back on the eye globe to tighten the muscle. A partial or marginal resection of an extrinsic muscle means that a small portion of the muscle has been excised and the muscle resutured. These operations should correct a mechanical defect of the muscles moving the eye.

The preoperative plan of care after surgery is that for any eye operation. Postoperatively it is preferred if the eye is left uncovered and bathed twice daily. Mydriatic eyedrops are instilled twice daily until any sutures are removed between the fifth and tenth post-operative day. A series of orthoptic exercises are arranged as an out-patient and the prescribed lens must be worn to improve the focusing ability of the affected eye.

NYSTAGMUS

Nystagmus is a disturbance of ocular movement in that the eyeball oscillates involuntarily in any direction, at any speed, and at any plane of possible movement. The disorder is either directly due to a disorder of eye movement, or to that of focusing. This uncoordinated oscillation may be due to a disturbance of either the third, fourth, or sixth cranial nerves which combine together to control eye movement. There is a common junction within the nerves and the brain stem.

Nystagmus is classified according to the part of the eye or brain which may be disordered, i.e., vestibular, cerebellar or retinal nystagmus.

Vestibular Nystagmus

Vestibular nystagmus is associated with the vertigo suffered in Ménière's disease, in which the apparatus for balance is diseased. It may also be seen in those patients who have had surgery of the inner ear.

Cerebellar Nystagmus

Cerebellar nystagmus is associated with the overdose of either barbiturate drugs or the anticonvulsant, phenytoin sodium, alcohol intoxication and multiple sclerosis. The co-ordinating mechanism of the three nerves in the brain stem are disturbed by all these factors.

Retinal Nystagmus

Retinal nystagmus will occur if the macula of the retina is impaired due to prolonged working in poor light. For example, due to persistent inadequate light, in the eyes of underground workers there may be difficulty in adapting the rods on the retina.

TRAUMATIC INJURY TO THE EYE (SEE ALSO ACCIDENT AND EMERGENCY NURSING)

Head Injuries

Fractures of the skull, or facial bones, and injury to the fascia may displace the orbital bones and cause a displacement of the eye

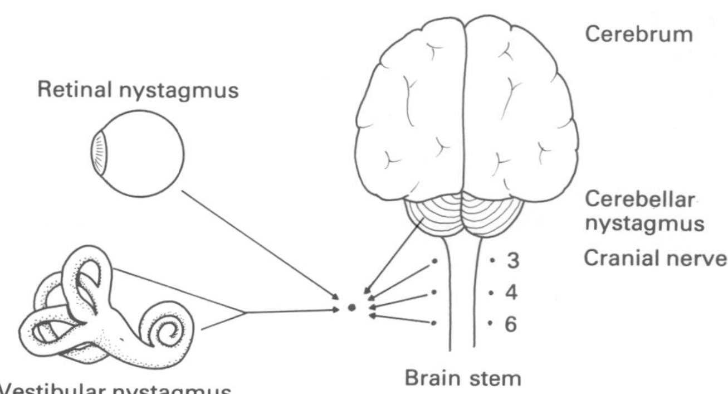

Fig. 61.2 Inco-ordination of eye movement.

globe with the immediate symptom of diplopia. If the orbital bones are 'blown out' it may force the eye down into the maxillary sinus causing an immediate increase in the intra-ocular pressure, i.e., papilloedema.

X-ray will demonstrate the site and severity of the fracture and an open reduction of the fracture is needed to restore the eye to its natural place in the orbit. This replacing of the eye, or elevation, may require that the eye rests on a piece of silicone or rubber for a short period of time.

Burns

Burns invariably result from chemical splashes. It does not matter if the burn is due to acid or alkali, the important principle is to irrigate the eye with copious amounts of water to remove the chemical. The eye changes which can occur, if first aid is not speedy, are corneal infection, scarring of the cornea and filtration angle and adhesion between the eyelids and sclera, and distortion of the eyelids. Alkalis are more dangerous as they tend to penetrate the coats of the eye with greater speed and damage the structure of the anterior chamber. The continued hospital treatment would be to continue the irrigations, instill atropine eyedrops, separation of the eyelids to prevent adhesions, and a course of steroids to limit the inflammatory effect of the chemicals.

Foreign Bodies

Minor irritations landing on either the conjunctiva or cornea can be either wiped off the conjunctiva with a wisp of cotton wool, or lifted off the cornea. After the foreign body has been successfully removed, the eye should be examined with fluorescin stain to ascertain if the cornea has been scratched or damaged. If so, then scarring or infection may establish itself, which can be treated by eyebathing and antibiotic therapy.

Perforating Injuries

Fragments of stone, metal or wood can enter into the eye. If entry occurs at great speed, the perforating object may lodge in the cornea and sclera, in which case a magnetic or forcep removal is carried out, followed by sutures. If the entry point is through the iris then a prolapse may occur, requiring an iridectomy, or if into the lens, a cataract may result.

Should the perforating object be metal, it will oxidise within the eye and deposit metal salts throughout the eye. It cannot be over-emphasised that the consequences of perforating injuries require expert treatment by an ophthalmologist if the complications are to be avoided and, where necessary, correctly treated.

Blunt Non-perforating Injury

A blow to the eye can cause bleeding into the anterior chamber, block the filtration angle, dislocate the lens, cause vitreous haemorrhage, choroid and retinal oedema, retinal detachment and avulsion of the optic nerve. Any disturbance of vision, however vague, therefore requires the expert opinion of an ophthalmologist before any treatment is embarked upon. The basic things which can be done are to keep the patient at rest and perhaps to apply antibiotics as a prophylactic measure until expert treatment is prescribed.

Laceration of Eyelids

Cuts, however minor, to the eyelids whether on the skin surface or of the conjunctiva require to be sutured within 24 hours of their occurrence. If the edges of the lacerated tissue are not correctly approximated and sutured with delicate expertise, a small cleft can develop through which the tears will constantly water. This is an intractable condition unless it can be prevented within 24 hours of injury.

Chapter 62
Structure of the Nose and Paranasal Sinuses

STRUCTURE OF THE NOSE (Fig. 62.1)

The nasal cavity boundaries extend from the roof of the mouth to the base of the skull in its midline. The nasal septum lies anteriorly, while the posterior nares form the posterior wall. The lateral walls of the nasal cavity are composed of the turbinate bones. Contributing to the structures of the nasal septum are a series of bones and cartilages. The principal bone is the vomer, a thin bone plate from which, extending backwards, is the ethmoid bone and, even further back, the sphenoid bone. Extending forward from the vomer is the septal cartilage which divides the nasal cavity into 2 chambers. The cartilage in fact gives shape to the external nose and, at the anterior nares, it possesses some muscle which allows the nares to dilate in respiratory exertion. Covering both the bone and cartilage is a rich vascular and mucous secreting membrane. Immediately above the nose the cribriform plate of the ethmoid bone is located and penetrating the many air cells of this bone

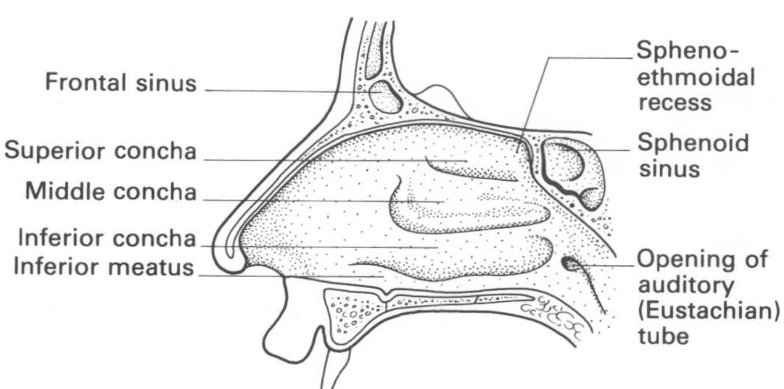

Fig. 62.1 Internal structures of the nose.

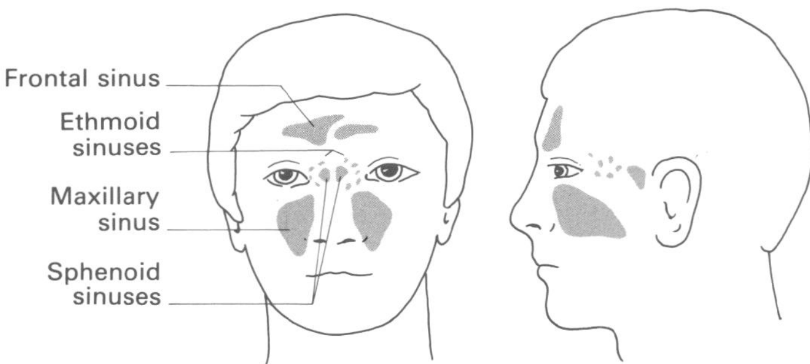

Fig. 62.2 The nasal sinuses.

are the terminations of the nerves for smell, i.e., the olfactory nerve.

On either lateral wall of the nasal cavity the turbinate bones or concha are arranged in a series of 3 ridges from below upwards. The space between each ridge is referred to as the meatus, respectively termed the *inferior*, *middle* and *superior* meati. It is into these spaces that the sinuses drain. The lacrymal duct drains into the inferior meatus. The middle meatus drains the ethmoidal air cells, the frontal and maxillary sinuses, while the superior meatus drains both the ethmoid air cells and the sphenoidal sinus.

The blood supply for the nasal cavity is derived from branches of the upper carotid artery, i.e., the ophthalmic and ethmoid arteries. A group of tiny vessels located at the Little's area, which is just behind the skin fold at the bridge of the nose, is very poorly supported and tends to rupture easily giving rise to epistaxis. In addition to the terminal branches of the olfactory nerve at the cribriform plate, the nose has further sensory appreciation from the sphenoidal and maxillary nerves.

The nasal cavity is the first part of the respiratory tract and has a number of important functions:

1. Inhaled air is filtered by the ciliated epithelium to remove dust particles.
2. Inhaled air is moistened by the mucous secreting cells.
3. Inhaled air is warmed as it passes over the capillaries invested within the mucosa.
4. Nasal resonance contributes to the quality of speech.
5. Affords drainage of the paranasal sinuses to the outside of the body.
6. Sensory appreciation of atmospheric odours.

CLINICAL EXAMINATION OF THE NOSE

The specific equipment which should be prepared for the doctor prior to the examination of the nose includes:

An angle-poise lamp
Forehead mirror
Various sizes of nasal speculae
Disposable and metal tongue depressors and tissues
Nasal cotton buds (orange sticks dressed at the tip with sterile cotton wool)
Post-nasal mirror
Spirit lamp with matches
Tilley's nasal forceps
Receiver for used instruments
Paper bag for used disposable items

For the examination the patient is seated facing the doctor. The angle-poise lamp is positioned behind the patient's left shoulder, its light beam directed at the aperture of the forehead mirror which the doctor will be wearing. In turn, the light will be reflected back from the mirror surface of the post-nasal mirror, if it is used, to inspect the nasal mucosa or posterior nares (Fig. 62.3).

The external nasal skin and structure are inspected for obvious abnormality of shape, size, contour, infection or inflammation. To test the patency of either nostril, the patient

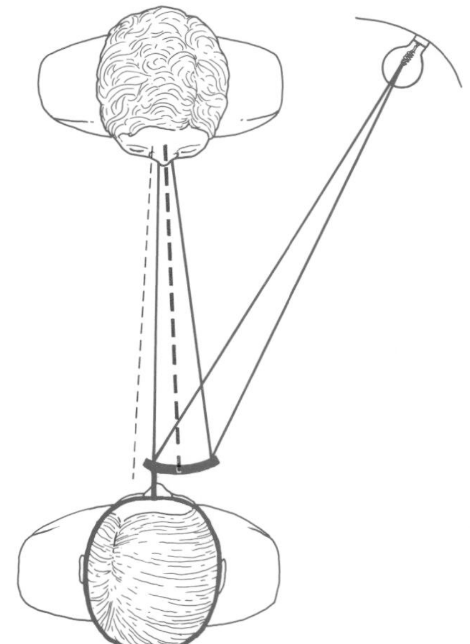

Fig. 62.3 Head mirror in use.

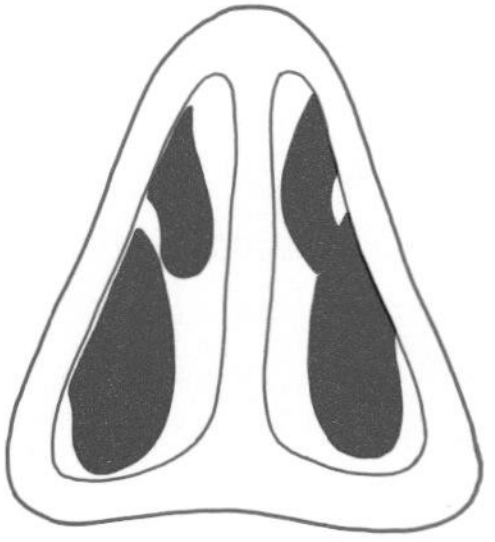

Fig. 62.4 Anterior rhinoscopy—the septum is slightly deflected to the left.

will be asked to breathe though only one nostril while the opposite one is sealed. An obstruction to inhaled air may be suggestive of sinusitis.

Prior to inspection of the interior nasal mucosa, it may be necessary to cleanse the mucosa using a sterile nasal bud or ask the patient to blow his nose. Should there be any oedema of the mucosa, this can be effectively shrunk by the instillation of a solution of adrenaline 1 in 1000 combined with cocaine to reduce the swelling. Nasal speculae are inserted to facilitate the inspection of the upper nasal mucosa. This is usually followed by an inspection of the posterior nasal space, using the angle-poise lamp and forehead mirror as the light source (Figure 62.4).

If local treatments are prescribed, e.g., nasal drops, the nurse should first ascertain if the doctor would like nasal swabs to be taken for culture and sensitivity tests. To instil nasal drops, the end of the pipette dropper is advanced into the nostril for 1–3 cm and at least 6 drops of the prescribed drug inserted. The patient's head is then tilted as far back as it will go, and kept in this extended position for at least 2 minutes. This will permit the drug to reach the post-nasal space. After the procedure, the patient should be provided with tissues to mop away excess nasal flow, and be offered a mouthwash to rid the mouth of any unpleasant taste which commonly follows the insertion of nasal drops.

THE PARANASAL SINUSES

No functions are attributed to the paranasal sinuses, except to say that since they contain air they may help to lessen the weight of the skull. If they became inflamed, infected, or blocked, the air in these spaces becomes stagnant leading to further infection. Interesting aspects of the sinus are as follows:

The sphenoid sinus is in direct relationship with the pituitary gland above. This gland, lying in the sella turcica of the sphenoid bone and the sinus itself, drains downwards. From a surgical point of view the pituitary gland can be approached via the sphenoid sinus, and operations on this gland have beome an ENT speciality.

The frontal sinus is not fully developed until about the age of 7, and until then it is in direct communication with the meninges surrounding the frontal lobe of the brain. The lining mucous membrane of the frontal sinus is continuous with that of the nose, and drains into the middle meatus.

The ethmoid sinus consists of three groups of air cells thinly partitioned from each other and located in the lateral area of the ethmoid bone.

The maxillary sinus (antrum of Highmore) extends from the upper maxilla to the turbinate bones and is closely related to the upper teeth. This close proximity makes the maxillary sinus prone to infection from decaying teeth, or tooth abscesses.

The mucous membranes of the nose and sinuses are affected and can be damaged by the use of antiseptics, alcohol, tobacco, snuffs and ointments. The use of drugs is very limited on or within the nasal cavity.

Chapter 63
Common Nasal Disorders

ACUTE AND CHRONIC SINUSITIS

The air-containing paranasal sinuses are in direct contact with the nasal cavity, via openings or ducts known as *ostia*. The ostia are not always at the base of the sinus, so drainage into the nasal cavity cannot be guaranteed. Additionally, the mucous membrane lining the sinuses is continuous throughout, although of a less complex structure than the nasal cavity. The size of the sinuses is also another predisposing factor to infection. The frontal and maxillary sinuses (antrum) are large, but superficially located, while the sphenoid and ethoid are small and deeply placed. This implies that the frontal and maxillary sinuses are more prone to infection. Like the nose the sinuses have mucous secreting cells and ciliated epithelium which sweep any particle debris along a moist surface towards the nose. Acute infection of the sinuses is due to a number of common factors:

1. Direct spread from the infected nasal cavity.
2. Septal deviation, preventing normal sinus drainage into the nasal cavity.
3. Dental caries of the upper mandible, infecting the maxillary sinus in particular.
4. Nasal polyps obstructing the sinus drainage into the nasal cavity.

As an acute infection develops within the sinus, this causes a series of changes which account for the more common complaints of headache, pyrexia, nasal discharge, tenderness and swelling over the frontal or maxillary bone. The changes causing these symptoms are:

Hyperaemia, or the increased blood flow into the sinus

Oedema of the sinus mucosa

Hypersecretion from the mucus producing cells

Leucocyte infiltration into the sinus causing the formation of pus

Treatment

In the vast majority of cases the simple treatment is bedrest, until the pyrexia resolves, an antipyretic drug, e.g., Aspirin, an antibiotic taken systemically, liberal oral fluids and repeated moist inhalations followed by the instillation of Ephedrine nasal drops $\frac{1}{2}$–1% into each nasal chamber. This will be sufficient enough treatment to improve the drainage of the sinus. Repeated attacks of acute sinusitis, however, will tend towards a chronic inflammatory condition. If this occurs, there will be irreversible loss of the mucosal lining of the affected sinus. With the loss of the ciliated epithelium, the tendency for a chronic infection is very high and the doctor may have to resort to a variety of treatments, these being to effectively drain the sinus. Three common procedures are:

1. Antral puncture and lavage (also known as a proof puncture since it confirms the presence of pus)
2. Intranasal antrostomy.
3. Caldwell Luc operation.

Antral Puncture (Proof Puncture)

The Antral Puncture procedure is both diagnostic and therapeutic. It is visually a rather unpleasant treatment, and the patient requires a great deal of reassurance throughout. The equipment normally required for this procedure includes:

A jug containing 1 litre of normal saline at a temperature of 37.8 °C.

An instrument tray containing

Lichtwitz antral trocar and cannula for a first puncture

Roses antral trocar and cannula for second treatments

20 ml syringe

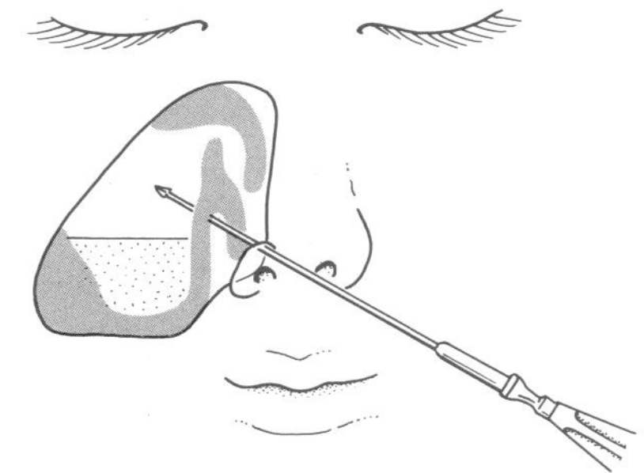

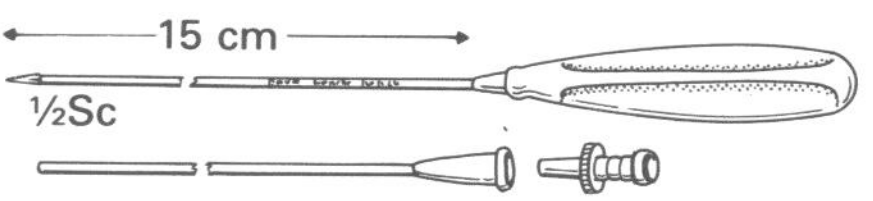

Fig. 63.1 Position of trocar and cannula in proof puncture of the right antrum with detail of the Lichtwitz trocar and cannula below.

Nasal speculae

Wool applicators

Higginson's syringe and adaptor

Cotton wool and swabs

A lotion tray containing

Local anaesthetic, e.g., nasal spray cocaine 5 and 10%, or lignocaine 4%, plus adrenaline or cocaine ointment

Mouthwash, already prepared

Emetic bowl and tissues

Lotion thermometer

Receivers for waste material and intruments

The patient's upper garments should be loose, and constricting clothing, i.e., jackets, should preferably be removed. The patient is then given a protective shoulder cape to wear to prevent soiling of his or her clothing. It is best if the local anaesthetic is applied to the nasal mucosa with the patient in the dorsal position. Once it has taken effect, the patient is sat upright and made comfortable, sitting slightly forward, and given a receiver to hold which will collect the drainage fluid as it escapes from the sinus washout. The anglepoise lamp is adjusted to enable the doctor to visualise the inferior turbinate area into which the antral trocar and cannula is directed until it punctures through into the maxillary sinus (antrum). The trocar is then removed and the Higginson's syringe is attached to the cannula using the adaptor. A well-fitting seal is absolutely vital. The normal saline is drawn into the syringe, checking that it is at a temperature of 36.6 °C. By regular compression of the bulb of the syringe the sinus is flushed out, removing debris trapped in the sinus. A great deal of the fluid will escape via the nose and should be collected into the receiver. The washout material is retained, if requested by the doctor, for a sample to be sent for culture and sensitivity testing, or cytology. After the washout the doctor may inject antibiotics into the sinus before removing the cannula. In some instances, when repeat antral lavage may be necessary, the doctor may elect to insert a polythene tube which remains *in situ* for the duration. It is secured in position by a piece of adhesive tape on the cheekbone. During and after this procedure the nurse should be aware of the following possible hazards:

1. Fainting. This risk is reduced if the patient is correctly positioned, seated with the head slightly tilted forward and the nurse standing at the side of the patient as a support in case of swooning or giddiness.
2. Severe pain. This results if the natural openings of the nasal cavity from the sinuses are blocked by mucosal oedema.
3. Accidental puncture of the occipital orbit, or injury to the malar tissues, may occur. The immediate application of a cold compress will limit the expected swelling.
4. Obstruction of a residual polythene sinus drainage tube. This is more likely if the tube is ever compressed by the inadvertent use of forceps or clamps to mistakenly stop free drainage.

The most common causative pathogens which are cultured from antral washout fluid are the *Streptococcus pyogenes*, *Staphylococcus*, *Pneumococcus* and *Haemophilus influenzae* and once identified the appropriate antibiotic may be prescribed. Even with systemic antibiotics it may be necessary to repeat the antral lavage once daily, for 5 days, to resolve a chronic infection.

Intranasal Antrostomy

In the event that a repeated antral puncture has failed to resolve the chronic infection, and the problem of an ineffective sinus drainage still remains, an opening can be created in the inferior turbinate bone. To achieve this the bone is either dislocated upwards or partially removed by punch forceps, and a 'window' created by a perforating instrument. Once enlarged by an antral chisel, the sinus should drain effectively. At the time of operation a great deal of pus tends to erupt from the sinus and this must of course be thoroughly mopped away and the sinus washed out. This is followed by the instillation of antibiotics, or by ephedrine to shrink the oedematous mucosa. This operation is quite successful in the younger patient aged between 10 and 14 years old.

Caldwell Luc Operation (Radical Antrostomy)

Caldwell (American) and Luc (French) simultaneously described this operation towards the end of the last century. Essentially it is reserved for those patients with chronic sinusitis, with irreversible loss of the mucous membrane of the maxillary sinus. These patients may have undergone repeated antral lavage without success and X-ray shows a dimming in the outline of the sinus and a persistent fluid level. The patient is prepared for a general anaesthesia and the preoperative care should include careful oral hygiene and a check for dental health of the upper teeth. An incision is made into the upper gum margin above the canine and the first and second molar teeth, after the general anaesthetic has been supplemented by local anaesthesia of the incision area. A gouging instrument or dental drill is then used to enter the maxillary sinus via the exposed bone. The hole is then enlarged by bone nibbling instruments which enables the sinus to be cleared of infected purulent material using suction apparatus. The dead mucous membrane is stripped out. A second hole is then made into the inferior turbinate bone which will drain into the nasal cavity. The original incision is closed with soluble catgut sutures.

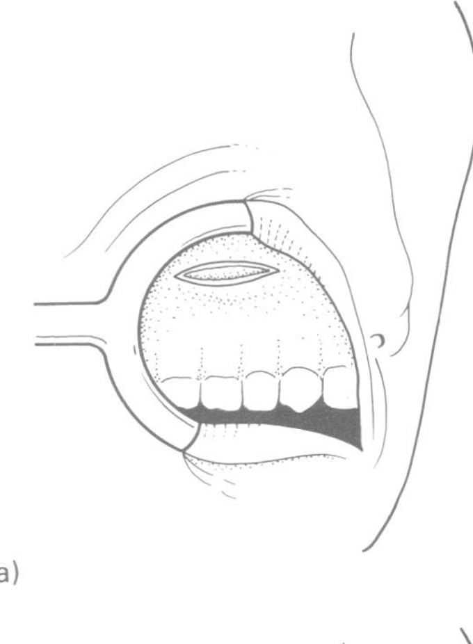

(a)

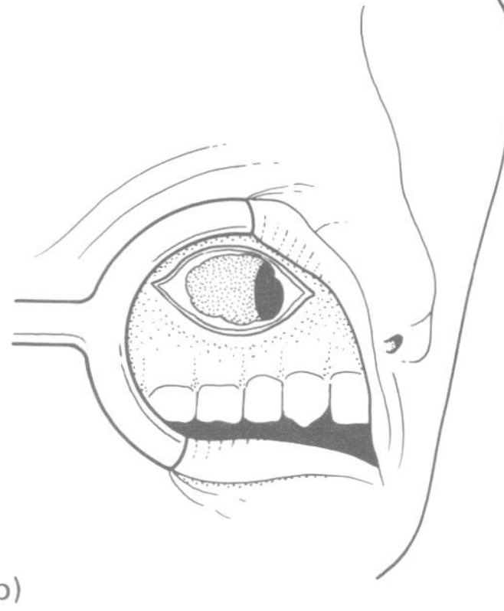

(b)

Fig. 63.2 Caldwell-Luc operation. An incision is made into the mucoperiosteum of the right canine fossa (a); a large window has been made in the medial wall of the antrum providing free drainage into the nose (b).

During surgery the oral cavity is loosely packed with light gauze to prevent any debris entering the pharynx and escaping down into the trachea. The nasal cavity may be packed to absorb any blood escaping from the maxillary sinus. On recovery from general anaesthetic the patient should be nursed in the upright sitting position to aid sinus drainage. The nursing plan should take into account the following measures to promote comfort:

1. Restlessness can be expected and in extreme cases may require a potent analgesic such as morphia.
2. Persistent headache may be relieved by giving a mild analgesic every 4 hours, e.g., 2 aspirin tablets.
3. Oral hygiene is of paramount importance and mild antiseptic mouthwashes should be given every 2 hours during the daytime.
4. The threat of infection is contained by the administration of a 5-day course of broad spectrum antibiotics.
5. If the nasal cavity has been packed, the earliest time the pack can be removed is usually 24 hours after surgery. Preferably, pack removal should be done by the surgeon or the most senior nurse. If bleeding is persistent, the nasal cavity may have to be repacked and, following pack removal, pulse and blood pressure observations for 12 hours should be implemented to detect any possibility of bleeding. Until the pack is removed, a nasal snuffler should be secured to the upper lip to absorb any nasal excretions.
6. Steam inhalations every 4 hours will help to shrink the nasal mucosa and aid drainage of the congested nasal cavity.
7. As soon as it can be tolerated, the patient should be encouraged to wear his or her dentures.
8. Any facial swelling over the malar area or near the occipital orbit may respond to applied heat, e.g., a warm dry towel placed over the area at regular intervals.
9. Smoking cigarettes should be absolutely forbidden, as this habit will increase nasal congestion and definitely spoil any chance of a permanent cure, i.e., the congestion tends to close the newly created drainage hole.

Ethmoidal Sinusitis

This condition causes a localised headache between the eyes and is accompanied by a nasal and post-nasal discharge. If the condition does not respond to conservative treatment the chances of a chronic inflammatory sinusitis increase. If of a chronic nature, the ethmoid sinus can develop polypoid growths. Surgery to strip out irreversibly damaged mucous membrane may be either by an intranasal or extranasal approach. For an extranasal approach the eyebrows may have to be trimmed, and immediately before surgery the eyelids are smeared with sterile petroleum jelly. Some surgeons will suture the eyelids together for the duration of the operation. The incision to reach the ethmoid is made between the nasal bridge and inner angle of the eye. Tissues overlying the ethmoid are separated until the bone is reached. After creating a hole through which some of the ethmoid air cells are removed, a second hole is created which leads directly to the nasal cavity.

Apart from the general care plan outlined for the Caldwell Luc operation, an additional point to note is that the incision wound requires daily wound toilet and a very small drain may have to be secured by one suture. This should be removed after 24 hours. Once the orbital swelling has receded, usually about 48 hours later, the wound area can be left exposed. The affected eye and orbit will be very bruised and usually requires antibiotic eyedrops, e.g., sulphacetamide 10% instilled every 4 hours for several days. The eye should be rested by applying a comfortable lightweight sterile eyepad.

DEVIATED SEPTUM

Another condition which effectively reduces sinus drainage into the nasal cavity is when the nasal septum is deviated, or deflected, either to the left or right. When a current acute or chronic infection has been resolved the surgeon may propose to correct this deformity by completing a submucous resection to prevent further attacks of sinus infections. This realignment of the septum will also improve nasal breathing and the tonal quality of speech.

Treatment

Preoperatively, specific attention should be given to the facial cleanliness, e.g., shaving off of a moustache and, if required, a nasal toilet. In addition to a routine premedication (e.g., omnopon 10 mg and scopolamine 0.6 mg thirty minutes prior to surgery) local

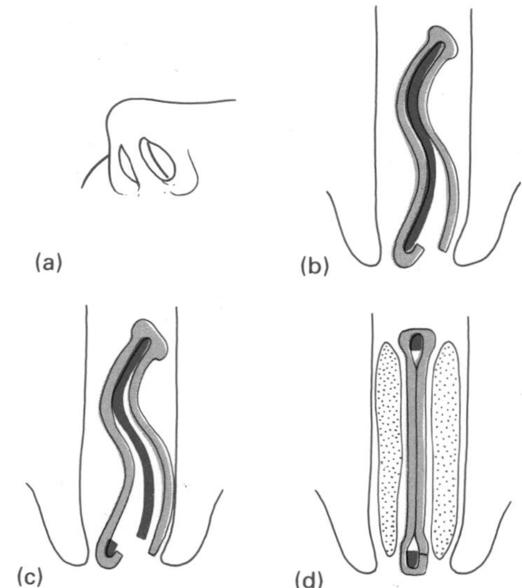

Fig. 63.3 Submucous resection of the septum. The incision (a) and diagrammatic transverse sections (b, c, d) showing the separation of mucoperichondrium (shaded) from the underlying cartilage and bone (blue). In d, the packs (stippled) have been inserted.

anaesthesia of cocaine 10% may be instilled into each nostril to complement the general anaesthetic.

When in theatre the general anaesthetic is further complemented by a second local injection into the nasal mucosa of either xylocaine or nupercaine. Although the operation can be done using local anaesthetic alone, it is fraught with unpredictable patient reactions and it is preferred to combine general anaesthesia with local anaesthetic. A longitudinal incision is made into the nasal mucosa of one side of the septum. The mucosa is then carefully elevated to reveal the underlying cartilage and bone. The second incision is made into the cartilage to gain access to the opposite side of the septum where the nasal mucosa is also freed from the septum. With the bone exposed the excess can be chipped away and the septum re-aligned and straightened. Before replacing the nasal mucosa over the bone and cartilage, the airway is double-checked and cleared if necessary by suction. No sutures are used, but the mucosa is fixed to the bone by either nasal packing or septal splinting. This will approximate the incised edges of the mucosa. The type of pack used is variable: ribbon gauze soaked in liquid paraffin or a rubber finger cot filled with gauze are two possible and typical examples. A nasal snuffler is applied to the upper lip and secured by adhesive tape to the facial tissues.

Postoperative Care

Postoperatively after full recovery from the general anaesthetic, the patient should be nursed sitting upright. This will aid drainage of the nasal sinus and cavity. The nasal pack is crucial to prevent a haematoma from forming between the mucosa and the underlying bone and cartilage. Hence, it can be regarded as a pressure pack. It is usually left in position for up to 48 hours to control any tendency towards bleeding. Problems arising from the pack, however, tend to be those of difficulty with swallowing, the sensory loss of taste and smell, and a dry oral mucosa from oral respiration. Until the pack is removed, these discomforts can be partially overcome by frequent oral toilet, and plenty of sips of clear, bland but nourishing fluid. Sleep can be a problem because of the nasal pack and also the localised pain. Analgesics are normally prescribed on an 'as required' basis, for at least 48 hours, along with tranquillisers or night sedation. Frequent changing of the nasal snuffler after each mouthwash, if possible, will also add to the patient's comfort.

Prior to the removal of the nasal pack the patient must be warned **not** to blow the nose in case of disturbing the incision edges and inducing any bleeding. After the surgeon has removed the pack, preferably with the patient under the effect of a mild sedation, the patient should be allowed to rest for at least one hour. The expected improvements will not occur immediately, at least not until the nasal mucosal oedema has resolved, and this may take up to 2–3 weeks. Steam inhalations (tincture of benzoin) preceded by instillation of ephedrine nasal drops are standard procedures after the pack has been removed.

Before discharge from hospital, the patient **must** be warned against taking part in any strenuous activities or sports, since either may cause an epistaxis. A quiet holiday would be most appropriate since the patient cannot return to work for at least a month. If a nose bleed does occur, the patient must seek hospital treatment immediately. The risk of a submucous haematoma remains high for some time and this may lead to an abscess.

NASAL POLYPS (Fig. 63.4)

Characteristically benign polyps can be described as tags of fibrovascular gelatinous tissue arising from oedematous nasal mucosa. These projections of tissue may be the result of either an allergy or chronic inflammation. Single polyps tend to multiply and can obtrude from the nasal cavity, when large enough. They can arise from the mucosa of the ethmoid sinus, turbinate bones and maxillary sinus. Their obstructive nature interferes with sinus drainage, nasal respiration and can be the cause of infections as well as inducing the typical 'nasal' speech. When both nasal cavities are obstructed in the posterior nares

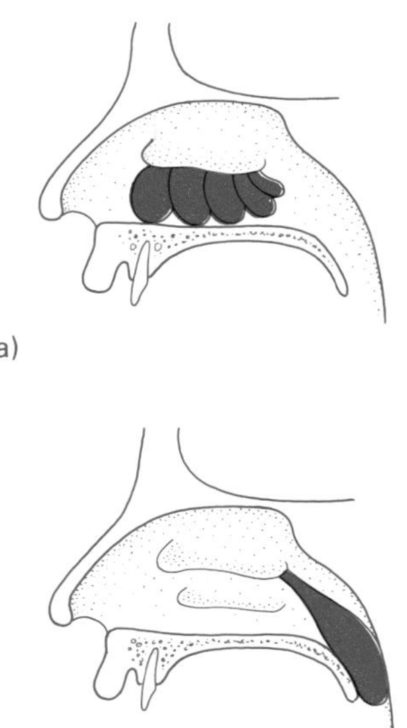

Fig. 63.4 Nasal polypi. Ethmoidal polypi (a) hanging beneath the middle turbinate and obscuring the inferior turbinate. A single antrochoanal polypus (b) filling the nasopharynx.

by the presence of polyps, it is described as *choanal polypi*. In this position, they are truly obstructive. If the surface membrane of a polyp ruptures, it will cause an epistaxis or, if infected, a purulent discharge. Occasionally a polyp will resolve spontaneously, or is blown out when the patient blows the nose vigorously. In the last resort, they can be removed by a snare instrument, i.e., polypectomy, when the polyp is divorced from the underlying mucosa. Some bleeding can be expected and may be effectively controlled with diathermy at the time of surgery. For the more severe cases of blood loss, a 24-hour pack may be required.

ALLERGIC RHINITIS (HAY FEVER)

Irritation of the mucosa of the upper respiratory tract is usually due to the pollens of grasses, household or industrial dusts, spray cosmetics, fungal moulds, and proteins from the furs of domestic pets. More rarely it can be due to food allergy. At first the patient is very conscious of a severe itching sensation at the anterior nares. This is followed by excessive watery nasal discharge, violent sneezing episodes and increased tear secretions. The causative agent in irritating the tissues causes the mucosa to release histamine. This chemical substance induces the reaction and as part of the process causes a mucosal oedema, usually of such intensity as to cause a nasal obstruction.

Immediate relief is usually obtained by taking one of the antihistamine group of drugs, e.g., piriton or phenergan. Otherwise there is little one can do at the time of the actual attack. If the offending substance can be identified from intradermal patch testing, a course of subcutaneous injections with the substance heavily diluted may gradually desensitise the patient. A programme of such injections, carefully planned to precede a seasonal increase in pollens, may be very effective. Each dose is increased until the programme of injections is completed.

EPISTAXIS (SEE ALSO ACCIDENT AND EMERGENCY NURSING)

By far the greatest cause of a nose bleed is that of trauma, but other frequent causes include:

Nasal polyps or tumours
Chronic nasal infection
Hypertension
Rhinitis
Blood dyscrasia, especially those related to deficiency of vitamins C and K
Prolonged anticoagulent therapy
Allergic reactions causing severe sneezing
Irritation of the mucosa from a foreign body
Congenital nasal deformity
Chronic and vigorous coughing

The greater majority of patients with epistaxis are treated in an accident and emergency department, where the initial therapy would be to contain the consequences of shock resulting from what at first appears to be a large blood loss. The patient is nursed in the sitting position with the head inclined forwards, the nasal cavity is cleared of blood clots by blowing the nostrils clear. Then the nasal alae are compressed together for at least 10 minutes while the patient is advised to breath though the mouth. Tight restricted clothing is released from around the neck and waist. If this fails to arrest the bleeding then the doctor may insert a nasal pack soaked

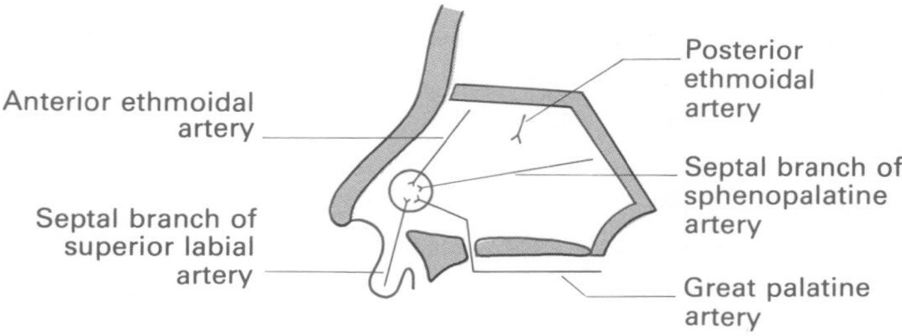

Fig. 63.5 The blood supply of the nasal septum. Little's area is within the circle.

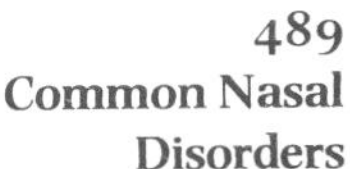

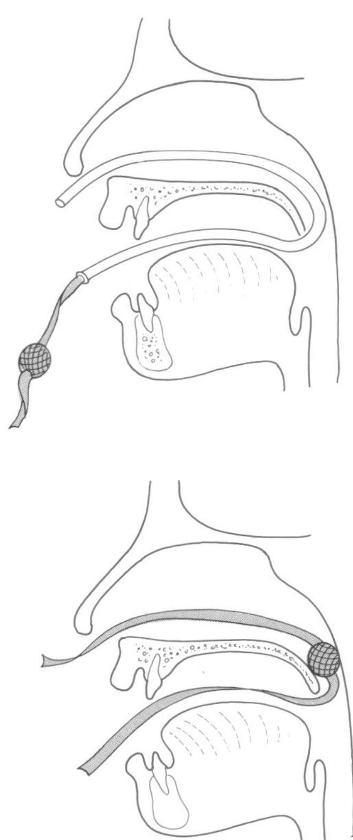

Fig. 63.6 Insertion of a postnasal plug with the catheter inserted (*above*), the leading tape, nasal plug and trailing tape are pulled into place (*below*).

with adrenaline 1 in a 1000 or cocaine 10%, and advise admission into hospital.

Once made comfortable in bed in the upright sitting position, an injection of morphine may be prescribed. This will reduce both the blood pressure and the restlessness of the patient. In addition to the nasal pack absorbing any blood, a nasal snuffler is applied to absorb excess seepage escaping from the nostrils. Repeated observations of blood pressure and pulse are vital to monitor the degree of 'shock', frequent swallowing movements should also be observed for and reported without delay as this means that blood is escaping from the posterior nares to the stomach. The period of bedrest is usually for 48 hours. This, combined with the nasal pack and sedation, may be sufficient to stop the nose bleed.

After the nasal pack has been removed it is important that the bleeding point is identified. If the point is unilateral, the bleeding may be due to a slight trauma, if however it is bilateral it suggests a constitutional disease such as hypertension. The point of bleeding may arise from either:

Little's area, approximately $\frac{1}{4}''$ within the nasal cavity. This point usually responds to an anterior nasal pack left in position for about 24 hours.

Anterior Ethmoidal bleeding tends to obstruct both the mastoid sinus and the eustachian tube, affecting the patient's hearing.

Posterior nasal space bleeding point is a very serious haemorrhage with a copious blood loss. Both the anterior and post-nasal space have to be packed in the first instance.

Either diathermy or silver nitrate cautery can be used to seal the bleeding point once the haemorrhage is under control.

A loss of blood is always difficult to assess by volume and therefore the patient will usually have both his or her haemoglobin and packed cell volume measured by a blood test. If these are below normal values, then grouping and cross-matching for 2–4 units of blood may be necessary for a transfusion, either immediately or at a later interval. When the patient has recovered from the initial epistaxis the doctor will usually proceed to investigate the underlying cause, requesting a variety of tests to eliminate any of the suggested causes mentioned at the beginning of this section. After recovery, the risk of fainting when first ambulated is very high and the nurse should take the precaution of remaining with the patient for several minutes until he or she is settled into an armchair. Useful measures to remember in caring for a patient recovering from an epistaxis are his or her appreciation of very cold drinks, frequent oral toilet, and ice cubes to suck. They also need a great deal of rest in a quiet atmosphere and, until treatment is concluded, night sedation is a prerequisite.

Chapter 64
Structure and Examination of the Ear

STRUCTURE OF THE EAR

In the study of the ear the nurse should constantly bear in mind its dual function of hearing and balance. The ear can be divided into three distinct compartments: outer, middle and inner ear.

Outer Ear

The outer compartment of the ear is formed of cartilage tissue arranged in a funnel shape so that it can collect sound waves. Generally the outer ear is referred to as the pinna or auricle, the outer edge being known as the helix while its lower edge is named the lobe or lobule. The cartilagenous funnel arrangement leads into the external auditory canal or auditory meatus. Hair follicles protruding from the meatus are derived from sebaceous glands, which also secrete sweat, and specialized cells which secrete a wax-like substance called cerumen. This wax-like substance has the function of keeping the ear waterproof, but is also often the cause of deafness when there is enough to occlude the external meatus. This skin of the external canal is tightly in line with the underlying bone tissues and any inflammation or infection is very painful since the area is well supplied by sensory nerves and blood vessels. The external ear is also drained by a considerable number of lymph vessels, which are placed behind, below and in front of the ear. The lymph glands and vessels enlarge in some infectious diseases such as mumps, but otherwise they are rarely involved in disease processes of the

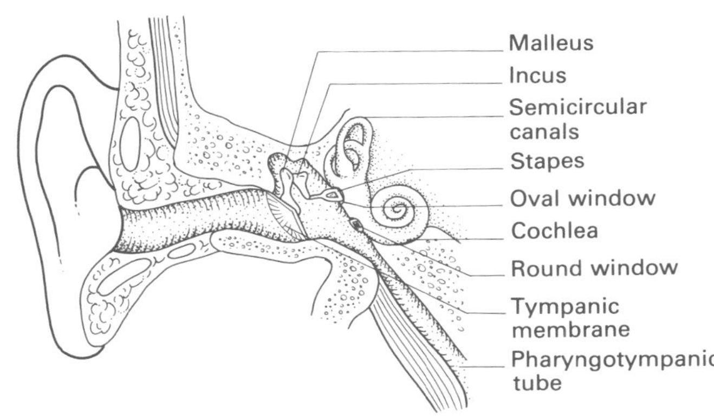

Fig. 64.1 Internal structure of the ear.

ear. The external auditory canal is about 4 cm in length and is S-shaped. The first third of this canal is composed of cartilage, while the last two-thirds is of bone, covered with mucous membrane.

Middle Ear

The middle ear is an irregular shaped cavity situated within the petrous portion of the temporal bone. Although of an irregular shape, for the purpose of study it can be regarded as a six-sided box.

Its entrance, or outer wall, is formed by the tympanic membrane, the only wall not to be formed from bone. The tympanic membrane is composed of three tissues:

1. An outer layer of stratified epithelium continuous with the outer ear.
2. A middle layer composed of fibrous tissue.
3. An inner layer composed of cuboidal epithelium continous with the inner ear.

The roof of the middle ear is formed from a thin plate of bone, also known as the tegmen, which separates the middle ear from the temporal lobe of the brain and is one possible source of infection up into the brain.

The floor of the middle ear separates the ear from the soft tissues and the great vessels entering and leaving the base of the skull.

The inner wall is made of a bony partition into which are built 2 openings covered by membranes. These are the 'windows' by which sound is transmitted onwards into the inner ear. The fenestra ovalis (oval window) leads to the vestibule, while the fenestra rotunda (round window) leads to the cochlea.

On the anterior wall, the pharyngotympanic tube (Eustachian) opening leads to the nasopharynx. In the act of swallowing, the tube opens to allow air to enter the middle ear from the nasopharynx. This ensures that the pressure is equal on both sides of the tympanic membrane so that the membrane can vibrate in response to soundwaves. Should the tympanic tube be blocked for any reason, the tympanic membrane loses the ability to vibrate, hence the deafness so often seen with patients suffering from catarrh.

The posterior wall communicates with the mastoid bone via a structure known as the additus (or tube), which delivers air to the mastoid air cells.

The middle ear is occupied by three tiny bones called the ossicles, and these can be remembered by the capital letters: M, I, S, in that order from the tympanic membrane to the oval and round window, i.e., malleus, incus and stapes. Once the sound waves cause the tympanic membrane to vibrate against the malleus, a chain reaction is set against the incus and stapes. The footplate of the stapes comes into contact with the oval window and the sound waves continue into the inner ear, stimulating the perilymph and endolymph of the cochlea and the semicircular canal. The 3 ossicles are held in place by small ligaments and moved by minute muscles. Since the tympanic membrane is larger than either the round or oval membranes, sound waves are much more concentrated before they reach the inner ear. To maintain the equilibrium within the middle ear during the transmission of soundwaves, the round window is pushed outwards while the oval window is pushed inwards.

The Inner Ear (Labyrinth)

The inner ear comprises 3 irregular shaped structures, each having its own distinct function, i.e., the vestibule, cochlea and semicircular canals. All 3 structures are contained within the petrous portion of the temporal bone.

Vestibule

The vestibule is a tiny irregular shaped cavity whose wall is interrupted with the oval and round windows. Leading from this cavity are the cochlea and semicircular canals. The cochlea is the organ of hearing, while the semicircular canals are the organ of balance.

Cochlea

The bony cochlea is similar in shape to a small shell, the bone turning upon itself $2\frac{1}{2}$ times from base to apex around a central column of bone known as the modiolus. Within this odd shaped cavity lies a membranous tube. In effect there is an outer bony tube and an inner membranous tube. Separating the bony tube from the membranous tube is a fluid known as the perilymph while the membranous tube contains a second fluid known as endolymph. These fluids are of the same composition as cerebrospinal fluid and arrive into the tubes from minute canals in the temporal bone. The spiralling cochlea has in fact 2 compartments within itself: the scala vestibule and scala tympani both containing perilymph. Within the membranous tube lies a basilar membrane known as the Organ of Corti, along the length of which there are fine hairs which move in response to soundwaves of a given pitch. These fine hairs transmit the soundwaves via the auditory or cochlear nerve to the hearing centre within the brain.

In summary the soundwaves stimulate the tympanic membrane to vibrate, creating a chain reaction along the ossicles within the middle ear. These, in turn, cause the oval and round windows to vibrate. The vibrations then stimulate the perilymph in the bony tubes, which in turn stimulate the endolymph within the membranous tube and the hairs on the basilar membrane conduct the sensory impulses of sound for further interpretation to the brain. Sound waves travel at 0.2 miles per second, or 1088 feet per second, and are conducted by air in the outer and middle ear and then by fluid (endolymph) in the inner ear. Finally, via nervous impulses, to the brain.

Semicircular Canals

These are 3 hoop shaped bones, each having a diameter of about 1 mm and set at right angles to each other. Each is at a different plane, and is associated with the balance of the body. At the base of the semicircular canals are the structures which communicate with the vestibule of the ear, these being the saccule, utricle and ampulla. Both the utricle and the saccule have fine hair cells and nerve fibres which together form the vestibular branch of the eighth cranial nerve, i.e., auditory nerve. The ampulla to each canal have their openings at the round and oval windows. Movement of the head causes movement of the endolymph and perilymph within the saccule, utricle and the canals. The vestibular branch of the auditory nerve passes to the cerebellum which registers the body's position (balance) in relationship to space. Equally important in the awareness of balance by the brain are the movements of the eyes, and the sensations from the sensory and motor nerves of the joints and muscles.

CLINICAL EXAMINATION OF THE EAR

Essentially two functions of the ear are routinely tested if the patient presents with any type of complaint, i.e., hearing or balance. Either of these functions can be affected singly or in combination. The following items of basic equipment should be available to the doctor to conduct a clinical examination:

Head mirror
Angle-poise lamp
Aural speculae of variable diameters
Battery or electrically operated auriscope (tested for function)
Applicators dressed with cotton wool buds
Angled aural forceps
Siegle's speculae and magnifier
Politzer bag
Eustachian catheter (soft metal silver)
Tuning forks of variable frequencies and pitch

If possible the patient should be seated sideways to the examining doctor and the light beam from the angle-poise lamp directed from behind the patient's head. If the patient is being examined in the dorsal position, the head should be turned onto the unaffected side. On those occasions when children are being examined, it is best to ask the mother to nurse the child on her knee. If necessary a restraining blanket can be offered to restrain the child's arm during the examination.

The auricle and pinna of the outer ear are visually examined for obvious abnormality, e.g., infection, discharge, inflammation, or oedema. Before inspecting the auditory canal it is a useful precaution to dry mop the external tissues of any debris using a dry sterile piece of cotton wool dressed on a disposable applicator. A suitably-sized aural speculae is attached to the auriscope for a lighted inspection of, firstly, the cartilagenous portion and then the bony area immediately before the tympanic membrane. To straighten the natural S-shape of the auditory canal the auricle of the ear is lifted upwards and slightly backwards. An improved view of the tympanic membrane is provided with the Siegle's speculae and magnifier. The speculae also has an attachment to provide for air inflation, if required.

Disease or obstruction of the Eustachian tube, the most common cause being cerumen or wax (see Ear Syringing, p. 494) which leads into the middle ear from the nasopharynx, will cause deafness. The following tests may be used by the doctor to confirm the presence of conductive deafness due to pharyngotympanic disease:

1. Valsalva's manoeuvre.
2. Politzer's method.
3. Eustachian catheterisation.
4. Hearing tests.
5. Balance tests.

Valsalva's Manoeuvre

An outward bulging of the tympanic membrane can be seen with the auriscope in the healthy ear if the patient is asked to pinch the nostrils together and blow air against the closed mouth. The air will not obviously bulge the tympanic membrane if the Eustachian tube is blocked. This manoeuvre is not used for children or those with traumatic injury to the ear.

Politzer's Method

Politzer's method is a test often used for children. The nozzle of the Politzer bag is gently inserted in one nostril and both nostrils pinched together. The child is then asked to swallow (in so doing, the Eustachian tube will open) and air is compressed into the middle ear and note is made if the tympanic membrane bulges outwards.

Eustachian Catheterisation

A Eustachian catheter is made of silver, being a soft malleable metal. It is passed along the floor of the nose until its tip reaches the opening of the Eustachian tube located in the nasopharynx. Once the tube tip is in position an air bag is attached to the tube and air compressed directly into the middle ear. If the Eustachian tube is patent, the doctor should be able to hear the rush of air into the middle ear via a stethoscope. If the air 'whistles' the tympanic membrane may be ruptured so accounting for an ineffective Eustachian tube. If the air noise 'bubbles' it may suggest a purulent infection. If the Eustachian tube is only mildly blocked, the air flow will clear the tube and therapeutically restore hearing.

Hearing Tests

Hearing tests using a tuning fork can indicate if the patient has either a **conductive** or **perceptive** type of deafness. The number inscribed on a tuning fork should indicate the vibrations per second of which it is capable when struck upon a firm surface. The greater the frequency of vibrations the higher the pitch of sound. While still vibrating, the tuning fork is held at a given distance from the ear being tested for air conduction of sound. If held against either the temporal or frontal bone, the patient is being tested for bone conduction of sound. The healthy ear can hear whispering speech from a distance of 3–4 m. A second hearing test would be to stand behind the patient and assess if whispering speech can be heard by either the left or right ear and then to measure the distance at which it was first heard.

Often in middle or inner ear disease the patient is relying solely on sound conducted via bone and therefore only loud speech will be appreciated. More precisely, hearing tests usually take the form of audiometric tests. In this test the sound is produced electrically, the patient being asked to respond to the quietest sound perceived at a given pitch. Each ear is tested separately and the results are depicted on a graph to indicate the severity of the deafness. The degree of deafness can be of a different intensity in either ear, and to distinguish this inequality the ear not being tested is masked by the noise from a Barany's box. While the Barany's box is masking one ear, the examining doctor asks the patient to repeat a series of words, phrases or numbers spoken into the unmasked ear.

Balance Tests

Balance tests are employed if the patient complains of vertigo, nausea, vomiting, or has evidence of nystagmus (fluttering eyeballs). With any of these symptoms the patient may have disease of the vestibule of the ear. Two of the tests are used to stimulate the inner ear (labyrinth), and thus the perilymph and endolymph of the semicircular canals: the rotation test and caloric test.

Rotation Test

In the rotation test, the patient is seated in a rotating chair and turned until nystagmus is induced. The actual test is to time the period it takes for the nystagmus to resolve, i.e., no longer than 2 minutes for a healthy inner ear. If no nystagmus occurs it is considered that the inner ear has lost the function of registering balance.

Caloric Test

The caloric test employs the same principle as for the rotation test, but uses hot or cold water as the stimulus. With the patient in a dorsal position and the head supported with one pillow, or at an angle of 30°, cold water (30° C) is introduced into the ear over a timed period of 40 seconds. The eyes are then observed for nystagmus. The duration of the nystagmus is carefully noted. The test is then repeated on the opposite ear after a period of 5 minutes' rest. The whole process is then repeated on each ear using hot water (44° C) and the nystagmus recovery time is recorded.

Nystagmus can now be measured electronically and with much greater accuracy, noting not only the recovery time but the speed, frequency and amplitude of the nystagmus, which are more important than duration.

Syringing the Ear

Ear syringing is a relatively safe, easy and reliable method of removing debris from the external auditory canal. It can be used as a method to remove wax, foreign bodies or infected material such as pus and dead epithelium. However, ear syringing is not done on those patients with a perforated ear drum, or where there is acute inflammation of the external or middle ear.

Removing Wax

Wax (hardened cerumen) may be removed by syringing after it has been suitably softened by one of the following techniques:

1. Instillation of warm olive oil or

paraffin liquid ear drops, twice daily for 3 days prior to syringing.

2. Instillation of 6% solution of sodium bicarbonate solution immediately prior to syringing.

3. Preferably, wax should be softened with one of the cerumenolytic agents 30 minutes before syringing, e.g., Cerumol, Waxsol, or Xerumenex.

Removing Foreign Bodies

Removing foreign bodies from the external auditory canal may be achieved by syringing. Impacted objects, providing they are rounded with a smooth surface, are readily loosened by this method but vegetable material (e.g., garden peas) will swell on contact with water and should, if possible, be removed by probe and forceps. If not, removal of this type of material should be done under general anaesthetic. Insects trapped in the ear require to be floated out using a few drops of warm olive oil followed by gentle ear syringing.

Removing Infected Material

To remove infected material, such as pus and dead epithelium, syringing must be done prior to an examination of the tympanic membrane.

Equipment Needed

The equipment required for ear syringing is set out below and should be assembled on a tray prior to examination:

A 50 ml metal aural syringe, or alternatively a Higginson's syringe

Tilley's forceps

A jug containing either plain tap water or a 1% solution of sodium bicarbonate at a temperature of 38° C

Protective cape and towelling for the patient's shoulders

Ear buds for drying the external canal after syringing

An auriscope and speculae to examine the external canal before, during and after syringing

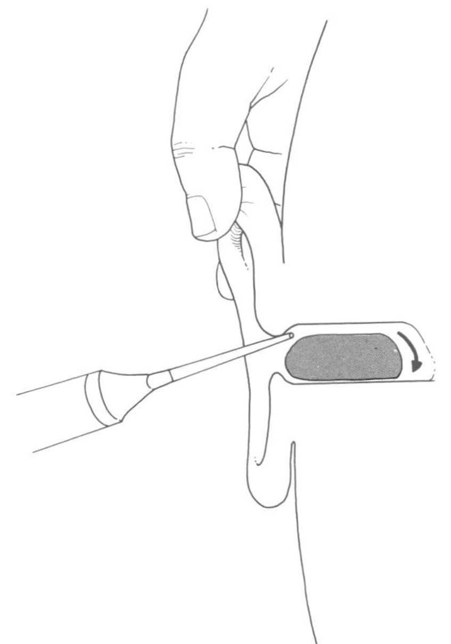

Fig. 64.2 Syringing the ear involves directing the stream of solution along the roof of the external auditory meatus.

A large receiver to collect the returned washout

Procedure for syringing

A good source of light is required to visualise the external auditory canal and assess the extent and depth of the impacted wax. After protecting the patient's shoulders with the waterproof cape and towelling, a careful explanation should be given to obtain their verbal consent and cooperation. The patient is given the large receiver to hold against the neck immediately below the ear. Once the syringe is filled with the solution, checking that the temperature is below 38° but above 36° C, the air is expelled from the syringe. A jet of the solution is directed against the posterior wall of the external canal from the tip of the syringe, which should be resting within the canal at a distance of about 2 cm. During this syringing the auricle of the ear is held upwards and backwards to straighten the S-shape of the canal. It is better to inject the stream of solution at interrupted intervals, rather than all at once. This means that the solution will get behind the wax and force it forwards and out of the ear. Occasionally the wax will occlude the ear and be visible. At such a time the wax can be gently removed with Tilley's forceps. Repeated examination with the auriscope should indicate the success and progress of the ear syringing. When the tympanic membrane can be seen, the syringing should be stopped. After dry mopping the external canal of excess solution, the canal should be inspected once again to ensure that all the debris has been removed.

Associated hazards

Associated hazards with this procedure are rare, except on those occasions when the forceful removal of very hard wax may cause an abrasion of the epithelial lining of the external ear. Similar abrasions can occur if the tip of the syringe is roughly inserted into the ear. Perforation of the tympanic membrane is a possibility if the jet of solution is too forceful, or if the syringe tip is advanced too far into the external canal. Otitis media can occur as a consequence of a perforated ear drum. If the solution is too hot or cold, it can overstimulate the perilymph of the inner ear and induce giddiness and nausea.

Chapter 65
Surgery of the Middle and Inner Ear

GENERAL PREOPERATIVE MANAGEMENT

The great majority of patients have all their preliminary tests and investigations completed in the out-patients department, and are usually only admitted as waiting-list patients. The precautions for any type of surgery are taken and, if admitted, it can be safely assumed the patient is to have surgery under the effects of general anaesthesia. Specifically the nurse needs to assess if the patient is taking any current medication, e.g., antidepressants, antiemetics, or steroid drugs. These particular groups of drugs must be brought to the attention of the surgeon, since the drugs can affect the outcome of surgery.

A nursing assessment should be made to exclude infections of the throat, sinus or trachea, and any suspicion of infection also needs to be reported as it is usually sufficient to cancel the operation until the patient has recovered. The skin surrounding the ear should be free of hair for at least 4 cm in diameter; long hair would of course be plaited and secured under a theatre cap. Some surgeons may request that swabs be taken from the external auditory canal for culture and sensitivity tests. If necessary, the canal should be cleansed by dry mopping.

Depending on the type of operation, the patient should be advised on what to expect in the immediate postoperative phase and have a clear understanding of the intention of surgery before signing the consent form. The more extensive the surgery the more likely it is that the patient will have a short course of broad spectrum antibiotics as a prophylactic measure against the risk of infection.

COMMON OPERATIONS OF THE EAR

Myringotomy

For a myringotomy a curved incision is made into the tympanic membrane with the myringotome to drain fluid from the middle ear (Fig. 65.1). Generally this simple procedure is reserved for those patients suffering from acute otitis media which has not resolved with the conservative measures of antibiotics and analgesics. At operation the exudate from the middle ear tends to spurt out through the incision, and a swab is taken for culture and sensitivity before the external canal is thoroughly cleansed.

'Glue Ear'

Myringotomy may also precede aspiration of the middle ear to relieve a condition known as *glue ear*.

This condition is associated with persistently enlarged adenoids, i.e., the lymph glands located in the nasopharynx. Their enlargement obstructs the entrance of the eustachian tube so that aeration of the middle ear cannot take place. This in fact leads to a vacuum within the middle ear. To compensate for this vacuum effect the sebaceous glands in the middle ear secrete serum. Ultimately this serum becomes extremely tenacious; a semi-liquid serous substance with the resemblance of glue. It contributes to a conductive deafness which will hamper the child's education and progress in learning because of a loss of hearing.

A similar condition occurs during a common cold when the Eustachian tube becomes blocked. However, in this situation, the 'deafness' is of a limited duration as the serous exudate will spontaneously resolve when the cold resolves. To bypass the obstructed Eustachian tube, a tiny tube made of metal, plastic, or polythene is inserted into the middle ear to allow it to be aerated. After aspiration of the glue-like substance, combined with artificial aeration, the Eustachian tube will gradually recover its natural function. The artificial tube is extruded and easily removed once healing is completed. Hearing should then return to normal.

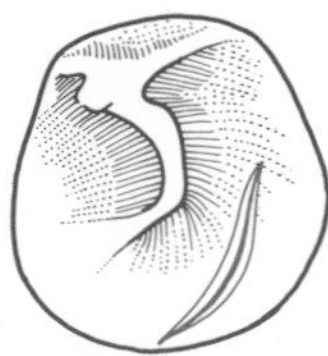

Fig. 65.1 Myringotomy with detail of the extent of the incision.

Myringoplasty (Tympanoplasty)

If the tympanic membrane is ruptured or perforated for any reason it can be repaired. If necessary, the ossicles of the middle ear can also be replaced by a prosthesis or a graft along with a repair of the eardrum. The operation can be used to eradicate chronic disease of the middle ear. The surgical incision may be either post-auricular (behind the ear) or from immediately in front of the ear. An operating microscope, i.e., Zeiss microscope, is required to visualise the operating field since the structures within the ear are of a miniature size requiring extreme magnification if they are to be manipulated.

Stapedectomy

The more simple of two possible operations is stapes mobilisation. This operation requires the eardrum to be reflected, which will expose the stapes bone, which is then gently rocked until it mobilises correctly so that it will vibrate against the oval window. A 'true' stapedectomy is the surgical removal of the sclerosed stapes bone, i.e., otosclerosis, and its replacement with a prosthesis. The prosthesis can be of teflon, stainless steel, or fat and wire. After the prosthesis is secured to the incus bone and the tympanic membrane replaced, the external canal is packed with ribbon gauze dressing for at least 24 hours. The success rate of this operation is very high, with a good improvement of hearing appreciation.

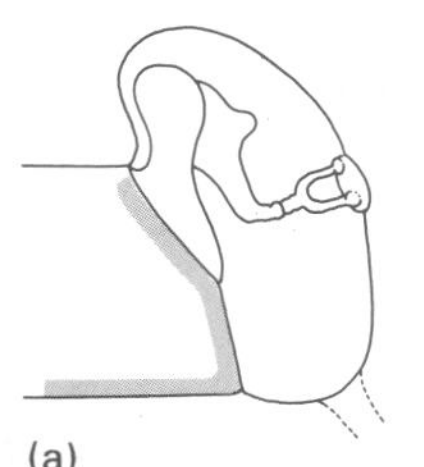

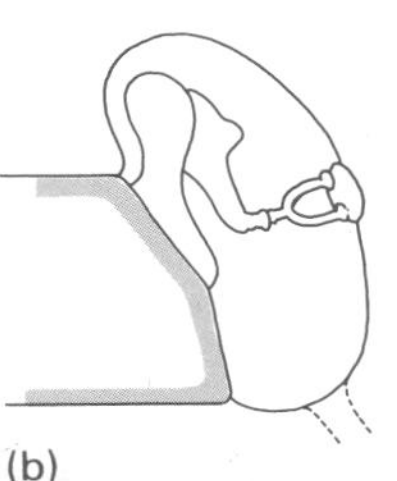

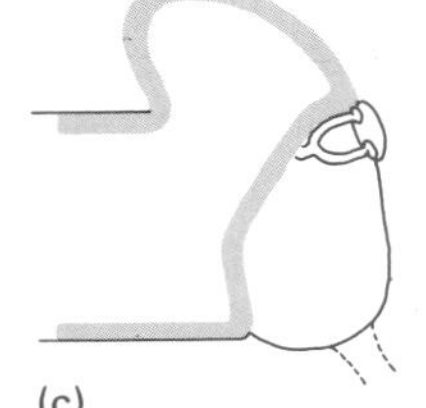

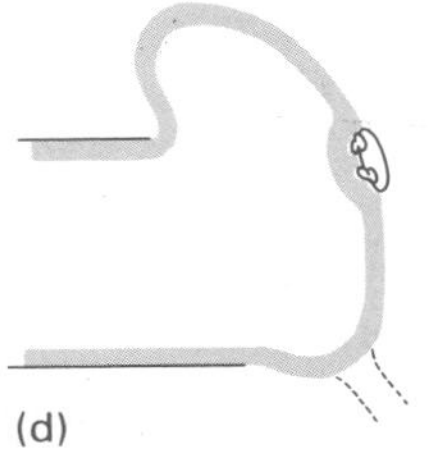

Fig. 65.2 Tympanoplasty. Depending on the degree of damage (a–d), vein or fascia grafts (blue) are used to reconstruct the sound conducting mechanism.

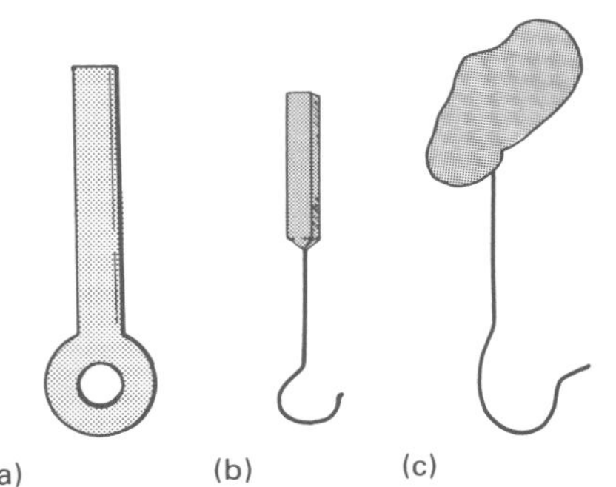

Fig. 65.3 Three forms of stapes prosthesis used in stapedectomy. Teflon piston (a), steel piston (b), fat and wire (c).

Mastoidectomy

Chronic disease of the middle ear usually involves the mastoid process and one of three operations may be done to remove irreversibly damaged structures from the middle ear and the mastoid bone:

Cortical Mastoidectomy

Refers to a resection of the superior mastoid bone air cell and the mastoid antrum via a post-auricular incision. The wound usually has a drain in position for 24–48 hours.

Modified Radical Mastoidectomy

Refers to the resection of the superior and posterior wall of the external auditory canal with wound drainage from this area taken via the external auditory canal.

Radical Mastoidectomy

Refers to the construction of a single chamber from the middle ear to the mastoid antrum, and requires major surgery which involves the removal of the posterior and superior wall of the middle ear along with the malleolus and incus bone and part of the external auditory canal. The related structures, i.e., semicircular canals, facial nerve, lateral sinus and stapes bones, are avoided but their relationship may cause serious postoperative side effects. The newly created cavity is protected by enlarging the external auditory canal with specially designed skin flaps and a light pack of ribbon gauze, e.g., bismuth iodoform and paraffin paste (BIPP pack), calcium alginate or penicillin.

Immediate Postoperative Care

As a general guide, patients with any type of surgery should be nursed flat and allowed one pillow only, with the head turned to the unaffected side. On recovery the patient should be persuaded to remain in this position until any feelings of nausea, actual vomiting, or vertigo have completely receded. If the operation has been of a prolonged nature, it should be remembered that the operating position requires the head to be fixed to a firm surface supported by sandbags. For those patients with short necks, the shoulders may also have required sandbag support. It is quite common for patients to complain of headache, neck stiffness and shoulder ache. These should not be confused with the actual operation, as they are usually caused by the operating position.

After a period of 4–6 hours, and if pain-free, the patient should be offered a second or third pillow, with the warning that sudden head movements are likely to induce unpleasant sensations of vertigo and headache, despite the administration of an antiemetic such as Stemetil. Any ear packs are observed at frequent intervals for signs of haemorrhage. If bleeding should occur, the pack is covered by a second sterile dressing and the surgeon informed. The removal of ear packs and post-auricular drains is normally done by the surgeon or a senior nurse. Subsequent dressings are completed by the nurse who must have a strict regard for the surgeon's instructions.

Persistent attacks of vomiting or vertigo implies that the vestibular apparatus of the inner ear is affected, which should respond to further rest and increased doses of analgesia and antiemetics. Facial paralysis may occur on the operated side. If this develops slowly, it means that the packing on the ear is too tight causing pressure on the facial nerve as it passes through the middle ear. This is one cause of Bell's palsy. If the paralysis occurs quickly, the facial nerve has been damaged during surgery.

Nystagmus (oscillating eyeballs) is rare, but should be reported immediately if it is observed for it implies a surgical irritation of the vestibular branch of the auditory nerve.

Continuing Care

The continuing care of the patient requires the nursing plan to take into account the patient's need for rest and sleep. If an ear pack is in place, night sedation should have been prescribed for at least 2 nights following surgery. Feelings of nausea should recede within a few days, but until they do the diet requires more than the usual consideration. Food should be bland, very light and easy to digest. Walking or even standing upright may present a problem following middle ear surgery. Often the patient is the best judge of whether it is feasible to get up and take a few steps. When ambulation is first attempted, a nurse should be available to remain with the patient because, apart from a feeling of giddiness, fainting is also a hazard at this time. When coping with his or her personal hygiene, the patient should be advised to avoid wetting the ear dressing. Blowing the nose also has to be avoided if prosthetic surgery has taken place, since vigorous nasal clearance will probably dislodge the prosthesis very easily in the first few postoperative days.

Prior to hospital discharge the surgeon will advise the patient on the potential hazards of swimming and high altitude work. The patient should also be warned that surgery to correct hearing defects does not offer an immediate improvement until the oedema within the ear has resolved about 1–2 weeks after the ear pack has been removed. Future appointments are absolutely essential to administer audiometric tests, but patients should be told to return without an appointment if there is any ear discharge. Excessive noise, e.g., discos, should be avoided, as should severe cold winds when the patient should wear a protective scarf or ear muffler.

Chapter 66 Common Conditions of the Middle Ear

MÉNIÈRE'S DISEASE

Ménière's disease (inner ear syndrome) or, *paroxysmal aural vertigo* is believed to be due to a retention of fluid within the cochlea and a subsequent distension of the balance mechanism, the vestibule of the inner ear. The group of symptoms classically associated with this disease combine to create the syndrome:

giddiness and vertigo preceded by tinnitus (noises within the ear)

sudden attacks of nausea and vomiting

progressive impairment of hearing

nystagmus (oscillation of the eyeballs) which occurs during an attack

Each attack is of a spontaneous nature, occurring without any warning with each attack becoming progressively more acute. Eventually the patient is totally incapacitated by the severity of the symptoms. The attack may last for several hours or several days. The distress of the attack prevents any testing or assessments being made until conservative treatment has taken effect. Some of these measures include administering one of the antiemetics such as prochlorperazine (Stemetil), a strong sedative at regular intervals, e.g., phenobarbitone 60–200 mg 3 times daily, or Largactil by intramuscular injection. The patient should be reassured that they are in fact suffering from a definitive disease, and not merely suffering from an attack of nervous exhaustion. This simple assurance will do a great deal to boost the patient's confidence and morale at a time of severe distress. Some otologists will prescribe a restricted salt diet, combined with a reduced fluid intake. However, even with drugs and dietary control of salt and fluid, relapses of the disease are quite common. During a symptom-free period the caloric test (see Chapter 64) is completed to demonstrate disease of the vestibule. Surgery to correct the disorder of the balance mechanism may be offered. Two operations are currently practised:

1. *Selective Destruction of the Vestibular Apparatus*. The vestibule of the inner ear is exposed via a mastoidectomy approach and is bombarded by ultrasonic soundwaves which destroy the affected part of the vestibule without any loss of hearing.

2. *Labyrinthectomy*. The membranous tube within the horizontal semicircular canal is destroyed. It is approached via a mastoidectomy and a burr hole of the bony semicircular canal. While the symptoms of vertigo are cured, the hearing of the operated ear will be lost. The postoperative care for this type of patient is as outlined earlier in this chapter with specific emphasis given to the need for bedrest for about 7 days because of symptoms of vertigo. Prior to being allowed out of bed, the patient may be involved in a series of exercises to control nystagmus (eyes) and head movements to improve coordination and balance.

Acoustic Neuromas

Fibroid tumours growing out of the auditory nerve are rare, but the symptoms are similar to those of Ménière's disease. However the symptoms are made complicated by the fact that the fifth and seventh cranial nerves are also involved, these nerves being compressed as they pass near the inner ear. Added to this is the risk of increased intracranial pressure, which gives rise to severe headache and papilloedema. Lateral X-rays of temporal and mastoid bone reveal structural changes, and the tumour itself may be detected by computerised axial tomography (CAT scan). A lumbar puncture will demonstrate a raised cerebrospinal fluid pressure. Surgical removal of this type of tumour is dangerous and hazardous requiring the combined skills of the otologist and neurologist.

Chapter 67
Structure and Examination of the Throat

The anatomical structures of the throat are the pharynx and its divisions, and the larynx and its parts. Related to these structures are the important functions of speech and swallowing.

THE STRUCTURE

The Pharynx

In the adult, the pharynx is a cone-shaped tube about 12–14 cm long which extends from the base of the post-nasal space until it terminates at the larynx. Its upper portion is parallel with the base of the skull; lying immediately in front are the nasal and oral cavities, while behind lie the cervical vertebrae. The pharynx can be divided into 3 parts; the nasopharynx, oropharynx and laryngeal pharynx.

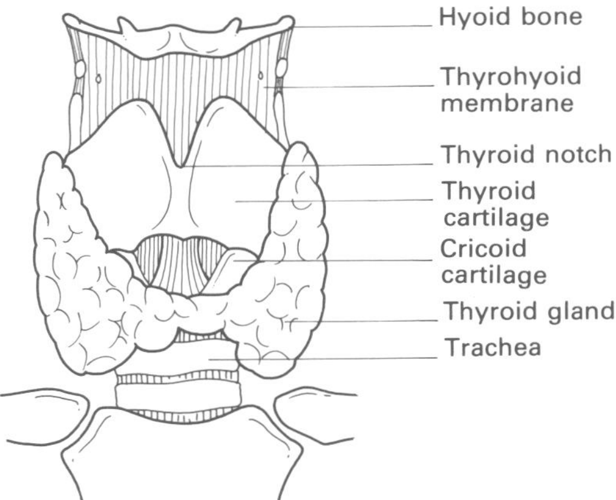

Fig. 67.1 Structures in the front of the neck.

Nasopharynx

The nasopharynx lies immediately behind the nasal cavity and contains 2 important structures: the adenoids, i.e., 2 lymph glands, and the opening of the Eustachian tube which leads to the middle ear. This tube allows air to enter this chamber to ensure that the pressure within the middle ear is equal to that of the external ear. Surrounding the entry of the Eustachian tube is the tubal tonsil.

Oropharynx

The oropharynx lies immediately at the back of the mouth. The lateral walls of the oral cavity blend with the mucous membrane of the soft palate to form a double membrane called the Pillars of the fauces, within which are housed the faucial tonsils. Hanging from the midline of the soft palate, almost guarding the oropharynx, is a small piece of muscle covered with mucous membrane called the uvula. The faucial tonsil is innervated by the ninth cranial nerve, which also branches to the ear. Therefore, it is possible to get a *reflex otalgia* from tonsillitis or after a tonsillectomy. The tonsils have a rich blood supply, which implies problems of haemorrhage after a tonsillectomy.

The combined effect of the adenoids, tubal tonsil and faucial tonsil is to create a ring of lymphatic tissue at the portal of entry to both respiration and digestion. This is referred to as Waldeyer's ring and is one example of a defence mechanism against infection.

Laryngeal Pharynx

The laryngeal pharynx contains the larynx and the vocal cords. The larynx commences at the hyoid bone, which is located at the root of the tongue, and continues downwards to meet the trachea. It lies parallel with the third, fourth and fifth cervical vertebrae. The larynx is composed of 4 irregular-shaped cartilages held together by ligaments and membranes. These are:

1. **Epiglottis**. This cartilage is leaf-shaped in adults and tubular shaped in children. It closes over the laryngeal opening of the trachea during the act of swallowing. The opening into the trachea is known as the glottis and it is into this space that the tip of an endotracheal tube has to be passed during anaesthesia.
2. **Thyroid cartilage**. This is fused at the midline, but open at its posterior surface. The fusion at the front creates what is commonly known as the Adam's apple.
3. **Cricoid cartilage**. This is of a signet ring shape, the ring lying back to front and forming the back and side walls of the larynx.
4. **Arytenoid cartilages**. These extend

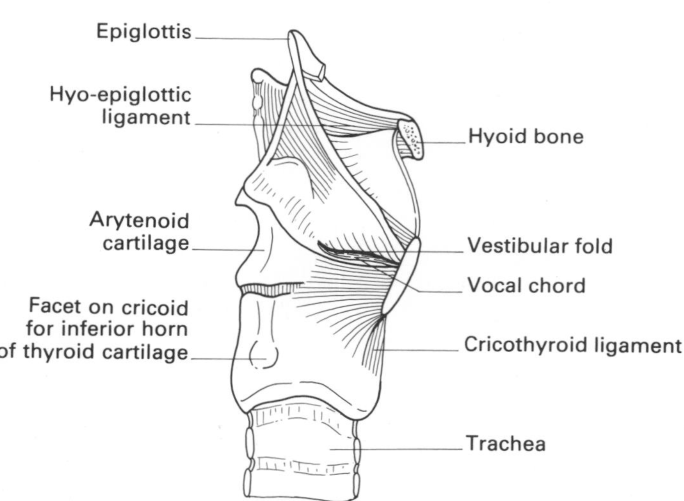

Fig. 67.2 The larynx seen from within.

round the back, and being of a pyramid shape, form the back wall of the larynx.

All these cartilages are held together by membranes and ligaments, their importance being the very limited movement they permit and the fact that any swelling is also minimal, both major considerations in surgery of the throat.

Within the larynx lie the vocal folds, which are pieces of membrane arising from the front wall of the thyroid cartilage and extending backwards to the arytenoid cartilages. The slit between the vocal cords (rima) depends on the tension of the arytenoid cartilages. When relaxed, air passes soundlessly between and around the vocal folds. When contracted, the air passes over a stretched vocal cord and causes it to vibrate and produce sound. The length of the vocal cords determines some of the qualities of speech. The pitch of speech is higher in females so the cords are longer. Loudness of speech is the force of vibrations on expiration of air, while the quality of speech involves not only the vocal cords but the shape of the mouth, position of tongue and lips, the facial muscles and the health of the sinus. The group of muscles which move the arytenoid cartilages, and so influence the length of the vocal cords, are the pharyngeal constrictor muscles which bring the vocal folds together to form what is known as the 'chink of the glottis'.

The functions of the pharynx and larynx combined can be summarised as follows:

1. Filtration of bacteria from food and air by the lymphatic Waldeyer's ring.
2. Equalisation of the air pressure between the middle and external ear via the Eustachian tube.
3. Deglutition (swallowing), the epiglottis reflexly covers the opening into the larynx when swallowing.
4. Respiration by the reflex relaxation of the epiglottis, permitting air to enter the trachea.
5. Speech by the constriction of the pharyngeal constrictor muscles stretching the arytenoid cartilages which pull the vocal cords together.

The blood supply to the pharynx and larynx is derived from the superior and inferior thyroid arteries. Venous return is via the jugular vein. The nerve supply arises from the motor nerves of the laryngeal and recurrent laryngeal nerve, while sensory appreciation is noted on the branches of the vagus nerve.

CLINICAL EXAMINATION OF THE THROAT

The patient should be seated facing the doctor during the examination, with a good source of light from an angle-poise lamp, further supplemented with a pencil torch for direct inspection of the throat. Dentures should be removed prior to the examination and temporarily stored in a dental carton. The tongue may be grasped with a dry gauze swab and brought forwards, but more usually it is depressed onto the floor of the mouth with a disposable wooden spatula (tongue depressor) to give a maximum view of the pharynx and larynx. Obvious abnormalities are noted, and these may include infection, exudate, redness, peculiar spots and oedema. The area on which the abnormality is located is also noted, being either the pharynx, faucial tonsil, upper larynx, vocal cords, or on the mucosa of the oral cavity.

Throat Swab

If a throat swab is requested, it should be taken before the commencement of any treatment, e.g., antibiotics. It is always better to take a throat swab in the morning and before the first drink of the day. The patient should be in a seated position with the mouth opened as widely as possible. The nurse, using a pencil torch, should be able to visualise the tonsil bed or actual faucial tonsil from where the swab is to be taken. The wool tip of the sterile swab stick is placed onto the tonsil and rotated several times until it is moistened. On removal, the swab should not be contaminated with the patient's saliva. Equally important, the moistened wool tip should not come into contact with the outer rim of its container, as it is being replaced.

During and immediately after taking the

throat swab the patient may gag and feel nauseated, which is one reason why patients often pull the head backwards and away from the nurse. However this can also indicate that the nurse is being too heavy handed. A sip of water will alleviate this minor discomfort.

The sealed swabstick and the pathology request form should be correctly completed with the patient's details before being despatched to the pathology department.

Examining the Larynx

Examination of the larynx is possible when the doctor uses the laryngeal mirror, after it is slightly warmed over the flame of the spirit lamp to prevent condensation on its mirror surface from the patient's breath. It is necessary to bypass both the soft palate and uvula to gain a view of the vocal cords. These can be tested by asking the patient to make a sound while the mouth is opened, in addition to looking for obvious inflammation. Detailed examination of the lower larynx, trachea, bronchus and oesophagus requires the patient to have a general anaesthetic.

Chapter 68
Tonsillitis, Tonsillectomy and Adenoidectomy

TONSILLITIS

The peak occurrence of infection and inflammation of the tonsil and adenoids is during childhood, between the ages of 5 and 10 years old. The adenoids within the nasopharynx begin to enlarge at about 3 years of age and remain enlarged until the age of puberty when they begin to recede in size and eventually disappear. The faucial tonsils start to enlarge from the age of 5 years, remaining enlarged until about 10 years old, and becoming much smaller after the onset of puberty. This enlargement is a natural physiological defence mechanism connected with the child developing his or her immunity system. While enlarged, however, they are more prone to infection, especially from micro-organisms such as the adenovirus, echovirus, influenza virus, but especially dangerous being the *Haemolytic streptococci*. The latter organism may be the forerunner of such diseases as rheumatic fever, acute nephritis and subacute bacterial endocarditis. Fortunately, these diseases are becoming increasingly rare.

A tonsillitis attack is associated with many uncomfortable symptoms, these being cervical adenitis, ear infections and earache, i.e., reflex otalgia, deafness, sinusitis, laryngeal oedema, loss of appetite, dysphagia, pyrexia, fetid breath, painful dry cough, and chest infections. Before conservative treatment can be given, however, a throat swab is usually obtained to identify the causative pathogen.

Antibiotics are the mainstay of treatment, even if the causative organism is a virus which does not normally respond to antibiotics. They will probably still be prescribed as a prophylactic measure to prevent further infections of other structures. Penicillin for 5 days is a very common treatment. Combined with this is the antipyretic–analgesic drug Aspirin, which the patient should gargle before swallowing, cleansing the tonsil area and reducing the temperature. Bedrest is advised until the temperature has returned to normal.

Recurrent tonsillitis predisposes to the formation of a peritonsillar abscess or quinsy. This is an excruciatingly painful collection of pus within the crypt of the faucial membranes, which can only be relieved by incision and drainage. The relief is almost immediate and, when combined with bedrest and conservative treatment, a full recovery takes a further 7 days.

TONSILLECTOMY AND ADENOIDECTOMY

The indications for the surgical removal of either the adenoids or the faucial tonsils, either in combination or alone are:

1. Recurrent tonsillitis after the age of 5; there should be a 6-week interval after the initial immunisation schedule, before the operation.
2. Recurrent peritonsillar abscesses (quinsies).
3. Cervical adenitis. This implies that the infection is not remaining localised but is invasive to other parts of the body.
4. If the patient is a 'carrier' of an infectious pathogen, e.g., diphtheria.
5. Persistently enlarged tonsils causing dysphagia.
6. To reduce the risk of the diseases caused by *Haemolytic streptococci*.
7. Excessive loss of time from either school or, in the case of adults, from work.

Preoperative care

Prior to the operation a careful assessment is made to ensure the patient has been free from tonsillitis in the last 6 weeks. For those with a history of recurrent attacks, they may still be taking oral penicillin on admission to hospital. Additionally, blood tests should have been completed to exclude haemorrhagic diseases, an extreme example being haemophilia. Finally, if there is a local epidemic of tonsillitis within the district, the operation may be cancelled.

The immediate preoperative care would specifically include attention to oral and dental hygiene, with examination of both the throat and the external auditory canal. In children the close relationship between parents and child should be encouraged by free visiting. Often play therapy is the best method by which to explain to a child the reasons for their being in hospital and what the treatment will involve, if their fears are to be overcome. Sedation for children is administered about 1 hour before surgery, an example being either Vallergan or Nepenthe at dosages commensurate with their body weight. In adults, some emphasis should be placed on the hazards of smoking before an operation on the throat, and this should be emphatically discouraged before a general anaesthetic. All patients should have had their blood grouped and crossmatched before surgery, in case of haemorrhage.

Removal of the tonsils and adenoids

The techniques used to remove the tonsils and adenoids (i.e., dissection, curettage and guillotine) are relatively quick, but they all carry a major postoperative risk, i.e., haemorrhage.

Dissection

Dissection is the most common method. The anterior wall of the faucial tonsil is held by a Wilson artery forcep, while an incision is made into the mucosa. Once the tonsil capsule has been widened with scissors, the tonsil itself is dissected from its bed. Although the pharynx will have been lightly packed with gauze, the area will require a great deal of suction to clear away the blood. The blood vessels are sealed either by diathermy or by ligation with sutures.

Curettage

In curettage the adenoids are removed from the pharyngeal position by the curette. This is a spoon-shaped instrument which scrapes away the lymphoid tissue. It is unusual if a great deal of blood is lost from this operation.

Guillotine

The guillotine method is rarely used today, but it involves trapping the tonsil behind a blunt-ended instrument which is then snapped shut against a firm edge, thus ripping the faucial tonsil from its bed. Bleeding from this technique can be quite profuse, since all the bleeding points cannot be tied off.

Postoperative Care

Postoperatively there are two immediate dangers: inhalation of blood into the trachea and continued bleeding from either the pharyngeal branch of the external carotid, the palantine branch of the internal maxillary, or the paratonsillar veins.

While every precaution is taken in theatre to seal these blood vessels by ligature and diathermy, or pressure packs, they may rupture from the rising blood pressure which occurs during recovery, i.e., reactionary haemorrhage. For this reason the patient should remain in the recovery room of theatre until they are fully conscious and the throat has been inspected by the surgeon. The recovery period is very short, since only light anaesthesia is normally used.

On return to a prepared bed in the ward, the patient should be nursed in the lateral position with the head resting on a covered waterproofed pillow. Observations should begin immediately and be recorded every 30 minutes for 12 hours, even if the patient appears to be making satisfactory progress. A falling blood pressure and a rising pulse indicate that 'shock' is developing and in this situation it is most likely to be from a tonsillar haemorrhage. Frequent swallowing, especially if the patient is asleep, is another indicator to observe for, undue restlessness can be caused by a slow but silent bleed. Any of these factors should be reported **immediately** to a senior colleague to enable surgical intervention as quickly as possible. This usually takes the form of further ligature or diathermy in theatre, followed by a blood transfusion.

Several hours after an uneventful recovery, the patient should be encouraged to use the throat muscles, i.e., the pharyngeal constrictors. This can be done by giving the patient sips of cool and refreshing fluids to drink, or mild antiseptic mouthwashes every 2 hours. Analgesia and sedation are essential for the first 24 hours, especially during the first postoperative evening when the throat can be acutely painful and sore. Aspirin gargles or a mucilage can be comforting, taking away the rough sensation felt at the throat. Anything which encourages swallowing after the 24-hour period is to be advocated, and which is to the patient's preference. Whether it be ice cream, blancmange, custard or soups does not really matter, the principle to grasp is that it is the swallowing movements which promote healing of the tonsil bed, not the substance swallowed. Therefore rough foods are totally unnecessary and are indeed quite barbaric.

For a further 3 days the patient usually continues to have penicillin to counteract the risk of a postoperative infection. Hospital stay is of a very short duration, perhaps no longer than 48 hours unless an unforeseen complication arises. Before discharge, the doctor will usually examine the external auditory canal to exclude any middle or external ear infection and question the patient about earache, which is usually due to reflex pain from the throat, especially when swallowing. Within 6 weeks of surgery the patient can expect to regain their normal weight and full relief from the many associated discomforts within the nose and ear.

Chapter 69
Tracheostomy

Tracheostomy is an elective surgical procedure in which an incision is made into the third and fourth tracheal rings to create a temporary or permanent stoma via which the patient can breathe. The stoma is held open by the insertion of either a plastic or metal tube. Apart from ensuring an alternative airway, the tracheostomy also provides for an adequate and repeated clearance of mucoid secretions by suction. It can also be used to administer intermittent positive pressure ventilation. The indications for a tracheostomy are mainly those which cause a respiratory obstruction above the trachea. For example:

1. Oedema of the glottis, i.e., a membranous obstruction.
2. Acute laryngotracheitis in children, e.g., croup.
3. Laryngeal diphtheria (rare).
4. Impacted foreign bodies within the larynx.
5. Traumatic injury of the glottis or the larynx.
6. Obstruction due to a benign or malignant tumour.

Tracheostomy may also be the preferred method of maintaining the airway of a patient who is in prolonged unconsciousness, usually due to a head injury. More rarely, it can be used in those patients with paralysis of the respiratory intercostal muscles as a result of bulbar poliomyelitis. More unusual still, it is used when the patient is suffering from paralysis of the recurrent laryngeal nerve.

Tracheostomy should wherever possible be an elective procedure, and can be completed under the effect of a local anaesthetic. In an

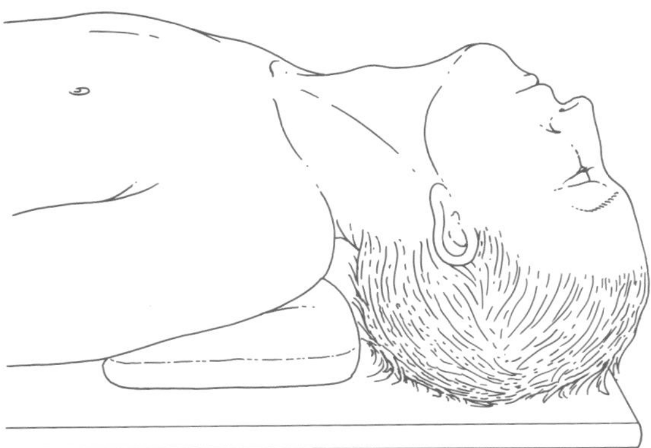

Fig. 69.1 Operating position for a tracheostomy.

emergency situation the first consideration should be to maintain the airway by endotracheal intubation. If this is impossible, it is quicker and easier to complete a pharyngotomy, i.e, an incision into the cricoid cartilage—such an incision is well away from the larger blood vessels and avoids the isthmus of the thyroid gland. During the procedure of tracheostomy, the position of the head and neck is that of extreme extension, with the shoulder supported on a sandbag (Fig. 69.1). The head is manually supported and held firmly while a vertical midline incision is made into the skin of the lower half of the neck. The underlying fascia are divided and the muscle retracted to reveal the thyroid isthmus and trachea. The thyroid isthmus is then divided and the related blood vessels ligated. An incision is then made into the trachea and there is an immediate escape of air from the stoma. The incision line is held open with retractors until a suitably sized tube in inserted and secured by cotton tapes taken around and tied to the side of the neck. The wound is then sutured and protected by a dry sterile gauze pad cut to fit immediately behind the shield of the tracheostomy tube.

The type of tracheostomy tube inserted can be any one of 13 types currently available, and the choice is made by the surgeon (Fig. 69.2). From the many types of tube there are 2 principles which the nurse must understand:

1. Metal tubes are made of silver, very expensive and made by hand. They come in 3 parts: an outer tube, a closely fitting inner tube, and an introducer. On the metal type tubes, there should be a stamped number which indicates its size and use, e.g.,

Size 1 = infant
Size 2 and 3 = children
Size 4 = adolescent
Size 5 = adult

2. Portex, nylon or plastic tubes are designed to last for about 6 months and are either uncuffed or cuffed. A cuffed tube has an inflatable ballon which secures the tube to the trachea. However the ballon must be deflated every hour for at least 5 minutes to prevent necrosis of the tracheal membrane from unremitting pressure. These tubes are invaluable in the administration of intermittent positive pressure ventilation.

NURSING CARE PLAN

In preparing to receive a patient into a general ward who has a tracheostomy tube in place, the following specific factors must be included in the care plan:

1. The bed should have an adequate number of pillows to nurse the patient in a semirecumbent or sitting upright position. If unconscious, the patient will have to be nursed in the dorsal and alternate lateral positions without a pillow.

2. Suction apparatus, either portable or wall mounted, should be tested. The suction jar is partly filled with a small volume of antiseptic lotion, e.g., 1% phenolic lotion. The tubing extending from the suction jars should preferably be of the disposable type, and because of its weight may require

pinning to the mattress. Sterile suction catheters sizes 10, 12 and 14 should be immediately available either at the suction point or on the bedside trolley.

3. Oxygen, whether from a wall mounted point or a cylinder, should also be tested and a spare oxygen cylinder be on standby. If requested, a humidification unit should be prepared with water and tested that its temperature control is operational to warm the water within the humidification unit.

4. A clean trolley for the individual patient's nursing care should be assembled to enable the nurse to carry out 3 essential features of care: tracheal suction, changing of the inner tube and wound toilet. This trolley should not be used for any other patient. Since all the procedures are sterile, it is suggested that the following layout would be most appropriate, but must be adapted to local hospital policy:

Upper trolley surface. This should be prepared as for a sterile dressing and left covered with a sterile disposable paper towel.

Lower trolley surface is equipped to meet the following needs:

Exchanging the inner tracheostomy tube:

duplicate tracheostomy tube immersed in antiseptic lotion

tracheal dilators in case of emergency

spare tracheal tube tapes

sterile test tube brush to cleanse the inner tube

solution of sodium bicarbonate to immerse the inner used tube

For tracheal suction:

disposable face masks

disposable sterile gloves

sterile suction catheters sizes 10, 12 and 14

distilled sterile water

For wound toilet:

dressing pack (basic)

scissors in antiseptic solution

antiseptic lotions according to hospital policy

5. A system of communication must be available to the patient, i.e., a buzzer or call-bell system in case of emergency, and a notepad and pencil or visual aid communication card for everyday communication. This should be within easy reach of the patient, perhaps on the locker top, and the locker should be positioned so that the patient does not have to struggle when reaching for personal items.

In the first few days of care the patient should not be left alone and should always be within direct visual view of the nursing staff who can deal promptly with any problem, whether it is one of obstruction of the tube or any feelings of panic and anxiety which the patient may experience. To deal with the frequent problem of tenacious mucous and sputum occluding the lumen of the trachestomy tube a method of tracheal suction is suggested.

Tracheal Suction

Even if the patient is unconscious, the procedure should be explained and the bed screened to give privacy for the patient and to reduce alarm in other neighbouring patients. The nurse must wear a face mask and the hands should be thoroughly washed and carefully dried. A suitably sized catheter is selected and the outer wrapping at the connection end is peeled back so that it can be secured to the suction tubing. The suction machine is then switched on and adjusted to reach a pressure vacuum reading of between 15 and 20 mmHg. The heavy suction tubing should be anchored under the nurse's arm to give better control over the catheter. Sterile gloves are put on before removing the outer wrapping of the suction catheter. A nipping pressure is applied to the catheter, while its tip is inserted into the tracheal opening and advanced as far as it will go. On releasing the nipping pressure the vacuum pressure will cause the mucoid secretions to be sucked up the catheter and into the suction jar. The tip of the catheter is rotated as it is withdrawn, rather than forcing it up and down. The minimum amount of time is used to actually clear away the mucoid secretions. After disconnecting the catheter from the tubing,

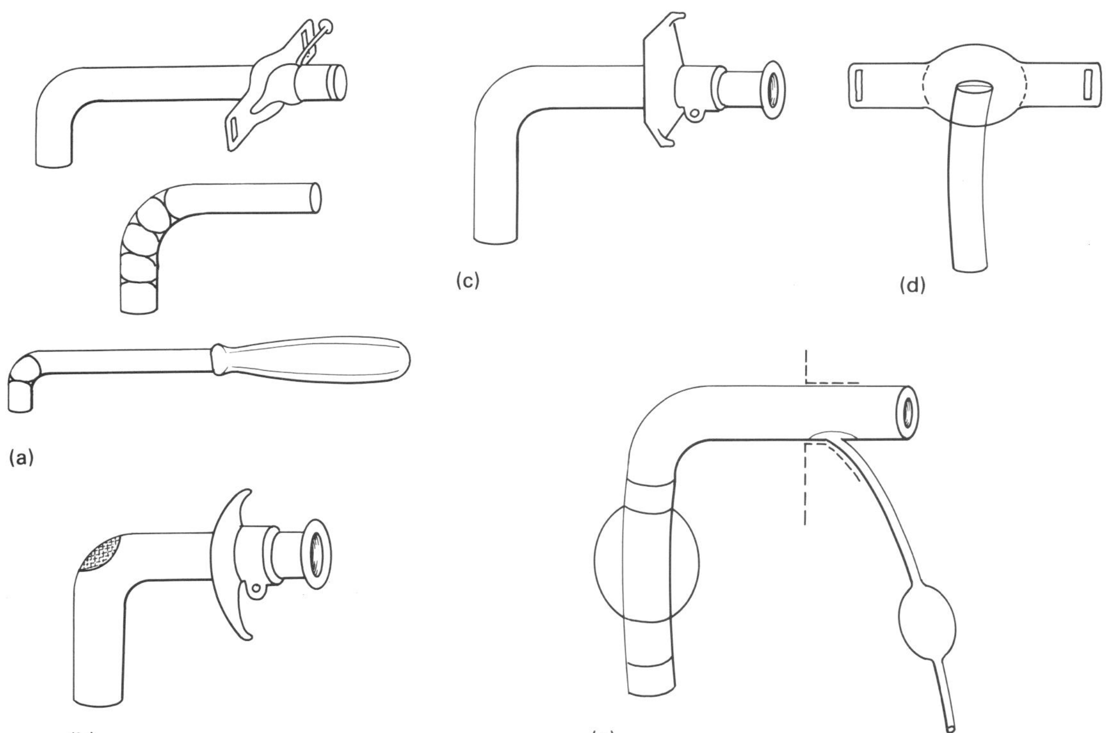

Fig. 69.2 Types of tracheostomy tube. Outer, inner and pilot introducer of Durham's tube (a); angled tube for laryngeal breathing (b) and with adjustable shield (c); portex tube (d) and with inflatable cuff reserved for use with intermittent positive pressure ventilation (e).

the catheter is retained in the hand and the glove peeled over it so that it is discarded within a covering surface. The suction tubing is then flushed through with distilled sterile water using the suction power to draw the distilled water up the tubing into the suction jar. The mask is worn to protect the nurse from the mucoid spray, which is inevitable during the suction procedure, and should be disposed of before washing the hands at the end of the procedure.

Care of the Tracheostomy Tube

The outer tube (silver) should not be touched by the nursing staff. The surgeon will indicate in the written instructions when this tube is to be changed or removed. However, the inner tube may require frequent changing, depending on whether the patient has a large or small volume of bronchial secretion. The inner tube is normally secured to the shield of the outer tube and requires a small rotation movement to release it from its retaining crevice. Being a sterile procedure the inner tube should be removed with a gloved hand, immersed immediately into a solution of sodium bicarbonate. The replacement inner tube is immersed in sterile water and smeared with a small amount of sterile liquid paraffin to make its insertion into the outer tube easier. It is positioned securely into the crevice of the outer tube shield. The used tube should be thoroughly brushed with the test tube brush both inside and outside before being immersed in a mildly antiseptic solution, e.g., Gluteraldehyde, which will chemically sterilise the tube so it is ready for the next change.

Changing the Outer Tube

When the surgeon has given explicit instructions, 2 nurses are required to change the outer tube. The replacement tube is double-checked to see that it corresponds with the one in position. After releasing the tapes and removing the existing tube from the tracheal stoma with a gloved hand, the assisting nurse immediately immerses the tube in a solution of sodium bicarbonate. The stoma edges and suture line are aseptically cleansed with a mild skin antiseptic and thoroughly dried with dry wool swabs. The replacement tube is fitted with new tape before it is inserted into the tracheal stoma. These tapes are taken around the neck and tied at the side. A keyhole dressing, e.g., Lyfoam, should also be prepared, along with a gauze swab which fits snugly behind the shield of the outer tube. Sutures along the wound edge tend to be left for as long as possible, usually 10–14 days. This is because the integrity of the wound is continually threatened by moisture from mucus secretion and is slow to heal. In male patients, a close skin shave is necessary every day by a skilled barber to reduce the discomforts of hair near the wound site. The used tube should be thoroughly cleansed and brushed before being returned to theatre or the central sterile supply unit.

Detubation (Permanent Removal)

Closure of the tracheal stoma can be achieved by reducing the diameter of the outer tube each time it is replaced every second day. This will allow the stoma to heal progressively. Alternatively, the lumen of the tube can be occluded by a piece of shaped cork for increasing periods of time each day. At first the patient tends to panic, often having adapted extremely well to tracheal breathing and having to relearn nasal respiration. However, one major advantage of the cork method is that the patient will regain the use of speech, even with a tube in place, and the nurse can do much to promote the patient's confidence by gentle encouragement to use the vocal cords. Once the tracheal stoma is of a small enough diameter, the tube can be removed altogether and the stoma covered by a seal dressing held in place by adhesive tape. The main problem related to detubation is that of stenosis or fibrosis of the stoma edge. This stubborn problem will inhibit any healing and therefore closure, and it may be necessary for the surgeon to refashion the stoma and close it by suture in theatre.

COMPLICATIONS OF TRACHEOSTOMY

Continuous assessment is made to detect any of the following complications which may arise immediately following the tracheostomy or during the course of care.

Surgical Emphysema of the Neck Tissues

On incision into the trachea, air escapes and may find its way into the surrounding tissues below the skin. This can also result from incorrectly sited tubes at the time of operation. The tissues appear swollen and crackle when touched. This emphysema may extend from the base of the neck across the chest wall to the axilla.

It is in fact only a minor discomfort and the air will be reabsorbed from the tissues within a few days, but occasionally may give rise to infection if the skin is roughly handled.

Laryngeal or Tracheal Stenosis

A stenosis, which means a hardening or fibrosis, may occur either at the stoma site or at the larynx. Either site indicates that the tracheostomy tube has been left in for far too long, allowing the tissues to fibrose. In those cases where a permanent tracheostomy is required, a fibrosis of the stoma is desirable. Otherwise it is necessary for the surgeon to refashion the stoma so that it can heal and close the stoma permanently.

Atelectasis

The collapse of a lobe or the whole lung may be due to one of the main bronchi becoming blocked by a plug of mucus. One aim of frequent suction is to avoid this very risk. The aid of specific physiotherapy exercises, always preceded by suction, will do much to prevent this complication. If, however, preventative and conservative measures fail to move the mucus plug, it may have to be aspirated via a bronchoscope while the patient is under the effects of general anaesthesia.

Wound Fistula

Since the wound around the stoma is persistently moist, the tissues tend to become infected easily and many necrose. The infection may track into the neck tissues and form a sinus wound which remains infected with copious exudate. Such a wound is very resistant to healing, despite the use of antibiotics and scrupulous aseptic technique. Often deeper surgical toilet and debridement in the operating theatre is required.

Chapter 70
Cancer of the Pharynx and Larynx

Primary tumours arising in either the pharynx or larynx tend to occur mostly in male patients, over the age of 40, who have been smoking cigarettes for a very long time. The very early symptoms of a tumour within the throat are vague, but disturbing enough to make the patient feel uneasy though without any definite reason for undue alarm. At first there is the sensation within the throat of a minor irritation, which is ineffectively relieved by persistent coughing. The tone of speech becomes thicker and, as the tumour increasingly involves the vocal cords, a hoarse voice becomes apparent. Should a patient complain of hoarseness for over a period of 4 months, it is highly suggestive of a laryngeal tumour. The symptoms increase in their complexity as the tumour infiltrates and spreads directly into all the structures of the larynx. Since the tumour can be regarded as an obstruction to both the airway and the oesophagus, both dysphagia and dyspnoea develop insidiously, becoming the focus of the patient's problems. The dysphagia prevents the patient from swallowing their own saliva, which means that they tend to expectorate very frequently requiring a great number of sputum pots. In an attempt to relieve the dysphagia, the patient coughs persistently and eventually may produce blood stained sputum. A second problem arising from the dysphagia is a marked loss of weight, since normal food cannot be taken. Reflex otalgia, i.e., earache, can be of an unremitting nature as the tumour presses on the ninth cranial nerve which also passes through the middle ear.

INVESTIGATIONS

Sometimes the diagnosis is relatively straightforward, since the tumour may be visually obvious with a direct laryngoscopy using a laryngeal mirror. The vocal cords can also be seen to be fixed, instead of vibrating as air passes over and between them. A series of investigations to determine the presence and extent of the tumour may include:

1. Lateral and anterior X-rays of the chest and neck, including tomograms to seek for unusual shadows or outlines.
2. Using a local or general anaesthetic the patient may have to undergo laryngoscopy, pharyngoscopy, bronchoscopy or oesophagoscopy to establish the primary site of the cancer and the extent of its invasiveness.
3. A biopsy is often taken for histological studies to prove that the tumour is derived from a malignant cell.
4. The neck and cervical lymph glands are involved as secondary sites, so these are usually examined in detail.
5. The tumour may of course spread directly to the lungs and an investigation would aim at excluding this possibility before local treatment commenced.

TREATMENT

Several possibilities of treatment may be considered, such as deep X-ray therapy to irradiate the primary site and the soft tissues of the neck. Following the initial treatment, the patient would have a rest period and then a block dissection of the cervical glands, i.e., a total removal of the lymph glands and vessels located between the larynx and the cervical spine. This may or may not be accompanied by a laryngectomy.

Laryngectomy

Laryngectomy is a major operation which may include the total or partial removal of either the pharynx, larynx, or upper oesophagus. It can be combined with the unilateral or bilateral removal of the cervical glands. Many of the investigations and tests will have been completed prior to hospital admission. The surgeon should also have given a considerably detailed explanation to the patient of what the operation entails. For such major surgery, a hospital stay between 3 and 4 weeks is usual. The principles of care involved when preparing the patient for surgery are set out below, but of paramount importance is the patient's familiarity with the ward environment and the nursing staff. This will instil into the patient a feeling of confidence. This feeling of trust would take between 3 and 4 days as the basic routine preparations are carried out as for any surgery. The commonly expressed fears with this type of operation include those of mutilation, the permanent loss of voice, and of work. The nurse can play a key role in alleviating these anxieties by explaining what is involved (see below).

Preoperative Counselling

Preoperative counselling must take into account 4 major considerations of postoperative care, the degree of counselling being adjusted according to what the patient has already been told by the surgeon:

1. Following surgery the patient will be dependent on respiration via a tracheostomy tube. Depending on the surgery performed, this may be either temporary or permanent. For a total laryngectomy the tracheostomy will be permanent. If the patient has a positive outlook, and can in the nurse's opinion understand the implications of a tracheostomy, it may be useful for the patient to handle or be shown a tracheostomy tube which will be used postoperatively. It is also useful to educate the patient regarding the plethora of equipment which will be around the bed in the immediate postoperative period. This includes the tracheostomy trolley, oxygen, suction, nasogastric feeding, oral toilet and intravenous therapy.
2. Since the swallowing reflex will be temporarily lost the surgeon will usually request nasogastric feeding for several days after surgery. Apart from giving liquified high protein, high calorie feeds every few

hours, the diet may be supplemented by intravenous infusions of Intralipid, Aminosol and Dextrose, i.e., parenteral therapy. Prior to the actual operation it will be a major task to correct any nutritional deficiencies so the patient is as nutritionally fit as possible for the proposed surgery. This will include persuading the patient to take a high protein diet, supplemented with vitamins and iron compounds to correct an expected anaemia. It may be necessary to tube feed the patient prior to surgery if dysphagia is a pronounced symptom. It is vital that the lower colon is empty of faeces before surgery. It is preferred that the patient avoids the desire to empty the colon for 3 days postoperatively to prevent any strain on the throat musculature.

3. A total laryngectomy implies a permanent loss of speech since the vocal cords will be removed along with the larynx. The restoration of some form of speech requires the expertise of a speech therapist, who should be introduced to the patient before surgery. From a nursing point of view a system of communication will have to be established, one for dealing with emergency situations and another for everyday nurse-patient communication. Whichever system is decided upon, e.g., note pad and pencil, picture cards, hand signals or lip reading, this should be known to all staff and relatives so that the patient is never placed under stress trying to determine whether the nurse is familiar with the system being used.

4. The relatives should be included in the preoperative counselling sessions, so they too are mentally prepared for what is going to happen. No matter how often the patient or relatives are counselled, the actual reality is both visually and physically harrowing for the layman. Preoperative counselling however does cushion the psychological stress and creates within the relatives a feeling of coping and also that they can positively contribute to the patient's care, even if it means no more than not displaying alarm and fear at the bedside when visiting.

Postoperative Care

The first 72 hours of postoperative care are the most critical, implying that the patient should not be left without a nurse for this period. The difficulties with which the patient has to cope include the repeated obstruction of the inner tracheostomy tube by excessive mucoid secretions, requiring very frequent suction and changing of the inner tube. Since the patient has to deal with a new method of respiration, there are frequent periods of minor panic arising from breathlessness. The patient has to be reminded not to try and breathe through the mouth or nose, as this will compete with tracheal respiration. In the event of oral or nasal breathing because of the tracheal tube, the air would not be able to reach the trachea. The difficulties of tracheal obstruction are reduced by the use of a portable humidification unit via which oxygen is supplied to the tracheostomy tube. The outer tube is not usually changed during the first 72 hours.

Another problem of which the nurse should be aware is that the restlessness of the patient may be due to severe headache and painful neck musculature due to the prolonged operation time during which the head and neck have been maintained in extension. The adroit use of pillows, not only maintaining the patient in an upright position but to cradle the neck and head, may ensure a more restful patient. The first postoperative night is a very frightening experience for the patient as he or she has to adapt to the new method of breathing and, apart from administering a potent analgesic, a large dose of sedation and an antiemetic will promote several hours of, albeit fitful, sleep.

In the first 24 hours tube feeding should be a low volume, low calorie value and delivered at a cool temperature, being neither too hot or too cold. Tube feeding may in fact threaten the pharyngeal suture line within the restructured laryngeal cavity. On the second day the patient should be encouraged to take small sips of clear fluid to begin the long process of regaining swallowing control. Until such time as the patient has complete control over swallowing, the nurse will have to offer oral toilet every 4 hours during the day. It is pointless offering mouthwashes, as the patient will not be able to gargle and has little power to expectorate.

Additional to the specialised care required for tracheostomy and nasogastric feeding, the general care is planned to meet the patient's needs for the next 7 days. This includes the discontinuation of any intravenous therapy, increasing periods of being allowed to sit out of bed, increasing periods of chest physiotherapy and gently leading the patient towards full independence. It is not unusual to teach the patient how to change their own tracheostomy tube, and to apply suction as and when they feel they need it. The surgeon would indicate the size and type of permanent tracheostomy tube most suitable for the patient, and detubation may begin once the surrounding wound shows signs of healing, the sutures remaining until 10–14 days later.

SPEECH THERAPY

Speech therapy should certainly be introduced before the patient is considered ready for convalescence, and it may be that the patient will be started on one of 3 types of speech retraining programme if a voice box is not to be used:

Alaryngeal speech
Oesophageal speech
Pharyngeal voice

The basic principle involved is to persuade the patient to inhale air and then to belch it up at the same time using the constrictor muscles of the anatomical area as air vibrators, and as the air is expelled from the mouth to also use the tongue and lips to shape words into sounds. It is vital for these exercises that the patient is totally relaxed and has a high motivation to repeatedly practice them. Much of this motivation can be derived from the positive approach of the nurses giving the direct care.

COMPLICATIONS

During the period leading towards detubation, the nurse should be constantly vigilant to observe for and report any of the following specific complications:

1. Salivary fistula formation, especially if the pharyngeal suture line threatens to break down. The local signs at the wound include increased exudate of actual saliva, which keeps the suture line of the neck tissues constantly wet. The neck tissues require protection against maceration.

2. If deep X-ray therapy has been completed, the soft tissues of the neck will not heal so rapidly and the blood vessels within the area may tend to rupture, this particularly applies to the carotid artery if a block dissection of the lymph glands has also been done.

Having adapted to the permanent tracheostomy and ultimately the detubation the patient may express concern about the cosmetic features and appearance of the neck. The wearing of a cravat during the day and replacing the tube at night is the easiest solution to the problem. The majority of patients with laryngectomy do extremely well, having an expected survival rate of between 10 and 20 years. They may also be put in contact with a Laryngectomy Club, several of which are to be found throughout the country.

Chapter 71
Structure and Function of the Skin

STRUCTURE OF THE SKIN

The outer layer of the fertilized ovum, i.e., the integumentum, gives rise to the development of the ectoderm, or the skin. During the development of the fetus the ectoderm becomes invaginated into the fetal body along the mid-dorsal line. Once absorbed, the ectoderm develops into the brain, spinal cord and sensory organs of the eye, ears, taste buds, olfactory bulb, temperature centre control and the endocrine glands. Thus, the basis of an extraordinary but harmonious relationship between the skin and the central and autonomic nervous systems is established before birth and continues throughout the

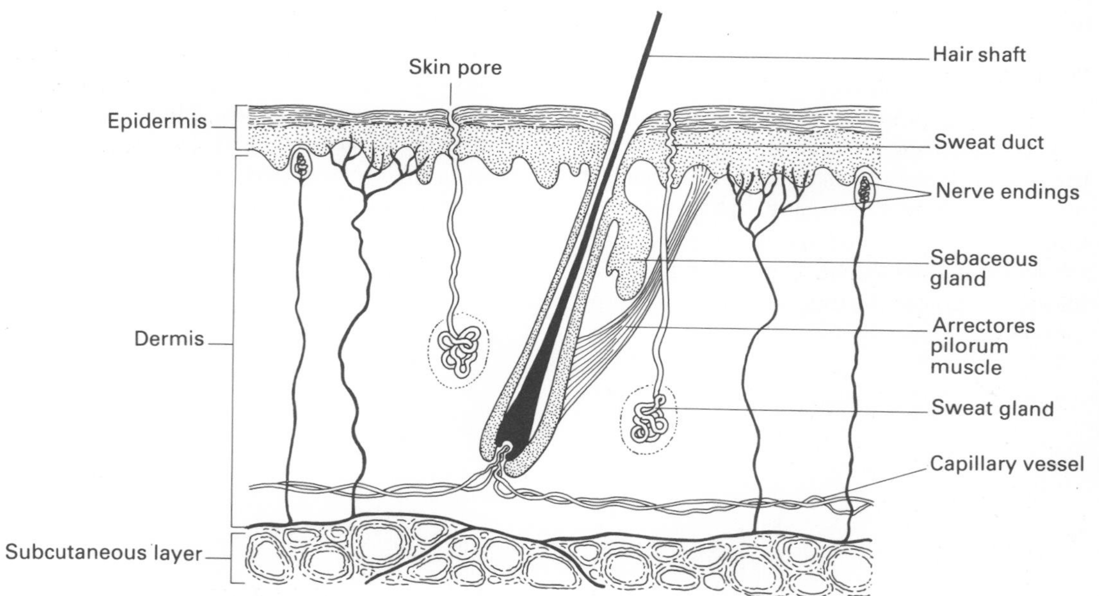

Fig. 71.1 Structure of the skin.

individual's life. Because of this close relationship, the skin is often regarded as the 'mirror of the mind', its condition often reflecting the state of the patient's thinking and general health at any given time. A depressed patient not only appears lethargic, but the skin sags and lacks any firmness of tone, whereas the excited happy individual positively glows with well-being, shown by the texture and tone of the skin.

The skin is the largest organ of the body, measuring between 1.6 and 1.9 sq. m. (M^2) or about 47 yards in area. In the average adult the skin would represent 6–10% of the body weight. Skin is divided into 2 distinct layers: (1) the upper and outer epidermis composed of stratified squamous epithelium, and (2) the deeper thicker dermis composed of fibrous connective tissue. Immediately below the dermis lies a connective layer of superficial fascia composed of areolar and fatty tissue (Fig. 71.1).

The epidermis is subdivided into two distinct zones: the lower germinative zone and an upper horny zone. These zones are each composed of various layers and working from the base of the dermis upwards they are as set out below (Fig. 71.2).

Germinative Zone

Stratum Germinativum or Basal Layer

Stratum germinativum constantly produce new epithelial cells to replace those being lost from the horny layer. As the new cells ascend to reach the upper zone, they become *keratinised* or hardened by the addition of protein to the cell structure. It takes about 14 days for a new cell to reach the horny layer, where it will remain for a further 14 days before being shed as part of the normal epithelial desquamation.

Stratum Spinosum or Prickle Cell Layer

The stratum spinosum is also known as the Malphigian layer and is composed of irregularly shaped columnar cells held together by prickle-like cell projections emanating from the cell wall. Scattered throughout this layer are the melanoblast cells which produce the pigment melanin that gives an individual his or her skin colour. Skin colour is determined genetically, but is strongly influenced by such factors as the capillary blood flow, and the melanocyte stimulating hormone (MSH) secreted from the pituitary gland.

The Upper Horny Zone

The upper horny zone can be made up of either 2 or 3 layers depending on which part of the body the skin surface is located.

Stratum Granulosum

The stratum granulosum is so called because of the presence of granules in the cellular cytoplasm. It is at this level that the new cells begin the process of being keratinised.

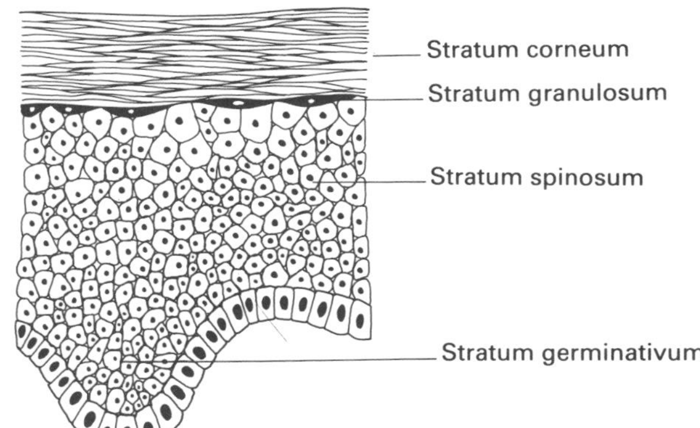

Fig. 71.2 Layers of the epidermis.

Stratum Lucideum

The stratum lucideum is present only on the thicker skin of the soles of the feet and the palmar surface. It has no hair follicles penetrating through its surface, but is interrupted by the coiled sweat glands and their ducts.

Stratum Corneum or True Horny Layer

The stratum corneum can be considered as a layer of dead epithelial cells converted into water repellant protein, i.e., keratin. This surface abounds with mainly commensal saprophytic micro-organisms. The cells are constantly being shed and replaced by newly keratinised epithelial cells.

Connective Tissue

The deeper dermis is a layer of connective tissue, mainly composed of fibrous protein collagen fibres embedded in mucopolysaccharide and supported by reticulum and elastic fibres. The undersurface of the epidermis is ridged and dented and provides the attachment for the dermis. Because of the unique ridging patterns seen clearly at the fingertips, fingerprints are widely used for identification purposes in police work. The dermis contains all the appendages for the function of the skin, these being the hair root and follicle, sebaceous glands, sweat glands and apocrine glands. Other structures permeating the dermal layer are the blood capillaries, lymphatic vessels, microscopic nerve endings, wandering tissue cells and the nail beds.

The Hair

Hair is widely distributed over the skin surface, being of dense growth in particular areas such as the scalp, axilla, pubes and perineum. The hair root is embedded in the dermis and the epithelial cells lying over this root, i.e., the papillae, ensure continuous new growth. Extending from the root is the follicle which, as it ascends into the epidermal layer, becomes keratinised. The hair visible on the skin surface is called the hair shaft. Similar to the epithelial cells, the hair shaft will also eventually be replaced by new hair and at a prolific rate if one considers how frequently a male has to shave, or how often a hair trim is required. Attached to each hair follicle is a fine muscle called the arrector pili. When this muscle contracts, it pulls the hair shaft upright. It is also the cause of so called 'gooseflesh'. The arrector pili muscle contracts in response to a fear reaction, 'hair standing upright', or due to intense cold in an effort to conserve body heat.

Hair colour is determined by the quality and quantity of the pigment melanin secreted from the melanoblasts in the prickle cell layer. White hair means the melanoblasts have stopped manufacturing melanin, which is associated with the aging process. Hair shafts emerging from the eyelids, nostrils and external auditory ear are protective in that they trap dust and other particles, but hair located elsewhere on the body seems to have no true function, perhaps a prehistoric vestige of helping to keep the body warm.

The Sebaceous Glands

There are at least 2 sebaceous glands to each hair follicle. They secrete an oily substance called sebum, which keeps the hair shaft soft and pliant. Sebum is a complex mixture of lipids and fatty acids and is mildly bacteriostatic and fungostatic in the healthy adult. Its oily consistency keeps the skin waterproof, but conversely also stops the skin excreting too much water via perspiration. It is a subtle point to note, but sebum does **not** protect the skin, only the hair shaft. This observation is borne out by the number of times a day a nurse washes the hands without any ill effect.

The Sweat Glands

The sweat glands are coiled tubes of cuboidal epithelium with a duct leading up to the epidermis, permitting sweat to escape onto the skin surface via a tiny opening, the pore, where the sweat will evaporate and by so doing help to maintain the individual's body temperature. Sweat is composed mainly of water minerals such as sodium, chloride, potassium and sulphate. There is a minute amount of nitrogenous waste product.

Each gland is surrounded by a capillary network which secretes excess tissue fluid into the gland for excretion as sweat. It permits the body one mechanism for keeping cool when the metabolic rate is raised as the result of hard physical labour or living in hot dry climates. The sweat has great difficulty in evaporating from the skin in hot, humid climates.

Both the sebaceous and sweat glands are under hormonal and nervous influences. If one imagines the 'cold sweat' of fear, or the 'acne' of teenagers, one can appreciate that the glands do not work in isolation from the other body systems.

The Apocrine Glands

The apocrine glands are specialised sweat and sebaceous glands located at the breast, perineum and axilla and are responsible for the odour characteristic to each individual. Certainly in certain species of animals these glands function as pherochemoreceptors to act as the attraction between male and female.

The Nails

Nails are derived from epithelial cells lying under the lunula or white crescent at the proximal end of the nail. These epidermal cells are rapidly converted to especially dense keratin and each nail has a phenomenal growth rate.

A FUNCTION OF THE SKIN

The blood vessels, lymphatic vessels, nerve endings and reticuloendothelial structures are best considered as follows:

1. **Protective.** The skin reacts and responds to the external environment by constantly adjusting the blood flow through its layers to conserve or lose body heat according to the external temperature. It is a natural water repellent structure which resists chemical, thermal and bacterial threats, providing the skin barrier remains intact.

2. **Sensory.** Scattered throughout the dermis are many diverse microscopic nerve endings which give a reflex response when stimulated by either pressure, texture, touch, temperature (both hot and cold) and in particular pain. These reflexes are protective in nature but are also good examples of reflex arc behaviours. The fingertips are especially richly endowed with nerve endings.

3. **Excretory.** The excretion of sweat containing water, minerals and some waste products once evaporated from the skin surface contributes to the control of body temperature and electrolyte balance.

4. **Secretory.** Sebum secreted from the sebaceous glands keeps the body hair supple and pliant. It also helps to keep the skin waterproof and because it is slightly acid has a bacteriostatic effect.

5. **Productive.** The action of the ultraviolet rays of the sunlight acting on ergosterol on the skin helps to produce vitamin D (calciferol).

6. **Attachment.** Appendages such as the hair, nails, subcutaneous fat and superficial fascia contribute to an individual's characteristics of body shape and contour.

7. **Absorption.** The skin surface has a very limited ability to absorb, the exception being topically applied creams, pastes, lotion or ointments containing an active drug ingredient, but even this is a limited local action.

Chapter 72 Dermatology Nursing Guidelines

The majority of medicaments applied directly to the skin are selected for their blandness and, as it is preferred that they be applied with the fingers, nurses should **not** wear gloves or fingercots, or apply pastes with a spatula. The only exceptions to this rule are the contagious conditions of which there are only a few, i.e., impetigo, herpes simplex, pediculosis, Norwegian scabies and syphilis. Since the nurse is constantly using the fingers and hands to apply various ointments and creams, the actual skin should remain supple and in good condition. Some attention should be given to keeping the fingernails short and well trimmed so that they never scratch a patient's vulnerable skin. Lotions with a known stain reaction, such as potassium permanganate, can easily be removed by washing the hands in a solution of Teepol, a well-known shampoo.

The nurse's uniform is protected from staining by wearing a plastic disposable apron, preferably the same colour as those sheets and towels used to protect the patient. A distinctive colour such as green or blue is normally used for all linen in the dermatology unit, or ward, to help distinguish it from the linen used in other parts of the hospital and from other clinical specialities.

An experienced dermatology nurse has an unparalleled knowledge of the many medications used in the treatment of skin conditions. A particular knowledge is needed of the active ingredient in the variety of lotions, creams and pastes which are in current use. It is equally important that the nurse has an appreciation of the possible side effects which the active ingredient can cause. This is more so with steroid creams and ointments. The same checking procedures are required as with any drug, particular note being made of the manufacturer's date of expiry and a thorough reading of any literature supplied with the drug to highlight any associated hazards with the drug prescribed. A particular skill related to patient care is the means and methods employed to communicate instructions about drug therapy and self-administered treatments. Many of the errors in dermatology are due to poor misunderstandings stemming from inadequate or poorly given instructions. For this reason, many departments have compiled instruction leaflets written in a clear and concise format to help the patient complete a course of prescribed treatment. Another important point is for the nurse to listen very carefully to the patient's own opinion about the drugs they are taking. Often the skin condition is of a chronic nature and the patient's knowledge about their condition often exceeds that of the nurse or the doctor, and the nurse should be humble enough to learn from her or his own patients.

During a therapeutic session, e.g., a medicated bath, the nurse should develop a rapport which allows the patient to express verbally their anxieties, worries, fears and frustrations. Careful listening may help both the patient and nurse to identify a specific psychological conflict which may often be the trigger of atopic skin conditions. It is often an assumption in dermatology nursing that a skin condition is a cause or a consequence of mental conflict. A caring mature approach which does not reveal any revulsion over the very disfiguring skin lesions may give the patient that confidence to begin explaining and talking through their own version of their problems. This type of conversation is of course confidential, but any relevant features should be given to the medical staff who may wish to pursue a particular point with the patient.

INITIAL EXAMINATION

An initial dermatological examination of a patient usually involves a total body examination of the skin surface in an excellent light source, in a warm environment, and in complete privacy. This is followed by a detailed history of the patient's symptoms and background to elicit as far as possible any familial, environmental, or allergic causes. To enable this first assessment the nurse should check that the room is suitably equipped with a low level examination couch which is protected by a disposable sheet.

Patch Testing

A microscope is an essential component of diagnosis, and glass slides and staining materials are needed to prepare a slide for taking skin scales or hair follicles for immediate examination. The equipment required for patch testing in suspected allergy reactions should be in a constant state of readiness. A trolley holding the following basic items should include:

- Small nail scissors
- Whitfield's hair forceps
- A one piece scalpel for skin scale specimen collection
- Comedo expressor to remove blackhead spots
- Several sizes of curettes
- Pointed and flat headed orange sticks and wooden spatulas
- A standard selection of skin antiseptics
- Rosaline dyes
- A standard selection of skin lotions, pastes, ointments, and creams
- Liberal supply of old but clean linen, wool swabs and gauze squares
- Tubular bandaging and stockinette
- Occlusive paste bandages

THE RULES OF BANDAGING

The clinical skill of bandaging is of major importance in dermatology and it is a useful exercise to review the rules of bandaging.

For Limbs

Commence from the distal inner aspect of the limb

Anchor the bandage with two turns

Ascend the limb, overlapping each turn by one third

Use a figure-of-eight turn at the principal joints

If possible, bandage the joint in slight flexion

Finish the bandage on the outer aspect of the limb

These rules are helpful when applying paste bandages to the limbs. Firstly they are occlusive and secondly the active ingredient in the paste will come into direct contact with the skin lesion being treated. Thirdly, they are often left in position for a prolonged period, hence the need to be very expert in bandaging. Paste bandages can be either:

Zinc paste BPC

Zinc paste and ichthammol

Zinc paste and coal tar

Zinc paste and iodochlorohydroxyquinlon

The active ingredients of these bandages may prove therapeutic in such conditions as chronic eczema, dermatitis and skin ulceration. In cold weather the paste bandage may have to be slightly warmed before it becomes amenable for application to the limb. After it is applied, the bandage will normally be covered with either tubigrip or stockinette bandage to protect the patient's personal clothing from becoming stained.

Tubular and stockinette bandaging and Netelast products are a positive boon in dermatology as they are easily applied to either a single digit, or to the whole body if a 'suit' is required for the patient. The skill of cutting and fitting is quickly learned and, in addition to being protective, such bandages also give considerable support to the limb or body surface and are excellent when dressing difficult areas such as natural flexures or skin creases. They also permit the individual joint to maintain optimal natural movement.

COMMON DERMATOLOGICAL TERMS

Alopecia. The absence of body hair from areas where it is normally present.

Bullae. Areas of elevated skin at least 1 cm in diameter containing serous or purulent fluids.

Keloid (Cheloid). A cosmetically disfiguring scar due to excess collagen being deposited during connective tissue healing.

Crusts. Hard horny masses of cells formed from an exudate.

Comedo. More commonly known as a blackhead, comedo is a plug in a secretory duct of the skin which is infected.

Erythema. Redness of the skin due to congestion of the local capillaries.

Furunculosis. Painful staphylococcal infected nodule, i.e., a boil.

Keratosis. A horny thickening of the epidermis due to increased rate of keratinisation or the deposit of protein.

Lichenification. A thickening of the skin (epidermis) which feels like leather.

Macula. For example, a freckle, or a flat small discoloured area.

Papule. For example, a pimple, which is a small raised solid area either flat topped or of conical shape.

Petechia. Red or purple spots disseminated over the skin.

Pustule. Similar to a papule usually larger and containing pus.

Plaque. An elevated area of abnormal skin.

Pruritis. Itching of the skin from any cause.

Scales. Collection of dead epithelial cells, adhering together to form a mass on the skin surface. They are derived from the stratum cornea.

Vesicle. Similar to a papule, but contains clear fluid, e.g., a small blister typical of chickenpox, allergic reactions and impetigo.

Weal (Wheal). The full skin thickness is elevated by a transient oedema, as seen in nettle rash which is an example of an inflammatory response.

Chapter 73
Common Skin Infections

IMPETIGO

This infectious skin condition is mainly caused by *Staphylococcus aureus*, but Streptococci may also be a causative organism. While the face is the area mostly affected, other parts of the body can be covered with the impetigo lesions. The affected skin becomes moist, developing red looking plaques and these in turn become covered by a yellowish dried exudate (Fig. 73.1). If the impetigo is the primary condition, the skin has probably been self-infected if the host has a high staphylococcal nasal count. A secondary impetigo can be induced by scratching a skin already

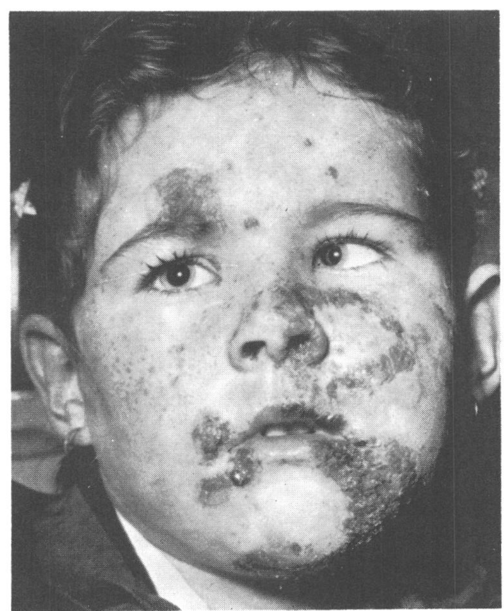

Fig. 73.1 Impetigo.

affected by either atopic eczema (dermatitis), scabies, or pediculosis capitis (head lice). It is usual practice to treat dermatitis after the impetigo has been dealt with, but scabies and head lice must be treated before the impetigo.

A swab is taken from the edge of the main lesion, before treatment is started with a systemic antibiotic such as Erythromycin or Cloxacillin. The crusts over the moist lesions are soaked 3 times each day with a skin antiseptic lotion such as Cetrimide 2%, and then the crusts are gently removed. Once the moist lesion is exposed, a topical antibiotic is applied, either Fuciden or Neomycin being the first choice. If the crusts prove to be excessive or very hard they can be softened with a boric and starch poultice every day, but this is unusual with modern antibiotics. Those patients who are self-infecting themselves should have Nasepten cream applied to the nasal skin and nostrils to reduce the staphylococcal count and it is a wise precaution to take nasal swabs of all the family (if applicable) and commence the same local nasal treatment if they too have a high staphylococcal nasal count. Impetigo occurring in institutions can usually be traced to the sharing of linen, soaps, towels in particular, and other toiletries. Apart from temporarily isolating the patient, the nursing staff should review any existing policies regarding sharing of personal articles. In maternity, children's and neonate units, the staff must be very diligent and implement the strictest isolation protocol in any case of impetigo since it can quickly reach epidemic proportions in vulnerable children.

Impetigo is a predisposing illness and is the cause of acute nephritis. It may also be the cause of a secondary eczema.

ERYSIPILAS

Erysipilas may occur as an acute single attack or be of a recurring nature. In the acute form the causative pathogens, i.e., streptococci, invade the deeper skin layers via inoculation through a tiny, almost imperceptible, crack on the skin surface. Before any skin changes appear, the patient becomes pyrexial and may suffer a rigor, as well as feeling extremely ill. The first discernible skin change is that of a patch of erythema of a well defined area, very hot to the touch, which spreads rapidly across one side of the face in plaques which soon become vesicular. The face is the one area most frequently affected and may involve the skin near the orbit, causing a marked oedema of the eyelids. Acute erysipilas responds quickly to a systemic course of antibiotics, e.g., benzylpenicillin 600 mg intramuscularly every 6 hours for 5 days, and then followed by a 7-day course of oral antibiotics. Skin vesicles also respond quickly when neobacrin cream is applied to the lesions.

Recurrent erysipilas is however far more difficult to treat, areas other than the face being affected. Lymphatic obstruction is one feature of the recurring erysipilas and this leads to lymphatic oedema of the eyelids, lips and, if affected, the limbs. The oedema may in turn lead to a cellulitis or inflammation of the tissues. Initially the portal of entry of the causative organism has to be identified, and a swab taken for culture and sensitivity, before being treated with either antibiotic or an antifungal cream. The more severe skin lesions may also require to be treated with a topical antibiotic cream. If the limb is affected by oedema, it is best to advise that it is rested in an elevated position with perhaps a compressive bandage supporting the limb. Oral penicillin 250 mg twice daily will normally induce a good response. For those patients with a history of repeated attacks over a period of years, the physician may elect to give the patient a standby prescription of antibiotics which they are advised to commence at the first indication of their recognisable symptoms, e.g., pyrexia, feeling unwell, or erythema. By anticipating the infection, the subsequent lesions are kept in control.

FURUNCULOSIS (BOILS, CARBUNCLES)

A boil can be described as a nodule containing pus or an abscess in a single hair follicle, while a carbuncle involves a group of hair follicles which are spread over a given area. Furunculosis can sometimes resemble acne in its appearance. The initial invasion of the deeper skin layer by the staphylococcus is via a friction injury such as a collar rubbing the neck or cuffs rubbing against the wrists, especially if the cuff or the skin is wet. Some conditions which predispose to furunculosis are eczema, diabetes mellitus and leukaemia. The patient may have a very high number of potentially pathogenic staphylococci in the nasal cavity and perineum and are self-infecting their skin. If the patient is in contact with a carrier, he or she may contract their infection during the winter months when nasal discharge from a carrier tends to be more of a problem. Nursing and medical staff who are proven to be carriers of staphylococci should not have any patient contact until their carrier state has been treated by antibiotics and a nasal swab taken to prove they are free from infection.

The treatment plan aims to reduce the staphylococcal numbers on the skin and to reduce their tendency to spread across the skin. All patients with boils should have their urine tested to exclude the possibility of diabetes mellitus. An increase in blood sugar does increase the likelihood of skin infections. Nasal swabs are routinely taken and despatched to pathology for culture and sensitivity to identify the causative organism. If the staphylococcus is positively found on these cultures, the nasal cavity is treated by applying an antibiotic ointment such as Chlorhexidine and Neomycin every day. The boil and the immediate surrounding area is treated by applying, for example, oxytetracycline ointment 3 times daily covering the lesion with gauze held in place by a lightweight bandage. Adhesive tape should not be used on the skin since it increases the risk of further infection from the site of the boil. If the lesion is located on a skin crease, this is better dealt with by an application of silver nitrate 2% in 50% spirit lotion which is allowed to dry before the clothing is replaced. Axilliary infection with or without boils is best treated with an antibiotic ointment such as Fucidin. The patient can be advised to cleanse his or her skin with an antiseptic soap and to dry their skin thoroughly before dusting lightly using an antiseptic talcum powder. If the patient has a very low resistance to staphylococci, a course of ultraviolet light will reduce the surface bacteria. Systemic antibiotics are only of value if there is a complication with the boil or furuncles, which includes cellulitis and lymphatic oedema. Furuncles which do not respond to antibiotic therapy and are fluctuant are incised and allowed to drain freely after a local anaesthetic has been given. Aseptic dressings are then completed daily until the indurated tissue has healed by granulation.

ACNE

Obstruction and inflammation of the pilosebaceous follicles of the face, neck, chest and back, appearing as crops of disfiguring spots, is quite common during adolesence, and is known as acne vulgaris (Fig. 73.2). There appears to be an equal distribution of this condition between the sexes. A well defined

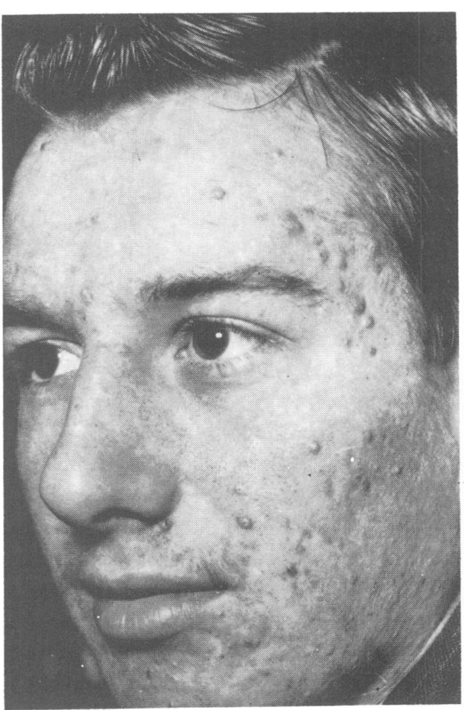

Fig. 73.2 Acne vulgaris.

series of changes occurs in the layers of the skin and follows a sequence of steps:

1. The hair follicle canal becomes blocked by a combination of dried sebum and a thickening of the horny opening at the opening of the hair follicle. This gives rise to the appearance of blackheads or comedos.
2. The sebaceous glands become distended, causing superficial papules.
3. In the deeper layers the tissue becomes inflamed causing the presence of painful nodules. The affected area may then become affected by cysts.
4. Any tendency to pick, squeeze or rub the blackheads, papules, or nodules may cause post-acne scarring.

The patient tends to have a greasy seborrhoeic skin, suggesting that this type of skin is more than usually prone. Acne can be induced by certain drugs such as the androgens, phenobarbitone, troxidone, phenytoin sodium, oral and topical steroids. An industrial form of acne can be caused by those processes which use chlorinated naphthalenes, e.g., in the rubber industry. A form of acne in middle-aged women known as *acne rosaecea* may occur during premenstrual oedema and is of a transient nature affecting the forehead, cheeks and skin over the lower jaw. Acne is rare in the negroid races and is far less common in sunny climates.

Prior to the prescribed treatment being given, the patient should have the benefit of a prolonged discussion to help place in perspective their natural anxieties, social isolation, and what can be for a teenager a major catastrophe in his or her own body image. Some guidelines which may help such a discussion would be to consider the following points:

Treatment, once started, may take from 4–12 weeks before there is any noticeable sign of improvement and it will require a great deal of patience on the patient's part. It is fatal to scratch, pick, or squeeze blackheads or other lesions. This in fact causes inflammation and will lead to scarring after the acne has resolved.

It is better to remove any blackheads with a proprietary abrasive remover such as Brasivol or a Comedome Stick.

Heavy clothing or activities which cause heavy perspiration exacerbate the condition, as will the wearing of high-necked pullovers.

Emotional distress worsens the condition and a state of depression or anxiety may require the appropriate drugs to lift the patient into a more positive, coping frame of mind.

Skin cleanliness is absolutely vital and hot soapy water should be used on each occasion of washing or bathing.

It has been noted by some researchers that eating chocolate, peanuts, bacon and pork fat has an adverse effect on acne by increasing the lipid content of sebum. These foods can be avoided if, when eaten, they obviously cause a worsening of the acne.

When taking holidays or short breaks away from home the patient should consider going to a dry warm sunny climate which will bring about an improvement, although it may be of a temporary nature.

During the counselling the nurse should note if there is any obvious emotional stress between the adolescent and the parent. If there is, this may delay recovery or reduce the chance of a successful treatment.

Treatment

The treatment follows 3 distinct avenues: relieving the pilosebaceous duct obstruction, reducing the skin microbial population, and decreasing the sebum excretion rate.

Relieving the Pilosebaceous Duct Obstruction

Application of tretinoin (vitamin A acid) lotion helps to relieve pilosebaceous duct obstruction by stimulating epithelial growth and reduces the tendency of any dried sebum to remain adherent in the follicle canal. The use of antimicrobial drugs also indirectly helps to release the duct obstruction.

Reducing the Skin Microbial Population

The control of any micro-organisms that may be present in large numbers, such as cornynebacterium acnes or staphylococci, can be achieved with the application of benzoyl peroxide (Panodyl Gel), cetrimide, neomycin or chloramphenicol. The micro-organisms can delay healing because they break down the triglycerides in the sebum to fatty acids, which then cause an inflammation. Antimicrobial therapy can be combined with ultraviolet light therapy at doses of E2 or E3, once weekly. If the acne is moderately severe or extreme in the area it affects, then a long-term course of oral antibiotics may be prescribed. The first choice is usually tetracycline 250 mg twice daily for 3 months. If the acne proves resistant, then the alternative drugs include erythromycin 500 mg daily, co-trimoxazole 2 tablets daily, or clindamycin 75–150 mg once daily. Antiseptic lotions such as Hibiscrub often prove useful if combined with systemic antibiotics.

Decreasing the Sebum Excretion Rate

The sebum excretion rate proves one of the more difficult avenues of therapy. Some patients may be tried with an oestrogen dominant hormone drug such as Minovlar or Ovulen, which may inhibit the hormone activity at the sebaceous gland level.

COMMON VIRAL SKIN INFECTIONS

The herpes group of viruses are the most persistent of the parasitic organisms, causing a considerable number of skin lesions. The most common of these are Herpes simplex, Herpes zoster, Molluscum contagiosum and warts.

Herpes Simplex

A parasitic virus which causes a minor but irritating lesion, when the skin erupts in smaller vesicular lesions grouped near the lips, at or near a body orifice such as the genitalia and anus. The incidence of genital herpes simplex has increased dramatically during recent times and is attributed to increased sexual freedom. The virus is usually contracted early in life and remains latent in the tissues until reactivated by any one of a number of stimuli, e.g., friction, trauma, heat, drugs or minor illness. About 60% of the population are carriers of the herpes simplex virus and cross-infection is inevitable. The primary infection takes between 10 and 14 days before the vesicular eruptions occur and in the vast majority of cases cause only a transient minor irritation and the lesion is self-limited. In the more severe forms recurring episodes make the patient's life very miserable. Scrapings from the vesicles are taken for cytology to confirm that the cause of the vesicular eruptions is in fact due to herpes simplex.

For mild attacks the patient can be advised to apply at regular intervals an astrigent lotion such as 70% alcohol directly to the lesion, or eau de Cologne. Recurring herpes simplex may be dealt with by prescribing herpid solution 5% (Diiodouridine) to be applied to the lesion every 4 hours each day for at least 4 days. Frequently recurring attacks may also benefit if the patient can attend hospital on a daily basis for superficial X-ray therapy.

In children, a herpes simplex may predispose to an aseptic meningitis or to a severe form of encephalitis, so the presence of the virus should never be underestimated and the child should be carefully observed until any lesions are cleared up. An associated pyrexia or irritated behaviour tantrum may be enough to suggest early meningism due to the herpes virus.

Herpes Zoster (Shingles)

The herpes zoster virus also causes chickenpox. Children between the ages of 2 and 6 years old contract chickenpox and on recovery the virus may remain latent in their tissues, particularly within the posterior horn root of the spinal cord. The latent virus can be reactivated at any time in later life, most commonly after the age of 45, by a variety of stimuli. The stimulus may take the form of trauma, drugs, leukaemia or a true psychiatric depression.

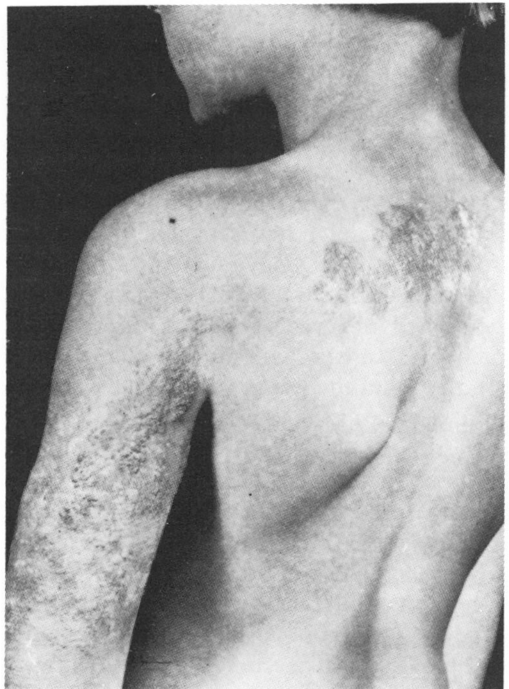

Fig. 73.3 Herpes zoster (shingles) (Institute of Dermatology, University of London).

On being reactivated the virus causes an inflammation and severe pain along the nerve track, extending from the particular level of the spinal cord affected. Hence, the zoster can appear across the abdomen, across the back and more commonly on the trigeminal nerve track over the face. Pain along the nerve track is the primary symptom and is usually severe enough for the patient to seek medical advice. The pain may last for 3 days before the first skin lesions appear. The lesion at first appears vesicular and classically will follow the nerve track. Eventually these vesicles erupt, becoming haemorrhagic, then purulent, and finally necrotic.

If the patient is young, that is over 16 but under 60 years old, the treatment is usually straightforward with a good response to analgesia, applying a skin antiseptic and remaining in bed until the lesions have resolved. The elderly, however, present many more problems. The principal problem is pain, and early treatment with potent analgesia is vital if post-herpetic neuralgia is to be avoided. The lesions are treated by applying topical idoxuridine 5% every 2 hours for 3 days. Alternatively the patient may be prescribed cytabarine intravenous injections once daily for 3 days. The patient is kept on bedrest, and nursing measures are introduced to reduce the associated pyrexia, nausea, anorexia and headache. Topical antibiotics are applied over the healing lesions to prevent any sepsis from occurring. If the nerve tract supplying the face, i.e., the trigeminal nerve, is involved along one of the branches supplying the facial muscles near the eye, this can lead to several ophthalmic complications such as conjunctivitis, iridocyclitis, photophobia and secondary glaucoma. If the eye is at all involved, an ophthalmic opinion should be sought to introduce treatment to control the likelihood of these complications.

After the local treatment has taken effect, the older patient may still be left with an intractable neuralgia due to the scarring which follows the inflammation of the nerve tract. Continuous analgesia, combined with an antidepressant and anticonvulsant, e.g., triptofen and phenytoin, may be required to overcome the patient's agitation and restlessness. The nature of the pain is such that all the normal daily activities are disrupted and any nursing assessment would have to measure to what extent this is causing physical neglect.

The risk of contracting herpes zoster is increased if patients have been prescribed either the steroid or immunosuppressive group of drugs. In these instances the physician may prescribe varicella hyperimmune globulin to prevent the occurrence of herpes zoster.

Molluscum Contagiosum

This viral lesion is caused by a pox virus and can resemble warts by behaving in a similar manner. The lesions are grouped together, usually over one area of the trunk, and appear as smooth, rounded, pearly coloured raised nodules. The virus is usually contracted in Turkish and public swimming baths. Treatment of these minor lesions is by any of the following methods:

1. Pricking the lesion with the pointed end of an orange stick which has been previously dipped into a phenol solution.
2. Freezing the lesions with liquid nitrogen.
3. Carefully curetting a small number of lesions in a series of treatments.

Warts

Warts are viral lesions which occur most frequently in the younger patient who has a moist skin. They may spread rapidly and can, on occasions, be contagious. Their appearance on any part of the body surface presents problems of selecting a suitable treatment from the many choices available. For the most part, warts are painless lesions except when they are located in awkward areas such as between the digits, on the soles of the feet, around the genitalia, or within a skin crease. In these circumstances, they will interfere with function because of friction. They are also cosmetically disfiguring, which detracts from a healthy body image. The variety of treatments available for children and adults are set out below.

In Children

Applying salactol (Dermal), a salicylic acid in a collodion preparation, directly onto the wart surface and repeating the therapy at regular intervals until the wart shrinks and falls away.

In Adults

The wart may be treated by a 'freezing technique'. A mixture of acetone–carbon dioxide, or liquid nitrogen, is applied directly to the wart with a cotton wool probe until the wart is frozen in appearance. It is then allowed to defrost and the treatment repeated. This is done every 2 weeks until the wart shrinks and falls away. If the wart is stubborn, it can be curetted out after being touched by a cautery probe.

Planter Warts (Verrucae)

Planter warts only appear on the soles of the feet. Normally, the weight of the body and the standing posture compress the wart surface into the thick skin of the soles of the feet, but they become obvious when the patient is at rest. They are treated by asking the patient to soak their feet every day in a solution of Formalin 3% for 10–15 minutes after they have abraded the wart surface with pumice. The healthy skin should be protected by a thin coating of paraffin gel. It may be necessary to continue this treatment for at least 6 weeks before any success can be achieved. Between treatments, the patient should be advised on the correct shoes to wear, i.e., low heel and leather to reduce the tendency to perspire, and pure wool socks if at all possible. Socks should be changed at least once a day.

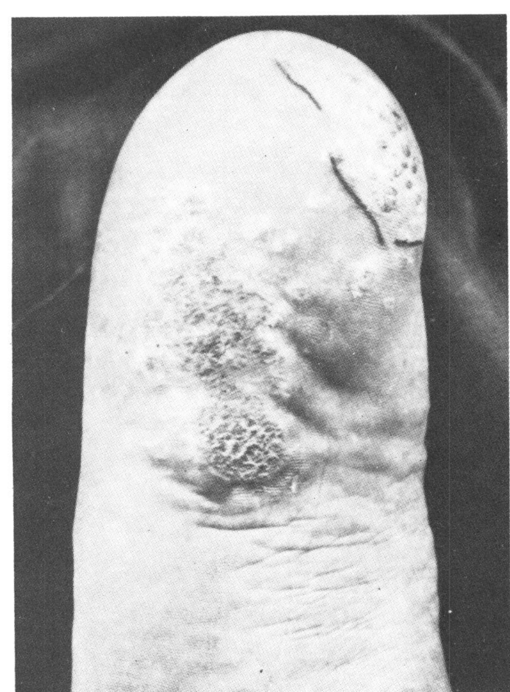

Fig. 73.4 Plantar warts.

Genital Warts

Genital warts are painted with podophyllin 5% in tincture of benzoin lotion, once-weekly. It is a highly irritant medicament and the patient should wash the lotion off after 4 hours. The virus causing such warts may be transmitted via sexual contact, and the patient's partner should also be examined and if necessary given treatment. Should the patient be pregnant a quick reference back to the obstetrician is most important.

Plane Warts

Plane warts are confined to the face and are cosmetically disfiguring. They are extremely difficult to treat, but may respond to applications of salicylic acid ointment 2%.

FUNGAL SKIN INFECTIONS

The species of fungi which are pathogenic to man are, by and large, confined to four groups from this widely distributed family of very primitive plant form:

1. Filamentous fungi which produce many different types of spores from their asexual reproduction.
2. Yeasts. These are single cells, round or oval-shaped and produce buds which enlarge into new cells.
3. Yeast-like fungi include the common pathogen Candida. While reproducing by budding, they resemble a mould.
4. Dimorphic fungi form a mycelium when growing in the soil and are saprophytic.

Generally speaking, fungi are opportunistic organisms which become pathogenic when the conditions are favourable. The following circumstances predispose to a fungal skin infection:

Heavy perspiration of the feet, groin, axillae and other crease folds, especially in the very obese patient

Chaffing of the skin surface from tight fitting clothing

Reduced immunity from any cause, e.g., debilitating illness

Occupations in which the hands are constantly wet

The two main fungal infection groups which the nurse may meet in the course of duty are those caused by *Candida albicans* and the *Dermatomycoses*.

Thrush (Monialisis)

Candida albicans is a yeast-like fungi present in the upper respiratory and alimentary tract. In normal health, its numbers are suppressed by other commensal micro-organisms. It may become pathogenic when these normal commensal bacteria are disturbed as in malnutrition, poor immunity, diabetes, leukaemia, or if the patient has been prescribed antibiotics. Once allowed to thrive it can cause a variety of disorders:

Oral Thrush

This, which mainly affects infants and the elderly, can be seen as a white patch that is very adherent to the oral mucous membranes. In the elderly, it can commence under a dental plate and may go unnoticed for some time. In the infant it can be very contagious and the child should be nursed in isolation until it is resolved. On adult wards, it may not be necessary to isolate the patient, but he or she should not be allowed to share cutlery or any type of crockery from the central pool. It would be better in this instance to supply the patient's meals on disposable crockery.

Vulvo-vaginitis

This appears as a white discharge from the vagina, with extreme itching and irritation of the labia and vulva. It may occur during pregnancy and would then of course require intense treatment. The sexual partner of the patient should also be examined to exclude transmission from another source.

Chronic Paronychia

Is a fungal bacterial infection of the posterior nail bed of those whose hands are constantly in water, or are kept wet for long periods. A careful assessment should be made of the patient's occupation to see if protective gloves or mittens could not be worn during the industrial or domestic work, e.g., housewives and fishworkers.

Dermatitis

Affects the warm moist surfaces of the skin wherever there is a skin crease or fold.

Bronchial Monialisis

Is rare and appears as a generalized lung infection.

Treatment and Care

The following treatments may be prescribed:

1. Nystatin is the most common drug used to treat fungal infections and is supplied and prescribed as either topical cream applications, which are antifungal in their effect when applied over the affected skin areas twice daily until the lesions are healed, or lozenges or suppositories which are systematically absorbed, each being 100 000 unit or 1 ml. The patient is advised to hold the lozenge in the mouth for at least 5 minutes until it dissolves, 4 times daily for not less than 7 days. Advice on thoroughly cleansing the dentures may need to be given. Vaginal pessaries, which can be inserted high into the vaginal vault each evening before retiring to bed and after careful vaginal toilet, may also be used.

2. Amphotericin is given as a lozenge (10 mg) for systemic purposes to be sucked orally 4 times each day.

3. Micnazole gel (Daktarin) is taken orally at frequent intervals to reduce the population of fungi in both the upper alimentary tract and gut.

4. Gentian violet lotion 1 % or penthrane lotion are both particularly soothing as topical applications, reducing itching and soreness. They also reduce any residual bacteria and fungal organisms lurking on the affected skin surface. When painted onto the lesion, a minimal amount only is all that is required and the nurse should consider taking measures to protect the clothing from being discoloured from both these lotions which are of a dark hue.

Chronic paronychia presents a difficult problem in that any proposed treatment may take at least 12 months to prove effective. Amphotericin B lotion applied every 6 hours and gentamycin ointment may prove therapeutic if combined with sensible measures to protect the affected fingers.

Dermatomycoses (Ringworm)

Fungi of the genera trichophyton, epidermophyton and microsporum are collectively known as the dermatophytes. The hyphae of this fungal group can cause superficial infections of the keratin layer of the skin, i.e., the corneum stratum, the hair and the nails. The term ‘ringworm’ dates back to earlier times when the circular skin or scalp lesions were thought to be caused by a worm. Fungal infections in this group are named according to the site of the body affected and the lesions may either appear as erythema with vesicular formation, or as a dry scaly lesion.

Tinea pedis, or, athlete’s foot is caused by the trichophyton, and is transmitted via the wet floors of showers, bathrooms, and swimming pools. Apart from advising of the correct care of the feet, an antifungal cream should be applied topically, e.g., micronazole 2% or clotrimazole 1% twice a day for 10 days over the lesions in the interdigits. Tinea corporis, i.e., of the body, and tinea crusis, i.e., of the groin, are treated in the same manner.

Systemic therapy is required for the more persistent fungal infections of tinea capitas (scalp ringworm), animal ringworm caused by the *Microsporum canis* which is transmitted via cats and dogs mainly to children, and onychomycosis, i.e., fungal infection of the nail finger plate. Griseofulvin 0.5 and 1 g is taken orally each day for at least 4 weeks. The drug acts by interfering with the metabolism of the fungi present in the corneum stratum layer of the skin.

Chapter 74
Common Skin Conditions and Emergencies in Dermatology

PSORIASIS

Psoriasis is a disfiguring skin disease with the appearance of clearly defined pink or red non-itching patches covered by silver scales which usually affects the scalp, elbows and knees, but its distribution may be generalised over the trunk and limbs. The causes of the eruption are variable. About 25% of patients have a definite familial incidence. Other noted factors which may trigger the skin reaction are streptococcal infection, e.g., tonsillitis in children, and emotional or social stresses. Hormonal changes at the menopause or during adolescence may also prove causative of psoriasis. Between 1 and 2% of the United Kingdom population are affected by psoriasis and it is mostly seen in the middle and elderly age groups. Sunlight is known to have a therapeutic effect on the disease and since it is virtually unknown to occur in the negroid races, it can logically be supposed that a lack of sunlight may also be a causative factor. Even with treatment psoriasis tends to be of a relapsing nature, the patient never being free of one or other symptoms for more than 5 years.

The treatment plan varies, depending on which part of the body is affected. In simple uncomplicated but generalised psoriasis the patient is prescribed the following:

1. Previously applied therapeutic pastes are cleansed from the skin, using nut oil, before taking a warm bath in the evening. Whilst in the bath the silver scales are removed with a soft nail brush and further descaling will occur when drying the affected areas with a warm towel.

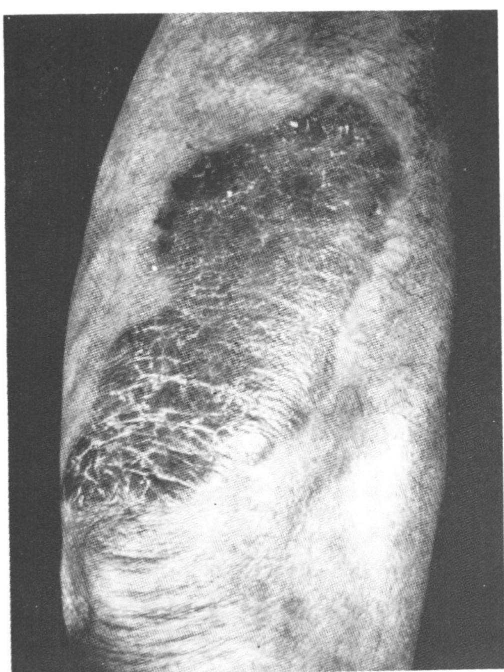

Fig. 74.1 Psoriasis.

2. A suberythema dose of ultraviolet light is given, lasting no more than 15 seconds initially but increasing in time with each subsquent treatment. During ultraviolet light therapy the patient must wear protective goggles to prevent any damage to the eyes.

3. A coal tar derivative dithranol in Lassar's paste 0.5 to 1–2% is applied carefully to only the areas affected by psoriasis. It is a very thick paste and stains the skin black. Therefore the nurse or the patient must wear gloves during its application. It is better to remove the paste from the jar with a spatula and smear it into a piece of clean linen, and then to apply it to the affected areas with a piece of gauze. The applied paste is then dusted over with a small amount of talcum powder, which will help to form a crust to prevent the paste from oozing onto non-affected skin.

4. To protect the clothing the skin is covered by a tubegauze suit, which can easily be cut from the larger diameter tubegauze bandages. This protective cover is worn until the next treatment on the following evening.

This course of therapy will usually successfully induce a remission of the skin eruptions within 2 or 3 weeks.

Scalp Psoriasis

Scalp psoriasis is far more difficult to treat as the epithelial scales are thickly matted into the hair strands. At the start of treatment it is best to advise the patient to have the hair cut short in an easily managed style. Each evening the scalp and hair are shampooed with Cetrimide solution 2% and then diligently combed through to remove as many scales as possible. The hair is parted in a series of logical but small steps from the crown of the head, working firstly to the right and then the left. Pyrogallol ointment is then applied to soften the remaining scales and the whole scalp is then covered with a tubegauze cap until the following morning when the hair is once again combed through to remove further scaling. When applying the ointment, the fingers are used to massage the ointment into each part of the scalp.

An alternative therapy that may be prescribed for scalp psoriasis is for the patient to shampoo each evening with Betnovate scalp lotion and to leave the hair damp. It is kept damp for as long as possible by encasing the hair in a polythene cap which is sealed down with sellotape at the forehead. In the morning the hair is thoroughly combed through to remove the softened scales. A course of ultraviolet light therapy may be combined with this latter treatment.

Psoriasis of the Face and Skin Creases

For psoriasis of the face and skin creases a corticosteroid ointment such as Betnovate or Synalar is applied 2 or 3 times daily until the condition regresses. Occasionally the psoriasis may become pustular and this is a very serious complication that requires hospitalisation. During his or her hospital stay the patient will be prescribed a defined period of bedrest with continued sedation. Oral methotrexate (cytotoxic drug) is usually prescribed to contain the rapidity at which the skin cells are dividing. A few patients have a psoriasis associated with rheumatoid arthritis, i.e., arthropathic psoriasis, and each condition requires to be treated separately, although the apparent relationship between the two remains a mystery.

ECZEMA (DERMATITIS)

Eczema is a skin disorder which is in reality a syndrome or a collection of symptoms reflecting several diseases within one patient. The one symptom common to all forms of eczema is that the skin is inflamed, itching and has a non-infectious vesicular eruption. This reaction may be due to either endogenous (intrinsic) or exogenous (extrinsic) factors, and may involve the patient, doctor, and nurses in detailed detective work to establish the true cause of the dermatitis. The term 'factor' is used deliberately to differentiate it from the term 'cause'. It is often found that a factor is the triggering mechanism to induce the changes in the skin.

Erythema or redness of the skin
↓
Localised oedema
↓
Appearance of vesicles
↓
Rupture of the vesicles with serous exudate escaping (weeping eczema)
↓
Drying of the affected area
↓
Descaling of the epithelium
↓
Fissure and cracking of the area
↓
Intense itching (pruritis)
↓
Lichenification or thickening of the skin

Endogenous Group of Eczema

The endogenous group of eczema is classified as being either atopic eczema, seborrhoeic dermatitis, discoid eczema, or varicose eczema.

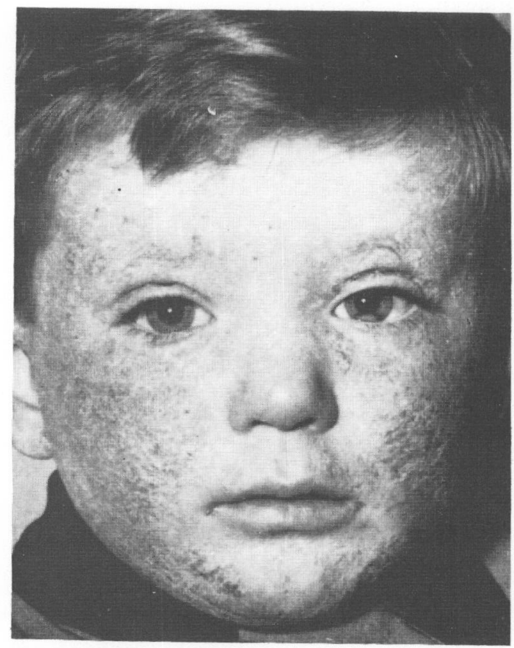

Fig. 74.2 Eczema.

Atopic Eczema

Atopic eczema, or simply dermatitis, is commonly associated with the allergies, i.e., asthma and hay fever. In infants it may occur at about 3 or 4 months of age, which suggests a genetic link and is often supported by a family history of atopy. A second factor often noted and commonly quoted by researchers is the emotional trigger in the child. Such children are observed as being overactive, curious about their environment, aggressive when being handled, insecure if deprived of affection, exceptionally sensitive to personalities and atmosphere, and are usually very intelligent.

A third triggering factor is that if the individual is prone to eczema, a sudden change in the temperature may induce an acute attack, e.g., the extremes of heat and cold. Many infants seem to go through a period of acute attacks with frequent remissions until they reach 3 years of age.

Seborrhoeic Dermatitis

Seborrhoeic dermatitis occurs more frequently in adolescents and adults, the areas of the body mostly affected being the scalp, within the ears, across the eyebrows and between any of the natural skin creases, i.e., axilla, groin, elbow, perineum. The cause of this form of eczema is unknown, but the eczema tends to be more sore than itchy and is easily infected. It responds well to emulsifying creams, or to diluted betnovate ointment once treatment begins.

Discoid or Nummular Eczema

Discoid or nummular eczema occurs in the middle and elderly age groups and takes the form of circular shaped lesions about the size of a coin. It is located only on the limbs and the cause is unknown.

Varicose Eczema

Varicose eczema is associated with both varicose veins and varicose ulcers. The latter conditions are mainly seen in elderly women who tend to obesity. The eczema is invariably located to the lower third of the leg and always excludes the feet. One of the more distressing features of therapy is the length of time it takes for a varicose ulcer to heal, being very prolonged, and this only exacerbates the emotional factor involved in the eczema.

Exogenous Groups of Eczema

The exogenous group of factors which contribute to eczema are subgrouped as being either contact dermatitis or sensitisation dermatitis.

Contact Dermatitis

As the term suggests contact dermatitis is when the skin comes into contact with an obvious irritant, e.g., an acid or alkali used in an industrial process.

Sensitisation Dermatitis

Sensitisation dermatitis occurs via the increased sensitivity of the immunological system of the body when it is repeatedly exposed to an 'allergen' or substances that it recognises as being foreign to the tissues. For an individual to become sensitised to an extrinsic factor, he or she, on first exposure, allows the *allergen* to mix with the tissue protein after being absorbed through the skin epithelium. Certain lymphocytes recognise the allergen as being foreign and sensitise the antibodies on the lymphocyte surface to the allergen. This sensitising process may take as long as 14 days to develop.

On the second exposure, the lymphocytes attack the allergen and in so doing cause an inflammatory response by releasing toxic substances such as histamine. The second exposure may in fact be an interval of 10 or 20 years, but the lymphocytes remember the allergen, the so-called lymphocyte memory. Allergens are very wide ranging in type and there does not seem to be a common denominator amongst them, e.g., nickel, zinc, chromate, dyes, chemicals, cosmetic ingredients, medication and plants are all quite commonly quoted allergens in susceptible patients with or without a history of atopy.

It is quite possible to be allergic to several allergens at the same time. During a period of remission the exact allergen to which the individual is sensitive can be identified by completing a *patch test*. A series of common allergens in dilute form and mounted on a small disc are secured to the patient's skin, usually the broad expanse of the back is selected. These discs are secured in place by non-allergic adhesive and allowed to be absorbed for 48 hours before being 'read'. Any note is made of a dermatitis response and a second reading is made again after a further 48 hours to exclude the chances of a false negative or false positive reading.

Planning the Care of Eczema

The plan of care for eczema will depend on the severity of the symptoms, the age of the

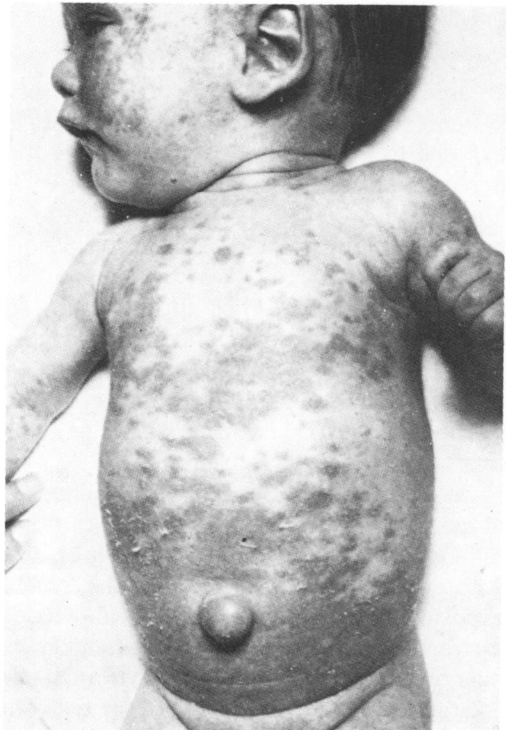

Fig. 74.3 Napkin dermatitis.

patient, and the locality of the area affected. In most cases the patient receives treatment as an out-patient, and in the department the nurse has a major role to play, not only as a clinician but also as a counsellor. Care of the infant, adolescent and adult are outlined below.

Infants

As a general rule the nurse, although clinically treating the child, will also have to educate and counsel the parents. It is not unusual for the parents to be exhausted, frustrated and to feel very guilty about their child's illness. They may have endured several sleepless nights due to the infant's persistent crying and restlessness. Guilt may be somewhat assauged by praising the parents for coping so well in very difficult circumstances. Their anxiety level will be definitely lowered by correcting any misconceptions they may have already been told by well-meaning friends. Misconceptions, such as that the baby is allergic to foods, can soon be authoritatively dispelled by assuring the parents that diet has absolutely nothing to do with eczema. Children with eczema are bright, lively and intelligent and, given a central figure of attachment for affection, they usually respond very well to therapy. However demanding the child may be, the parent must not spoil or over-discipline the child during its formative years. Absolute cleanliness is vital if the eczema is to be contained, e.g., the infant may be more prone than usual to nappy rash and this can be avoided by the use of disposable nappies and frequent toileting. If there is a history of atopy in the family, then it may mean that moderate reinforcing to control things such as house dust and to avoid having pets with fur may be all that is required.

While the eczema is dry and crusty, it is best to avoid the use of any soap when bathing the infant. As the infant grows older the parent will have to advise the health visitor, school nurse and general practitioner of the history of eczema, since the child suffers a severe reaction if ever given smallpox vaccination or tetanus toxoid immunisation. The local treatment is based on the following principles:

1. Encourage sleep and relieve the infant's pruritis with an evening dose of Benadryl Elixir or Phenergan Elixir at paediatric dosage, given during the acute phase of the eczema. Hydrocortisone ointment 1% is applied sparingly over the affected areas, usually the scalp and face, 3 times each day. Fluorinated hydrocortisones such as Betnovate and Synalar may be used but only in severe cases and for a short period of time. A simple emollient, e.g., calamine lotion or Cetomacrogel cream, can be applied to supress any mild itching. If the child is itching furiously, it indicates the treatment is inadequate. Restrainers should **not** be used to prevent scratching. Should the itching and scratching be causing concern, the child's hands should be dressed with tubegauze mittens and the treatment reviewed.

2. If the eczema has spread to the limbs, a coal tar dressing (Tarband) may be

applied and an occlusive covering of tubegauze left in place for 1 week may prove effective.

3. Infective eczema may occur from scratching, and it is usually staphylococcal in type; local or systemic antibiotics may be prescribed to treat such infection.

Adolescents and Adults

A similar plan of treatment as that for infants may be used in adolescents and adults, except that the eczema may be due to an extrinsic cause. Investigations to establish the cause may have to wait until the condition is in regression. Such treatment may include the following, especially if there is a serous exudate:

1. Painting the affected area with Potassium Permanganate Solution 1 in 1000, followed by an application of Paté à l'eau lotion, which contains equal parts of talcum, zinc oxide, glycerine and lime water.
2. Application of calamine liniment lotion 6.6%, which contains calamine, lanolin, olive oil and lime water.

These lotions should sufficiently dry out the affected skin to allow, at a later date, the application of Lassar's paste bandages which should remove the crusts when the bandages are taken off a few days later.

When healing has taken place the dermatologist may do a series of tests which can include a skin biopsy, blood serum to measure the level of immunoglobulin E, which is usually raised in intrinsic eczema, or a patch test. If the latter test proves positive to an allergen, then there is no other resource but to avoid that allergen in the future.

Often the patient is suffering from indefinable psychological or social stresses, and a period in hospital may offer some respite to enable the stress to be placed in perspective. This perspective, however, can only be achieved by talking rationally to someone with a sympathetic ear and an empathic attitude. Such a person is usually the nurse who can, during the giving of treatment by simply listening, help the patient achieve some kind of ease in mind and body.

If the eczema is due to a contact dermatitis it may be necessary to check on the place of employment to assess if the industrial process or atmosphere is such that it could contain a common allergen. As a passing remark, if the industrial process is causing contact dermatitis then the patient may claim compensation under the Industrial Injuries Act, but nurses should **not** take part in discussions leading to any type of industrial claim.

In adolescents, schooling can be dramatically curtailed and this in turn has implications for future education and career development. Often a quiet word with the school nurse or school psychologist can benefit the youngster so that they have access to professional help at any time if emotional stress is the trigger mechanism to their eczema.

PARASITIC INFESTATION OF THE SKIN

Although the skin can be affected by a wide range of insects, including fleas, only the acarus and the louse are actually parasitic on the skin.

Scabies

Scabies is an infestation which is caused by the eggs or mites of the *Sarcoptes scabiei*. When pregnant, the female lays her eggs in the horny layer of the skin by burrowing through the upper epithelial layer. She lays only a few eggs per day and over a period of 2 or 3 weeks the eggs hatch and the larva feed on or near the orifices of the secretory glands. On average a patient may show between 5 and 10 burrow lesions, which appear as small greyish white lines with a shadow at one end where the mites are sited. The common sites of these lesions are in the skin flexures, the interdigital clefts and on the genitalia. If a baby is infested, the lesions may appear on the face or scalp. Transmission of the mites, or the adult acarus, is by direct skin contact and therefore it is not unusual for a whole family to be affected.

After about 3 weeks the host becomes sensitive to the secretions of the mites and this allergy causes intense itching that is especially bad at night when trying to sleep in a warm bed. The diagnosis is sometimes made by needling the shadow end of the lesion to extract a mite and examining the point of the needle with a magnifying glass to confirm the presence of a parasite. Absolute certainty of the diagnosis is essential before advising any patient that they are infested, since the common reaction of most people is that they are dirty and socially unacceptable. However, they can be reassured that if they follow the treatment plan to the letter, they will soon be rid of the scabies. The whole family requires to be treated whether they have any clinical signs or not.

Treatment

As a first step the patient should take a very warm bath in hot soapy water, staying in the bath for about 20 minutes. During the bath the skin should be mildly abraded with either a rough flannel or a soft nail brush, which will open up the entry to the burrow lesions. After drying the skin, the patient should apply the supplied acaracide (such as emulsion of benzyl benzoate 25%) from the neck to the toes and to include the soles of the feet. No area of the body should be omitted and to be absolutely certain a friend or relative should apply the lotion. The emulsion takes about 20 minutes to dry, which means the patient requires to stay in a warmed bathroom for this period before redressing in their normal clothes. There is no need to treat clothing in any special way as the mite cannot survive without human contact. The skin may then be left without further treatment for 48 hours or alternatively the physician may recommend that the skin be emulsified each evening for 3 nights. Benzyl benzoate stings as it is being applied, and is not recommended for the treatment of babies or infants. Benzene hexachloride 1% is applied to the body, and if the face and scalp are affected, crotamiton (Eurax) lotion is used in the treatment of infants.

The patient should be warned that the itching will persist for some days after the first treatment, but will recede and the temptation to scratch should if possible be resisted. To help with the intolerable itching, the doctor may prescribe calamine lotion to be applied over the emulsified skin.

Norwegian Scabies

A non-itching variety of scabies referred to as Norwegian scabies may occur in geriatric, psychiatric and mental-handicap institutions. Since there is no itching response, the lesions progress to a thick brown crusting of potentially infective material over the flexures and skin creases of the body. There may be as many as 5 million burrows covering the skin with a single mite in each burrow. Dissemination of this type of scabies throughout the institution can reach epidemic proportions through vigorous activities such as bedmaking. The treatment in this instance is to apply DDT cream to the skin after a very warm bath.

One complication which may occur after contracting either type of scabies is that of post-scabetic eczema which may be due to unremitting scratching or infection. This would indicate that the treatment for the scabies is ineffective.

Pediculosis

The louse is about 2–4 mm in length with an oval body from which extend 6 legs, each having a claw. It literally sucks blood through its proboscis after injecting an anticoagulent into the host's skin. Lice have a persistent presence at all levels of society, and can reach epidemic proportions in schools or in the poorer parts of industrial cities. They are mainly detected by the presence of nits attached to the hair follicles and are visible to the eye as shiny pearly coloured oval bodies which have a cuff surrounding the hair follicle.

The louse is often associated with the transmission of such diseases as typhus, trench fever and relapsing fever, especially in war-time conditions and in extreme poverty.

Apart from their tendency to wander over

the skin, the 3 types of louse tend to be quite specific as to the body area they infest.

Pediculosis Capitis

The pediculosis capitis louse is specific to the hair of the scalp, and those people with long hair are more prone to carry the parasite. The intense itching seems for the most part to be confined to the side and crown of the skull. A secondary infection, such as impetigo, may be caused by the intensity of scratching. In every case of scalp impetigo, the patient should be examined for head lice. The lymph glands at the back of the neck may be obviously swollen. The treatment is to shampoo the hair with malathion 0.5% (Prioderm) and leave the hair to dry naturally. This lotion is alcohol-based and highly inflammable. Therefore the patient should not go near naked flames, or use a hairdryer. After 12 hours the hair is carefully and thoroughly combed through using a Derbac narrow toothed comb to remove any nits. The treatment is repeated 1 week later to ensure complete success. There is no need to cut the hair, nor should this be insisted upon by the nursing staff. If there is a secondary infection, the patient may be prescribed an antibiotic cream. N.B. Prioderm should **not** be used as a shampoo preoperatively due to its flammable nature.

Pediculosis Corporis or the Body Louse

The pediculosis corporis louse is commonly found on vagrants, the elderly self-neglected, and eccentrics. Apart from the parasitic infestation the skin may be covered with scratch marks, be excoriated, and be infected with papules or scabs. Once the patient is undressed, the seams of the clothing when searched and examined reveal the familiar shiny eggs lying in rows. The nurse should of course wear a protective plastic apron and disposable gloves when dealing with these clothes. The patient is given a very warm bath and, after being dried, the skin is treated with calamine lotion with 1% phenol. The clothing is dusted with DDT powder (dichloro diphenyl trichlorethane) and bagged before being sent for disinfestation. If available it is more appropriate to dust the clothes with Gammexane. Many hospitals will prefer to burn the clothing and issue the patient with new clothes.

Pediculosis Pubis

The pediculosis pubis are commonly known as crabs and are considered as a paravenereal disease, often being transmitted by direct body contact. The intense itching of the genitalia and the feelings of shame often cause the patient to employ extreme methods to rid themselves of the infestation, e.g., using paraffin or Dettol. Washing the area each day with Lorexane shampoo for 3 days should remove the louse successfully without any need for extreme measures.

EMERGENCIES IN DERMATOLOGY

Of concern to determatology, but which can be seen in any clinical speciality at any time, are the rare emergencies of, angioneurotic oedema, acute anaphylaxis, multiple wasp or bee stings, and malignant melanoma.

Angioneurotic Oedema

Angioneurotic oedema is an allergic reaction to a variety of stimuli, e.g., a drug reaction, which is the sudden development of an urticarial rash combined with an oedema, usually of the tissues of the throat and lips which threaten with a rapid laryngeal obstruction. The degree of shock is immediate with a noticeable tachycardia and an ever deepening hypotension. The treatment for shock is of paramount importance, i.e., to keep the patient in a dorsal position, to keep him or her warm, to loosen the clothing and to apply a cold compress to the oedematous lips and throat until medical aid can commence the vital treatment of giving:

adrenaline 1/1000 0.5 to 1 ml immediately by subcutaneous injection, and a repeat injection in 10–15 minutes to restore the blood pressure;

hydrocortisone 50–100 mg intravenously or intramuscularly is also given immediately to act as anti-inflammatory agent.

The degree of shock is such that, once it is seemingly under control, the continuing anxiety may pose a threat to the restored blood pressure. This is prevented by giving:

ephedrine 30 mg

an antihistamine, e.g. chlorpheniramine (Piriton)

phenobarbitone 30 to 60 mg

If the angioneurotic oedematous attack is sustained, then a further dose of Piriton may be given and an emergency tracheostomy prepared if hospital treatment is not immediately available.

Acute Anaphylaxis

Acute anaphylaxis is due to an antigen sensitivity and can be to some degree prevented if the patient is always asked about their past medical history to elicit if there has ever been an allergy to any substance or drug. In this instance a positive allergy would indicate the need to avoid the normal procedure and opt for an alternative drug or safer vaccine method. The anaphylactic reaction is one of sudden shock, collapse and there may be an urticarial reaction or local skin reaction. As with angioneurotic oedema, the treatment of shock is of paramount importance to maintain the blood pressure until medical treatment can be given. This may include:

artificial respiration if there is any respiratory arrest

adrenaline 1/1000 1 ml subcutaneously and repeated in 15 minutes

oxgen via an Ambubag until advised otherwise

hydrocortisone succinate 100 mg intravenously, if necessary via a cutdown into a vein

antihistamine therapy, e.g., Piriton

admission to hospital as rapidly as possible

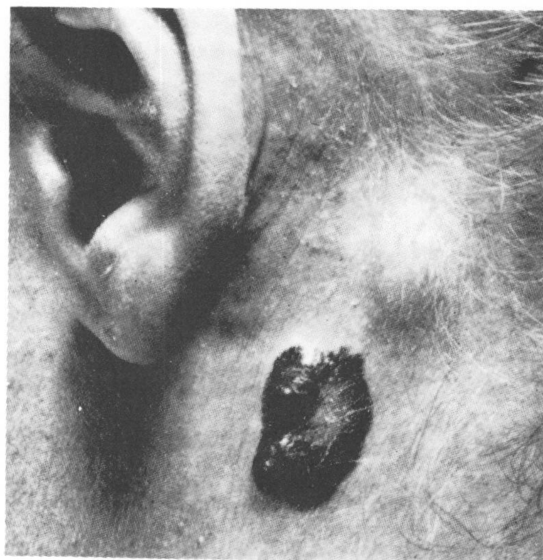

Fig. 74.4 Malignant melanoma (Institute of Dermatology, University of London).

Multiple Wasp and Bee Stings

Multiple stings from bees or wasps are very rare but the 'sting' causes an immediate inflammatory response, setting off a massive urticaria of the area affected, usually the face, neck and hands. Stings to the face and neck are particularly dangerous as they may also cause angioneurotic oedema. If the victim has a history of allergy of any kind, then anaphylactic shock may also occur.

The emergency nature of the treatment is to deal with the 'shock' mainly by resting the patient in the dorsal position and keeping him or her warm until a medical regimen of substantial sedation can be administered, combined with a course of antihistamine drugs.

Malignant Melanoma

Malignant melanoma is a primary lethal cancer arising from melanocytes located in the basal layer of the epidermis. Its 'emergency' nature is that it can metastasise very quickly to other areas of the body via the lymphatic system. Therefore, the patient requires immediate referral to the radiotherapy department for extensive investigations to exclude lymphatic spread and a large surgical

Table 74.1. Common topical applications to the skin

Lotions	Suspensions of insoluble powder in water	
	Calamine	A mixture of zinc carbonate and ferric oxide, its main effect being antipruritic. After being applied it evaporates and cools the skin. If applied to a weeping skin, e.g., eczema, it has a drying effect
	Copper and zinc sulphate (Dalibaur)	Used as the 'wet' agent of a wet dressing when applied to a very dry skin
	Crotamiton (Eurax)	Both antipruritic and an acarocide, it is also available as a cream containing hydrocortisone 25%
	Formaldehyde 3%	Sometimes used to treat planter warts
	Amphotercin B (Fungilin)	Local application for the treatment of candidiasis, i.e, thrush
	Corticosteroid	Useful for the scalp and other hair growing areas of the body, e.g., betnovate, dermovate and synalar
Creams	Mixtures of oils and fats in water, the droplets being dispersed within each other and immiscible. A preservative is normally added to prevent the growth of fungi or bacteria within the water content of the cream. Creams are used to carry an active ingredient which will specifically treat the skin lesions of a given disease. Zinc remains the most popular to all dermatology creams	
Ointments	Thicker than creams, base being either a natural fat or oil. All ointments leave the skin feeling greasy and act as an occlusive cover which promotes skin contact with the active incredient added to the ointment	
	Wool fat	Basis of many 'cold creams' used in cosmetics
	Lanolin	Derived from wool fat, and water is then added to make the ointment
	Wool alcohols	Extracted from wool fat and is a simple type of ointment to which an active ingredient is added
	Cetyl alcohol	Is obtained from whale fat and is used as an emulsifier in the ointment preparation
	Lanette wax	Contains fatty alcohols and is used as an emulsifying wax
	Arachis	Just as effective as the more expensive oil, it is mainly used as a skin cleanser to remove previously applied pastes
	Yellow and white soft paraffin	Inert fat forming an impervious greasy layer over the skin and the active ingredients added are usually tar or salicylic acid which are easily emulsified into a paraffin base
	Polyethylene glycols (carbowaxes) (macrogols)	Synthetic wax bases used to carry active ingredients such as the steroids
Medicated baths		
	Emollient	Prescribed where a soothing effect is required, being achieved by using one of the bathing oils currently available. A typical water dispersible emollient is made up from liquid paraffin, anhydrous lanolin, emulsifying wax and cetomacrogol wax. Two tablespoonfuls (40 g) are blended with hot water and then added to the bath water. Soaps should not be offered or be used by the patient during this therapeutic bath
	Tar	Used to treat such conditions as eczema and psoriasis and the tar is also emollient in its effect. Two capfuls of the emollient, e.g., polytar, are added to a 30 gallon bath

Table 74.1 (*continued*)

	Potassium permanganate	Useful if an antiseptic effect is required for conditions such as impetigo and infected eczema. Two teaspoonfuls 10 g of the potassium permanganate crystals are dissolved completely in a bowl of hot water before being added to the prepared bath water. The crystals are caustic to the skin so the nurse must ensure that they are completely dissolved. The patient should soak in the bath for about 5–10 minutes to achieve the best effect. Unfortunately the dissolved crystals stain the patient's skin a light brown: the bath and towels are also stained. The bath can be protected by a layer of polythene sheeting, while old towels should be used to dry the patient
Pastes Powders combined with an ointment which, when applied to the skin, dry to form an impervious layer. If the powder is combined with a natural oil it will both dry and cool the skin		
	Zinc oxide	A cooling agent
	Zinc gelatin (Unna's paste)	A drying agent
	Zinc and salicylic acid (Lasser's paste)	Exceptionally thick paste requiring a wooden spatula for its removal from the container jar. It is possible to have it supplied in half strength
	Zinc peroxide (Meleney's paste)	Forms an impervious layer over the skin enabling direct contact between the peroxide and the lesion
	Metanium and titanium	Dry pastes that protect the underlying skin
	Zinc combined with vioform	An antimicrobial agent. Apart from being supplied as a paste, it can be incorporated into bandaging material into which is incorporated an active ingredient such as coal tar, or ichthammol. Whenever a paste is applied to the skin the patient's overclothing should be protected from staining by covering the treated skin with stockinette bandage. When it is due for removal the skin is cleansed with arachis (nut) oil saturated cotton wool balls
Specific agents		
	Benzyl benzoate lotion	Specific for the treatment of scabies infestation
	Dithranol (antharolein)	Extensively used in chronic psoriasis. Unfortunately it stains the skin and clothing and can cause conjunctivitis if accidentally rubbed into the eye
	Gamma benzene hexachloride	An insecticide which is the preferred method of treating pediculosis (body lice) rather than DDT, which is now restricted in its use because of harmful effects to the ecology systems
	Phenol 1% or 2%	Sometimes used as an antipruritic agent
	Rosaline dyes	These include gentian violet, brilliant green, magenta and Castellani's paint, and are employed as antifungal agents, or skin antiseptics
	Antifungal agents	Proprietary substances available in creams, ointments, pastes, pessaries, lozenges, etc. Include, nystatin, amphotocerin B, clotrimazole 1% (Canesten), microazole 2% (Daktarin), tolnaftate, natamycin (Pimafucin)
	Antiviral agents	Supplied as creams, include herpid which is usually prescribed for the local treatment of herpes simplex and herpes zoster

	Cytotoxic agents	5% fluorouracil (Efudix) may be prescribed for the treatment of some early skin cancers, but is reserved for hospital treatment only. Podophyllin 25% is a cytotoxic cream used in the treatment of genital warts, providing the patient is not pregnant
	Steroids	May be supplied alone, or in combination with antimicrobial preparations. Basically their action is anti-inflammatory and helps to assuage the soreness and itching often seen in eczema. Long-term prescription is unusual, as these drugs tend to sensitise the skin very quickly. Examples include hydrocortisone cream 1%, betamethasone 0.5% and dermovate (Clobestasol)
	Salicylic acid 20–40%	Added as an active ingredient to pastes, paints, ointments and in plasters to soften the horny layer of the skin
	Tars	(a) Bitumenous, e.g., ichthammol BPC (b) Wood extracted from beech, pine and birch trees (c) Coal tars are a complex mixture of paraffin hydrocarbons and are the active ingredient in lotions, creams and ointments The cruder the tar the more effective it seems to be as an antipruritic, and in the treatment of eczema and psoriasis
	Sulphur	Recommended for use in either acne or seborrhoeic dermatitis
Skin antiseptics	Wide ranging, a few examples should already be familiar to the nurse:	
	Benzyl peroxide (panoxyl gel)	May be recommended to help cleanse the skin of an acne sufferer
	Chlorhexidine	Commonly used antiseptic used on the skin prior to needling procedures. It is effective against gram positive organisms but is ineffective in combination with soap
	Cetrimide	Is both a detergent and a mild skin antiseptic
	Eusol	If combined with liquid paraffin is a very useful skin cleanser before applying dressings to venous ulcers and infected eczema
	Hexachlorophane	Useful antiseptic if the patient has gram positive organisms present on the skin lesions
	Hydroxyquinolones	Are both antibacterial and antifungal and useful in the treatment of infected eczema
	Phenoyethanol	When added to half strength Lasser's paste is effective against the pseudomonas organism

removal of the tissues involved, perhaps combined with a course of cytotoxic drugs.

Other tumours of the skin include epitheliomia which are slow growing tumours arising from warts or papules that lead to a nasty, foul smelling ulcer. Rodent ulcers are a cancer of the basal cells of the epidermis, usually confined to the face and not a metastasising tumour. This type of tumour normally responds well to either surgery or radiotherapy treatment given daily for 10–14 days, combined with, or separate from, a course of cytotoxic drugs.

Chapter 75 Overview and Investigation of the Nervous System

The most senior of the two controlling systems of the body is the nervous system, the other being the endocrine system, their dual relationship being important for coordination of all other body systems. A logical sequence of study is vital for any understanding of the nervous system and it is proposed here to look briefly at the following:

1. The neurone, which is the basic unit of the nervous system.
2. Reflex arc and the synapse.
3. Brain structure and the principal functional areas.
4. The spinal cord and peripheral nerves.
5. Autonomic nervous system.

THE NEURONE

A neurone is the basic functional unit of the nervous system and is composed of 3 basic elements: a cell body, an axon and the dendrites. The cell body is composed of cytoplasm within which are scattered Nissl's granules, thought to contribute to the cell's metabolism. Within the centre of the cell body is the very important nucleus which if damaged means that the cell and its other elements will die. Once fully developed, a nerve cell cannot regenerate. The cell membrane is semi-permeable allowing for the exchange of sodium and electrolytes. These 2 electrolytes ensure the property of electrical conductivity, once the cell is irritated by the exchange.

Extending from the cell body are the dendrites. These small multiple branching nerve fibres receive information into the nerve

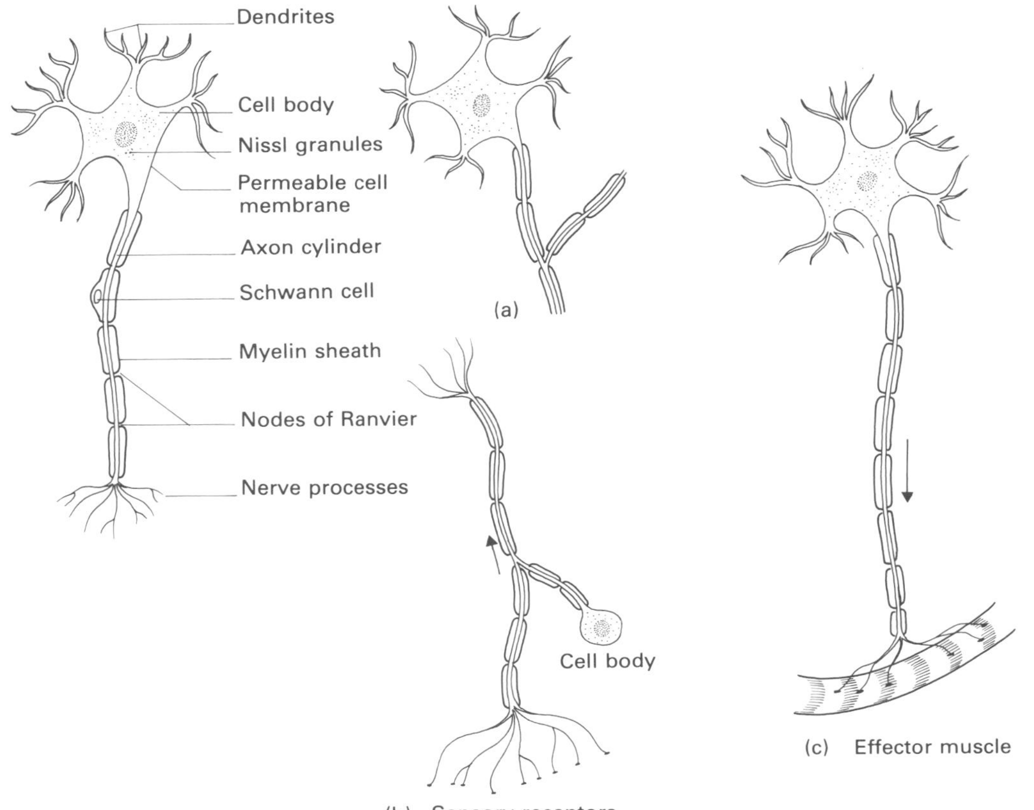

Fig. 75.1 Myelinated neurone (*left*) with details of an interneurone (a), a sensory neurone (b) and a motor neurone (c).

cell. The impulse irritates the cell body into movement and the message is then relayed onto the axon which conveys the impulse away from the cell body. An axon can vary in length from 1 mm–90 mm and may be covered by a protective insulating sheath, i.e., the myelin sheath. This sheath is mainly composed of lecithin, a fatty substance which gives the myelin its white appearance hence the term *white matter* which denotes that an axon is medullated. Along the length of the sheath are regularly placed indentations called the *nodes of Ranvier*. Their presence will increase the speed of electrical conductivity of the impulse, the average impulse speed being 0.08 seconds along the axon. Apart from insulating the axon, the sheath is also a nutrient source. Covering the sheath is a fine membrane called the neurilemma which contains the Schwann's cells vital for the regeneration of the axon should it become damaged or injured. Schwann's cells are the centre of healing and growth. Many nerve fibres, especially in the autonomic nervous system, are nonmyelinated, i.e., without a myelin sheath, and these are referred to as *grey matter*. In general terms, nerve cells form most of the grey matter at the periphery of the brain and in the centre of the spinal cord. Otherwise, all other nervous tissue appears white.

There are 3 types of neurone, each having a distinct function;

1. Interneurones are found in the brain and spinal cord and connect one nerve fibre to another. They are also known as *association neurones* linking impulses in the complex structure which is the brain.

2. Sensory neurones convey messages from the periphery of the body and internal organs towards the brain; sensations, such as pain, touch, temperature, texture and proprioception, travel from the skin, joints and muscles to reach the posterior root of the spinal cord before ascending to reach the sensory appreciation area of the brain.

3. Motor neurones transmit impulses from the brain to the peripheral muscles and other organs in response to sensory stimuli. On descending through the brain and spinal cord the impulse synapses in the anterior horn of the grey matter in the spinal cord with an interneurone. The impulse then travels from the spinal cord to terminate at a junction within the muscle fibres, known as the *motor end plate*. Usually the impulse will cause the muscle fibres to constrict, thereby causing movement of the muscle which has been innervated.

REFLEX ARC AND THE SYNAPSE

A reflex action is an automatic motor response to a sensory stimulus without the brain being involved. Reflex responses reduce the amount of work the brain would otherwise have to do in keeping the body coordinated. The incredible speed at which the reflexes work is also protective. Examples of reflexes include:

1. Light reflex of the cornea of the eye, i.e., the pupil contracts when light is directed into the eye.

2. Temperature and pain receptors located in the skin, if massively stimulated, cause reflex contraction of local muscles causing the limb to 'withdraw', this being a protective mechanism to protect the person from further harm.

3. Receptors in the joints and muscles help to reflexly maintain body posture and balance, being complemented by information from the eyes and ears. This is known as *proprioception*.

4. Vital centres located within the medulla oblongata reflexly control aspects of body function vital to survival. These are blood pressure, cardiac function, respiration, coughing, swallowing, sneezing and vomiting.

Because of their importance, many physiologists regard the reflex arc as the basis of our physical behaviour, responding as people do to many crisis situations. For example, reaction to shock, injury or bad news will cause many reflex responses and ensure a better chance of survival. Many reflexes are conditioned by social learning, e.g., the infant overcoming the reflex emptying of the bladder and bowel by toilet training. A reflex arc is composed of:

a sensory fibre (posterior nerve root)
posterior horn of the spinal cord
interneurone in the spinal cord
anterior horn of the spinal cord
motor fibre (anterior nerve root)

For a reflex arc to respond in a coordinated manner, the brain does exert an 'inhibitory' effect over the motor response after it has been briefly analysed by the sensory stimulus. This influence, however, is

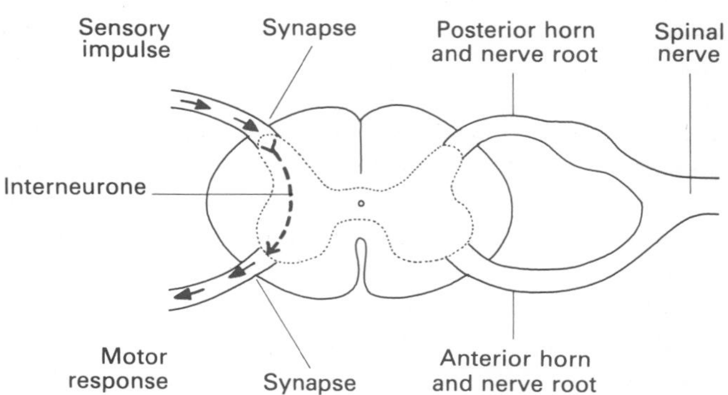

Fig. 75.2 Spinal reflex arc.

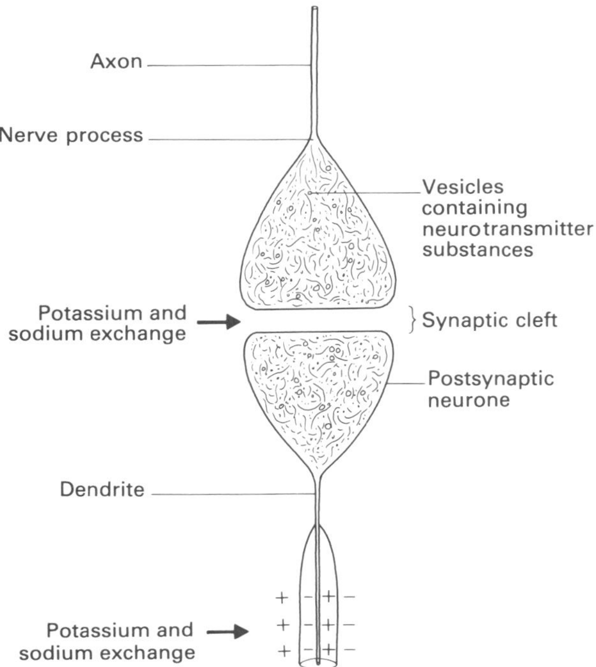

Fig. 75.3 Synapse.

only partial to ensure the speed of response at spinal level.

Nerve Impulse and Synapse

The nerve processes at the end of an axon have, at their terminations, small vesicles containing a neurochemical transmitter substance. Since these nerve processes are not in direct contact with the dendrites of the next neurone, all messages are transmitted over this junction or synapse by the release of transmitter substances released by an electrical impulse. The action of these released substances is short-lived, since as soon as they are released they are quickly negated by an enzyme (cholinesterase). Otherwise, the impulse would persist long after it was of any value. The commonly known neurochemical transmitters at the synapses are:

1. Noradrenaline, found in the sympathetic system, influences the level of blood pressure.
2. Dopamine, found at the synaptic junctions in the brain, influences motor coordination.
3. Prolactin, which is related to dopamine.
4. Serotonin (5 Hydrotryptamine), found in the central nervous system but has an obscure function.
5. Histamine, which is released when tissue is damaged. It also stimulates the pain pathway.
6. Acetylcholine, which is found in all synapses of the central nervous system.
7. Gaba (gamma amino butyric acid), which inhibits amino acids.
8. Prostaglandins, found in the synapses of the central nervous system.
9. Endomorphins are recently discovered neurotransmitter substances released in the brain itself.

Many of these transmitter substances can of course be opposed by neuromuscular blocking agents commonly used in anaesthetics, e.g., tubocurarine, flaxedil, scoline and valium. Noradrenaline, which is found in the sympathetic system, is the transmitter essential to control the diameter of the blood vessels, hence blood pressure. If the blood pressure is too high, the excess secretion of noradrenaline can be blocked by drugs such as serpasil, betanidine and ismelin used to treat hypertension.

These transmitter substances are released by the action of electrical conductivity, which is the essential property of the nerve fibre. This property is due to the exchange of sodium and potassium along the axon sheath, section by section, until the impulse is fully transmitted. The consequences of an electrolyte imbalance will affect the nervous system and partly accounts for some of the discomforts felt long after an acute illness has effectively been dealt with.

BRAIN STRUCTURE AND THE PRINCIPAL FUNCTIONAL AREAS

The brain is encased within the bones of the cranium and weighs between 3 and 4 kg. On average there are 8 billion nerve cells and their axons are held together by connective tissue called *glia*. Glial cells come in many different shapes and sizes and are called oligodendrocytes or astrocytes, the names referring more to shape than to connective function. In gross structure the brain is divided into 2 hemispheres or halves, being joined at its base by a bundle of nerve fibres known as the corpus callosum thus ensuring coordination between the right and left hemispheres. In the majority of individuals one hemisphere is more dominant than the other, usually the dominance refers to muscle (motor movement) and to speech. If an individual is said to be right-handed, then the left hemisphere of the brain is more dominant since the nerve fibres from the left half of the brain cross at the medulla to supply the right side of the body.

Each hemisphere is roughly approximated into lobes by fissures or grooves and each lobe is named after the overlying cranial bone. The frontal lobe is, in evolutionary terms, the most recently developed part of the brain (forebrain) and is responsible for abstract learning, memory and behaviour. The temporal area has 2 main functions, that of hearing and of speech coordination. A very extensive area at

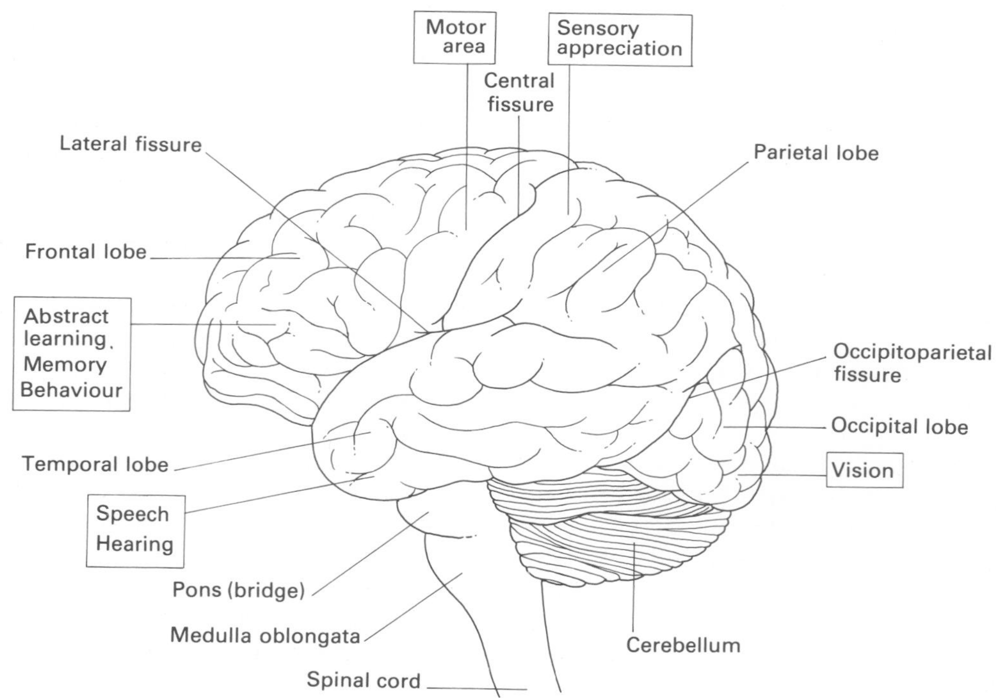

Fig. 75.4 Side view of cerebral hemisphere.

the occipital lobe is designated for vision, while the parietal lobe contains specific areas for sensory appreciation and motor response. At the base of the brain, 3 important functional areas are the pons varolii (bridge), the cerebellum which coordinates fine movements, and the medulla oblongata possessing groups of cells which control and coordinate the vital functions of respiration, blood pressure, cardiac function, vomiting, coughing, sneezing and swallowing.

The cortex or outer surface of the brain is mainly composed of nerve cells which give the exposed surface its grey appearance (grey matter). In the deeper layers of the brain, where the nerve fibres branch downwards towards the spinal cord, the brain colour is mainly white due to the fibres being encased in myelin sheath. Interspersed between the nerve fibres, deeper in the brain substance, are many specialised functional groups of nerve cells influencing the coordination of many of the body's functions. The principle areas which the nurse would find useful to study are the:

basal ganglia
thalamus
hypothalamus and pituitary gland
brain stem
cerebellum
ventricles, cerebrospinal fluid and meninges
cerebellar blood supply

Basal Ganglia (Basal Nuclei)

Lying within the cerebral hemispheres are a series of highly specialised nerve cells whose function it is to receive incoming information from many sources, e.g., the eyes, ears, thalamus and cerebellum, and to organise the received information which will contribute to modifying the total body response to all sensory information. These groups of specialised cells lie close to the lateral ventricles and are named the *corpus striatrum, amygaloid body* and *claustrum*. Their ability to organise sensory information allows for a coordinated motor response and is the basis of the extra-pyramidal system.

Thalamus

The thalamus consists of 2 oval-shaped masses of nerve cells which lie just below the lateral ventricle and on either side of the third ventricle, and are part of the basal ganglia's organising system. Mainly the thalamus is a relaying station through which all sensory information passes to reach the cerebral cortex. The thalamus conveys sensory information of pain, temperature, touch, some sensory information from the cranial nerves, and from the receptors of muscles and tendons. It has association fibres which link it to all the basal nuclei and with the cerebellum, and sends all its information to the cerebral cortex via the internal capsule. This is a most important area where ascending and descending fibres meet and form a channel. It is easily affected by any pressure which may arise as the result of a cerebrovascular accident, hence paralysis and the sensory depreciation of a stroke.

Hypothalamus and Pituitary Gland

This specialised group of nerve cells is linked to the posterior lobe of the pituitary gland by nerve fibres, and to the anterior lobe of the pituitary gland by a complex system of blood vessels. The hypothalamus therefore controls the posterior lobe by nerve impulses and the anterior lobe by blood flow, a unique biofeedback mechanism. Secretory nerve cells in the hypothalamus produce two hormones: the antidiuretic hormone and oxytocin. These pass to the posterior lobe of the pituitary gland for storage and for use as and when demanded by their target organs, i.e., the kidney and the uterus in childbirth. The anterior lobe is influenced by a releasing factor secreted from the hypothalamus, one factor for each hormone released, i.e., adrenocorticotrophic hormone and gonadotrophic hormone. Other functions attributed to the hypothalamus include those of hunger and its satiation, thirst and its relief, control of body temperature and the mechanisms of fear or rage which are defensive physiological states expressed through emotional means. In

Table 75.1. Cranial nerves. The majority of the cell bodies originate in the medulla oblongata

Number	Name	Nerve type	Function
1	Olfactory	Sensory	Smell
2	Optic	Sensory	Vision
3	Occulomotor	Motor	Eye muscles
4	Trochlear	Motor	Oblique eye muscles
5	Trigeminal	Mixed	Facial muscles Scalp muscles Mastication muscles
6	Abducent	Motor	Rectus eye muscles
7	Facial	Mixed	Muscles of expression Taste buds
8	Auditory	Sensory	Balance Hearing
9	Glossopharyngeal	Mixed	Muscles of pharynx Parotid glands
10	Vagus (to wander)	Mixed	Thoracic and abdominal organs
11	Accessory	Motor	Neck muscles
12	Hypoglossal	Motor	Tongue movement Hyoid bone

either fear or rage, the hypothalamus stimulates not only the endocrine system but also the medulla oblongata to enable the body to deal with the crisis. An area of the brain known as the reticular formation extending from the brain stem upwards, is a group of cells responsible for two opposing functions: those of sleep requirement and its opposite, being alert. This area is also influenced by association fibres from the hypothalmus. The hypothalamus lies immediately behind the pituitary gland below the third ventricle and is immediately behind the optic chiasma.

Brain Stem

The brain stem contains the following specialised areas:

Midbrain
Pons Varolii
Medulla oblongata

The area as a whole is important for two reasons. Firstly all the cranial nerves, with the exception of the olfactory and optic nerves, arise here (Table 75.1). Secondly, all the vital centres which sustain life below our conscious level are located in the medulla oblongata. Ascending from the medulla to the thalamus is a stretch of nerve cells called the *reticular formation*, which has the primary function of keeping the cerebrum alert. If damaged, a coma may result.

The midbrain consists mainly of fibres, both motor and sensory connecting the cerebrum to the cerebellum and the medulla oblongata. Within this area is the *red nucleus* which is a relay station for messages from the basal ganglia and hypothalamus to the pyramidal system. It also receives information from the ears and eyes and plays an important part in the reflex action of both these sensory organs.

Pons means 'bridge' and nerve fibres pass from the pons to the midbrain, cerebellum and medulla oblongata. The fifth, sixth and seventh cranial nerves arise from this area which is also a part of the respiratory centre in conjunction with the medulla. Nerve cells within the pons are sensitive to blood levels of carbon dioxide, which is the stimulus to respiration.

Both nerve cells and nerve fibres are to be found in the medulla oblongata. This very crucial area lies at the base of the skull, just above the foramen magnum and joins the pons to the spinal cord. The arrangement of nerve cells make up what are known as the vital centres, i.e., those vital for life. These include maintaining the involuntary control and coordination of the following:

Rate and depth of respiration (in conjunction with the pons)

Heart rate

Diameter of the blood vessels and as a result the blood pressure is determined

Swallowing reflex

Cough reflex

Vomiting centre

Sneezing reflex

Yawning reflex

As the nerve fibres pass through the medulla from the pons, they cross or decussate, implying that the nerve fibres from the left hemisphere of the brain control the right side of the body, and vice versa. The eighth and twelfth cranial nerves arise in the medulla, but also receive a great deal of information via association neurones from the cortex, caudate nucleus and the cerebellum which tends to calm down or 'inhibit' the action of the pyramidal system.

Cerebellum

The cerebellum is separated from the cerebrum by a piece of dura mater called the tentorium cerebelli and like the cerebrum it is in 2 hemispheres joined together by a small wormlike structure called the *vermis*. Similar to the cerebrum, the nerve cells are arranged on the cortex of the cerebellum with the nerve fibres flowing through the cerebellar substance. The nerve fibres enter and leave via 3 pathways:

1. Superior cerebellar peduncles from the midbrain and cerebrum.
2. Middle cerebellar peduncles from the pons varolii and medulla.
3. Inferior cerebellar peduncles from the medulla and spinal cord.

The principal function of the cerebellum is to coordinate voluntary muscular movement and body balance. It does this by receiving information from many sources such as the eyes, inner ear, skin, receptors in the muscles and joints. All this information arrives in the cerebellum simultaneously and can therefore be modified immediately, adjusting the body's position and balance from second to second so it remains a functionally coordinated unit. This function is carried out below the level of conscious awareness, the messages entering and leaving the cerebellum via the pyramidal and extra-pyramidal tracts.

Ventricles, Cerebrospinal Fluid and Meninges

The brain is not a solid structure, as deep within each cerebral hemisphere is a cavity known as the *lateral ventricle*. These 2 cavities are joined by a foramen to a narrow centrally placed cavity called the third ventricle. From here an aqueduct flows through the midbrain and then widens to form another cavity called the fourth ventricle. This fourth ventricle lies behind the pons varolii and medulla oblongata, and in front of the cerebellum.

In the roof of each ventricle are tufts of capillaries known as the *choroid plexus* which, although covered with pia mater, secrete cerebrospinal fluid into the ventricle directly from the cerebral blood flow. Only small molecular substances can cross through these fine semipermeable walls of the capillary tufts, giving one example of what is known as the *blood brain barrier*. From the lateral ventricles the cerebrospinal fluid flows down the aqueduct to the fourth ventricle and escapes via small openings (foramina) into the subarachnoid space to circulate over the brain and down around the spinal cord.

About 130 ml of cerebrospinal fluid is in circulation at any one time, although over 500 ml is produced every 24 hours. Apart from being protective to soft brain tissue by acting as a cushion, it is supportive to the meninges as it exerts a uniform pressure between the subarachnoid and middle meningeal coat. Cerebrospinal fluid is alkaline in reaction, being between 8 and 10 pH. Its specific gravity is about 1004, near to that of water. In composition the smaller molecular substances that are secreted as cerebrospinal fluid are water, amino acids, glucose and sodium. Carbon dioxide content influences the respiratory centre in the medulla oblongata. After circulating over the brain surfaces and spinal cord the fluid is reabsorbed into the venous circulation via tiny villi which feed

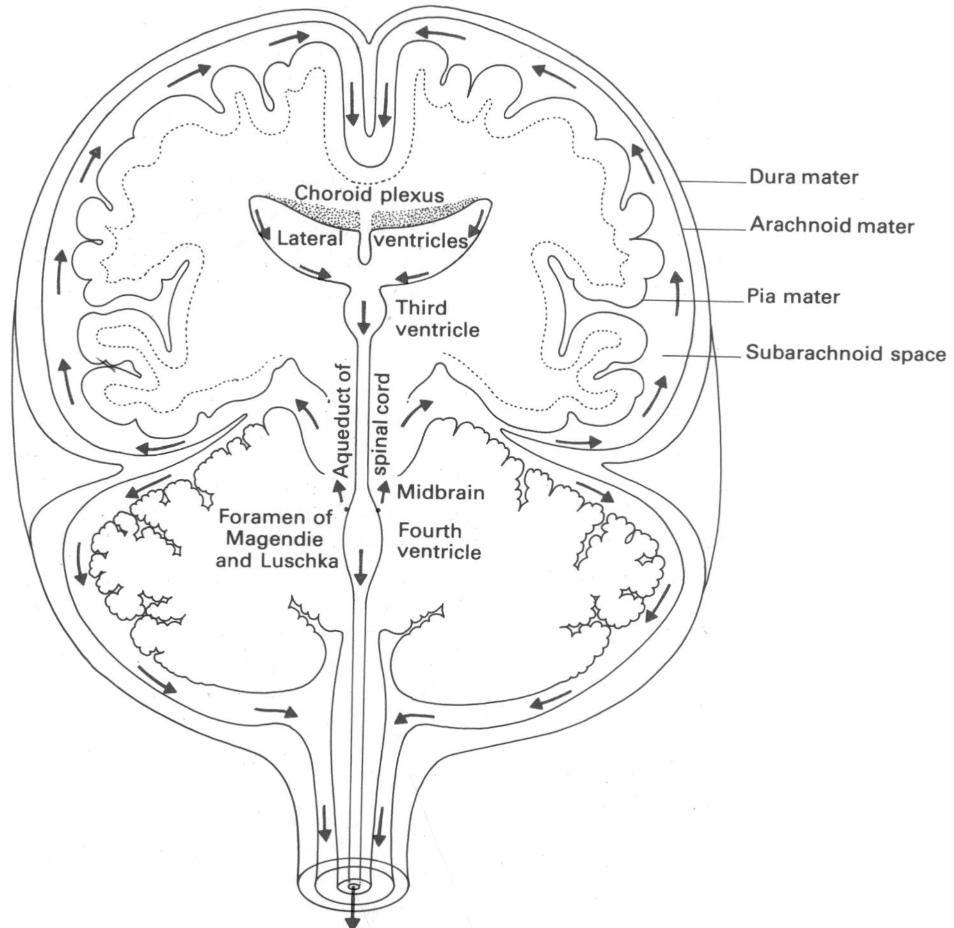

Fig. 75.5 Ventricles and flow of cerebrospinal fluid.

into the venous sinuses which remove venous blood from the brain into the jugular veins.

The Meninges

The brain and spinal cord are covered by 3 membranes, referred to as the meninges. From outer to inner, these membranes are:

dura mater
arachnoid mater
pia mater

Dura Mater

The dura mater consists of 2 layers of dense fibrous tissue. The outer or parietal layer takes the place of periosteum on the inner surface of the skull bones, while the inner or visceral layer of dura is a protective fibrous covering for both the brain and spinal cord. At several points the dura mater folds to dip into deep fissures such as the falx cerebri separating the 2 hemispheres, and at the tentorium cerebelli separating the cerebellum from the cerebrum. The dura mater extends beyond the terminal portion of the spinal cord to reach the level of the second lumbar vertebra.

Arachnoid Mater

The arachnoid mater (or spider's web) is a serous avascular membrane separated from the dura mater by a potential space, i.e., the subdural space. This membrane is loosely

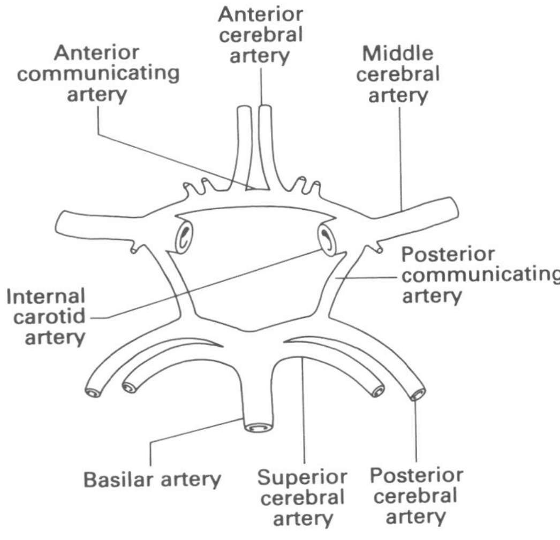

Fig. 75.6 Circle of Willis (base view).

invested over the brain tissues, but where it stretches over irregular parts of the brain it forms cisterna (cisterns) which contain a larger than usual volume of cerebrospinal fluid, e.g., the cisterna magna at the base of the occiput. The space between the arachnoid mater and the pia mater, i.e., the subarachnoid space allows for the circulation of cerebrospinal fluid over the brain surface and spinal cord.

Pia Mater

The pia mater (tender) is a fine vascular membrane which supplies the surface of the brain with many small blood vessels. It is closely adherent to the brain and spinal cord, dipping into all the fissures or sulci. Where it dips into the ventricles of the brain, it forms small tufts of specialised capillaries, i.e., the choroid plexus from which cerebrospinal fluid is derived.

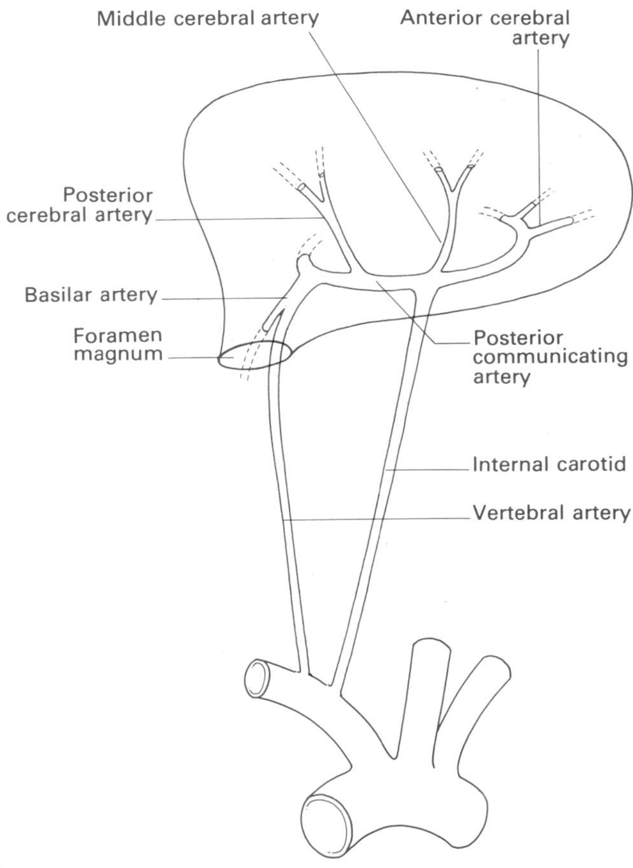

Fig. 75.7 Half circle of Willis (side view)

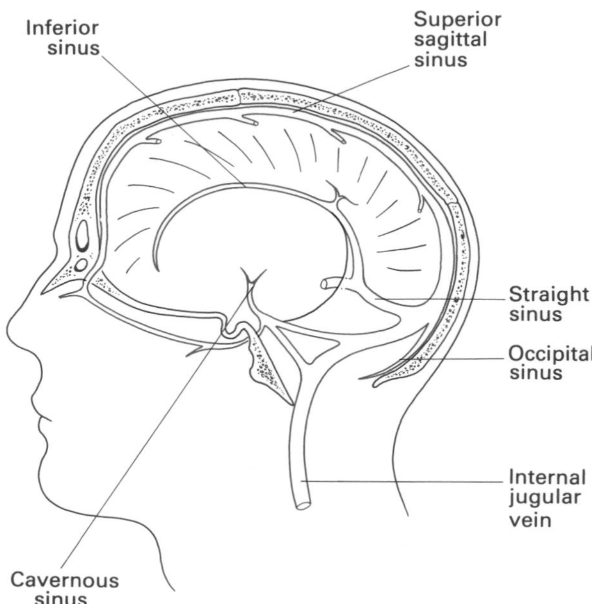

Fig. 75.8 Cerebral venous sinuses.

Cerebral Blood Supply

The brain requires a continuous high blood flow for its activity. Deprived of oxygen, the brain cells begin to die within 3 or 4 minutes. For each 100 g of brain tissue, it has been calculated that the blood flow needs to be 55 ml per minute to satisfy oxygen needs. To meet this requirement, blood is conveyed to the brain by the 2 internal carotid arteries anteriorly and the 2 vertebral arteries posteriorly. Each internal carotid artery divides to form 3 principal cerebral arteries: the anterior, middle and posterior cerebral arteries. As their names suggest, they supply those parts of the cerebrum. The 2 vertebral arteries entering at the base of the skull through the foramen magnum join together to form the basilar artery which sends branches to the brain stem and cerebellum. Further subdivision of the basilar artery gives rise to the 2 posterior cerebral arteries which supply the occipital region. The carotid artery is joined to the cerebral artery by a communicating artery. Likewise, the 2 anterior cerebellar arteries are joined together by a communicating artery. In this way a circle of vessels creates a continuous blood supply at the base of the brain, more commonly known as the circle of Willis.

Venous blood is drained away from the brain by large collecting cavities known as sinuses, which lie between the layers of the dura mater. These spaces or sinuses are all linked together, the most prominent being the superior saggital sinus which drains the anterior part of the brain, the cavernous sinus which lies proximate to the sphenoid bone and the pituitary, while the transverse sinus drains the occipital region. Eventually all venous blood drains into the internal jugular veins.

THE SPINAL CORD AND PERIPHERAL NERVES

The spinal cord lies within the neural canal of the vertebral column, being continuous with the medulla oblongata and extending from the upper border of the atlas (the first cervical vertebra) to the lower border of the first lumbar vertebra. It is approximately 45 cm in length and about as thick as the little finger. Like the brain, it is protected by the meninges and the cerebrospinal fluid. In the spinal cord

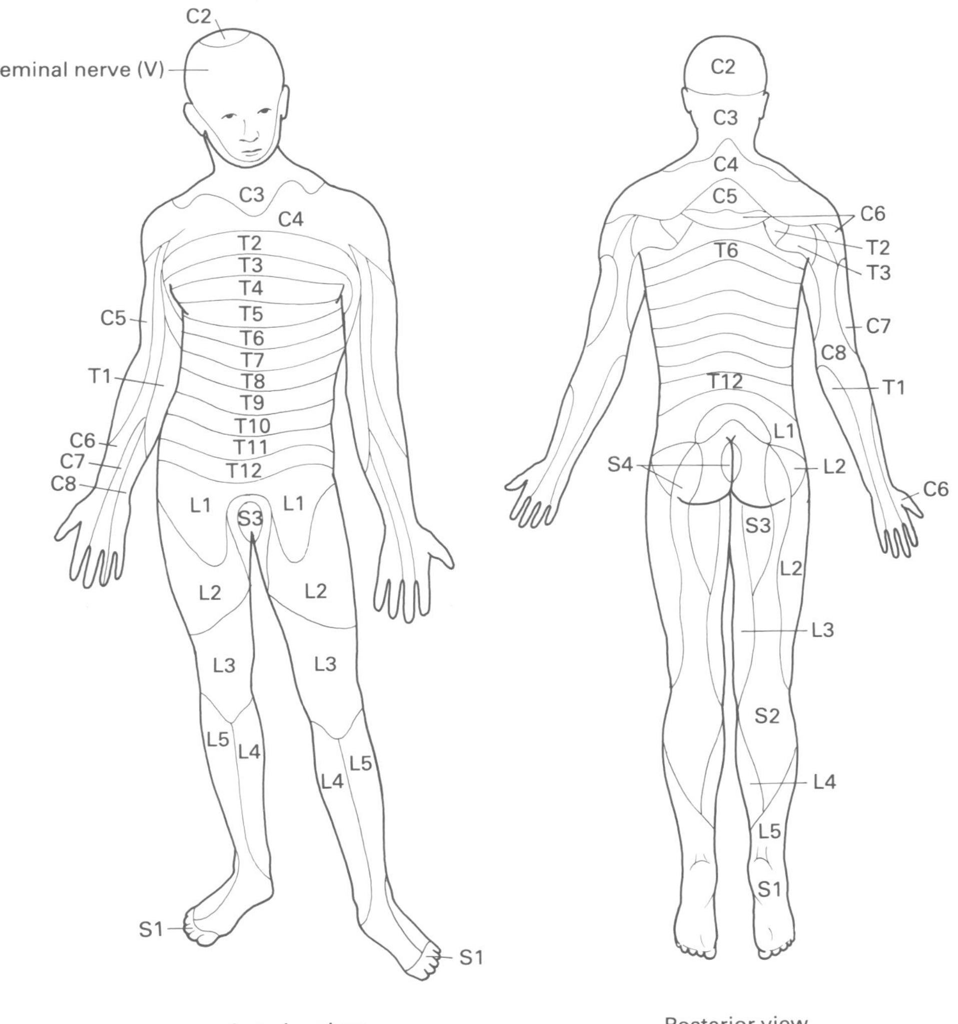

Fig. 75.9 Distribution of peripheral nerves. C = cervical segments, T = thoracic segments, L = lumbar segments, S = sacral segments.

the grey cell matter is on the inside and the white fibrous matter on the outside, and is of course the nervous link between the brain and the organs of the body. There are 31 pairs of nerves arising from the spinal cord which are divided as follows:

- 8 pairs of cervical nerves
- 12 pairs of thoracic nerves
- 5 pairs of lumbar nerves
- 5 pairs of sacral nerves
- 1 pair of coccyxygeal nerves

At the cervical and lumbar regions, the cord enlarges due to plexus, which are areas where the nerves interlace into a large network.

The white matter contains the nerve fibres arranged to form pathways up and down the cord, respectively referred to as **ascending** and **descending pathways**. The ascending pathways or tracts carry sensory messages, while the descending pathways carry motor responses which travel to the muscle groups of the limbs or the organs. Within the centre of the cord the nerve cells are arranged in an H-shape and here there is a complex aggregate of

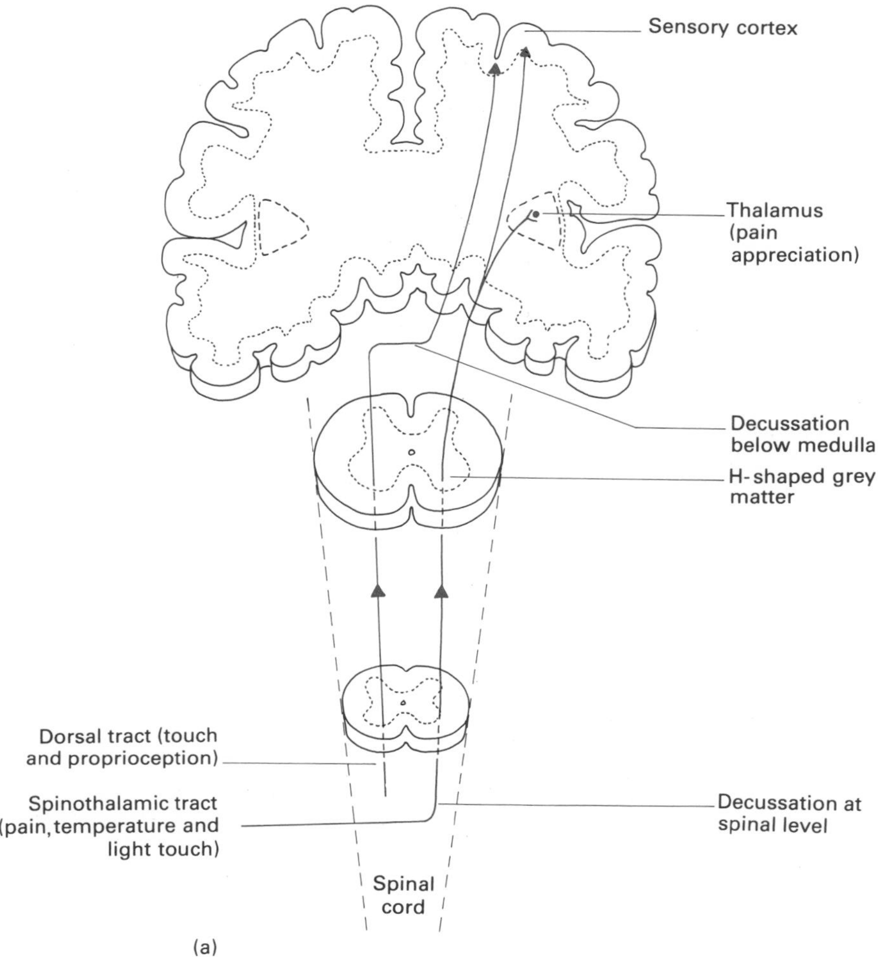

Fig. 75.10 (a) Sensory pathways (ascending), (b) motor pathways (descending).

sensory and motor cells and association neurones. The sensory nerve cells tend to be located in the posterior roots of the H-shape, while the motor nerve cells are found in the anterior root. The majority of spinal nerves enter and leave the cord as mixed nerves travelling together through the foramen in the vertebral column. Where the spinal cord terminates at the first lumbar vertebra, the lumbar sacral and coccyxygeal nerves continue to form a sheath of nerves known as the *cauda equina* (horse's tail).

Ascending Pathways (Sensory Tracts)

The peripheral senses of proprioception, pain, touch and temperature travel via afferent neurones towards the spinal cord, and ascend by one of two tracts, the dorsal and lateral (spinothalamic). Ascending and passing through the brain, some fibres cross at the medulla but all fibres pass through the thalamus before reaching the sensory area in the cortex of the brain. Association neurones in the brain will also relay sensory information at the basal ganglia, the cerebellum and the medulla. The first neurone of the ascending pathway at spinal level is part of a reflex arc,

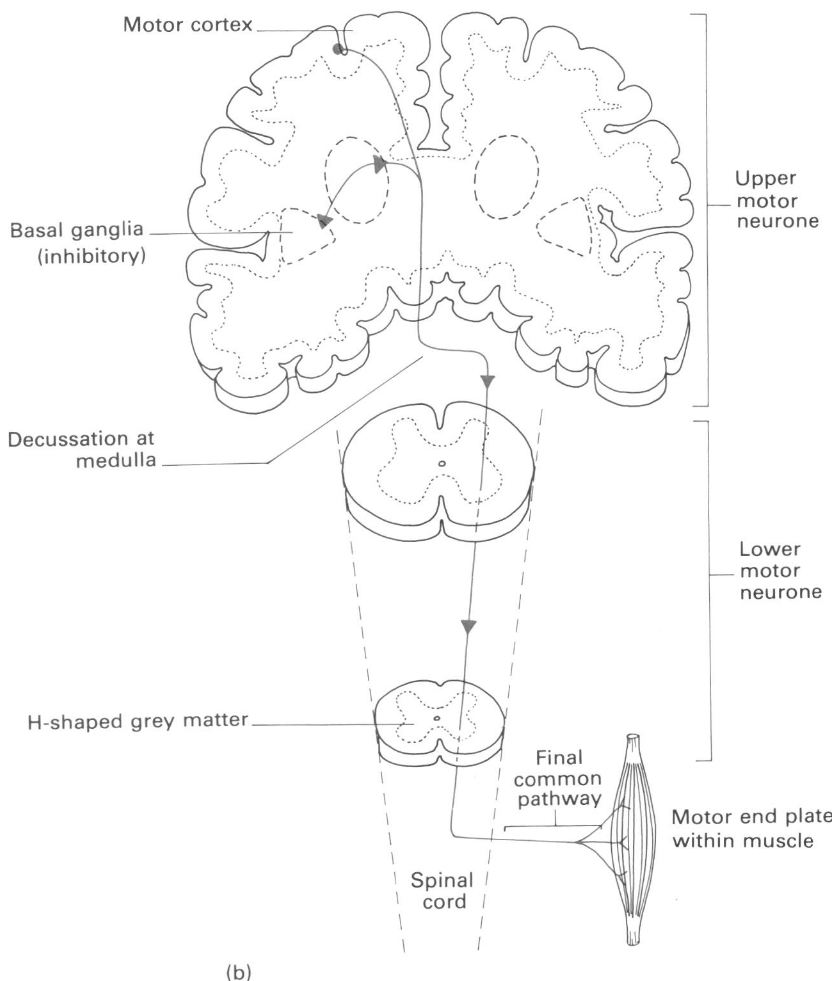

Fig. 75.10. *(continued)*

and the motor response will, in many cases, arise at spinal level before being influenced by the brain.

Descending Pathways (Motor Tracts)

For muscular movement to occur, the nerve impulse has to descend from the motor cortex of the brain via either a direct pathway, the pyramidal tract, or indirectly via the extrapyramidal tract. This latter tract has the effect of inhibiting or influencing the nerve impulse and by so doing makes for a smoother more coordinated muscular contraction and total movement. Each of these 2 tracts consists of an upper motor neurone, a lower motor neurone and a final common pathway. In descending through the brain, the nerve fibres pass through a very important area of the brain known as the *internal capsule* which is surrounded by the basal ganglia and the thalamus. On reaching the medulla, the motor nerve crosses or decussates so that the right hemisphere controls the left side of the body and the left hemisphere controls the right side of the body. In descending through the spinal cord the motor neurones synapse in the anterior horn of the spinal cord before each leaves as a spinal nerve to reach its target muscle in the motor end plate where the nerve ending has a junction with the muscle fibre.

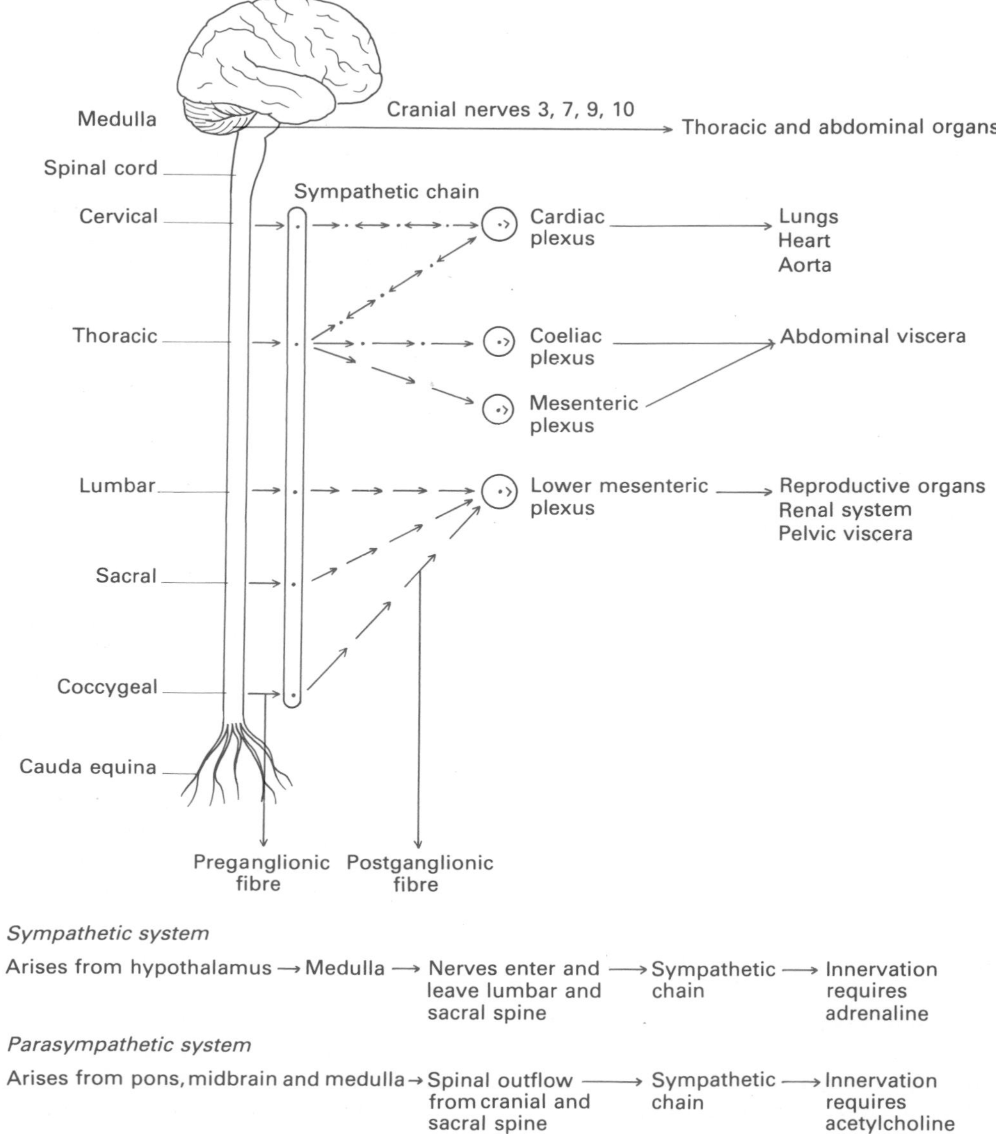

Fig. 75.11 Autonomic nervous system pathway from spinal level.

AUTONOMIC NERVOUS SYSTEM

The autonomic nervous system controls all those activities which are not under conscious control. Basically these are the involuntary muscles of many internal organs, the secretory cells within the organs, and the heart. It is important to emphasise that the system is automatic but is reliant on a biofeedback mechanism from the endocrine system, especially from the hypothalamus. These automatic functions are subdivided into 2 subsystems, being the sympathetic, or accelerating, system and the parasympathetic, or decelerating, system. (Table 75.2).

Sympathetic System

The sympathetic system is a 3 neurone system. The first neurone is derived from a cell

Table 75.2. Autonomic nervous system

Involuntary organ	Parasympathetic system	Sympathetic system	General total effect
Pupils	Constriction of diameter	Dilation of diameter	Control amount of light entering the eye
Ciliary eye muscle	Constrict muscle fibre	Relax muscle fibre	Accommodation of eye to distance
Blood vessels	Relax muscle fibre	Mixed response	Constant adjustment of blood pressure
Spleen	Relax blood vessels	Contrict blood flow	Adjust circulatory blood volume
Heart rate	Reduce	Increase	Adjust to body need for oxygen
Bronchioles	Constrict muscle fibre	Relax muscle fibre	Adjust respiratory rate to oxygen need
Sweat glands		Increased secretion	Contributes to control of body temperature
Adrenal glands		Increased secretion	Reinforces all sympathetic responses
Peristalsis of bowel	Increased activity	Decreased	Regulates digestion, absorption and elimination
Sphincters	Relax	Constrict	Control of emptying of bowel and bladder
Digestive organs	Increased secretions	Decreased activity	Adjusts the speed of digestive processes

in the brain, hypothalamus or medulla oblongata; its fibre travels in the spinal cord. The second cell is in the lateral horn of the spinal cord lying between the fifth thoracic and the fifth lumbar vertebra. The fibre leaving from this cell travels to and terminates in the sympathetic ganglia which lies outside the spinal cord. This type of fibre is known as the preganglionic fibre and is very short in length. Arising from the ganglia is the third cell and its fibre which travels towards an organ or an involuntary muscle, and is known as the postganglionic fibre. The sympathetic system accelerates all involuntary activity and for this it requires adrenaline, which is the basis of its other name the *adrenergic system*. Increased adrenaline and noradrenaline, when secreted from the medulla of the adrenal gland, increase the body's ability to cope with either 'flight' or 'fright', which is the easy way to remember how the body would cope in a situation of shock or fear.

Parasympathetic System

The parasympathetic system is a 2 neurone system with the nerves emerging only from the cranial or at the sacral level of the vertebral column.

1. The cranial outflow of preganglionic fibres have their originating cells located either in the midbrain, pons varolii or the medulla oblongata, and the postganglionic fibres innervate respiratory involuntary muscles, the heart and the aorta.
2. The sacral outflow refers to the preganglionic fibres having their originating cell body in the sacral vertebral region of the spinal cord. The postganglionic fibres innervate the lower mesenteric, reproductive organs and the kidney.

In effect the parasympathetic system decelerates body activity. It slows down all involuntary muscle activity, but increases cellular secretions which can only come about if secretory organs, such as in the intestinal system, are in a relaxed state.

In normal health the total effect of the 2 systems is to achieve a balanced activity of physiological mechanisms, i.e., balancing the heart and respiratory rate after a period of strenuous exercise.

Chapter 76
Care of the Neurological Patient

NEUROLOGICAL INVESTIGATIONS

To elicit and clarify the wide variety of neurological signs and symptoms arising from disease, the physician may spend a great deal of time examining 3 components of the nervous system:

1. Sensory responses to various stimuli, which test the discriminating ability of the ascending pathways within the spinal cord.

2. Motor responses, mainly the principal reflex arc to test the coordination of the lower motor neurones, and the influences of the upper motor neurone and cerebellum.

3. Autonomic responses of the cranial nerves of which the greater majority are mixed nerves arising from the brain stem.

In further investigations the physician may request:

Invasive and noninvasive radiological tests

Lumbar puncture

Specimen collections

From the patient's point of view, this can mean a bewildering battery of tests and careful explanation and reassurance is necessary to ensure that the patient realises the vast majority of tests are painless and without risk or any harm. The main role of the nurse will be to coordinate the patient's nursing needs to match the timing of the tests, and to be available to help the doctor during the tests. For the physical neurological examination (often completed by a specialist) the nurse should ensure that the previously taken medical and social history in the form of case notes are available, as should be the reports of any previous tests. Preferably the patient should be dressed only in their undergarments and a tie back cotton gown. The examination room should be well lighted, warm and free from draughts.

On first meeting the patient, the physician will visually assess the patient's posture in both the standing and sitting positions and look for strengths or weaknesses of the various groups of muscles. Simple questioning should help to assess the patient's speed of verbal delivery, and their word and sentence structure. In addition, the same type of questioning should identify if the patient is orientated to time, place and event as well as the quality of recent memory.

Sensory Responses

Sensory responses to test discrimination of the ascending pathways are pain, touch, temperature and vibration.

Pain

A sharp pointed needle or pin is used to prick the skin surface along a defined pathway towards the spinal cord. The patient should be able to discriminate when the pin prick is felt. It is possible to map the sensory pathway on the skin with indelible pencil.

Touch

The nerve receptors, i.e., Miessner's, Krause and Pacinian corpuscles, located in the dermis, should appreciate the textures of various items when touched. Usually the patient is asked to close the eyes and identify the size and shape of a coin, e.g., the difference between a 5 and 10 pence coin. Equally the patient should be able to feel the touch of a wisp of cotton wool taken over the skin surface.

Temperature

Both hot and cold appreciation can be tested by asking the patient to discriminate between these two when holding a glass tube of either hot or cold water.

Vibration

Vibrations of a very minor nature should be appreciated over the skin covering the smaller joints of the ankles and wrist. A vibrating tuning fork is placed over these areas and the patient asked to say what he or she can feel.

Motor Responses

Motor responses discriminate the reflex response of the lower motor neurones. A reflex arc is composed of a sensory fibre, an interconnecting neurone or synapse within the spinal cord, and a motor neurone, the latter also being referred to as a lower motor neurone. This motor response to a local sensory stimulus is also influenced by the upper motor neurone and the cerebellum. A damaged upper motor neurone will exaggerate the normally smooth reflex response, while damage to the cerebellum will prolong the time of the reflex arc. Initially the right and left limbs are compared with each other to note if there is any obvious wasting in any groups of muscles. If necessary, the muscles can be measured and contrasted for greater accuracy. Muscular strength can be tested by either a hand grip, or by opposing the patient's hands with that of the palmar surface of the physician, and asking the patient to push as strongly as they can. The principal reflexes tested are:

1. Elbow. With the arm flexed, the point or side of the elbow joint is tapped to test if the arm will straighten.
2. Knee. The point immediately below the patella, i.e., the tendon, is tapped. This should cause the thigh muscles to contract and thereby flex the knee. It is the best example of a simple reflex arc.
3. Planter. The inner aspect of the sole of the foot is stroked and the toes should point downwards. If they point upwards and spread outwards, in the adult this would indicate upper motor neurone disease, although it should be noted that an upward

toe movement is normal in infants, i.e., Babinski's sign.

4. Abdominal. The lower or middle abdominal muscles are lightly stroked, which should cause an immediate contraction of the muscles in the area. This is also a good example of a superficial reflex arc.

Autonomic Responses of the Cranial Nerves

Autonomic responses of the cranial nerves are tested as follows:

1. The olfactory nerve is responsible for the sensation of smell. While one nostril is occluded, the other is tested by watching and asking the patient to sniff the aroma of easily identified substances such as oil of cloves, peppermint and lavender. The absence of smell, i.e., amnosia, is of itself not significant.

2. The optic nerve, unlike the other cranial nerves, does not arise in the brain stem but in the occipital lobe of the brain. Standard tests for vision are completed using the Snellen's chart. The retina is examined to exclude any swelling of the optic disc, i.e., papilloedema, and the visual fields are tested either by perimetry or by asking the patient to count the number of fingers he or she can see when the physician's hand is held to the side of the eye.

3. The occulomotor, trochlear (4) and the abducens (6) are simultaneously tested by asking the patient to move the eyeball in every direction to test the eye muscles, noting if there is any nystagmus and if the pupil reaction to light is normal.

4. The trigeminal nerve is tested by assessing the response to a pin prick gently placed into the facial skin, and by testing the corneal reflex with a wisp of cotton wool.

5. The facial nerve is not tested.

6. The auditory nerve is responsible for both hearing and balance. The outer canal should firstly be inspected to check that there is no ear wax. The tympanic membrane is also inspected to ensure that it is healthy before any of the standard hearing tests are carried out. Vibration tests with a tuning fork will help establish if the patient is either suffering from perceptive or conductive deafness.

7. The glossopharyngeal nerve is responsible for the sensory appreciation of tastes, mainly these are salt, sour, sweet and bitter. The tongue has firstly to be cleansed and then blotted with paper before asking the patient to identify the four specific tastes of prepared solutions as they are dripped onto the tongue.

8. The vagus nerve has branches extending into the soft palate, as well as to the heart and lungs and many abdominal branches innervating internal organs. It is usually sufficient for the physician to examine the throat as the patient makes a vocal sound. The movement of the soft palate is noted. Vocal changes in the last 4–6 months are of interest, as is the ability to swallow fluids and foods.

9. The spinal accessory nerve is tested by asking the patient to shrug the shoulders and noting if there is any disparity between the right and left shoulder muscles during movement.

10. The hypoglossal nerve innervates the tongue, and any abnormal movement or wasting can be detected by asking the patient to obtrude the tongue as far as possible.

Proprioception Test

Nerve receptors located at the joints, tendons and muscles combine with those of balance to give the individual his or her sense of gravity, and thus an awareness of body position at any one time. This sense of proprioception is influenced by vision. Total body coordination can be tested by a variety of methods, e.g., by asking the patient to close his or her eyes and placing the tip of one finger onto the tip of the nose. Alternatively, the patient may be asked to walk in a straight line so that the gait may be observed. This is commonly used in alcoholism testing. Thirdly, the patient may be asked to place the heel of one foot on the shin of the opposite leg and move it up and down, and fourthly he or she can be asked to stand upright and close the eyes, and the posture observed for any distinctive wavering, i.e., Romberg's test. The inability to coordinate any of these movements, especially with the eyes closed, would indicate some damage to the ascending sensory pathways within the spinal cord.

Invasive and Noninvasive Radiological Tests

Plain X-rays of the skull at various angles will identify previous or existing bone lesions which may account for some neurological symptoms.

Air Encephalography

Air encephalography will outline the contours of the ventricles of the brain which are situated in the midline of the brain. About 30 ml of air are injected into the subarachnoid space via a cisternal puncture. Alternatively the air can be injected directly into the ventricles via a burr hole operation. Any displacement or distortion of the ventricles from the normally placed midline would suggest altered intracranial pressure.

Cerebral Arteriography

Cerebral arteriography is the injection of an opaque dye directly into the carotid arteries, or indirectly into the vertebral arteries, or via the femoral artery. The dye should outline any displacement of cerebral vessels caused by tumours, aneurysms, angioma, thrombosis, or indicate the degree of any cerebral atheroma.

Isotopic Encephalography and CAT Scan

Isotopic encephalography and computerised axial tomography (CAT scan) are two investigations which can record any alteration in the density of soft tissue. The serial X-rays are retained by the computer's memory and used as a basis for further investigation or as a means on which to base treatment.

Myelography

Myelography demonstrates the flow of cerebrospinal fluid between the meninges of the spinal cord and involves injecting an opaque dye (myelodil) into the spinal theca. Minor obstructions or lesions on or within the spinal cord will interrupt the flow of cerebrospinal fluid, increasing intracranial pressure.

Electroencephalography

Electroencephalography is commonly used in the diagnosis of epilepsy and records the electrical wave patterns discharged as the result of cerebral neuronal activity. A specialist spends some time studying the wave pattern, i.e., alpha, beta and theta waves; too many slow waves from one focus may suggest the presence of a tumour, or epilesy.

Electromyography

Electromyography is the measurement and recording of electrical discharges given from contracting muscle. It measures the conduction time to assess if there is any degree of wasting or weakness in a group of muscles.

Lumbar Puncture

There are 3 main reasons why a physician may wish to perform a lumbar puncture:

1. Diagnostic. Between 5 and 8 ml of cerebrospinal fluid is removed from the lumbar meninges and despatched to pathology, with a request for it to be cultured to find the causative organism for such infections as meningitis. The protein level is measured, which is very high in cerebral tumours, and the specimen is tested for the presence of blood. During the puncture, the pressure under which the cerebrospinal fluid is flowing can be measured.
2. Therapeutic. After inserting the needle into the lumbar meninges, drugs can be injected into the spinal cord, e.g., antibiotics, cytotoxic agents; or by removing cerebrospinal fluid, the intracranial pressure can be lowered.
3. Radiological. Opaque dyes, such as myelodil, can be injected which will outline the shape and contours of the subarachnoid space and meninges.

Sites for Lumbar Puncture

There are 3 sites from which cerebrospinal fluid can be taken:

1. Most commonly from between the fourth and fifth lumbar vertebrae, where the meninges continue beyond the spinal cord.

2. From the cisterna magna below the base of the skull. The point of the needle will be near the medulla oblongata and therefore great care is required in correct positioning of the patient.

3. Immediately below the lateral ventricle in the brain, usually only reached by drilling burr holes through the cranial bones. The needle is passed through the brain tissue and the cerebrospinal fluid drawn off. This is an emergency operation, the procedure confined to those patients who urgently require fluid to be withdrawn to reduce an extremely high intracranial pressure, It is also known as ventricular tapping.

Procedure for Lumbar Puncture

The anxiety levels of a conscious and cooperative patient will only be reduced with a careful explanation of the procedure. Outlining what is required of the patient by way of maintaining an awkward position, small details such as when the lumbar puncture will be done, and by whom, should not be forgotten and timing is important if the patient is worried about visiting relatives.

The bed should be prepared with only one head pillow, preferably a small firm one. Some doctors also prefer fracture boards to be placed beneath a soft mattress. The bedclothing is arranged to cover the patient at half body length, while the adopted position is to place the patient on his or her side with the knees towards the chest and the head flexed towards the chest. This position will open the spaces between the vertebral spine. The vertebral column should be parallel with the edge of the bed. A small cotton blanket should be placed over the upper half of the patient, only leaving the lumbar and lower thoracic spine exposed. One nurse should be sitting at the head of the patient, to maintain eye to eye contact and, if necessary, to hold the patient's hands during the procedure. A second nurse should have already prepared a sterile trolley and both the nurse and physician should use an aseptic technique. The suggested procedure can be modified with local policy:

1. With the aid of a nurse, the physician should prepare his or her own sterifield.

2. The nurse pours out those lotions identified by the physician as being needed, e.g., lotions used to cleanse the skin.

3. A 2 or 5 ml syringe is prepared with the requested local anaesthetic, which the nurse double-checks is correct before it is injected into the skin over the lumbar vertebra.

4. Needling of the spine is the physician's responsibility and it is best done if he or she is in the sitting position. Once the tip of the needle enters the subarachnoid space, the nurse can assist by supporting the manometer which is attached to the needle. This will measure the pressure of the cerebrospinal fluid, the normal range being 100–200 mmHg. The nurse may at this point be requested to assist with the Queckenstedt test, which involves the nurse compressing the jugular veins. If the venous sinuses, i.e., venous cerebral drainage system, are congested then the pressure on the manometer will rise above the normal range.

5. It is usual for 3 specimens to be collected, 2–3 ml in each specimen bottle, which the nurse passes to the doctor, already uncapped. Immediately following the procedure, these specimens are correctly labelled and despatched to pathology with the signed request forms.

6. On withdrawal of the needle the puncture wound is sealed either with a collodion soaked cotton wool swab or a small seal dressing.

During the whole procedure a second nurse should be supporting the patient's position and immediately report to the physician any untoward signs of facial or visual distress.

Once the procedure is complete, the patient is allowed to rest in the recumbent position with only one pillow. If a headache is complained of, the foot of the bed should be raised. Hourly observations should be taken of the pulse, respiration and blood pressure. The patient should be questioned as to the severity of any headache and appropriate action taken to nurse him or her in a quiet area of the ward with dimmed lights. Any paraesthesia of the hands and feet should be reported to a senior colleague, as should any leakage from the puncture wound. Some patients recover very quickly, while others may require as long as 24 hours to recover from headache and a reduced cerebrospinal fluid pressure.

It should be noted that cerebrospinal pressure will rise if the patient is frightened. It will also be raised in obese patients. A genuinely high pressure due to a cerebral tumour, which is causing papilloedema, will rule out a lumbar puncture as a safe procedure. If carried out when the patient has papilloedema, there is a risk of cerebral herniation.

The dangers to take precautions against include any sudden movement while the needle is in place, as the needle point if displaced could damage the cauda equina. A poor aseptic technique not only risks infection of the puncture wound, but also places the spinal meninges at risk. The removal of too much cerebrospinal fluid will induce shock, causing the pulse to become rapid and the blood pressure to fall.

These days it is unusual for a cisternal puncture to be performed, but it may be necessary if the patient has a spinal deformity. The same procedure as for lumbar puncture is adopted, except to say that resuscitation equipment should be on hand in case of collapse which may occur because of being so near the medulla oblongata. The point of the needle is inserted between the first and second cervical vertebra, while the patient's head is in full flexion.

Specimen Collections

Contributing to the diagnosis of neurological disease are those measurements of the waste products found in the urine. A 24-hour urinary specimen may be requested to assay the amount of albumin, protein, creatine, creatinine, hormones and, more rarely, the waste products of any drug which has been taken over a long period of time.

Similarly, 24-hour collection of faeces may be asked for to confirm the diagnosis of excessive fats in polyneuropathy, parasites in encephalitis, viral culture in the case of poliomyelitis and blood if there is a primary growth in the bowel which has caused a secondary cerebral tumour.

Chapter 77
Pain and Migraine

PAIN

Pain is by definition the uncomfortable motor response to a sensory stimulus which is either noxious or an irritant. The stimulus is either appreciated at the pain nerve ending receptors lying in the epidermis, or within the involuntary muscles surrounding the majority of organs. Peripheral nerve endings of the skin transmit the sensory appreciation of pain via the central nervous system, while internal organs transmit pain sensation via the autonomic nervous system. This will inevitably produce an overlap of symptoms since the response to the pain will involve a reaction from both nervous systems. Also, since the endocrine system is an integral part of the autonomic nervous system, this gives a third response. This triple response to pain is then heavily influenced by the patient's personal psychological outlook.

Pain can be classified into various stimuli. For example, a mechanical pain implies the boundaries of a structure are under some form of stress, such as an obstruction. Chemical and toxic irritants upon the skin, or if taken internally, cause an immediate oedema and the scarring effect induces severe pain. Thermal burns either by extreme heat or severe cold irritate the nerve pain endings to an intolerable degree, as will electric shock. Psychological pain is now a well recognised feature in psychiatry. If there is fear or anxiety in the situation, and there usually is, then the intensity of the motor response to pain becomes more intensified. This latter fact underlines the importance of reassurance. If given with a positive outlook and phrased correctly reassurance increases the patient's coping skills in tolerating the pain and thereby reduces the pain without actually removing it.

TYPES OF PAIN

Ache

An aching type of pain is usually localised and often involves a muscle or group of muscles. Headache, tummy-ache and tooth-ache all imply a localised area. The more intense the ache, the less ability there is to deal with activities of normal daily living.

Acute Pain

Acute pain is of an intense unremitting nature. It too tends to be localised, e.g., the appendix; the muscles surrounding the area go into spasm and 'guard' the area. Terms such as 'stabbing' or 'probing' should be pursued, by asking the patient to point directly to the area affected. A basic knowledge of anatomy will help the nurse identify the structures involved.

Colic

Colic is an intense intermittent acute pain which travels along a well defined pathway, e.g., renal colic travels from loin to groin when a stone is irritating the involuntary muscle of the ureter. Its excruciating nature causes the patient to double up in posture and to clutch the affected area. Such pain is usually relieved by pethidine when combined with an anti-spasmodic drug such as probanthine.

Neuralgia

Neuralgia describes the pain of an irritated nerve fibre, as opposed to the stimulus of a nerve ending. It is usually chronic in nature and should not be confused with neuritis, which is the inflammation of the nerve fibre and its myelin sheath.

Referred Pain

Referred pain is acute in nature and implies that the stimulus is travelling along an associated branch of the main nerve affected. The acute pain of coronary thrombosis can also be referred to the left arm and up to the jaw. Splenic pain may be referred to the shoulder blades. Naturally the patient can be confused when the location of the pain is some distance from the affected site, and a brief explanation may be required to describe a shared-nerve pathway.

Phantom Pain

Phantom pain should be distinguished from *limb phantom*. Following the amputation of a limb the patient may still be able to feel the limb, although it has been removed. This limb phantom may not be painful and indicates that the patient has not been able to adjust the persisting whole body image. Phantom pain, on the other hand, is due to a damaged nerve fibre from poor surgical technique, and the cut nerve fibre has developed a neuroma which is causing unremitting chronic pain at the site of amputation. If the pain persists for more than 6 months, it is called *causalgia* and requires a further operation to restructure the damaged nerve fibre.

Intractable Pain

Intractable pain is invariably chronic in nature, and does not respond to conventional analgesia or other therapies. Osteoarthritis of the smaller joints such as the jaw can cause excruciating unremitting pain. Similarly, rheumatoid arthritis can also affect the shoulder and spinal joints, causing intractable pain. In cancer nursing, intractable pain caused by a tumour is in fact a very late symptom, but combined analgesia therapies are proving increasingly successful.

Psychological Pain

Psychological pain is best explained by considering the physical deterioration seen in those suffering from a true endogenous depression. This is a psychiatric emergency, for such is the degree of mental pain that the patient is often suicidal. Those suffering a

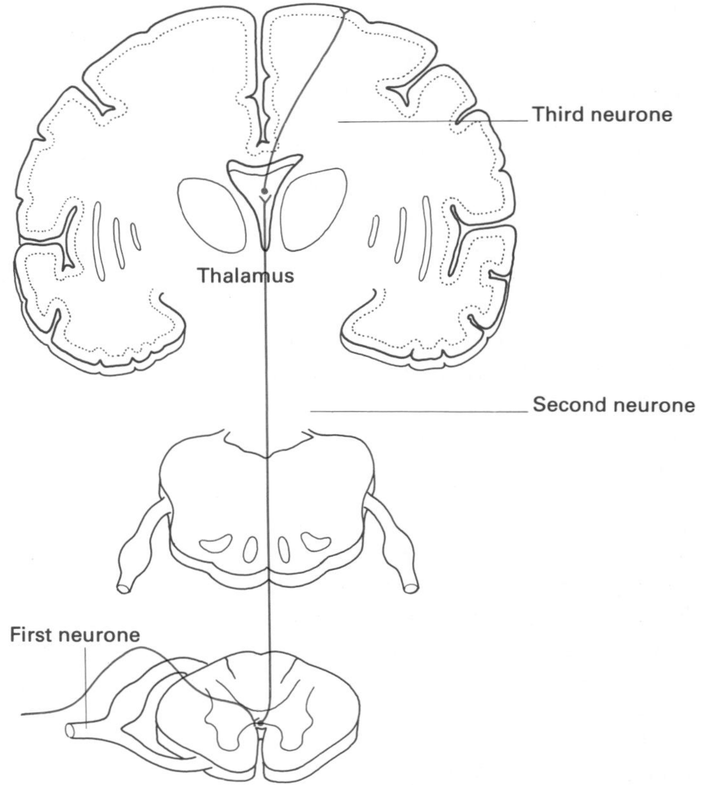

Fig. 77.1 Pain pathway 'gateway' theory. Lateral spinothalamic tracts with three 'gateways'.

bereavement may also have psychological pain of a persistent nature, especially if they have not been permitted a period of mourning and adjustment.

The 'Gateway Theory'

The 'gateway theory' attempts to explain the dominance of the sensory message of pain as it travels towards the cortex of the brain. At a local level the neurone conveys the message to the spinal cord (first gateway) and induces an immediate reflex by causing the local muscles to contract. To interrupt this motor response, the physician may prescribe and administer either local or regional anaesthesia. An uninterrupted pain message will then ascend up to the brain via the lateral spinothalamic tract to reach the thalamus (second gateway). This message can be interrupted by the administration of a spinal (epidural) anaesthetic. Travelling from the thalamus the message is then conveyed to the sensory appreciation area of the frontal lobe, and is influenced by parts of the limbic system (third gateway). It is transmitted to the motor area, which induces a muscular contraction response at the local area (Fig. 77.1).

This third gateway can be interrupted by the administration of cerebral opiates. At each gateway or synaptic junction the sensation of pain takes dominance over every type of sensation, regardless of the size or diameter of the neurone. Apart from causing a muscular contraction, which can be regarded as a protective reflex, the brain tissue may also secrete a recently identified substance known as endomorphin. This substance has similar properties to morphine and may explain the phenomena often seen in severely injured patients who seem to be euphoric, despite their injuries.

ASSESSING PAIN

As shown, there are many types of pain and the nurse, when assessing pain, should have a clear understanding of some of the more common terms used to describe a type of pain. Technical terms are not usually used by patients, so the nurse may have to persist with reasonable questioning to obtain a clear idea of the type of pain and its duration. This is also a situation when the nurse's own observations are a valid part of any assessment. During any assessment, it is **vital** to ask pointedly if there is any pain. Many patients in fact do not complain of pain, as they expect pain to be part of the process of being ill.

The assessment of pain or of its relief is a very difficult area of nursing as a personal judgement can be clouded by the nurse's own feelings about the total situation, or by his or her relationship with their patient. Regardless of what a nurse may feel about the situation or the patient, it is important to believe what the patient is saying about their pain. Any implied doubts will destroy the relationship and make it very difficult to achieve an accurate assessment with any objectivity. The nurse can assess the following features:

1. Facial expression and the appearance of the eyes. This often indicates internal distress, especially if the features can be compared before and after the giving of any drugs.
2. Body and limb posture. This often describes the area and intensity of the pain. The tone of muscles around the affected area are often extremely tense and may feel very warm. Apart from muscular tension the area may be slightly oedematous and discoloured.
3. Pyrexia and vomiting can cause pain or be the result of pain. When it is present it increases the intensity of existing pain and requires separate treatment.

Pain tolerance is very subjective. It has long been the subject of research, but as yet there is no clear answer as to what factors confer tolerance since it is confused by individual psychological strengths and weaknesses in individuals' characters. However, the following features may help the nurse make some objective measurement. Intractable pain is all consuming and the patient is usually disorientated to **time**.

The **first priority** of someone suffering severe pain is immediate relief and all actions are to this end

All the normal **coping skills** are subservient until the pain is relieved

The normal known **sleep pattern** is grossly disturbed

The patients **self perception** of their body image is that of degradation.

Tolerance to the usual **social interactions,** even with relatives and loved ones, is reduced. Indeed, one may witness anger accompanying pain.

Relieving Pain

One or several of the factors outlined previously are sufficient to justify relieving the pain immediately. A nursing plan to deal with a patient's pain is firstly to be positive in approach showing that the methods used to relieve pain do work in most situations, and to convey this belief to the patient. Reassurance not only in manner but also verbally will reduce the anxiety factor in the patient's suffering and reduce the intensity of the pain. Changing the patient's position, although a minor step, may be sufficient to support the affected area. Increased support can be given by the use of firm pillows or actual splints. If the area is positioned in natural alignment, it should help to relax any muscles in unusual tension. Hot or cold applications to the painful area alter the blood flow through the affected part, and although a simple remedy should not be denigrated as many patients find a great deal of comfort, if not actually total relief of their pain, from these applications. For instance, superficial areas respond well to cold compresses such as an ice pack, while deeper areas relax when a hot poultice is used.

Drug Therapy

The principal conservative measure in the relief of pain is the administration of analgesics such as pethidine or morphia, although many patients respond well to the simpler compounds such as codeine. An important point about analgesics is that having once achieved control over the pain the intention should be to **prevent** further pain by regular administration. The best example of this is when dealing with postoperative pain. It is equally important to remember that traditional regimens such as the 4- or 6-hourly prescriptions may not work in every case, and that some patients in fact do not necessarily respond to classical drugs such as pethidine. Analgesic drugs of themselves may prove insufficient, and secondary features of pain such as vomiting, anxiety or insomnia may require the appropriate antiemetic, tranquilliser or sedative. If the patient has a history of taking self-prescribed medication, this factor may influence the success of any prescribed regimen and may be the cause of confused states in the elderly if there is any overlap between the prescribed and self-prescribed medication. Constant checking, i.e., by direct questioning, of the effectiveness of an analgesic should be made every hour until the patient has no further complaint of pain. Apart from drugs, other methods of achieving pain relief are being currently researched before their use is totally accepted: acupuncture, hypnosis and surgery.

Acupuncture

Acupuncture is gaining popularity with both patients and medical practitioners working in some pain clinics. If it is successful, it obviates the need of drugs which many patients do not like relying on because of uncomfortable side effects.

Briefly, acupuncture is the stimulation by sterile needling massage of recognised pain points in a defined area of the body. It operates on the principal of reducing pain dominance along a sensory fibre, allowing the other sensations to reach the brain. There still remains a great deal of research to be done before this method can be universally accepted.

Hypnosis

Hypnosis is a second technique currently being researched. There are recorded successes with patients suffering from persistent low backache, causalgia, asthma, skin lesions, and of course in obstetrics. There is the suggestion that it would be of value in psychological pain.

The procedure involves inducing a trance-like state in the patient. The first stage of hypnosis is marked by a complete relaxation of the voluntary muscles. During the trance-like sleep certain suggestions or instructions are made which should increase the coping skills of the patient's ability to control his or her symptom of pain. On being brought out of the trance, the patient should have an unconscious mechanism implanted so that when pain occurs his or her coping mechanism comes into operation. Several sessions are usually required to reinforce the technique, and from experience it has been found that those with a degree of imagination can be taught to self-induce a trance-like state through which they gain complete control over their pain.

Surgery

Several surgical techniques are available to relieve the more persistent intractable forms of pain. For example, these include:

1. Rhizotomy, or the cutting of the posterior sensory nerve at the point where it enters the spinal cord.
2. A chordotomy is the cutting of the anterolateral ascending tract within the spinal cord.
3. Lobotomy, a rarely performed technique to destroy the sensory neurones in the sensory area of the frontal lobe via a prefrontal lobotomy.

MIGRAINE

To distinguish classical migraine from a transient headache the term *paroxysmal unilateral headache* is more commonly used in medical terminology. A transient headache would be caused by the increased tension of scalp muscles, which arises when the individual has or is enduring overwork, extreme anxiety, or prolonged periods of concentration. Transient headache may also be symptomatic or be a consequence of many illnesses such as hypertension, hypoglycaemia, after an epileptic attack, meningitis, electrolyte imbalance and increased intracranial pressure. A classical migraine however refers to the spasm of one or a group of arteries, which is followed by a dilation of the blood vessel and which is paroxysmal in nature.

The actual reason why one of the cerebral vessels should go into spasm in the first place in the absence of any disease evades the current research. Key factors common to many migraine sufferers are:

1. There is some evidence that it is heriditary, especially in families where there is a history of allergies.
2. The ratio of migraine sufferers is 3 females to every 1 male.
3. Migraine tends to commence in adolescence and continues into adulthood.
4. The menstrual cycle and menopause is a constant factor in the associated symptoms. Allergies to certain foodstuffs such as chocolate and cheese can cause migraine. If removed from the diet, this can induce a cure in some individuals.
5. The taking of oral contraceptive pills may be causative and a trial period with an alternative method of contraception should be attempted if this seems to be the case.

On close questioning the patient may relate that the headache is preceded by a warning or *aura* during which there is some sensory disturbance. In the majority of cases this sensory aura is a disturbance of vision, either a double vision or flashing lights, that warn the patient that a migraine attack is imminent. Other sensory disturbances which the patient reports include nausea or vomiting.

This aura phase usually lasts for about half an hour, and its cause is the blood vessel in actual spasm. The second phase is that of the actual chronic disabling pain localised to one part of the skull and is the result of the vessel becoming dilated after a short period of spasm. The resulting pain may last for a period of hours. If the pain follows a set pattern recurring at the same time of day over a period of days or weeks, it is called periodic migrainous neuralgia and this severe form of migraine is accompanied by photophobia and marked prostration.

Neurological examination and tests using X-ray and scanning techniques, and radioactive isotopes, may highlight the specific artery affected. For example if the retinal arteries are in spasm, apart from causing migraine, they will cause a transient blindness which many lay people who witness the attack assume to be hysteria. Spasm and then dilation of the middle cerebral artery would cause paraesthesia of the limbs for the duration of the attack. If the basilar artery is also affected the patient would most likely faint. If the migraine is followed by a systemic oedema, and then followed by a diuresis, the patient may be suffering from an endocrine or metabolic disorder which would require further investigations in hospital.

Therapy

Those who experience these attacks seek relief by resting in a darkened room, preferring not to be disturbed, and to avoid all distractions. They are readily irritated and feel worse if there is any noise. Examples of therapy which offer relief but not a cure in the absence of a proven cause are set out below.

Prophylactic Drugs

Ergotamine tartrate (Bellergol)

2 mg tablet to be taken sublingually when the aura stage begins. It is effective within 30 minutes and may prevent the migraine attack. Since it has serious side effects, this drug should not be repeated twice in the same day.

Methyosergide (Sansert)

1–3 mg 3 times daily for a precisely defined period, as the side effects of this drug are serious.

Dihydroergotamine

1–2 mg twice daily combined with clonidine 0.025 to 0.075 mg twice daily is a third alternative therapy.

Antiemetics

Prochloroperazine (Stemetil)

5 mg 3 times daily in maxolon syrup are usually prescribed to control the sensation of nausea and to prevent vomiting.

Tranquillisers

Amytriptyline

Is a useful drug if the migraine is associated with either anxiety or depression, especially so at the menopause.

Chapter 78
Epilepsy

Translated from the greek, the word *epilepsy* means 'seizure', but it is a generic word which includes 'convulsions' and 'fits' in its meaning. Epilepsy is regarded by medical research to be a symptom rather than a disease, and the working definition most frequently referred to is that by Hughling Jackson who describes epilepsy as 'an occasional, sudden, local, excessive discharge of the grey matter'. This physiological definition does not however clarify the cause, the presenting features, or the consequences of a seizure.

There are about 300 000 known epileptics in the United Kingdom, or 6.5–6.9 per thousand of the population in Europe and America. A rough guide to the scale of incidence of epilepsy by age group shows that:

17% occur within the first 2 years of life

13% occur between the ages of 2 and 5 years old

34% occur between 6 and 14 years of age

13% occur during adolescence

21% occur between 20 to 59 years of age

2% occur in those over 60 years of age

N.B. The majority of epileptics have their first convulsion before 20 years old, i.e., 70%.

In addition to these figures, a further 5–15% of the population are suspected of having abnormal EEG patterns without any clinical manifestation of epilepsy.

CLASSIFICATION OF EPILEPSY

Epilepsy is classified into 2 main groups:

Idiopathic Epilepsy

In idiopathic epilepsy no true cause can be found. There may be some familial tendency, but epilepsy does not follow the genetic rules of inheritance which precludes a genetic predisposition.

Symptomatic Epilepsy

Symptomatic epilepsy has an established cause in which there is a definitive cerebral lesion brought about by either injury, infection, inflammation, or infarction. The lesion takes the form of scarring of the grey matter, which comes about from healing. For example in conditions such as head injuries, birth trauma, alcoholism, meningitis, encephalitis and a pyrexia, especially in infants all may predispose to convulsions either at the time of the illness or at a later date.

A seizure or fit may be a minor or major convulsion, and an accurate nursing observation of a convulsion may help to define the convulsion. The types of convulsions which have so far been classified are as set out below.

Petit Mal

Petit mal is a momentary loss of consciousness without any significant muscle tremor. It usually starts in childhood and may persist until adolescence when the incidence spontaneously resolves.

Jacksonian fit

Jacksonian fit is a twitching movement of a localised area, e.g., the toe or thumb, which spreads firstly down one side of the body and then crosses to involve the opposite side. This type of convulsion is due to scarring of the cerebral cortex which, by its irritation, is creating abnormal electrical discharges from a focus of the brain and spreads to involve both cerebral hemispheres and thus both sides of the body.

Focal Epilepsy

Focal epilepsy is a form of a Jacksonian fit when the muscle tremor remains localised to one area of the body, e.g., an arm or leg. It indicates the specific area of the cerebral cortex which is being irritated by a lesion. Accurate nursing observations should be able to differentiate a focal epilepsy from a Jacksonian fit.

Grand Mal

Grand Mal or a major convulsion, comprises all the classical stages associated with epilepsy. It is usually idiopathic. The stages are:

1. Aura, or the warning stage, in which the patient has a specific sensory stimulus particular to the patient; it may be either a sound, smell, taste or a visual stimulus. The experienced epileptic recognises the warning sign and will prepare him or her self for a fit, advising the nurse of its imminence.
2. Tonic phase, identifies the second phase when there is marked muscular rigidity with a temporary arrest of respiration, which causes the tissues to become cyanosed.
3. Clonic, or the convulsive, phase when all the muscles go into spasm, alternating with relaxation, and causing rapid and dramatic jerking movements. These jerking movements may appear violent, but as often as not are of short duration and limited in their arc of movement, i.e., they are not thrashing or wild in their degree. The teeth are clenched tightly together and the salivary glands excrete an excessive amount of saliva, causing the socalled 'foaming' at the mouth. The duration of this type of convulsion rarely exceeds 1 minute, although at the time it does seem much longer. Urinary incontinence is quite common.
4. Sleep or comatose phase identifies the actual phase of recovery from the convulsion, but many patients want and prefer to have a sleep after their ordeal. Their behaviour is one of a confusional state and bewilderment, and the patient must not be left alone.

Myoclonic attacks

Myoclonic attacks are described as jerking movements of the muscles early in the morning and are typical of diagnosed epileptics. It would indicate that the drug regimen requires reviewing. If this type of convulsion occurs during a subacute encephalitis, it may indicate that the inflammation is causing irritation of the grey matter.

Psychomotor Epilepsy

Psychomotor epilepsy describes a grand mal convulsion accompanied by sudden behavioural changes or violence without any recall of the event by the patient. This form of epilepsy has important medico-legal implications, since the inability to recall the post-epileptic behaviour known as *automatism* may have involved the patient in a criminal act without his or her own knowledge. With this type of convulsion the patient may have a psychiatric history.

Post-traumatic Epilepsy

Post-traumatic epilepsy may occur between 6 months and 2 years after the patient has suffered from a head injury. A patient with scarring of the brain tissue, especially after an open head wound and accompanied by a depressed fracture of the skull, or a patient with a penetrating head wound followed by a period of unconsciousness, is a prime candidate for the complication of epilepsy. With medication there is a 50% chance of complete recovery from the epilepsy 3–4 years after the head injury. The compulsory wearing of protective helmets for motorcyclists is an example of a legal reform to reduce such complications from head injury.

Temporary Epileptiform Seizures

Temporary epileptiform seizures can occur if the blood pH (7.35–7.45) is disturbed because of either biochemical or metabolic disorders which cause an acidosis or alkalosis, e.g., diabetic ketosis or uraemia.

Status Epilepticus

Status epilepticus is repeated grand mal convulsions at frequently spaced intervals while the patient remains unconscious. These convulsions are accompanied by hyperpyrexia and quickly lead to cerebral anoxia and utter physical exhaustion. They are precipitated by the cessation or unsupervised withdrawal of prescribed anticonvulsant drug therapy.

Status epilepticus, if it occurs, usually seems to be most frequent 3–4 days after the withdrawal of anticonvulsant drug therapy. It represents a medical emergency and apart from the drugs outlined in Table 78.1, the nurse should plan for the care of an unconscious patient, who is best nursed in the semi-upright position. Once the sedative drugs have established control over the frequently occurring seizures, the doctor may prescribe intravenous mannitol 50% to relieve if not prevent cerebral oedema. Oxygen and suction therapy are both required in between the seizures. Recovery is usually slow and is not really complete until the medication has restored the previous blood serum level.

ASSESSMENT, CARE AND EVALUATION

When the epileptic is admitted to hospital for investigation, or for stabilising his or her medication, the nurse has a multiple role in the care of this type of patient:

Initial Assessment

At the initial assessment interview the nurse will have to explain the likely course of events to placate the patient's natural anxiety. The bed should be so located in the ward that the patient is under continual observation at all times, so should a convulsion occur nursing care and observation will be immediate. The patient is never left alone. The previous medication should be known to the nursing staff and the actual drugs returned to the pharmacy.

Since the group and type of epilepsy may not be exactly known, the features of the patient's immediate environment should emphasise that of safety. Sharp-edged furniture and electrical gadgetry should be removed and the surrounding bed area always kept clear and not cluttered with unnecessary furniture. The only time the safety rails of the bed need to be in the upright position is following an actual convulsion.

Plan of Care

The nursing staff should be familiar with the specific observations requested by the physician and have a working knowledge of the patient's previous medical history. A closer examination of the observation charts should highlight the exact points to be noted during a convulsion and these usually include the following features:

1. If the convulsion was preceeded by any stimulus or aura, such as an odd smell, visual disturbance, auditory stimuli or hallucinatory behaviour; this may indicate the focal area of the brain from where the excessive discharge is originating.

2. Was it obvious that the convulsion started at the periphery and then spread to involve the whole body? Alternatively, was it a generalised convulsion? If it remained a focal convulsion, the area of the body affected should be clearly noted. The time and duration of the convulsion should be timed with the second hand of a stop watch, if possible. It is equally important to log if the convulsions occur at specific periods of the day, especially myoclonic convulsions which tend to occur early in the morning. Differentiation should be made between the period of unconsciousness of the convulsion itself, and the period of sleep following the convulsion.

3. Note should be made if the patient was actually incontinent. This is often used to differentiate between a true epilepsy and a hysterical fit. The hysterical patient does not usually lose control of his or her bladder.

4. Following the convulsion, the axilliary temperature should be recorded. It is usually raised. The nurse should try to describe the patient's post-convulsion behaviour, especially noting the degree of disorientation: if amnesic, if violent, or if the patient can respond to simple questions so as to be able to clarify if there is any speech defect.

5. Eye changes should be recorded following the convulsion. The degree of any deviation and size of the pupils and their reaction to light may indicate the actual depth of unconsciousness.

6. If despite normal precautions the patient has sustained any injury, the nurse should immediately inform the physician so that the normal procedure to deal with the hospital policy regarding accidents to patients may be implemented.

The observation chart should assist the nurse in making a chronological observation of the convulsion, so that little of the actual convulsion is missed, and will prove a most valuable tool in diagnosis of the group and type of epilepsy.

Implementation of Care

During a grand mal convulsion the clinical skills of the nurse, as well as their observational ability, will be required to:

Remove the patient from any danger at the first sign of a convulsion. Lie them down on the bed surface, or on the floor, and screen the area to avoid alarming any nearby patients.

The head should be cushioned with one firm pillow, dentures be quickly removed and any tight clothing around the neck and waist loosened. If time permits, the shoes or footwear should be removed.

The airway is maintained by supporting the lower mandible at its upper third, and either a padded wooden spatula or a piece of soft material is wedged between the teeth to prevent the tongue being caught between the teeth when they become clenched.

During the clonic phase, i.e., the convulsion, the limbs are guided rather than restrained, any forcible restraint risks injury, e.g., a fracture, such is the force of the convulsion.

Once the convulsion is over, the patient requires to be reassured about where they are and that they will not be left alone. Allow the patient to rest for a few moments before cleaning away excess saliva and changing the patient's clothing if they have become incontinent. The patient is then settled comfortably in bed and allowed to sleep. Nursing observations are continued until the patient recovers.

Diagnostic Tests

EEG

Assisting the physician with diagnostic tests includes preparing the patient for an electroencephalogram (EEG). This test requires the physician to ascertain if the following features are present before the test is done, as they may adversely affect the results: menstruation, insomnia, current medication, and the duration of symptoms are examples of those features which can alter an EEG rhythm and should be known to the technician conducting the test. While an EEG can detect gross lesions, infections and cerebral damage, it cannot identify biochemical or metabolic disorders, even if they are suspected of being the cause of epilepsy. EEG is usual for confirming if a patient has a suspected brain pathology, but is of limited value in cases of idiopathic epilepsy. However it is normal practice to investigate a first convulsion with the EEG before any treatment is initiated.

Cerebral Angiography, Brain Scanning, Air Encephalography and Lumbar Puncture

May all be attempted to exclude or confirm the presence of cerebral scarring or tumours. The *Wasserman* and *Kahn blood test* are routinely done to exclude undiagnosed syphilis or untreated gonorrhoea.

The witnessing of a convulsion by any member of the family can be crucial evidence and the relatives may give confidences to the nurse which should be passed on to the physician if the details are relevant to the diagnosis. Nursing observations of a convulsion may also help exclude differential diagnosis such as hysteria, vasovagal attacks and, very rarely, tetany.

Evaluation of Care

Drug Therapy

Once the diagnosis of epilepsy is confirmed, the patient is invariably started on a regimen of anticonvulsant drugs for a prolonged period, the aim being to achieve a blood serum level without inducing any side effects (Table 78.1). Anticonvulsant therapy, even in children, is usually a combination of drugs, e.g., phenobarbitone and phenytoin, as an initial therapy. Each particular drug however has its own side effects, particularly when it is taken over a prolonged period.

Phenobarbitone

Taken over a period of months can induce skin rashes, ataxia, persistent drowsiness and hypertrophy of the gums which interferes with dental development. Therefore the prescribed medication needs frequently reviewing. These side effects may be countered by giving the patient folic acid 5 mg daily with the phenobarbitone.

Troxidone

While a useful anticonvulsant, can cause serious disorders of the eyes, nephrotic syndrome, agranulocytosis and aplastic anaemia. Sudden withdrawal or cessation of anticonvulsant therapy can precipitate status epilepticus. Therefore when it is decided to alter therapy, the drug regimen should be reduced slowly with a warning given to the patient that there is a 50% chance of recurrence of attacks within 6 months of either altering or concluding a therapeutic regimen, and that precautions may be necessary.

Counselling

Counselling of the patient and their relatives depends to a great extent on the age at which

Table 78.1. Anticonvulsant drugs in common use

Grand mal and focal epilepsy
Sodium phenobarbitone (Luminal) 30–60 mg twice daily
Phenytoin sodium (Epanutin, Dilatin) 100 mg twice daily
Primidone (Mysoline) 250–2000 mg twice daily
Carbamezapine (Tegretol) 20 mg 3 times daily
Clonazepam (Rivotril) 1–8 mg once daily
Sodium valproate
Suthiame (Ospolot) 200 mg 3 times daily
Phenyl ethylacetylurea (Benuride) 200 mg 3 times daily
Petit mal
Ethosuximide 250 mg twice daily
Clonazepam (Rivotril) 1–8 mg once daily
Sodium valproate
Troxidone (Tridione) 60–1200 mg daily
Status epilepticus (to prevent cerebral oedema and anoxia)
Diazapam 10 mg intravenously every 15 minutes up to a level of 60 mg, i.e., 0.25–0.75 mg per kg bodyweight, until control of convulsion is achieved. It has a rapid sedative effect
Combined intramuscular injections of sodium phenytoin and phenobarbitone
Slow intravenous infusion of thiopentone (Pentothal) providing anaesthetic equipment and resuscitation techniques are available
Paraldehyde 2% solution by intravenous injection which is rapidly disseminated via the pulmonary circulation and maintains a continuous sedative effect

the epilepsy is first diagnosed. In the case of children there will be a natural concern for the educational development of the child and the main difficulty may centre on the bias and prejudice, if it exists, in the local school authority. There is no evidence to suggest that an epileptic child cannot benefit from a normal education, provided that the seizures are well controlled.

The parents, however, should be advised that the drug regimen may affect the child's natural abilities in swimming, cycling and climbing until the physician is satisfied that the drugs have achieved complete control of the tendency to convulsions. If there are behavioural problems, then a deeper consultation is usually required to establish if in fact there is a brain lesion, as opposed to the drugs or epilepsy causing the problems.

In young adults, some attention should be given to their understanding that prolonged physical endurance or emotional turmoil, which causes exhaustion, may precipitate a convulsion even if they are controlled by drugs, the exhaustion utilising the existing blood levels of the drug. The patient's preferred activities, especially those relating to contact sports, should be re-assessed in the light of the diagnosis. Alcohol excess can also precipitate a convulsion and is best avoided until such times as the medication is discontinued. The patient should be given a medicare card and a bracelet, which he or she should carry at all times in case of an accident. If possible the current medication should be identified on the card. The British Epilepsy Association may have a local branch in the vicinity and the patient should be given the telephone number to make personal contact from which they may obtain a counselling service and a friendship group which they can join.

Surveys in both the United Kingdom and America show that epileptics continue to experience problems in several areas. For instance, obtaining employment in a suitable job is a major difficulty. A guiding rule is that the patient must not be a risk to his or herself or to others if he or she were to suffer a convulsion while at work. This of itself precludes many jobs such as heavy industry, climbing, electrical work and driving. This limitation of itself puts many employers in a dilemma, creating a reluctance to employ someone at risk. The current legislation states that for an epileptic to be able to drive he or she must be able to produce a medical certificate showing that there have been no convulsions in the previous 3 years or show that he or she has not had a convulsion in the previous 12 months without any medication, and this is to be proved by a doctor.

A great deal of the social stigma associated with epilepsy may be the cause of the personality difficulties the patient experiences, as he or she cannot freely discuss personal feeling and attitudes to the handicap. It is a frequent observation that many epileptics tend to have an introverted personality, prefer social isolation, have intellectual limitations, are egotistical and are garrulous when held in conversation. This should not however be paralleled with mental illness.

Chapter 79 Common Motor Dysfunction

MULTIPLE SCLEROSIS (DISSEMINATED SCLEROSIS)

Multiple sclerosis is the principal disease from a group of chronic disorders known as the demyelinative diseases. It is of very obscure aetiology and results in the patchy loss of some of the myelin sheath encasing the nerve fibres in the white matter of the brain and spinal cord. Current research is exploring several suggested causes, these proving that there are some 50 000 sufferers in the United Kingdom and the ratio is 3 women to every 2 males. One third of those affected are grouped as the young chronic sick who require fuli-time nursing care in residential disabled units.

Causes

Causes which are being investigated include:

1. Deficiency of linoleic acid (i.e., a fatty acid) which is an essential component of the myelin sheath and is regarded as being protective in function. The main dietary source is from sunflower seeds, but an increased intake does not in fact resolve the symptoms of a sufferer.
2. Slow but progressive viral infection of the myelin sheath which continues long after a contact with a common childhood infection, such as measles.
3. Auto-immune response related to repeated exposure to an allergen to which the patient is hypersensitive and which is specific to the myelin sheath.

Signs and Symptoms

Common to many patients is that immediately preceding a first attack they have endured a minor trauma, or have been subjected to some psychological stress. The patchy loss of myelin from the nerve sheath interrupts the conduction of both motor and sensory impulses in a single or multiple nerve pathway. It is usual for the nerve sheath to heal, providing that the cell and its axon are intact. However with repeated attacks the myelin sheath becomes fibrosed and scarred and is ultimately unable to convey nerve impulses. The patient therefore has a disease which will usually remit (heal) and some time later will suffer a relapse. This remitting and relapsing nature of the disease occurs over a period of 20 or 30 years. In its severity it is extremely variable, affecting perhaps only one pathway with a mild but residual handicap, or alternatively it may be widely disseminated throughout the brain and spinal cord and is inexorably progressive leading to spastic paralysis and incontinence.

From the patient's point of view the symptoms are bewildering, are without a rational explanation and most frightening. Early explanations are usually made by trying to explain 'neuritis', but the physical changes hardly match the meaning of the word. In the first few attacks only a few doctors would feel justified in giving a detailed explanation, as the disease is so unpredictable, but a nurse should of course convey some optimism and be positive when giving physical care. The earliest classical symptoms are:

1. Visual disturbance.
2. Paraesthesia of limbs.
3. Sensory symptoms.
4. Brain stem involvement.
5. Altered emotional response.

Visual Disturbance

Odd and peculiar visual changes are experienced. These range from blurring, dimming and double vision, being due to retrobulbar neuritis which causes atrophy of the optic disc. These first symptoms are transient in nature, lasting from a few hours to several days, and then completely remitting. With each attack, however, the visual acuity is reduced and therefore, in the later stages of the disease, the nursing plan of care has to take into account the needs of a partially-sighted or blind patient.

Paraesthesia of Limbs

Weakness of the muscles of one or all the limbs is a distinct discomfort, leaving the patient exhausted after the most minimal physical effort. An upper limb weakness (monoparesis) will leave the hand with little or no power of grip, the patient constantly dropping even the most lightweight articles and feeling clumsy.

Lower limb weakness (hemiparesis) means that posture and walking are very uncoordinated, i.e., ataxia. The patient tends to trip easily and to fall with the effort of walking.

Physical examination may reveal brisk reflexes and a positive Babinski sign. In this case it means that the pyramidal tracts within the spinal cord are partially demyelinated. These symptoms may also remit after a short time, only to occur at a later date. After several such attacks the incidence of paralysis increases.

Sensory Symptoms

Tingling and numbness of the affected muscles are a constant distraction and lead to the classical picture of someone with the 'useless hand' syndrome. The appreciation of touch perception with a loss of position and joint sense on the same side as the body supplied by sensory nerves entering the spinal cord, i.e., Brown-Séquard syndrome, is sometimes noted on physical examination. Although this particular symptom may remit within weeks or months, further relapses will exaggerate the loss of sensory appreciation. Pain can be felt in the later stages of the disease if there is spinal compression of a sensory tract, nerve or root. All the muscles supplied by the affected pathway are tender to touch when handled.

Reflex emptying of the bladder replaces

previous control over the need to void urine, and is replaced by urgency and frequency to micturate, which implies that unless regular toileting is offered to the patient they will be incontinent.

Brain Stem Involvement

Demyelination of the nerve tracts in the white matter of the brain stem leads to quite severe symptoms of headaches, vertigo, vomiting, facial anaesthesia and ataxic nystagmus. The remitting and relapsing nature of these symptoms often frighten and bewilder the patient, often presenting features of confused behaviour.

Altered Emotional Responses

In the early phases of the disease it is quite common for the patient to exhibit hysterical behaviour, which may in fact mask the true symptoms of multiple sclerosis. Alternatively the patient may be quite euphoric and happy, despite the seriousness of his or her handicap. Either emotional response defies explanation. Later a marked depression sets in as a reaction to his or her symptoms. This may last for a long period and can only be overcome with the use of antidepressant drugs which may also help the patient make the psychological adjustment to his or her altered body image. A small number of this group of patients suffer from a progressive dementia which will require institutional care.

Diagnosis

The diagnosis of the disease is based upon the clinical signs and symptoms. If a lumbar puncture is done it is usually to exclude other causes of demyelinative diseases, e.g., encephalitis. An extensive neurological examination will identify the nerve pathways affected and may help the nurse to identify the exact problems the patient will have, and establish the aims and priorities of care in the nursing plan.

Medical treatment is somewhat limited. During a relapse one of the steroid drugs, e.g., adrenocorticotrophic hormone (ACTH) is given by injection. Being mainly an anti-inflammatory drug, it reduces the severity of the symptoms. Physiotherapy techniques are of positive benefit during a remission, helping to tone up muscles affected by transient paresis. During a relapse the joints should be put through a range of movements at frequent intervals and these passive movements should be quite vigorous.

Diazapam if prescribed will help to reduce any joint spasticity, thus enabling physiotherapy techniques to be of more value. To reduce urinary frequency and painful bladder spasm, propantheline (an anticholinergic drug) may prove useful.

If the muscular spasm and spasticity is painful, the physician may elect to administer intrathecal injections of phenol in glycerine to dull the pain fibres. In the very long term some of these patients will eventually become bedfast because of widespread paralysis and incontinence. When ultimately the patient is bedfast, the complications of bedrest pose the major problem. To some extent they are overcome by prophylactic antibiotic therapy, but are mainly contained by vigilant nursing care to prevent urinary tract and respiratory infections and pressure sores.

Nursing Plan of Care

The nursing plan of care is highly individualistic, being centred on meeting the specific problems analysed at each nursing assessment. The physical needs are usually quickly established and in the early stages it is more positive to assess the social factors around the patient so that the future prognosis can be met. The majority of patients are young females who have a crucial position in the family unit, being a mother, housewife and possibly contributing to the family income with her own job. The anxiety therefore of the husband and children, as well as the patient, is often centred dramatically around altered family roles. This reorientation of a whole family illustrates the need for nurses to involve the immediate family in the care plan. Requesting a home assessment will be an essential feature of future care. The patient will need a telephone. Aids such as a wheelchair for mobility during periods of relapse may require some adaptation of the home. If the patient has dependant children, the usual means of taking them to school, for outings and normal care will have to be assessed and perhaps some help sought from the local authority to help the handicapped mother to cope with these everyday activities. Normal activities such as cooking, shopping and cleaning become major problems which also require such help as can be offered from the local authority social welfare department, e.g., a home help for several hours a week. The marriage partner will need to be counselled from the very outset and, if possible, persuaded to assist in the nursing skills required to care for the patient when he or she is at home. What seems a simple task such as lifting or feeding someone can be a major difficulty for the novice, until they learn how to do it correctly. Some marriage partners will ask for either genetic or sexual counselling, and this is best undertaken by the physician in charge of the patient.

In assessing the physical problems the nurse should be systematic, dealing with each body system in turn and then placing a priority on the patient's actual needs:

1. Nutritional needs are calculated firstly by assessing the patient's calorie requirement per day and then by ensuring that he or she does not need help with feeding, and is proficient in the handling of crockery and cutlery. If necessary the patient is fed. If obesity is a problem, then a long-term reducing diet is planned. Obesity will increase the problems of prolonged bedrest. Equally malnutrition must be avoided for the same reasons.

2. Locomotor function during a remission is best enhanced by regular attendance at the physiotherapy department, and also by walking without causing undue exhaustion. Indeed long slow walks should be a daily feature of the care plan. If suffering paresis the patient may benefit from correctly fitting shoes with a low heel, and wearing warm clothing. Simple splint devices may create feelings of confidence in the ability to grip, and to put the whole affected limb through a series of passive or active movements. The paralysed patient will need regular and exacting care to prevent pressure sores from developing, i.e., either 2-hourly turning or using devices to ensure adequate capillary circulation through the skin, e.g. ripple beds, air mattress, water bed, pillow support and sheepskins. The limbs should be so placed that their alignment follows their natural anatomical position.

3. Excretory function, especially if he or she has urinary tract frequency and urgency, will require detailed assessment. In the early stages regular toileting, perhaps as often as 2-hourly, may be of benefit to avoid incontinence. Often the patient will reduce his or her fluid intake in a deliberate effort to control micturition, but this will risk dehydration and the nurse should ensure that the patient drinks at least 2 litres of fluid per day. A high fibre diet, fruits and roughage will do a great deal to prevent constipation, but in the later stages of the illness it may be necessary to rely on either oral aperients or suppositories. As a last resort, evacuation of the lower colon by simple enemas may be required. If the patient has a tendency to retain urine, and this is a possible side effect of anticholinergic drugs, then bladder training may prove to be the best answer. Catheterisation is the last resort and should be reserved for when the patient is actually bedfast with paralysis. It will then help to reduce the risk of pressure sores.

4. Integumentary risks are mainly that of pressure sores over the dependant areas of the body and the risk is reduced if the nurse follows the principles outlined in dealing with locomotor function.

5. Sensory handicaps of visual loss, sensory depreciation of touch and joint sense implies that the nurse should assess the patient's environment for any hazards. Any aids used in giving care should be tested and assessed for their safety. Wheelchairs or armchairs should also be viewed

with some concern; not only will the patient be at risk from falling forward from the seat but if there is not a brake system and a safety bar the patient may well sustain injury without realising the actual danger. Such an assessment of environment and potential hazards would also have to be made in the home. The occupational therapist may have some useful tips to aid the patient, and advice should be sought. Speech therapy is a positive benefit if it can be arranged. Dysphasia, aphasia, dyslexia and agraphia are some of the difficulties the patient may have, and regular sessions with a speech therapist will help the patient to improve his or her communication skills.

During periods of remission the patient should be encouraged to become an active member of the Multiple Sclerosis Society. This organisation has over 300 branches in the United Kingdom and like other specialist groups is keen to develop research into multiple sclerosis, methods of care, be supportive to other sufferers, and provide a counselling service to both patients and their relatives. The society gives many useful tips on such matters as holidays, organising journeys and trips to places of interest, aids from local authorities, social benefit entitlement for the chronic sick, the legal aspects of car driving, and dietary information.

PARKINSON'S DISEASE (PARALYSIS AGITANS) (SHAKING PALSY)

Parkinson's disease is caused by a decreased secretion of the transmitter substance, an amino acid called dopamine, from the nerve cells of the basal ganglia. These specialised groups of cells are located in the midbrain and include the substantia nigra and caudate nucleus in which 80% of the dopamine is concentrated. Dopamine, when secreted, inhibits the nerve impulses travelling through the corpus striatum and works in harmony with the excitatory transmitter substance, acetylcholine. The total effect of these transmitter substances is to achieve a smooth coordinated muscular response to a sensory stimuli. The decreased secretion of dopamine causes the acetylcholine to become dominant and thus increases the activity of the corpus striatum leading to the cardinal symptoms of tremor, rigidity and facial immobility.

Possible Causes

The cause of Parkinson's disease is unknown, but several factors have been exhaustively researched and are common to the majority of sufferers:

1. The highest frequency of Parkinsonism occurs in the elderly between the ages of 64 and 74 years. It affects both sexes equally and the degeneration of the nerve cells, especially of the substratia nigra, seems to be initially triggered off by extreme fatigue, emotional stress, or severe cold. The incidence of Parkinsonism is expected to rise above the present figure of 60000 sufferers as longevity becomes a social norm.
2. Cerebral arteriosclerosis associated with hypertension in the elderly may initiate this chronic disease.
3. It can be induced by carbon monoxide poisoning, head injury and the drugs, reserpine, chlorpromazine (Largactil) and haloperidol.
4. Very rarely, if ever, will a patient develop Parkinsonism as the result of encephalitis lethargica, which has almost vanished as a disease entity. This would also apply to neurosyphillis, which has almost been eradicated by natural deaths or by medical progress.

Signs and Symptoms

The signs and symptoms can vary in their severity and are quite different in their complexity in each individual sufferer. No two patients are ever the same, and this is important in planning their nursing care. If untreated the symptoms do become progressive and lead to the following:

1. Mask-like facial expression. The facial muscles remain immobile and the eyelids unblinking. In the later stages, involuntary

excess salivation may occur with constant dribbling from the mouth.

2. Speech is very slow, quiet in tone and monotonous in quality.

3. Body movement is increasingly difficult to initiate, i.e., akinesia, and could be described as being 'frozen' when the patient is observed trying to start a movement from a seated to a standing posture. Each movement is slow, deliberate and performed only with the greatest difficulty. There is rigidity in the flexor and extensor muscles of the joints, but this should not be equated with spasticity.

4. The shoulder girdle is tilted forwards, causing a stooped appearance, and the walking gait is composed of short shuffling steps in an effort to overcome the feeling and sensation of falling.

5. The handwriting becomes very small and increasingly so when contrasted with earlier ability.

6. There is a coarse tremor, especially noted of the hands and feet and the head. Often the pin rolling movement between thumb and first finger is quite pronounced.

7. Disturbance of the autonomic nervous system causes increased salivation, perspiration and retention of urine.

8. It is important to appreciate that although the physical appearance of the patient is distressing, the intellect is not impaired and is one contributory factor to the psychological changes noted since the patient cannot convey or truly express his or her feelings.

Diagnosis and Treatment

The majority of patients are diagnosed on the presenting of clinical signs of tremor, rigidity and facial immobility. More than 90% of those affected are cared for at home. Hospitalisation is mainly reserved for medical assessment, review of treatment and, if necessary, to give exhausted relatives a break and to take a holiday.

The aim of treatment is to replace the depleted stores of dopamine in the basal ganglia and this is achieved by the dopamine group of drugs. Secondly, the aim is to eliminate the cardinal symptoms with the use of anticholinergic agents. Levodopa (L Dopa) has revolutionised the outlook and treatment of Parkinson's disease, but when given at high doses it produces untoward side effects of which the nurse should be aware and be able to assess and report to medical colleagues.

To exclude the risk of postural hypotension the physician will usually request blood pressure readings, an electrocardiograph and make a detailed examination of the cardiovascular system to ensure the patient will be able to tolerate the therapy.

When commenced, the drug dosage is minimal and gradually built up, e.g., 250–500 mg daily up to 2–8 g daily, until the clinical signs are completely controlled. In evaluating the effect of levodopa, the nurse apart from noting the expected benefits should be able to report on the following:

1. Gastrointestinal. Early reactions include nausea, vomiting, loss of weight and constipation. These effects can be minimised by giving the drug immediately after meals and ensuring the patient has at least 2 litres of clear fluids to drink during the day. Vitamin B6 (pyridoxine hydrochloride) reverses the effect of levodopa and therefore foods which yield a high amount of this vitamin should be excluded from the diet.

2. Cardiovascular. The blood pressure and pulse should be recorded 4-hourly for several days, when the drug is increased to note for postural hypotension, tachycardia and palpitations. The patient should be kept under visual observation in case of fainting attacks.

3. Neurological. If the drug dose is increased in those patients with an existing organic brain disease, then they may become confused, disorientated and suffer from insomnia. Eliminating the evening drug dose may prove effective in reducing these untoward effects. Involuntary movements may become exaggerated, especially those of the head, lips and tongue. Swinging of the arms, if exaggerated, is a strong indication that the dose of the drug needs to be reduced.

4. Psychological. Changes of mood, coloured by increased agitation, aggression, depression and nightmares can be expected with ever increasing doses of the drug and implies that the nurse needs to increase the supervision of the patient.

It is usual to combine levodopa with an anticholinergic agent. The latter drugs will improve the tremor, rigidity and facial immobility as well as the autonomic disturbances. The following anticholinergic drugs are in common use:

Amantidine hydrochloride (Symmetral) 100–300 mg daily

Beperiden (Akineton) 3–6 mg daily

Benzhexol hydrochloride (Artane) 2–20 mg 3 times a day

Benztropine methanesulphone (Cogetin) 2 mg twice daily and at night

Ethopropazine (Lysivane) 200–500 mg daily

Phenglutarimide (Atarbane) 20–50 mg daily

Prozilidine hydrochloride (Kemadrin) 5–20 mg 3 times daily

Bromocriptine (Parlodel) and levodopa is a relatively side effect free compound which enhances the effect of dopamine and its usual dosage is between 40–100 mg daily

This combination therapy is prescribed at ever increasing doses until control is achieved over tremor, rigidity and akinesia. As with levodopa, the nurse should regularly evaluate the effect of the anticholinergic agents to detect if they are causing blurred vision, dryness of the mouth, nausea, vertigo and urinary retention. Until a satisfactory balance has been achieved, this is usually determined by blood levels and neurological examination.

Nursing Plan of Care

The nursing plan of care for those admitted to hospital should evolve from a detailed assessment of the typical common problems of:

1. Degree of immobility.
2. Nutritional needs.
3. Psychological changes.
4. Urinary retention.

Degree of Immobility

Assessment should be made regarding the degree of immobility due to the tremor, rigidity and akinesia which give rise to the difficulties in dressing, handling cutlery, poor posture and incorrect gait, impoverished handwriting, and toileting. However, the drug regimen, coupled with intensive physiotherapy over a period of weeks, should resolve many of these problems.

The aim of physiotherapy is to encourage the patient in performing stretch exercises of all the joints at least 20 times per day. These should improve if not also prevent postural defects, joint contractures and deformities. The shoulder girdle should also become less stooped. Occupational therapy would correctly assess the coping skills with dressing and self-feeding skills, and implement exercises to be performed each day to improve on the existing ability. Since there is a tendency for hand tremor, large handled cutlery and deep centred plates can be used at mealtimes. For drinking fluids, a straw is more useful than struggling with a cup or beaker. It may prove necessary to complete a home assessment to ensure that the safety features of the home are examined in some detail. The fear of falling and the typical shuffling gait increase the likelihood of tripping over loose floor-rugs, door-steps and steep staircases. Unguarded fires and gas or electric ovens may require to be fitted with safety guards. Akinesia may make the patient prone to hypothermia, if the home is inadequately heated. There is no obvious need for bedrest and the programme of care should highlight specific periods of the day devoted to walking exercises. If very immobile the nursing plan would have to counter the risk of pressure sores by insisting on movement every 2 hours and utilising those aids which would relieve pressure on body areas subject to constant pressure.

Nutritional Needs

Nutritional needs are often a problem if the patient abandons any attempt to feed him or herself because of the frustration of their tremor. This is coupled with the need for the nurse to exclude from the patient's diet those foods which are rich in vitamin B6. In the early stages of care the patient may need to be fed to ensure both an adequate intake of calories and fluids. Relatives should also be involved in discussions with the dietician regarding the patient's future diet once their drug regimen is established, and they should be given a list of those foods to avoid which are rich in vitamin B6. Adequate roughage in the form of fruit, vegetables and fibre foods is essential if the tendency to constipation is to be corrected. It may be necessary to use a simple aperient to aid the patient with bowel evacuation in the first instance. Obesity must be overcome by dietary control. If this is not corrected it will exaggerate the clinical symptoms of rigidity and possibly increase the patient's depression.

Psychological Changes

Parkinsonism sufferers are prone to severe psychological changes, often becoming over-demanding and obstreperous, making their relatives increasingly intolerant towards them. Relationships therefore are prone to stress, anger and disruption. This can be partially overcome by offering several teach-in sessions to enable the relatives to express their frustrations with attempting to cope. If explained, an understanding of the disease process and the intention of therapy may increase their tolerance until the drugs have a chance of controlling the worst of the symptoms.

The patient's intellect is not impaired, and exclusion of the patient from general conversation and not encouraging them to be generally interested in everyday matters is in fact inviting the patient to express anger in response to being rejected.

Urinary Retention

Urinary retention is a problem both of Parkinson's disease and a side effect of the anticholinergic drugs. It can be prevented by regular toileting and by ensuring the patient has at least 2 litres of fluid each day. To help in monitoring the effectiveness of this suggestion, an incontinence bladder training chart and a fluid balance chart should be maintained for several days or at least until the drug regimen is finally established when the urinary retention problem should be resolved. The drugs do tend to alter the patient's skin pigmentation and the colour of the urine, and they should be warned that this is an expected effect and is not a sign that the disease is becoming worse. With good nursing care there is rarely, if ever, a need to resort to catheterisation.

Both the patient and family will find support, advice and encouragement if they are put into contact with a local branch of the Parkinson's Disease Society. The principal aims of the society are to educate, offer welfare to those in desperate need, fund raising for research, offer social activities and a platform for discussion on topics relevant to Parkinson Disease sufferers. Typical of some of the problems facing the patient at home is the type of bed best suited to someone who has great difficulty in turning or sitting upright, adapting to work conditions with a chronic disease, the most advantageous home adaptations, and whether or not they are allowed to drive a car.

MYASTHENIA GRAVIS (MOTOR END PLATE DYSFUNCTION)

Myasthenia gravis is a chronic progressive muscular weakness with excessive fatigue of the skeletal muscle fibres which may be either mild, moderate or severe.

Causes

Its true cause is unclear, but it is thought to be due to:

1. Deficiency of the chemical neurotransmitter, acetylcholine, at the neuromuscular junction, i.e., at the motor end plate where the nerve innervates the skeletal muscle. Why the acetylcholine is deficient is uncertain. It may be due to a deficiency of a precursor metabolite, or excessive and rapid

destruction by the enzyme cholinesterase. In the event, without the appropriate innervation, the muscle fibres are unable to contract at their normal strength and tone, leading to both muscle fatigue and to wasting from a lack of use.

2. There is the suggestion that the fault may lie within the muscle fibres themselves or possibly in the post-synaptic junction.

3. There is a strong relationship between myasthenia gravis and enlargement of the thymus gland. The thymus gland is related to immunity development in the early years of life and should naturally recede in adulthood once the body has developed its immunity. However it tends to remain enlarged, giving rise to the assumption that it may be the cause of autoimmune disease which is destroying the receptor neurones in the muscle fibres. In those instances where thymectomy has been done, there is a 70% chance that the myasthenia gravis will remit within several months or in 2 years.

4. There is evidence to show a relationship between cancer of the bronchus and thyrotoxicosis, both of which may precede myasthenia gravis.

The disease is not inherited, it tends to occur more in women than in men and can occur at any age, the larger number of known cases however reveal that it tends to occur more frequently in women under 50 years of age. The disease does not spontaneously remit, but may either remain of a mild nature affecting only one group of muscles or become increasingly progressive to involve many groups of muscles.

Signs and Symptoms

The principal muscles affected are the occulomotor muscles of the eye, which leads to a ptosis or dropping of the eyelid. Other muscle groups, which become weak and can lead to serious problems with everyday activities, are the muscles of speech (glossopharyngeal) and swallowing. Later the muscles or respiration become weak, affecting the ability to breathe deeply and also making the patient more than usually prone to chest infection.

If the neck muscles are affected, the patient tends to be unable to hold the head still and to tilt the head backwards so they can actually see what is going on around them. The generalised fatigue worsens as the day progresses, and in a severe case the nurse would observe a patient with facial immobility who has ptosis, resting with the head tilted backwards, unable to chew or swallow. When speaking, he or she will be barely audible with the respiratory effort which speech requires. If there is any emotional stress, beyond that normally experienced, the symptoms are quickly exaggerated and the patient becomes even more prone to infection.

Diagnosis

Diagnosis of the disease is by stimulating the ulnar nerve with high amplitude electrical shocks, and observing the muscles at the hypothenar eminence. These would record little if any activity of muscle contraction. A test dose of an anticholinesterase drug such as neostigmine 1.5–2 mg is given intravenously and the electromyograph repeated. The second test should show a dramatic improvement within 30 minutes of the drug being given.

A second drug, edrophonium 2 mg given intravenously, will produce a dramatic change in muscle strength and tone within 30 seconds.

However, because myasthenia gravis is associated with the thymus gland, cancer of the bronchus and thryotoxicosis, these diseases would also be investigated to confirm or exclude their existence. Although the disease is not inherited, the newborn child of a myasthenic mother would have some of the symptoms for several days, implying that the placental barrier can be crossed by whatever is causing the disease in the mother.

Treatment

The treatment is mainly by the prescription of anticholinesterase drugs. These are mainly palliative and are required continuously, i.e., for life. An anticholinesterase drug would reduce the effect of the enzyme cholinesterase, which is normally secreted at the neuromuscular junction. In reducing its effect, it gives the acetylcholine a chance to bridge the synaptic gap and the innervation of the muscle to be complete, allowing contraction.

1. Neostigmine (Prostigmin) is generally accepted as the most effective cholinesterase inhibitor.
2. Pyridostigmine (Mestinon) while having the same effect as neostigmine produces less serious side effects, particularly diarrhoea and abdominal pain, and is preferred by many patients. It is supplied in slow release tablets and less frequent prescriptions are therefore needed.
3. Ambenonium (Mytelase) is similar in effect to pyridostigmine.

With either drug, the nurse should observe and report on not only its therapeutic effects, but what can be the serious side effects of increased peristalsis causing abdominal pain and diarrhoea, perspiration, nausea, vomiting and twitching of the skeletal muscles. These observed effects imply the drug requires to be adjusted in a dose. These drugs may also cause a hypokalaemia (low potassium level) and supplements may be required if the level of potassium is outside the normal range of 3.6–5.0 mmol/litre.

Nursing Care Plan

The nursing care plan must take into account the severity of each possible group of muscles which can be affected. If there is ptosis, it is useful to either fit the patient with an eye patch or have the glass lens of the affected eye fitted with a frosted lens. This will help with the diplopia suffered as a consequence of the ptosis. Habits such as smoking or taking alcohol exacerbate the symptoms and should be reduced if not stopped altogether until the symptoms are under control. Prolonged heat or extreme cold also worsen the symptoms and therefore the ward and nursing environment needs to be monitored especially at night time. The wasting of muscles would have to be assessed and a programme returning the patient to full mobility and coping with every day simple tasks of dressing, eating, toileting and correct posture is welcomed by the patient. However, too much enthusiasm must be contained to avoid further stress from failing to meet goals which are not set at an achievable level. This is most important if the patient has endured a prolonged period of bedrest. Dysphagia can be a problem for some time, until the drug regimen is established. This may require the nurse to adapt the diet as the patient improves. In the severe case, nasogastric feeding may be necessary and all medication given in a syrup base. The metabolic requirements of the patient have to be graduated in calories and substance as improvement is achieved.

Since many of these patients are nursed at home from the outset the family should be involved in the care plan so that they can share in the gradual improvement, having perhaps been coping with the patient over many months if not years of the patient's dependance. A young patient would perhaps require advice about pregnancy, and the future prognosis of the disease with his or her marriage partner.

In general, the prognosis of the disease is very good provided that the prescribed medication is taken without fail and that the patient reports regularly for medical checkups. The drugs, it should be pointed out, are palliative and not curative. Therefore they are required for life. In recent years, trials with cortisone drugs are holding out the promise of cure. Prednisone, given on alternate days, in a high single dose prescription is currently being tried in the United States.

The patient should be put into contact with a branch of one of the Muscular Dystrophy groups who are only too ready to offer help on very basic issues and to keep the patient up-to-date on current research.

Chapter 80
Care of the Unconscious Patient

Unconsciousness is a temporary or prolonged loss of arousal and protective reflexes due to damage of or pressure upon the reticular activating and hypothalamic system. This group of nerve cells extends from the base of the medulla up towards the third ventricle of the brain. It is chiefly concerned with the level of arousal during and after a period of sleep. During natural sleep the reticular activating system is sensitive to those reflexes that will readily arouse the individual from sleep, if life or survival is threatened. For example, the system is susceptible to nerve connections related to pain reflex, sound, smell and temperature. It is also responsive to all the specialised nerve cells that go towards protecting the individual, i.e., the vital centres in the medulla oblongata. In unconsciousness, or coma, it is impossible to innervate these reflexes by the most dominant of all reflexes, the pain reflex.

CAUSES

The causes of unconsciousness are legion, a few of the more common examples being:

Injury to the brain, especially from impact fractures of the skull

Infection of the meninges or brain substance, e.g., meningitis, encephalitis and brain abscess

Malignant or benign tumours with or without cerebral oedema

Toxicity from drug overdose, alcohol intoxication, carbon monoxide poisoning, anaesthetic accident and hypothermia

Metabolic disorders such as diabetic

coma, Addisonian coma, chronic renal failure, severe electrolyte disturbance such as sodium depletion, water intoxication, hypokalaemia and hyperkalaemia, and cirrhosis of the liver

Cerebrovascular haemorrhage, embolism and thrombosis, especially if associated with systemic and cerebral hypertension

NURSING CARE PLAN

Regardless of the cause of unconsciousness, the nurse on being notified of an admission would need to prepare a bed which is positioned in a quiet area of the ward and permits constant observation both during the day and at night. Oxygen and suction equipment must be available at the bedside, but all other items of furniture which would impede access to the patient should be removed. Articles and equipment necessary for nursing procedures should be arranged on a portable trolley which can be removed at a moment's notice. The environmental temperature should not be below 28° C (75° F), especially if the patient is elderly. The majority of those patients who are admitted into hospital unconscious are from the elderly population, and are prone to hypothermia. Therefore the environmental temperature is an aspect of care which should not be overlooked.

The bed should be equipped with safety rails and the linen covering the mattress be protected by a drawsheet. No pillows should be used for a deeply unconscious patient. Once admitted, undressed and placed in a lateral position, the first priority of care is to ensure that the patient's airway is patent. Dentures should be removed, the oral cavity inspected for any debris which may impede respiration and suction applied to remove any viscous sputum or vomitus. The head should be flexed forward to enable the tongue to fall forward so that it is not occluding the pharynx. Deeply unconscious patients may require to have either a Guedal airway placed in position, or an endotracheal tube if there is severe damage to the respiratory centre.

Once the patency of the airway is guaranteed the nurse may then consider the nursing care plan which would best meet the contingencies of prescribed therapy. However a general plan of care should already be formulated in the mind of a senior learner, and one which meets all exigencies to reduce nursing care by crisis. To this end the nurse should know which observations are relevant, why they are being done, and be able to assess the priorities of physical care an unconscious patient would need. Finally, a working background knowledge of the patient's social and family history should be known.

Essential Observations

It is a wise precaution if the same nurse over a span of duty accepts the responsibility of recording and reporting on the observations made. It should be borne in mind that changes may be either quite dramatic, or slow and insidious; either way it requires constant vigilance. The essential observations during the first 24–48 hours are best done every 15 or 30 minutes, and reviewed by medical staff at least once every 12 hours if not asked to do so more frequently by the nurse. Observations should be noted on a single chart, preferably a neurological chart, and so recorded that any changes can be seen at a glance. Each chart should cover a period of 24 hours and medical advice should be sought if 2 consecutive readings are at a marked variance, e.g., if the pulse and blood pressure show radical change.

Levels of Consciousness

Levels of consciousness are graded as being:

1. Comatose with absolutely no response to painful stimuli, i.e., rubbing the sternum with a clenched fist in vertical strokes.
2. Stuporose, responding only to vigorous painful stimuli, i.e., the sternal rub.
3. Drowsy, but responding to mild painful stimuli.
4. Confused, disorientated to time, place and event on simple questioning, and remains sleepy for long periods.
5. Orientated to circumstances and easily aroused from a light drowsy state.

Pupillary Reflexes

The following abnormalities should have been ruled out by the physician: trauma to the eye, previous eye disease, damage to the ciliary muscle, and injury to the third cranial nerve. Once these have been excluded, any other eye changes are a useful diagnostic aid to the condition within the brain, especially any indication of increased intracranial pressure or brain death.

Pupil size, on average, measures between 4 and 8 mm in diameter. If, however, the eye is dilated, pinpointed or of an irregular shape, it would immediately suggest altered intracranial pressure. If both pupils are unequal, or if very dilated, it may be suggestive of extradural haemorrhage.

The reaction to a beam of light from a pencil torch should indicate to the nurse if the reflex is brisk, sluggish, or absent. Both eyes are tested, as one may be normal when contrasted with the other. Light shone into the eye should cause the pupil to become smaller, then reflexly return to normal size once it has adjusted to the light source.

Ocular movements can be tested to measure for nystagmus, but this is done by the physician and is one of the tests which, if negative, may prove that brain death has occurred.

Respiration

Respiration should be counted and assessed before taking the pulse or blood pressure as these latter activities even on the unconscious patient influence the outcome of the respiration. Movement of the rib cage and diaphragm should indicate the depth of respiration. Evidence of apnoea, alternating with sighing respiration (Cheyne Stokes breathing) should be reported immediately as it indicates increased pressure on the medula oblongata with a risk of respiratory arrest. Breath odour should be noted, as it has particular characteristics in alcohol intoxication, diabetic coma and uraemia. Odd respiratory sounds should also be reported, as these may indicate the imminence of a chest infection. Blood gas levels to determine Po_2 and PCo_2 levels are estimated in all undiagnosed cases of unconsciousness.

Pulse and Blood Pressure Readings

Pulse and blood pressure readings will reflect whether the heart and cardiovascular system are involved, and any changes are usually related to altering intracranial pressure. A tachycardia with a low blood pressure would always suggest shock, while a bradycardia and a rising blood pressure is almost diagnostic of increased intracranial pressure and should be reported to senior staff at once, when it can be checked and treatment commenced to relieve such pressure. Fluctuations in the pulse count, coupled with increasing restlessness, may suggest either improving arousal or a deterioration and need to be assessed along with other observations.

Temperature Recordings

Temperature recordings are taken either from the axilla or the rectum, never from the mouth of an unconscious patient. For those patients requiring intensive care the core temperature may be monitored constantly by an electronic disc placed in the rectum or attached to the skin. Unconscious patients are prone to the extremes of temperature. If there is increased intracranial pressure, the temperature regulating centre in the hypothalamus will be severely disturbed. If there is an underlying infection, then pyrexia may be symptomatic. Alternatively, if the metabolic activity is very low then the patient is prone to hypothermia. In each case the nurse requires to be flexible to meet the requirements of the patient on a day-to-day basis.

Abnormal movements

In the unconscious patient, abnormal movements are of extreme importance as they may help to localise the area of cerebral irritation and are also diagnostic:

1. *Opisthotonos*, or acute arching of the spine with the body resting on the heels and

occiput is sometimes seen in tetany, meningeal irritation and subarachnoid haemorrhage.

2. *Neck stiffness and rigidity* noted by resistance when rotating the skull is a typical finding in meningitis and encephalitis.

3. *Tetanic hand*, or spasm of the wrist, fingers and toes sometimes preceded by repeated clutching and release of the bedclothes is a sign of tetany.

4. *Paralysis* is accompanied by an obvious loss of muscle tone and girth. The flaccidity of an affected limb or its spasticity should be assessed by attempting to put the limb and its joints through their normal range of movement. This assessment may determine specific needs of the patient for correct positioning of the body.

5. *Convulsions* are typical of epilepsy, but may result from cerebral tumours or from hyperpyrexia. They should be assessed as for any type of epileptiform seizure, bearing in mind that the cause is not necessarily epilepsy.

The majority of these observations are to indicate to the physician if the intracranial pressure is increasing. The conservative medical treatment of cerebral oedema is based on the principle that water and oxygen cross from the cerebral capillaries into the brain cells with great ease, but the electrolytes sodium and chloride move very slowly. This is referred to as the barrier effect, or blood brain barrier. The barrier is thought to be the glial cells or the supportive connective tissue of the brain cells. If injury destroys or disturbs the glial cells, electrolytes can now pass freely through the barrier increasing the pressure within the brain, as sodium in particular will hold onto water. The bones of the skull limit the potential of the brain to expand, so the pressure is reversed into the brain itself, the actual pressure being caused by excess water. This increase in pressure will limit cerebrospinal fluid circulation and increase the pressure on the reticulating activating system, causing a deeper level of unconsciousness and eventually press upon the vital centres of the medulla oblongata. Any destruction of cells at this level may lead to an irreversible coma and cerebral death. The aim of treatment therefore is to reverse the water content of the brain, and this may be achieved by either:

1. Administration of intravenous hypertonic solutions of normal saline 25% or sucrose 50%.

2. An intravenous infusion of mannitol 50% solution in 0.2% normal saline up to 400 ml. While this may reduce the pressure by as much as 40 or 50%, there is an increased risk of cerebral bleeding.

3. Steroids such as dexamethasone are especially useful if the cerebral oedema is localised to one part of the brain. It is also reparative in its effect.

Physical Care

A plan of care in the absence of patient cooperation should cover all the systems of the body, placing each system in a priority order to meet the patient's most obvious needs first.

Airway

Patency of the airway at all times, which always takes first priority and has already been discussed.

Skin Care

The care of the skin has as its over-riding aim the prevention of pressure ulcers on the weight bearing dependant areas of the body. A firm mattress is more appropriate than either a water or ripple bed. If the patient is nursed on a full length sheepskin and turned every 2 hours, this in itself will do much to prevent skin redness and sores from developing. Basically the patient can be turned onto right and left lateral positions and supine, only rarely is the prone position used. A prepared chart showing the required positions at the appropriate time is one of the best methods of ensuring correct turning procedure. Skin cleanliness will do a great deal to prevent perspiration, and incontinence from excoriating the skin and a daily bed bath is a prerequisite of any care plan. Many unconscious patients are nursed naked, with only pelvic modesty clothing. A covering sheet and heavy-weight blankets are avoided if possible, or their weight supported by a bedcradle. The correct method of lifting and rolling the patient when used avoids friction on the skin. If the patient is pulled into position, the skin will easily abrade. To reduce excoriation from urinary incontinence an indwelling urinary catheter is recommended for the deeply unconscious.

Nutritional Needs

In the unconscious patient, assessing nutritional needs is quite difficult since the metabolism of the body is often disturbed as a consequence of adrenal shock, a mechanism in the unconscious patient as yet not fully understood. However the mechanism does delay gastric emptying and intestinal absorption. The main disturbances can however be fairly assessed by fluid balance charting, electrolytes assessment and comparing the age, weight and sex of the patient with standard nutritional graphs which will indicate the required calorie intake per day. A typical plan of care is as follows:

1. After 12 hours, a nasogastric tube is passed and the stomach contents aspirated. Feeding should then commence by giving small volumes (no more than 400 ml) of either glucose or ½ strength milk with glucose and water. The total fluid volume should not exceed 3 litres in 24 hours, implying the patient should have at least 8 feeds per 24 hours on the first day of care.
2. After 48 hours the calorific value should be increased to at least 2500 calories in the 24 hours with the same fluid volume as before. For each kilogram of body weight the patient should be given 1.5 g of first class protein to compensate for negative nitrogen balance, e.g., a 70 kg patient requires at least 105 g of protein in a liquidised form, usually made up from milk, eggs, Complan and 'Build up'. It is usual practice to add several drops of multivitamin complex to one feed per day. Regular assessment is required of weight loss and a daily urinalysis to test for excess proteinuria. A knowledge of the patient's allergies, if any, would help to eliminate from the liquidised preparations those foods to which the patient may be sensitive. Excess milk or sugar and broad spectrum antibiotics may induce a faecal incontinence.
3. Intravenous feeding is reserved for those patients who go into negative nitrogen balance, or for those with prolonged coma.
4. At each feed the nurse should inspect the oral cavity and the throat, and cleanse the mouth before giving a feed, even if this seems not to be required.

Urine Excretion

Excretion of urine is best controlled by the use of an indwelling catheter. Apart from giving a very accurate fluid-balance record and contributing to the prevention of pressure sores, its use does have a constraint since it risks a urinary tract infection. Regular catheter specimens should be despatched for culture and sensitivity testing, in addition to a very high standard of genital toileting and catheter care.

On the third day of care a small oil or soap and water enema should be administered to evacuate and cleanse the lower colon, and thereafter repeated every third day. Aperients or suppositories should not be used on an unconscious patient.

Care of the Special Senses

Special senses, particularly the eyes, require regular attention. They require protection against injury from, for instance, dust particles. If the eyelid remains open the sclera of the eye is prone to keratitis and ulceration of the cornea. The eyelids should be massaged daily to promote natural tear flow and also swabbed in an aseptic manner with sterile normal saline to remove any mucus from the conjunctiva. If required, soft eye pads should be taped over the eyeball should the lids not reflexly close. Mucus from the nasal cavity can usually be easily removed by nasal bud sticks. If not, then sodium bicarbonate may be required to soften hardened mucus to facilitate its removal. The ears should be inspected for the presence of wax at the outset of care.

Care of the Locomotor System

Care of the locomotor system involves an assessment of both the muscular system and the joints, as both must be maintained at their optimal function. Passive movement of all the limb joints will prevent contracture and muscle spasm if the exercises are done frequently and routinely, e.g., 3 times each day. Without this type of exercise the shoulder, hip, elbow and knee joints are at risk of contracture. The ankle, wrist and finger joints are prone to flexor spasm if they are not exercised. Spasticity of the muscles and joints may precede contractures and these spasms can be overcome by:

Stretching the opposing group of muscles

Tapping the muscles above the area of spasticity

Applying palmar pressure to the soles of the feet if the lower limbs are affected

Half-rotation of the head to deal with spasm of the cervical area

Cold packs applied for a few minutes over a spastic muscle will help relax the muscle

Soft lined splints can be constructed to house an affected limb and prevent a contracture from becoming worse, e.g., a padded plaster of paris which is bivalved

The longer the period of unconsciousness, then there is increased calcification of the principle joints which should be expected. This will contribute to the likelihood of contracture in the absence of passive movement exercises.

Preventing damage to the peripheral nerves from any type of indirect pressure is an essential component of planning care of the locomotor system. Pressure upon the radial or ulnar nerve causes wasting of the muscles of the hand and can be prevented by correct alignment of the upper limb. Irritation of the sciatic nerve may occur from giving badly sited injections into the gluteus maximus muscle. Injury to a motor nerve will cause paralysis, soon followed by atrophy or wasting of the muscles. Correct lower limb positioning will reduce the risk of injury and pressure, ensuring that bed-aids, the patient's own body weight and safety rails never trap or pressurise a limb. Restlessness requires the patient to be nursed in a bed with the safety rails raised and secure. Soft pillows should pad the rails. Direct physical restraint does not work and it may well be that a mild sedative drug is all that is required to reduce the risk of self-inflicted injury from exaggerated limb movements.

Psychosocial Aspects of Care

Psychosocial aspects of care should, from the very outset, involve both relatives and friends. Relatives especially should be encouraged to take part in the direct giving of physical care. They can be taught and supervised to do small simple tasks and be reassured that a nurse will always be available if anything untoward should happen.

Being involved, the relatives gain two advantages: firstly some of the guilty feelings which many people feel, even if there is no fault to be apportioned, are lifted by active participation and secondly the patient may recognise a familiar voice, even if unconscious.

In giving care such as sponging the patient's hands and face or hair brushing, relatives must be encouraged to talk to the patient. As a general rule hearing is the last sense to go and the first to return in the unconscious patient. It is often noted in those with prolonged unconsciousness that the playing of favourite music, or a tape recording of a favourite voice repeatedly played, may be the one stimulus to a recovery. No harm can come from trying.

On recovery many patients are violently sick, vomiting the gastric contents quite forcibly. Many are bewildered, confused and troubled by amnesia until familiarity restores memory recall. The plan of care alters to emphasise increasing independence from nursing skills, at first being supervised and then encouraged to self-determine the self care required, this being achieved over a defined period of time. All nursing care should go hand in glove with the prescribed medical regimen.

Chapter 81 Peripheral Nerve Conditions

PERIPHERAL NEURITIS

Inflammation of the peripheral nerves may be either acute, subacute, or chronic in nature. The site of inflammation will render the nerve fibre eventually incapable of conducting impulses either to the brain (sensory) or from the brain (motor), the motor nerves mainly being the type of nerve affected.

Acute Polyneuritis (Guillain-Barré Syndrome)

Acute polyneuritis is invariably due to a viral infection, causing an allergic reaction to the motor component of a nerve fibre. The causative viral infection may be mumps, herpes zoster or glandular fever, affecting adults between 30 and 50 years old. It may also be a consequence of an allergy to tetanus toxoid. The inflammatory process is usually allergic in type, but also may cause degeneration of either the cranial or peripheral nerves.

Since acute polyneuritis only affects the motor component of the nerve fibre, the main symptoms are weakness, paresis, or paralysis of the muscles supplied by the affected nerve. Sensory appreciation usually remains intact, if not actually exaggerated, especially temperature and pain sensation. Should the seventh, eighth or ninth cranial nerve be affected, the motor responses from the medulla oblongata become ineffective and result in a transient paralysis of swallowing, speech and possibly respiration. The inflammation is of a temporary nature, lasting between 2 days and 2 weeks with a full recovery in 18 months being the usual course of events.

The Guillain-Barré syndrome is diagnosed by examination of cerebrospinal fluid obtained from a lumbar puncture. The red and white cell counts are both raised and the precipitation of the protein from the white cells is quite pronounced. Although the medical regimen is usually palliative to control the worst of the symptoms, the nursing skills are quite important in dealing with any temporary paralysis, especially if affecting the cranial nerves.

The 3 risks which may occur are:

1. Respiratory arrest, which means that skills should be focussed on maintaining the airway.

2. Speech may be affected, so some means of communication may need to be implemented, e.g., pad and pencil, picture cards.

3. Swallowing difficulties. If this is the case, the patient should be nursed near to a suction point.

Subacute Polyneuritis

The term subacute polyneuritis describes an inflammation of the motor neurone cell located in the anterior horn of the spinal cord. The inflammation and degeneration of the peripheral nerves are caused by damaging toxic substances, the most common toxic substance being alcohol (alcoholic polyneuritis). More rarely, lead, arsenic and fortified wine may be the cause. Dietary deficiency of either vitamin B1 (aneurin) also known as the antineuritic vitamin, and deficiency of vitamin B12 (cyanocobalamin), if uncontrolled can lead to subacute degeneration of the spinal cord, a well recognised complication of pernicious anaemia.

An uncontrolled mature onset of diabetes mellitus will ultimately lead to a peripheral neuropathy, the toxic substance being excess blood glucose. Athough the damage is at the anterior horn cell in the spinal cord, the first effects are felt at the terminal portions of the peripheral nerves with the effects gradually moving towards the centre of the body. The initial symptoms begin with muscular cramp-like pain of the lower limb, the gait and posture are uncoordinated, the muscles begin to atrophy and appear wasted as the result of increasing weakness and paresis.

Retention of urine is a particular problem of subacute polyneuritis, if it is left untreated. Later symptoms include a marked depression and, in alcoholism, it may proceed to dementia. The principles of treatment include bedrest, correcting nutritional deficiencies and relieving both the physical and psychological pain. Those who suffer from alcoholism are usually referred to specialist units within a psychiatric hospital.

Chronic Polyneuritis

The more rare group of chronic inflammatory peripheral neuritis tends to affect the Schwann cell and segments of the myelin sheath. It is presumed to be due to the toxic metabolites of malignant tumours, notably lung cancer, which may affect the brachial plexus and the related nerves causing a motor and sensory deficit of either arm. Should it affect a sensory nerve, the resulting pain will be of a chronic nature requiring the advice of a consultant in a pain clinic.

The nursing care plan should direct its first priority to caring for the consequences of any paralysis of the cranial nerves. Attention should be focused on skills required to maintain the airway should the patient require artificial respiration either via an endotracheal intubation or temporary tracheostomy, these being essential to avoid respiratory arrest. If speech is affected, an appropriate means of communication either by pad and pencil or picture card should be implemented to help the patient's needs to be more quickly anticipated. Swallowing difficulties require the patient to be nursed near to a suction point so that excess saliva can be promptly removed.

Motor paralysis or paresis is, in the majority of cases, of a transient nature and requires an assessment to be made of the dependance the patient will have on nursing skills until the medical investigations and treatment have a curative effect. It can be expected that full mobility will be achieved, providing that in the meantime steps are taken to prevent any muscle atrophy from becoming worse by using passive physiotherapy, combined with correct positioning techniques, whether on bedrest or being nursed in an armchair. A period of immobility will subject the skin to increased risk of pressure ulcers and basic measures such as skin cleanliness, frequent turning, and a nourishing diet will minimise this risk.

Any loss of the swallowing reflex will require a plan to meet the dietetic needs of the patient. The correct calorific and fluid volumes should be calculated for each 24-hour period of dependance, during which the patient may need either nasogastric or intravenous feeding. Injections of vitamin B12 are vital to correct the peripheral neuritis caused by pernicious anaemia, such injections being for life. Diabetic patients require a carbohydrate controlled diet, and perhaps their diabetes stabilising with one of the sulphonureas or biguanides. In some diabetic patients the peripheral neuropathy may not resolve, requiring the patient to be referred for the specialist opinion of a surgeon. Often the neuritis is a precipitant signal to peripheral gangrene. Alcoholic patients have great difficulty responding to any dietetic regimen until they have been 'dried out' and their vitamin deficiencies corrected by massive doses of vitamin B1 and B12.

Urinary excretion may be a problem for some patients with subacute polyneuritis, although of a temporary nature it may require an indwelling urinary catheter to relieve urinary retention. Daily urinalysis would be done in any case, and catheter specimens of urine are useful in that any test can exclude renal tract infections and other minor abnormalities.

In all types of polyneuritis the patient has a degree of anxiety coupled with depression, often needing reassurance that their muscular paresis or paralysis will get better. In the vast majority of cases, such a reassurance can be given providing that the diagnosis is accurate and the patient can be persuaded to wait for a few days to see the obvious improvement which results from treatment. Any measure which encourages the patient to take an interest in their cosmetic appearance should distract and reduce the misery of depressing thoughts. Relatives should be counselled if the underlying cause of the peripheral neuritis is a chronic disease such as pernicious anaemia, alcoholism, or diabetes, as the treatment and after care services are usually required for life.

Rabies (Hydrophobia)

Rabies is a rare disease that is transmitted to animals and humans via the bite of a rabid animal, usually a dog, fox, or a bat. Once inoculated through the broken skin, the rabies virus travels along the nerve fibres to reach the brain where it is infectious. From the brain the virus then travels to the salivary glands, where it multiplies in number. This series of events takes between 2 weeks and several months before the first symptoms appear, the incubation period being shorter if the victim is bitten on the face.

At first the patient feels apprehensive and is easily irritated by noise or other sensory stimuli. Cerebral symptoms of headache accompanied by pyrexia and insomnia are quite pronounced. The area bitten begins to tingle and sensations of numbness or pain are usual. From 24 hours after these initial symptoms the victim begins to suffer from laryngeal and pharyngeal spasms which will cause sensations of choking, dysphagia, and hoarseness of speech. In the following 48 hours a period of 'excitement' occurs in which the patient is hyperactive and every action is associated with fear. The laryngeal spasms become more violent, forcing excessive volumes of saliva from the salivary glands and mouth. Any offer of water increases the fear reaction and the violence of the laryngeal spasm, i.e., hydrophobia. As time passes the spasms become more generalised to include peripheral muscles, the most extreme spasm causing an opisthotonos, followed by convulsions which are associated with delirium. The final stage occurs within 5 days of the initial symptoms and is one of paralysis, coma and respiratory failure.

All patients reporting to the accident and emergency departments with a history of an animal bite must be questioned about the animal, especially if it is known that the animal has been vaccinated against rabies, or if in fact it showed any signs of a rabid infection. The wound itself should be thoroughly douched with an antiseptic lotion. The period of incubation is such that no rabies symptoms will be apparent, but if the animal is wild then precautions should be taken by offering the patient a daily injection of antirabies serum each day for 14–21 days. At a later date if cerebral symptoms occur, the prevention of the 'excitement stage' should be dealt with by intensive nursing techniques and anticonvulsant therapy. Any laryngeal symptoms would require a tracheostomy, repeated laryngeal suction, oxygen therapy and artificial respiration via a ventilator. The patient would have induced muscular relaxation with either injections of tubocurarine or succinylcholine. Although rabies is not transmitted from human to human, the patient will require to be nursed in isolation with the strictest control of infection until advised otherwise by the public health authorities, i.e., the environmental medical officer.

The prevention of rabies is particularly strict in Europe and America. The quarantine period for domestic pets is on average 6 weeks before it can enter another country and the penalties are quite severe for those who attempt to bring animals into the country illegally. The immunisation of domestic pets has practically eradicated this disease, but it is still occasionally reported in America and Northern Europe. Wild animals which are sick or dead should be handled with the greatest of care, certainly never with an ungloved hand. If a live animal has rabies then it must be destroyed as soon as possible.

Tetanus (Lockjaw)

The anaerobic spore forming organism tetanus bacillus (*Clostridia tetani*) can gain access to the tissues via a deep penetrating wound contaminated with either soil or manure. On multiplying, the organism produces an exotoxin called tetanospasmin which travels along the nerve sheaths and is further disseminated via the blood vessels. The exotoxin interferes with the inhibitory influences exerted on the spinal reflex arc. This means that on the lightest sensory stimulus the muscles will suffer an intense spasm. The incubation period varies between 2 and 21 days before any symptoms appear in an untreated wound.

Symptoms are progressive, perhaps beginning with difficulty in opening the jaw (trismus), dysphagia and neck rigidity. Later there can be tonic spasm of masseter, pharyngeal and laryngeal muscles, when combined they produce the typical 'risus sardonicus' of the face. Abdominal rigidity and spasms of the limbs may be followed by convulsions. Cerebral irritation is intense, any noise provoking the spasms into an opisthotonos. The spasms progressively extend to involve the intercostal muscles and the effort to breathe is extremely desperate causing dyspnoea and cyanosis, the respiratory effort being accompanied by profuse perspiration, tachycardia, heart failure and utter exhaustion.

With previous immunisation the tetanus infected wound will produce less severe symptoms. A booster injection after any injury will almost eradicate the risk of tetanus. Those who are hypersensitive to horse serum (from which tetanus toxoid is derived), or who are prone to allergies, may have the alternative tetanus immune globulin derived from human tissues. The circulating exotoxin can be neutralised by the administration of tetanus antitoxin 60 000–10 000 units, half the dose given intravenously and the other half intramuscularly. It is usual practice to also give benzyl penicillin 2–4 g daily in divided doses every 6 hours, if the wound is very mutilated. The wound itself may require excision to facilitate debridement and exceptional toileting of the damaged deeper tissue.

If admitted with the symptoms of tetanus the patient requires intensive therapeutic care based on:

1. Tracheostomy, suction and intermittent positive pressure ventilation.

2. Complete muscular relaxation induced by either injections of tubocurarine or succinylcholine.

3. Chlorpromazine (Largactil) to reduce any muscular spasms.

4. Nursing measures to reduce hyperpyrexia and sensory stimuli (e.g. noise or visitors).

Tetanus is a notifiable disease and while it is not transmitted from human to human the patient will require strict isolation nursing since he or she is prone to other infections. International travellers should always take the precaution of having a booster injection several weeks before making any journey.

Huntington's Chorea (Huntington's Disease)

Is a rare heriditary disease carried on a dominant autosomal gene with a 50% chance of being transmitted to either a daughter or son. It does not miss a generation. The first symptoms do not, however, appear until the patient reaches 30–50 years old. Although the cause of the disease is still being researched, its effects are the degeneration of cells and nerve fibres of the cerebrum, cerebellum and the brain stem with an ultimate atrophy of the areas affected. These changes result in classical choreiform jerking movements of the muscles, akinesia and mental deterioration. Huntington's chorea is one cause of pre-senile dementia.

Initially the patient undergoes mental changes or periods of depression and temper outbursts for no obvious reason. His or her posture and gait becomes noticeably odd and bizarre as the ability to coordinate voluntary movement is lost. Speech becomes slurred and noticeably dystharric leading to difficulty with communication. Jerky movements, at first of the facial muscles and then of the upper limbs and finally the whole body progress, and ever worsen in their purposelessness and also in their violence, often to such a degree that the safety rails of the bed require to be padded to avoid self-injury by the patient. It should be noted that physical restraint is quite useless as the violence of the movement if restrained may actually cause a fracture. Over the next 10–20 years the disease becomes increasingly worse and chronic in nature and will eventually rob the patient of the power of speech. He or she will become physically totally dependant on others for all care. During this period the personality changes are also quite dramatic. Such patients can be irritated by any personal slight; they are irascible, hostile and have frequent periods of depression which may be the reason for the high suicide rate amongst this group of patients. As they become more and more irresponsible in their personal care, the question of legal supervision eventually arises, often being the reason for their admission into psychiatric institutions. If the choreiform movements are untreated and are severe, the patient usually dies either from exhaustion, pneumonia, or heart failure.

Diagnosis is principally from the clinical signs and a detailed family history, as one parent also has the disease. Air encephalography may be completed to detail the areas of the brain suffering from atrophy. Unfortunately there is no known cure at this time, and all treatment is aimed at dealing with the symptoms to make the patient more comfortable. Several drugs do lessen the severity of the involuntary movements and, combined with mood controlling agents, the quality of life can be considerably improved. Such drugs as Librium (chlordiazaposide), Haldol (haloperidol), Prolixin (flupherazine), Largactil (chlorpromazine) and Imipramine (Tofranil) in suitable assessed dosage given at frequent periods will control the worst of the symptoms.

When the time comes for admission into a protected environment, the nursing staff would require to assess the amount of visual supervision that would be required to detect behaviours that would disrupt the smooth running of the unit or ward. The risk of attempted suicide should be borne in mind and obvious hazards may have to be removed from the patient's vicinity. Increasingly communication will be difficult, but this does not imply the intellectual ability is in any way diminished, and although the patient's speech is slurred and unintelligible he or she may well be capable of understanding normal conversation, read newspapers, listen with appreciation to the radio and television and continue to play table games with dexterity. For as long as he or she is able, the patient should be encouraged to look after personal physical needs such as dressing, toileting, cosmetics, hair care and eating, and be encouraged to remain mobile.

Although a psychiatric institution can be helpful to the patient, the amount of support and help the relatives need in coming to terms with this horrendous disease may require repeated explanations to assuage the guilt that many families feel, and to remove any feelings of stigma. The children of such parents do need genetic counselling; with a 50% chance of carrying the disease, either a son or daughter would perhaps be best advised not to have children but rather consider adoption, if they would like to have a family. Often it is found that the relatives are so distressed by the physical changes of the patient that they are reluctant to visit the hospital, but by merely having a telephone contact with them they may be of some reassurance to the patient.

Anterior Poliomyelitis

There are 3 known viruses which cause poliomyelitis: the Branhilde, Leon and Lansing, the latter being the most virulent of all three. The virus may gain entry into the body either via the nasopharynx or via the gastrointestinal tract, and exists in contaminated water such as one might find in escaped sewage or contaminated swimming pools. Poliomyelitis classically occurs in epidemics in the summer and autumn months, affecting children and young adults who have not been immunised. On gaining access to the body it travels through the tissues via the blood stream until it reaches the nerve fibres where it then moves along until it reaches the nerve cells in the anterior horn of the spinal cord. In multiplying it destroys the nerve cells and since the anterior horn supplies the motor nerves which innervate the muscles, the consequence of poliomyelitis is flaccidity of the muscles affected, i.e., paralysis. The virus may also spread up the spinal cord to invade the meninges, brain, cranial nerves and base of the brain.

The incubation period of anterior poliomyelitis is between 7 and 14 days before the first symptoms appear. The virulence and site of inflammation determine the severity of illness, and are classified by stages:

Stage 1: Subclinical stage where there are no manifest symptoms, except a mild pyrexia and a feeling of being unwell. Without further symptoms the patient goes on to develop a natural immunity to the infection.

Stage 2: Abortive stage, the symptoms of pyrexia, nausea and vomiting are mild in degree but last several days, almost as though suffering from influenza. The symptoms recede leaving the patient with a life long immunity against the disease.

Stage 3: Non paralytic stage, the signs of meningism, i.e., rigid neck, cerebral irritability, severe headache, marked pyrexia, vomiting and a sore throat persist for 2–4 days. Virology of the cerebrospinal fluid would demonstrate one of the causative viruses, while the cerebrospinal fluid would also show increased protein, leucocytes and lymphocytes. After this uncomfortable period, the patient may either get better with immunity established or proceed into stage 4.

Stage 4: Paralytic stage. The inability to move the voluntary muscles of the lower limbs is a most frightening experience, and fear is the paramount symptom which is the most difficult to resolve unless sedation is used. In the early stages the lower limbs are affected, but gradually the upper limbs may also become flaccid with absent reflex. The muscles become wasted very quickly and during the initial stages of paralysis are painful to the touch because of spasms, and the nursing care requires very gentle lifting and handling techniques. Urinary retention may also occur and must be tested for at periodic intervals in the early stages and requires to be relieved by catheterisation. If the patient's speech becomes staccato in style it should be taken as a warning sign that the muscles of speech and possibly respiration will soon become paralysed and that the upper limbs are also threatened.

Diagnostic confirmation of poliomyelitis is made by lumbar puncture and the obvious clinical signs; being a notifiable disease a careful social history is required for the environmental medical officer to locate and contain the source and any contacts, if the disease is becoming epidemic.

Isolation nursing is a paramount importance, even if the staff have been immunised, until the acute nature of the infection is over and some assessment can be made of the extent of the residual paralysis. Each symptom has to be assessed on its own merit and severity. In the early stages when polio may not be expected the patient is nursed in isolation as though suffering from meningitis. As the limbs become flaccid it may remain limited only to the lower limbs and the paraplegia will then require intensive physiotherapy after the acute phase is over to prevent muscular wasting. Should swallowing become impossible then without hesitation a nasogastric tube should be passed into the stomach for nutritional purposes and the patient should have regular suction of the larynx and pharynx as saliva and bronchial secretions cannot be swallowed and may enter the bronchial tree. If the diaphragm and intercostal muscles become paralysed the patient will require a tracheostomy and intermittent positive ventilation on a respirator combined with frequent periods of postural drainage and suction.

After the acute phase a detailed assessment is made by the remedial physiotherapist to ascertain the exact degree of paralysis and what passive and active exercises are required to place the patient into a positive phase of recovery.

Fortunately this is now a rare disease in western society due to the mass population immunisation schedule with the Sabin oral polio vaccine, which is given in 3 doses. Being a weakened live virus it confers good immunity which may require a booster dose for those who are international travellers. Other features of prevention include a protected and treated clean water supply, a closed system for dealing with sewage, the control of the domestic fly and good social standards of hygiene in the community at large. During epidemics, when sore throats may be a common complaint, hospitals should cancel their plans for routine tonsillectomy operations until the epidemic is over.

Part 8
Primary Health Care Team

Chapter 82
Hospital and Community Liaison

HOSPITAL DISCHARGE

Coordinating a patient's discharge from hospital to home can be quite complex if the patient has experienced a prolonged or serious illness. Any type of chronic illness may require extensive community nursing help, this being a basic need to the other requirements of statutory and voluntary organisations. Within the hospital itself the nurse should be cognisant with the communication network and liaison between professional peers and various departments. There is however an obvious uncertainty to any communication system existing between the 'hospital' and 'community' staff when, as is most likely, there is no face-to-face meeting but a reliance on letters or telephone calls.

The doctor or surgeon on taking the

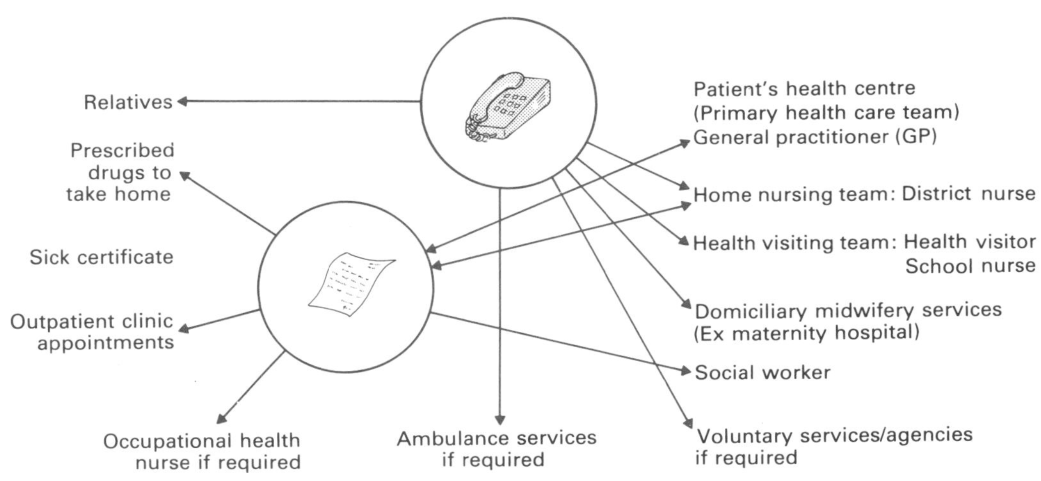

Fig. 82.1 Coordinating a patient's discharge from hospital.

decision to discharge the patient from the hospital must write to the general practitioner indicating the patient's diagnosis, investigations, prescribed treatment and give a prognosis. This first letter may be either sent by post or, more usually, given to the patient to hand in to his or her own doctor's health practice. The complementary nursing care however usually requires many more contacts, for nursing also possesses a social dynamic which must not be overlooked when returning the patient home or to convalescence.

As an initial step the relatives should be advised of the patient's imminent discharge from hospital and arrangements made to transport the patient home either by car or ambulance. Patients are not usually allowed to leave hospital premises on their own and should always be accompanied by either relatives or a friend. Travel by public transport should also be avoided. Since the required ongoing care can be quite complex it is sensible to take time and explain to the relatives the arrangements which have been made regarding outpatient appointments, medications, and home visits by specialist nurses. Any liaison with professional groups will be ill-received by the relatives if they are not forewarned of the likely visitors to their home. Instruction should also be given in writing as in the excitement of going home, verbal instructions can be forgotten.

Ward administrative techniques ensure that the patient is issued with a sick certificate if the convalescent period goes beyond 5 working days. Generally, hospital practice is to issue these certificates for a 1-week period only; further certificates must be obtained from the general practitioner. Likewise prescribed medication will be sufficient for only one week. The patient needs to be warned of this limited issue, which also pertains to surgical supplies such as colostomy and ileostomy appliances, syringes, needles and surgical dressings. If a clinical nurse specialist, e.g., mastectomy nurse or stoma nurse, is part of the hospital staff, the problem of liaison and supplies is minimal as the nurse will have arranged future home visits.

COMMUNITY LIAISON

Initial contact with professional colleagues in the community nursing team is usually by telephone. Where clinical care is the priority then the district nurse or domiciliary midwife (for maternity patients) will be contacted in the first instance. In paediatric and children's nursing the health visitor or school nurse may require to be contacted. All these community nurses are based in the Health Centre servicing the geographical area in which the patient lives. Information sent by telephone can however lead to errors if the ward nurse has not clearly thought out the essential information required by the community nurse to initiate the ongoing care from the first home visit.

A second problem with telephone information arises when it is connected to a message recorder. Without human contact error is more likely, causing bemusement with its very one-sided conversation. The essential information in a recorded message required by the community nurse to ensure that a first home visit is successful is:

The patient's forename and surname, unusual names should be spelled out clearly.

Give the patient's title, i.e., whether Mr, Miss, Mrs or Ms, and age.

Emphasise the home address, the street number and house name, spelling out awkward names or words clearly.

Give an updated diagnosis as it often alters once treatment has begun and a basic outline of the treatment given and the specific nursing care required.

List the drugs which are currently prescribed for the patient.

The name of the patient's general practitioner.

Finish by giving the ward name or number and hospital from which the patient is being discharged.

On listening to the message the nurse in charge of the home nursing team is in a position to delegate the visit to the district nurse allocated the particular area in which the patient lives. A reasonably good clear message should ensure that the visiting nurse takes along any essential equipment which is not ordinarily included; this is most important for the first home visit. Many of the errors experienced by community nurses means time wasting, when they are sent to the wrong address, given the wrong diagnosis, or are unaware of present medication.

An outline of the responsibilities and roles of the various community nurses is given to enable the learner to gain more insight into how the primary health care team coordinate their work, liaise with each other, and communicate with statutory and voluntary organisations.

Chapter 83
Role of Team Members

THE HEALTH VISITOR

The mid-nineteenth century is regarded as the beginning of British social reform to deal with poverty, squalor and deprivation of the lower and working classes. The great reformers such as Shaftesbury, Fry and Nightingale drew attention to the particular needs of the poor. One predominant need was for 'education' not only in its formal sense, but more particularly in an applied social sense to everyday living. The recognition of the need to teach women in their own homes took firm root in Manchester and Salford with the 'Ladies Sanitary Reform Association'. The members, usually middle class educated ladies, visited the homes of the poor to teach the women in particular about the basic rules of cleanliness. This work from 1857 till 1890 was always on a voluntary basis, but their work was finally recognised with the offer of a salary for those who did the 'visiting' on a full-time basis. The first training course was offered by North Buckinghamshire in 1891 to ladies who were referred to as 'health missioners'. Between 1897 and 1908 the concept of health visiting spread to Worcester, Huddersfield and then London, and finally to other major cities in the country. Until as late as 1945, health visiting was mainly identified with infant welfare. Even today the largest group remains pre-school children and their parents.

Formal statutory requirements for health visitors were first issued in 1909 by London Councils, but by 1915 with the enactment of the Notification of Births Act the role of the

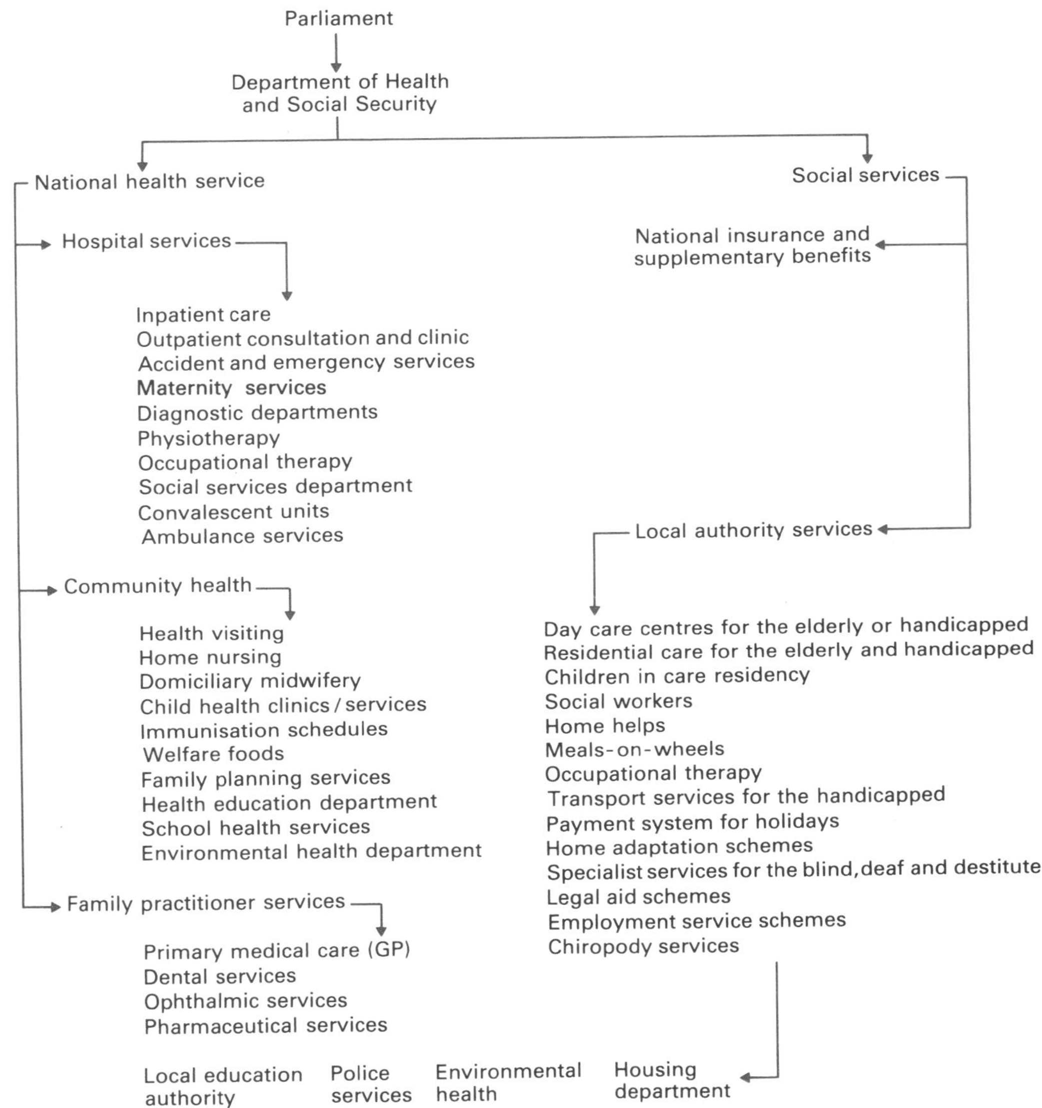

Fig. 83.1 Hospital, community and local service liaison.

health visitor was firmly established. More importantly from 1915 the health visitor could organise visits soon after the birth of any child since it had to be notified to the local authority. The Maternity and Child Welfare Act of 1918 made it a duty of Local Authorities to provide health visiting services for their citizens. Naturally this Act increased the formality of the qualification of a health visitor. Training regulations became more stringent and formal national examinations were held in London, organised and conducted by the then responsible body, the Royal Sanitary Institute. Under the regulations of the School Health Act 1945 the role of the health visitor was extended to include the health and welfare of the schoolchild, and indeed school nurses had to hold the qualification of a health visitor. From the many reports on the role of the health visitor during the last 40 years, it can be said in many general terms that the health visitor is a health educationalist, counsellor and advisor to the family unit as a whole.

It is usual for a health visitor to hold a dual qualification as a registered nurse and a midwife or to have undertaken an obstetric course. These basic statutary nursing qualifications may be sufficient for a nurse to apply for 1 of 5 possible courses to gain the Health Visitors Certificate awarded by the Council for the Education and Training of Health Visitors (CETHV). More recently the Nurses, Midwives and Health Visitors Act 1979 enables the National Boards of the United Kingdom Central Council for Nurses (UKCC) to regulate and control health visitor training.

The aims of health visiting and teaching are fourfold:

1. To promote health.
2. To prevent mental, physical and social ill health.
3. To detect abnormality and refer for diagnostic screening.
4. To influence attitudes and behaviours which will improve environmental physical, mental and social well-being.

To achieve these aims the health visitor is trained to appreciate and understand, within a given cultural context, the health needs of individuals and their families. There are many predisposing factors to ill health, each requiring detailed assessment. Poverty in all its guises is readily appreciated as a major cause of physical ill health, but oddly enough the affluent are equally prone to certain illnesses. The opposites of unemployment and overwork can directly lead to many physical and emotional stresses. Social habits of smoking and drinking are a proven direct cause of many diseases, some of which are preventable by health education techniques.

Apart from assessing risks to health, the health visitor is regarded as expert at implementing procedures which will prevent diseases. These techniques are immunisation and vaccination schedules, health surveillance screening, and monitoring the health status of infants and school children.

Although based in a health centre, the concept of 'visiting' remains paramount to the success of preventing ill health. There are many avenues open by which the public can be reached: e.g., schools, churches, voluntary groups, the press, television, pamphlets and health education departments. Visiting means communicating, it also means teaching, either on a one-to-one basis or to small groups and the skill here requires a deeper than usual knowledge about sociology and psychology. Increasingly there is a need for specialist health visitors based in hospitals who concentrate on the particular needs, e.g., diabetic children, the physically handicapped, or as a paediatric liaison officer between hospital, home and the general practitioner.

The nature of health visiting lends itself to research and an appreciation of research methodology will give the work far more challenge and meaning. Liaison with many groups includes contact with statutory bodies, educational departments, voluntary groups and professional organisations at both a local and national level.

DISTRICT NURSING

The earliest evidence of district nursing can be traced to Liverpool where a nurse was employed in 1859 to care for the sick and the poor in their own homes. In subsequent years Manchester and Salford also recruited nurses, and by 1868 the London Bible Women and Nurse Mission formed the East London Nursing Society. Eight years later the first training school for district nurses was opened and the concept rapidly spread to many cities in the United Kingdom, reaching the Scottish highlands by 1912. As part of Queen Victoria's Jubilee celebrations the Institute of Nurses was established during 1887 and granted the Royal charter in 1899. This organisation eventually became known as the Queen's Institute for District Nursing.

The Maternity and Child Welfare Act 1918 enabled local authorities to employ district nurses with a special remit to help in the detection and control of common infectious diseases. Training in these years was jointly organised by the Royal College of Nurses and the Queen's Institute. After the 1946 National Health Act the local Health Authorities were the main employers of district nurses. From 1955 onwards there has been extensive development in the clinical role, training regulations and specific curriculum aims in the now statutory course which leads to the District Nurses Certificate, to which both the registered and enrolled nurse can apply.

The district nurse has an expert role in providing the clinical care for both the acute or chronically ill in their own home. Using the nursing process philosophy the district nurse has to develop a keen sense of anticipatory care, being able to identify problems as either actual or potential, plan the required care and implement such care effectively. Emphasis is also given to dealing with the emotional stress often experienced by the patient and the immediate and extended family. Since many patients tend to be elderly, the nurse has a particular need to be able to deal with the terminally ill and console the relatives. The majority of district nurses are attached to or based in a health centre covering a specific geographical area. Liason with other members of the primary health care team is paramount in the successful management of what can be a very heavy case load. Other contacts of great value in everyday work include those with local hospitals, statutory bodies and voluntary organisations.

DOMICILIARY MIDWIFE (See also Obstetrics)

The earliest efforts to provide a formal training for the midwife were attempted by Florence Nightingale in 1862. However it was only in 1865 that socially suitable ladies were given an instruction course on midwifery at the Ladies Medical College in London. From this start there followed a tremendous amount of legislation dealing with training and development of the midwifery services. From the first Midwives Act of 1902 there followed 6 further Acts culminating in the 1979 Nurses, Midwives and Health Visitors Act. On the basis of several of these acts the midwife has certain clinical freedoms, especially important in home deliveries, i.e., the right to prescribe and administer certain controlled drugs and to deliver a child without the direct supervision of medical staff.

During the last 20 years the reports from various working parties on the midwifery services, i.e., Stocks, Cranbrook, Mayston and Peel Reports, have made recommendations culminating in the centralising of domiciliary midwifery services in maternity hospitals. The majority of births occur in hospitals; recent figures for England and Wales suggest that only 2% of childbirths occur in the home. Social changes however may reverse this trend as mothers are more frequently expressing a wish to have the choice of either hospital or home birth.

The domiciliary midwife, like her hospital counterpart, would be expert in antenatal and post-natal care. Special emphasis would be given in health education to the parents if the child were to be born at home, particularly in parentcraft. Education of the mother should reflect any concerns arising from being a single parent, or if the abuse of drugs, smoking or alcohol exists. All the foregoing are threats to the fetus and the baby when it is eventually born. After the baby is born the mother may then require detailed advice on family planning. Supervision of the mother may continue for up to 6 weeks, after which time the health visitor would assume responsibility for the health of both mother and baby.

OCCUPATIONAL HEALTH NURSING

British legislation does not require an employer to provide specifically for the health provision of their employees. However there are many acts of Parliament which provide for the safety and welfare of many groups of workers whilst at their place of employment (see list at end of chapter). In general terms those who employ large numbers of people find it a possible advantage to have an occupational health department in liaison with a personnel department to monitor the health status of their employees. Currently there are some 9000 nurses working in industry and about 23% of this number have trained specifically as occupational health nurses (OHNCerts).

Depending on the type of industrial process and the number of employees, a nurse may have a narrow remit or a wide all-embracing contract of employment. Professional colleagues such as doctors, dentists, chiropodists, diagnosticians and screening agencies tend to have a fee contract with the employers, leaving the nurse as the only full-time health consultant.

The occupational health nurse on completion of the course of study, would have a wide knowledge of the health dangers associated with many industrial processes and service industries. Apart from having a specific knowledge on the particular industry in which the nurse is working, a typical remit usually includes:

1. Pre-employment health screening of job applicants and their physical and mental suitability for the particular job. Certain jobs require specific manipulative skills or aptitudes which may require testing in some detail. In some industries, e.g., food processing, the employee may in fact be a hazard to the process, such as a 'carrier' of a pathogenic organism, and is excluded on health grounds.

2. Health supervision of those currently in employment. This may be quite intensive. Some firms have a clear policy of health screening their employees every year not only for health reasons but for insurance and safety purposes, e.g., air pilots. Such screening is not a threat, but in fact very reassuring to the worker and one of the best preventative health measures, detecting disease very early which can be readily treated.

3. Monitoring for possible health hazards in the working environment. This is a double check not only in risks to health but to those for safety.

4. Offering health advice to employees and arranging referrals to specialists if the need arises. This is often best achieved using informal methods during a 'welfare clinic', during organised 'teach-ins', or during in-service training sessions.

5. Ensuring that there is first aid provision within the working premises and arranging training for those appointed as safety representatives in basic first aid. Nurses do need to know the provisions set out in the Health and Safety at Work Act, regardless of which industry employs them.

6. Arranging for the resettlement of those who are returning to work after an illness or injury and checking on those who are currently ill or incapacitated. A general knowledge of injury benefits and insurance schemes is an advantage to the nurse as often an industrial worker may be seeking financial help during the illness and may be entitled to compensation.

7. Promoting positive health standards, especially in those industrial processes with established risks. This often means encouraging workers to wear the safety or protective clothing provided, using the safety devices to protect eyes or ears or simply following basic rules of personal hygiene.

8. Liaising with members of Health and Safety Committees appointed by management to monitor illness or injury within the working premises. Records should be kept of all accidents and investigated to see if prevention is feasible, and then implemented.

9. Liaising with specialists, welfare agencies and management to secure and maintain a safe working environment for all workers on the premises.

10. Where required by the industrial process, to have a contingency 'major disaster' plan ready. This applies to all processes where the risks of fire, explosion, flooding or accident could occur. The plan should include details of ambulance, fire and police services, details of local accident and emergency departments and the location of emergency first aid equipment and trained personnel.

11. Maintaining health records is an essential component of health screening, particularly if follow-up is necessary. Apart from a managerial interest, such records are useful for insurance benefits, claims and injury benefits. They are naturally confidential to the medical officer who signs

them, and in the custody of the nurse should not be released except on the authority of the doctor who signs them. Records of this nature are also useful as the basis of research.

12. The clinical role of the nurse is several fold, assisting medical staff during examinations and providing a 'medical centre' for initial care of the injured or a 'treatment centre' for minor dressings and medications.

SCHOOL NURSING

The first school nurse was appointed by a school in London in 1892. Six years later 5 school nurses established a School Nurses Society to formulate future plans and needs. In part, this led to the London County Council creating a financed local School Nursing Service. Later in 1907 the service was extended and renamed the School Medical Service.

One provision of the Education Act of 1918 required local authorities to create a system whereby children's minor ailments could be treated and dealt with on school premises. Apart from the need to extend the medical service for school children, it meant that more school nurses had to be recruited. The major and reforming Education Act of 1944 made it compulsory for all education authorities to create and maintain a school health service. Several sections of this Act specified the need of schools to take medical advice and to promote the hygiene not only of school premises but of the children. During 1945 a further Act of Parliament required that school nurses should possess the Health Visitors Certificate, an indication of the increasing importance given to the need to detect disorders at an early stage. To meet this policy change the role of the health visitor was extended to be clinically expert not only in infant welfare but in school child health. Until 1973 the school health services were managed by local education authorities of the local councils. They are now, however, managed by local district health authorities. School health services are within the remit of the district medical officer of health, and for nurses this means that their contracted employment is with the local health authority.

Each health authority provides a child health service of which the school health team is an integral part. Usually the doctor within the team has an interest in child health, and when employed by the health authority is then appointed to several schools within the district. The overall aims of the school health service of which the nurse should be aware and support are to:

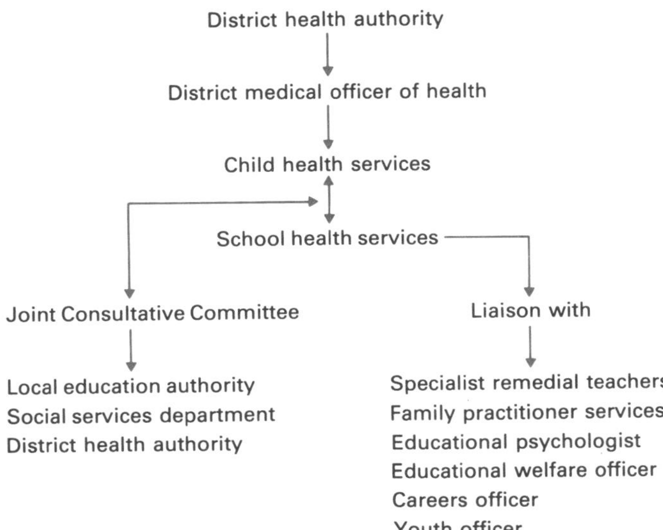

Fig. 83.2 School health team liaison.

1. Offer a health provision for each child attending primary and secondary school.

2. Monitor that the special needs of the physically handicapped child are being met.

3. Detect and correct common childhood health problems which would otherwise interfere with academic learning or social development.

4. Develop and monitor the effectiveness of health screening programmes.

5. Implement immunisation schedules to prevent and control infectious disease.

In pursing these aims the school nurse has to develop an awareness of the structure and organisation of each school in which she works. To achieve effective liaison when there is a problem, the nurse should know the names and location of specialist remedial teachers, educational psychologists, educational welfare officers, careers officers, youth officers and family practitioner services, e.g., ophthalmologists, dentists, speech therapists and general practitioners. If a notifiable infectious disease should occur within the school population, the nurse needs to be aware of the liaison system between the school and the local Department of Environmental Health.

From surveys completed in the early 1970s, it is a statistical assumption that for every 250 schoolchildren there are about 17 who will need the services of the school health team. The circumstances requiring help are mainly that the child will have a psychiatric, physical or social problem of such dimensions that it interferes radically with either academic learning or social development. Detecting these problems is a major role assigned to the school nurse. Apart from routine health screening the nurse should note the referrals made to her by teachers, if the child is absent a great deal from school, or if parents express undue anxiety about their child.

The clinical expertise of the school nurse will be utilised to its best extent during routine health checks. Basic skills in visual testing, detecting, hearing loss, dental decay, postural problems and enuresis are undoubted assets in the early detection of problems. Monitoring those children with diagnosed conditions such as diabetes mellitus, epilepsy or physical handicap often prevents complications and ensures that prescribed treatment is being taken. Detection and treatment of hair infestation remains a major problem in all schools. Immunisation and vaccination schedules are also a prime preventative measure organised via the child health services and carried out via child clinics and the school health team. A clinical knowledge of first aid is essential. Many health authorities have the schoolchildren's health status recorded on computerised programmes which, if constantly updated, make the management aspects of child health more pertinent and somewhat easier than manual record-keeping. The teaching and counselling roles of the school nurse are most important, considering they are in a prime position to advise individual or groups of children on health hazards such as smoking, abuse of alcohol, venereal disease and the advantages of contraception and family planning.

LEGISLATION INFLUENCING COMMUNITY HEALTH SERVICES

1848 First Public Health Act
1858 Medical Act (I)
1866 Sanitary Act
1870 Education Act
1875 Second Public Health Act
1885 Housing Act
1886 Medical Act (2)
1890 Housing Act
1893 Buckinghamshire finances first training for health visitors (Act of Parliament)
1899 Infectious Disease Notification Act
1902 Midwives Act (created Central Midwives Board)
1907 Notification of Birth Act (Permissive) i.e., optional
Education Act created the School Medical Services
1908 The Children Act
1911 National Insurance Act
1912 Notification of Birth Act (compulsory to notify births within 48 hours to the Local Authority)

1916 Public Health Venereal Disease Regulations
1918 Midwives Act (introduces medical aid procedure by midwives)
Maternity and Child Welfare Act (Local authorities required to provide health visitors and midwifery services)
Education Act (3)
1919 Nurses Registration Act created General Nursing Council
Ministry of Health formed
1920 Employment of Women, Young Persons and Children Act
1921 The Tuberculosis Act extended the 1912 Act
1926 Third Midwives Act
1929 Local Government Act specified the required qualifications of public health team members
1933 Children and Young Persons Act
1936 Fourth Midwives Act created a domiciliary midwifery service.
1936 Public Health Act consolidating previous public health acts
1938 Young Persons (Employment) Act
1944 Fourth Education Act creating among many things a compulsory school health service
Disabled Persons (Employment) Act amended again in 1958
1945 Family Allowance Act creating child benefit payments
Handicapped Pupils and School Health Regulations
1946 National Health Services Act, basis of the present National Health Service
National Insurance Act
1948 Children Act
National Assistance Act, basis of unemployment benefits and payments
Industrial Injuries (Insurance) Act
Nurseries and Child Minders Regulation Act
1951 Midwives Act consolidating the legislation of previous Midwives Acts
1954 Mines and Quarries Act
Baking Industry (Home and Work) Act
1956 Agriculture (Safety, Health and Welfare Provisions) Act
1957 Occupiers Liability Act
Nurses Act
1959 Mental Health Act
1960 Professions Supplementary to Medicines Act
1961 Factories Act
1962 Health Visiting and Social Work Act combined the training of health visitors and social workers
1963 Children's and Young Persons Act
Shops, Offices, Railway Premises Act
1964 Industrial Training Act
1965 Redundancy Payment Act
1968 Health Services and Public Health Act
1969 Children and Young Persons Act
Employer's (Compulsory Insurance) Act
1970 Local Authority Social Services Act
Nurses Act
Chronically Sick and Disabled Persons Act
Equal Pay Act
1971 Industrial Relations Act
Mines Management Act
1972 Contract of Employment Act
Redundancy Payments Act
1973 Employment of Children Act
Education (work experience) Act
Local Government Reorganisation Act
National Health Services Reorganisation Act
1974 Health and Safety at Work Act
1975 Children Act
1976 Fatal Accidents Act
1978 Employment Protection (consolidation) Act
1979 Nurses, Midwives and Health Visitors Act. This created the United Kingdom Central Council for Nurses enabling the formation of the Boards for each country in the kingdom and also gives the Conduct Rules for Nurses which were implemented by 1983.
1983 Mental Health Act (amended)

Part 9
Professional Responsibility and Ward Management

Chapter 84 Organisation and Communication

'Let whoever is in charge keep this simple question in mind, not how can I always do the right thing myself but how can I provide that the right thing shall always be done.' (Florence Nightingale)

FEATURES OF NURSE MANAGEMENT

Conventional professional wisdom allows for the fact that the shifting pattern from learner status to that of a fully fledged qualified nurse takes about 6 months following registration. In this period, the registered nurse is expected to accept a staff post, usually in her or his training hospital, so that they can develop and consolidate what they have been studying and learning during their years of training.

In addition to this consolidation, the nurse has to begin to develop her or his ward managerial role. Familiarity with ward organisation begins with an appreciation of the organisation of the hospital itself and the district health authority within which the hospital functions.

Nursing officers in these higher levels of authority set the policy pattern and framework within which the newly qualified nurse has to work. The larger and more complex the hospital the more features there are which will parallel those of industry in general. These features are the basis of bureaucracy, without which the aims and intentions of the hospital would not be achieved. The features to note are that larger hospitals have:

1. Specialised units within the structured framework which tend to work in isolation.

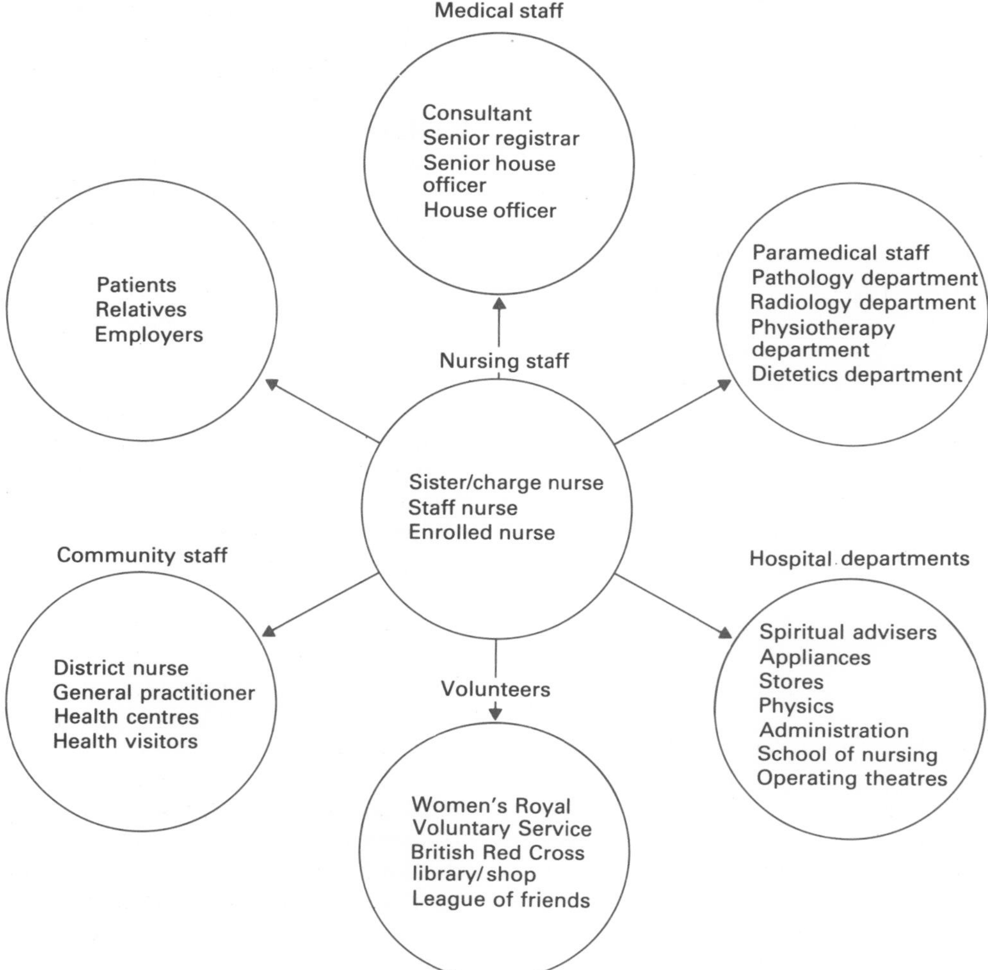

Fig. 84.1 Coordinating role of nursing staff.

2. Areas of responsibility and authority of individuals working in the structure are exactly defined.

3. Policies, regulations and procedures are precisely defined and are part of the contractual obligations of every employee.

4. There is impersonal efficiency with little obvious kinship between the various working groups.

5. Different staff groups are treated equally and are all represented usually in staff working groups, hence the need for more than the usual number of committees.

6. Different work groups tend to be stereotyped into having certain behaviours because of their uniform or colour coding. Behaviours tend to be hierarchical in a hospital setting.

7. Although the hierarchy is formal in its outward aspects, it always possesses an informal structure with unwritten rules and expectations.

In the smaller hospital, and indeed in a specialised unit of a large hospital, the managerial features tend to be far more informal. Staff are allowed to use their own initiative with far more freedom. Intuition and experiment is much easier and personal endeavour not only is expected but is more appreciated in human terms. While large units make economical sense, they are perhaps wasteful of talent and fail to exploit those individual touches which try to make working conditions more attractive and rewarding. The larger the hospital the more need there is for the nurse to have a clear idea of her or his expected role. Some unit managers will specify quite clearly the job description along with the contract of employment. A typical job description for a staff nurse is given here, and is a worthwhile detailed analysis as it forms the basis for discussion of those elements of management which the nurse is expected to develop. Additionally, it can be used as a basic appreciation for student nurses in their management studies. As can be seen, the job description is divided into 5 main areas, and these are discussed in detail.

Job Description for Staff Nurse (Day Duty)

Role: to be a skilled member of the nursing team providing the highest standard of care for the patients. In addition, the staff nurse should participate in the organisation and management of the ward and delegate such duties as necessary to take total charge in the absence of the sister or charge nurse.

Grade: Whitley Council Scale Grade

Accountable to: Nursing officer

Reports to: Sister or charge nurse

1. *Ward organisation and management.* To:

Maintain at all times a high standard of nursing care for all patients

Ensure that junior members of nursing staff receive adequate support and guidance

Contribute towards the smooth administration of the ward and to assume responsibility for the ward in the absence of the more senior qualified nurse

2. *Clinical Role.* To:

Lead a team of nurses in assessing, planning, implementing and evaluating nursing care of the highest possible standard

Administer prescribed treatments according to hospital policy

Supervise and encourage learners to acquire clinical nursing skills

Ensure that the patients' dietary requirements are met by supervising the serving of meals

Ensure that the junior ward staff are conversant with equipment in use having regard to the safety of staff, patients and themselves

Cooperate with medical staff to ensure that prescribed treatments are carried out correctly, and to report on patients' response to therapy

Report immediately to the most senior nurse on duty within the unit if untoward/unexpected changes are being experienced by the patients

3. *Administration and coordination.* To:

Assume responsibility for the ward in the absence of the senior member of nursing staff and in doing so accept responsibility for the ward

Ensure that accurate records of observations, treatments and progress are maintained

Ensure the safe custody of patients' belongings and valuables, according to hospital policy

Be aware of and ensure that junior colleagues also know the position of fire appliances, instructions for fire drill, and cardiac arrest trolley

Liaise with heads of departments, e.g., domestic supervisor, dietician, physiotherapy, etc.

Arrange overnight accommodation for relatives, if and when required

Maintain ward stocks and supplies, requisitioning with due economy when provisions, supplies and replacements are required

4. *Professional communication.* To:

Receive patients and their relatives courteously into the ward in a calm and reassuring manner

Give and receive regular reports on the progress of patients

Give and receive regular reports to and from medical staff on the patient's progress and the efficacy of prescribed therapy

Ensure that medications, solutions and lotions are correctly stored, administered and recorded in accordance with hospital's policy

Ensure that controlled drugs are correctly stored, administered and recorded according to hospital policy, which is based on legal requirements

Participate in the teaching of student nurses on the ward

Participate in the orientation and supervision of new members of the nursing staff in their duties

Attend organised conferences, study days, or in-service training, as arranged, to remain conversant with any changes in current practice

Exercise discretion with confidential notes and information about patients in care.

5. *Personnel coordination.* To:

Cooperate and liaise with members of staff of all other departments within the hospital

Participate in the training and supervision of newly qualified nursing staff in ward management, helping to develop their skills

Participate in the induction and in-service training of other grades of ward staff

Contribute to the written assessment of progress of training of student nurses allocated to the ward during their training

Contribute to the promotion of good relationships between nursing colleagues in other units and with those on night duty

WARD ORGANISATION AND MANAGEMENT

The geographical layout of the ward is the first constraint on actual day-to-day ward management. The Nightingale type of ward, with its double row of beds separated by a tremendous width of floor space, very similar to a dormitory, is still the more popular design with both nurses and patients. This type of layout derives its popularity because the nurse can see at one glance what is going on, even the most distant areas of the ward can be scrutinised with some detail, and patients are able to develop a keen interest in each other. In a subconscious way, patients can become supportive of each other during their illness. There are disadvantages:

1. The nurse can expect to walk at least 7 miles a day on such a ward.
2. Equipment layout has to be highly organised if time is not to be wasted fetching and carrying.
3. The ward can be rather noisy and draughty at night, and the toilet facilities can be rather Dickensian.

The Bristol-designed ward layout contains bays holding 4, 6 or 8 beds, and with modern fabric is made visually very attractive. Equipped with the latest designs in furniture and technical equipment, with everything immediately to hand, it can be a pleasure to work in such an environment. Certainly the distance walked by the average nurse is much less than for a Nightingale ward (in theory), but the design requires a higher ratio of nurses to manage the whole ward. The senior nurse on duty has to rely a great deal on the junior nurses to report sudden changes, since only a few patients are visible to direct view at any one time. This type of ward is often used as a mixed sex ward, males in one cubicle and females in the other, but surveys show this is not popular with the elderly patient. Morale may be low among patients, due not to the nursing but rather to the reduced contact with other patients and if the ward is run as a mixed sex ward.

There are a number of factors in the ward environment which may detract from giving good care and should be scrutinised carefully, for often a minor change can reap great benefits. These factors include:

1. Ventilation
2. Noise
3. Decor, i.e., tone and colour scheme, soft furnishings
4. Common hazards, e.g., used needles, infected dressings, etc.
5. Ward routine
6. Record-keeping
7. Philosophy of nursing care
8. Duty rota

Ventilation in the Ward

Ventilation, whether natural or via extractor fans, should ensure a complete change of air every 20 minutes. Offensive odours can be very noticeable at night and early in the morning when windows are closed tight against uncomfortable draughts. A simple carpentry adjustment of the window casement, however, may be enough to have the window open without the inconvenience of a draught.

The abundant use of aerosol air freshener is not an answer to the problem of poor ventilation. It rather implies the ward manager does not know how to requisition for the maintainence staff to inspect and repair structural defects.

Noise

Noise can be controlled, but it requires a disciplined approach during an average working day. A great deal of ward noises come from telephones, trollies, vacuum cleaners, loud radio volume, and swinging doors. These noises are further intensified by the hustle and bustle of nursing, domestic, paramedical and medical staff as they go about the multiplicity of tasks, usually all condensed into a few hours during the morning. Ward telephones are notoriously busy during the first period of the morning and it is a useful idea to have these equipped with a light-up button rather than the usual ringing tone bell.

A good ward manager will insist quite firmly on a quiet period during the day so that the patients can rest and have some respite from the noise and distraction of normal ward activity. Night noises are often exaggerations of the day noises which have gone unnoticed during the day and nursing staff should remember that while they may accept a great deal of background noises inherent in their working environment, such noises are anathema to the patient. Noises emanating from high technology machinery are a case in point.

Decor

Colour schemes, the tone of decor and soft furnishings of a ward make a considerable difference to creating a calming atmosphere. Soft pastel shades, contrasted for visual interest, have a calming effect. Large areas of one colour are boring, and garish colours tend to actually raise the blood pressure. Although the colour schemes may not be the actual remit of the nurse, the staff need to be aware that colour plays an important part in the psychology of the working environment. The ingenious use of interesting or humourous posters can often break the bleak prospect of huge areas of single colour, However, it is bad policy to have official bulletin boards in the patient's direct vision.

Common Hazards

The hazards which are common to many acute general wards are listed below, but the qualified nurse should be aware of the Health and Safety Act 1974 and the amendments made in 1982. This act requires that both employers and employees draw any identifiable hazards in their working environment to the attention of the Health and Safety Officer. This official is also employed in the same building and his or her name should be known to permanent staff. This officer also has the right to inspect any ward at any time to check for the presence of hazards.

A hazard, in this sense, implies a risk to anyone's health or safety. In hospital, a greater dimension for any hazard would be in addition to a patient's illness. Staff cannot use ignorance as an excuse for not dealing with a known hazard or ignoring a potential hazard. Equally they cannot claim ignorance of the existing hospital policy with regard to health and safety.

Visitors to hospitals are often advised or guided by directional signs such as 'No Smoking', 'No Entry', 'Restricted Area–No Visitors' and 'Isolation Nursing–No Visitors'. These signs are in fact protecting the visitor against potential risks to their own health and safety. Table 84.1 details the hazards to staff and patients in an acute ward of a general hospital.

In specialised units the hazards may be

Table 84.1. Typical hazards to staff and patients in an acute ward of a general hospital

Hazard	Risk	Prevention
Used needles	Hepatitis	Disposal in Sharps box
Used scalpel blades	Cuts and hepatitis	Disposal in Sharps box
Infected dressings	Cross-infection	Disposal for incineration
Unlabelled drug containers	Incorrect medication	Return to pharmacy
Electric plugs	Shock and burns	Frequent checks
Oxygen points	Combustion	No smoking or naked flames
Infusion fluids	Infection	Insist on checking system
Locked fire doors	Suffocation by smoke	Clear access at all time
Confused patient	Accidental injury	Cotsides, nursing supervision
Floor spillage	Accidental fall	Immediate mopping
Radium, radioactive needles	Anaemia, etc.	Protective portable lead screens

related to the type of patient, e.g., paediatric, geriatric, obstetric, psychiatric and mentally handicapped. The qualified nurse must then apply common sense to the situation and assess environmental risks to the patients and themselves. In addition to working on this problem the nurse should also be aware of the hospital's policy in the event of an accident. This usually requires the patient or staff member involved to be examined by the doctor on call and to have any investigations or X-rays to confirm or eliminate diagnosis of an injury. An accident or 'unusual incident' form should then be completed, signed by the doctor and a nurse witness, and sent to the nursing officer of the unit. It is usual for the incident to be investigated to see if such accidents can be prevented in the future.

Routine

The typical pattern of the day on the ward revolves around fixed 'times'. The patient's day, even in a typical, chaotic busy ward has fixed time for meals, medical rounds and visiting when nursing activity is at a minimum. From such fixed points a great deal of the actual nursing work has to be fitted in, and direct physical care planned, so that it dovetails with the demands of imposed organisational times. Many argue that the nursing care can be equitably spaced over the whole working day, but this in fact ignores several realities. For instance, hospital departments usually arrange that their workloads are concentrated in the morning, leaving the afternoon free for outpatient commitments. Logically, therefore, the nurse may well find that the patients for theatre, physiotherapy, X-ray, discharge, admission, and other investigations, are all timed for the morning. This leads to a greater nursing workload being concentrated in the morning, whether the nurse likes it or not. It also means that the majority of nurses are required to be on duty in the morning. Therefore, it is obvious that there are very few nursing duties that can be spaced over the whole working day. Trials show that patients much prefer their bedbaths in the morning, not in the afternoon, so even this aspect of care cannot be readily shifted to a quieter part of the day.

Record-keeping

Nursing responsibility for records is quite exacting, even where a ward clerk is in post. In the final analysis it is the nurse that accepts responsibility for good records. The typical array of documents with which the qualified nurse should be familiar are:

- Nursing care history sheets
- Nursing care plans
- Observation charts
- Diet sheets
- Medication charts
- Requisition forms for ambulances, district nurse services
- Request forms for all investigations
- Bed state status

With regard to a patient's file, the nurse should appreciate that these are in fact doctors' notes about the patient. The notes do not belong to the patient, but to the examining physician, and as such are confidential to the employing authority and the doctor. Such records as are compiled during a patient's stay in hospital may be retained for up to 10 years, even after the patient's death. Equally, documentation relating to actual admissions and discharges, or pharmaceutical requisitions are also kept for several years and should only be discarded on the advice of the unit nursing officer.

Philosophy of Nursing Care

An experienced nurse should be quite clear about the underlying philosophy which determines the approach to and the giving of nursing care. The majority of newly qualified nurses would expect the nursing process philosophy to be in operation. This particular philosophy meets the demands of 'total care' in that the nurse looks at the patient as a person, *not* as a disease or a fracture or whatever causes the person to require nursing care.

In this process of nursing, the patient is carefully assessed to assist the nurse in planning the kind and amount of care that is needed. The delivery, or implementing, of care follows the plan. The nursing care is evaluated at regular intervals to determine whether the expected goals are being achieved or whether the care plan must be revised to achieve those goals.

Social, psychological and spiritual needs have equal importance to physical distress. To ensure 'total care', nursing management has to shift away from task allocation to nurse–patient allocation, with the intention of tailoring a care plan to meet the individual needs of each individual patient.

Duty Rota

One ward managerial task which requires careful planning is the duty rota; a poorly planned rota leads to a great deal of contention. To promote an atmosphere of fairness to both permanent and learning nursing staff, some basic principles related to shift-type work may be followed. These principles are common to all types of hospital and all nursing specialties, and integrate a number of important philosophical issues:

1. Inexperienced or learning staff should **never** be left unsupervised, though they may be left alone. For example, a student nurse may be left alone for short periods, but must be directly supervised by a fully qualified nurse within the unit (if not actually on the ward). This often occurs on night duty.
2. If student nurses are to learn, then they must actually work with a staff nurse, preferably in a team arrangement. This can be reflected in the duty rota.
3. The duty rota can be markedly influenced by the nursing style practised on the ward. If, for instance, primary nursing is practised, then several patients are assigned to a staff nurse and his or her team from admission to hospital until discharge. The team's duty rota would reflect their continuous commitment to their group of patients. Alternatively, if team nursing is practised then 1 of possibly 2 ward teams would accept responsibility for a given number of beds or rooms. In either case, however, primary or team nursing would mean that the staff nurse leading the teams would have the authority over the plan of nursing care implemented. To this extent, the duty rota may be plotted around their commitment.
4. Job, or task, allocation is now unusual in acute wards of general hospitals because of the adherence to the nursing process. The former, however, may still have some relevance in high dependency units where 'tasks' may be highly specialised and only possible for those trained in expert techniques.

Guidelines for Implementing a Rota

Several principles which may help the newly qualified staff nurse to negotiate a duty rota and to understand its structure are contained in the following guidelines:

1. A registered nurse must be in control of each shift.

2. There should, as far as possible, be an equal distribution between staff and student nurses working on each shift.

3. There should be a balance between experienced and inexperienced nursing staff working on each shift.

4. Busy days, such as admission days, operation days and major medical rounds, require a higher proportion of nursing staff on duty.

5. Weekend and evening 'on duty' should be fairly distributed among full-time nursing staff; certainly weekends off should be rotated, and it is usually possible to ensure 1 weekend off in 4.

6. To calculate a fair distribution of days off, the total number of days off required by all full-time staff in 1 week is divided by 7, the resulting figure is the number of nurses that can be off at any one time. If at all possible, days off should be taken together and be preceded by an evening off and followed by a morning off. This is not always possible for qualified staff who must be the first to accept unpopular off duty, as they are ultimately responsible for the welfare of patients and are accountable for the ward.

7. There should be a continuous policy, whenever possible, of honouring 'special requests', providing they have been submitted for consideration well in advance of finalising the duty rota.

8. It is unusual and undesirable that nurses are made to work overtime, but nurses are expected to accept unsocial hours, for which they are paid.

9. The duty forecast should be completed one month ahead of schedule to allow nursing staff to organise their personal and social life and to remove any excuses for unnecessary requests, i.e., dental checks, optician visits, which staff are expected to organise in their own time. Permanent ward staff should have any holiday requests and entitlements at least planned, with a 3-month forecast to permit long-term planning with the unit nursing officer.

The following example may help potential staff nurses to familiarise themselves with planning a week's duty rota. It is suggested that a pencil be used, as there are on average over 12 changes before a reasonable rota which meets all the principles outlined above is achieved.

Exercise in Planning a Week's Duty Rota

As the most senior qualified nurse, you have to stand in for the ward sister who is ill. The unit nursing officer requests the duty rota for the following week. The nursing staff on the ward includes:

3 staff nurses
2 enrolled nurses
2 third-year student nurses
2 second-year student nurses
2 second-year pupil nurses
3 nursing auxiliaries who are contracted to work:

(a) Full-time 08.00–16.30 hrs Monday to Friday

(b) 09.00–15.00 hrs Monday to Friday

(c) 18.00–22.00 hrs Monday to Friday

The following circumstances have to be taken into account when formulating the duty rota:

One enrolled nurse has a long-standing request for the weekend off.

A second-year pupil nurse is owed 2 days off for working a recent bank holiday weekend.

The total hours worked by each nurse must not exceed $37\frac{1}{2}$ hours in 1 week, and it is ward policy that nurses do not work more than 2 evenings per week (excluding auxiliaries).

It is ward policy that days off are preceded by an evening off and followed by a morning off.

A third-year student nurse has a pre-arranged hospital admission scheduled for Tuesday, with hospital discharge on Friday.

A trained nurse must be on duty for each shift, i.e., learners are not left alone.

Table 84.2. Duty rota

Ward:	Week commencing:						
	Mon.	Tues.	Wed.	Thurs.	Fri	Sat.	Sun.
Sister	M	E	M	E	M	DO	DO
Staff nurse	DO	DO	E	M	E	M	E
Staff nurse	E	M	Rm 1–4 M	DO	DO	E	M
Rooms 1–4							
Staff nurse	M	E	E	M	M	DO	DO
3rd year student	M	DO	DO	E	E	M	E
2nd year student	E	M	E	M	M	DO	DO
2nd year pupil	E	M	M	DO	DO	E	M
Introductory course student	M	E	M	E	M	DO	DO
Nursing auxiliary	DO	DO	E	M	DO	E	M
Nursing auxiliary	Rm 5–8 07.30–13.30	07.30–13.30	DO DO	DO DO	16.30–21.30	07.30–13.30	DO DO
Rooms 5–8							
Enrolled nurse	E	M	E	M	M	DO	DO
Enrolled nurse	DO	17.00–21.30	07.30–13.00	DO	DO	17.00–21.30	07.30–13.00
3rd year student	M	DO	DO	E	E	M	E
1st year student	DO	E	E	M	DO	E	M
1st year pupil	M	M	DO	DO	E	M	E
Nursing auxiliary	DO	DO	07.30–13.00	07.30–13.00	07.30–13.00	DO	Rm 1–4 16.30–21.30
Nursing auxiliary	16.30–21.30	16.30–21.30	DO	16.30–21.30	16.30–21.30	DO	DO
Totals	7 5	6 6	6 6	7 5	6 6	5 5	5 5

M—Morning: E—Evening; DO—Day off; Rm—Rooms.

The ward has 36 beds, deals with general surgery and has admissions days on Monday and Thursday, with operating days on Tuesday and Friday.

Night duty is not applicable, as this is done on a separate staff basis by the night nursing officer.

Taking Table 84.2 as an example, on a blank sheet of paper first pencil in the facts that you do already know from the above list, and then finalise your duty rota.

CLINICAL ROLE

Clinical expertise in a given field of nursing is a continually developing aspect of the nurse's career as a professional. The preference or choice of a nursing speciality is usually made during training and does determine the specific skills which the nurse will want to develop. The model for clinical expertise should be the ward sister/charge nurse or an attached clinical nurse specialist.

Nurses should neither think of themselves as 'administrators' nor try to imitate the worst of all 'sins', which is to sit behind the nursing station directing the traffic through the ward doors. What is important to understand is that the nurse is in fact the *model* for the junior nurses.

Much of the learning of practical skills is done at the bedside, not in the school of nursing. Therefore, if junior nurses are to learn well, they must, of necessity, model their

Table 84.3. Nursing auxiliary training schedule

Admission, discharge and transfer of patients	Taking observations of
Care of patient's property	weight
Assisting with	pulse/temperature/respiration
bedmaking	Obtaining simple specimens
lifting	Basic urine testing
bedbathing	Deal with official telephone messages
toileting	Domestic duties related to
ambulation	locker tissues
hygiene	sluice areas
serving meals	stock cupboards
last offices	linen stock
Chaperone duties	correct disposal of rubbish
	basic clinical equipment
	patient's drinks

efforts on what is observed at the bedside. If bad habits are absorbed, especially in the first year of training, they will be difficult to unlearn, and will be transferred to other areas of work throughout the whole period of training.

The term *highest standard*, which is repeated in the job description, is deliberately used to draw attention to the fact that in the real situation, many factors may compound to prevent 'excellence'. Underlying any clinical procedure or care given, however, the term *safe* must, at least, be used. 'Safe' is the minimal standard which is acceptable for a learner. For the professional nurse, the standard expected should always be towards *excellence*.

In carrying out this major aspect of caring, the nurse also needs to appreciate the roles of all nurses and others on the ward team. Many hospitals employ a considerable number of auxiliaries. They may represent at least one-third of the total nursing staff. Nursing auxiliaries have no statutory training scheme, but are prepared for their duties by in-service training, organised by a training officer within the hospital. A typical training programme is shown in Table 84.3 to highlight those areas in which an auxiliary can be expected to function and make a contribution to the ward team.

The basic training programme outlined in Table 84.3 usually takes 5 days, with a further day's release for additional study as the auxiliary gains experience. As a permanent member of staff, an auxiliary nurse is a very stable influence and, correctly employed, can make a significant contribution for the staff nurse who is seeking to achieve a harmonious team effort.

In determining the clinical role, the staff nurse should also remember that the role of medical staff is quite specific, that is to diagnose, prognose and prescribe. Beyond helping with these three aims, the nurse should not continue to accept a subservient role as has been the habit in the immediate past.

ADMINISTRATION AND COORDINATION

The newly qualified nurse must develop leadership and communication skills, and coordinate the various aspects of patient care instigated from many sources in the health care team.

Leadership

The morale of the nursing team of any ward or department is a reflection of the style of leadership in current practice. A happy, cheerful *and* tidy ward reflects the efforts of the person in charge who while maintaining discipline:

Is approachable by all junior members of the ward staff

Table 84.4. Achieving a balanced leadership

Dos	Don'ts
Have a consistent attitude	Be temperamental
Set the example	Stay in the office
Communicate with staff	Ignore junior colleagues
Plan well ahead	Wait till the last minute
Delegate whenever possible	Do it all yourself
Be approachable	Appear flustered and overwhelmed
Involve the staff in decisions	Give orders without explanations
Say 'thank you' for a job well done	Accept hard work without acknowledgement
Request rather than order	Demand without grace or manners
Criticise constructively in private	Criticise destructively in public
Encourage team decisions	Impose personal decisions
Be supportive of all staff	Have favourites
Be impartial and fair	Be overfamiliar
Listen and assess	Listen and then ignore

Values and correctly ascertains the endeavours of the permanent ward staff

Interacts with colleagues in a professional manner

Defines the goals to be achieved and determines the priorities

Accepts the ultimate responsibility for standards of nursing care

Sets aside time to integrate new members of staff, to create a feeling of belonging

Has clinical expertise and standards of excellence in the speciality of care of the ward

Has a sense of justice *and* also of humour

Supervises the planned care, delegates according to ability, and sets aside time to teach the junior nursing staff

Attitudes

It is now generally accepted that patient care can be achieved only by the team approach, which involves all professionals in the health care team. Extending from this premise is that the style of leadership on the ward must follow democratic attitudes and principles. The days of the 'dragon' ward sister are long gone since the concept of team work was introduced.

Authoritarian and *laissez faire* attitudes in their extreme form are not suitable for nursing at ward level. The majority of individuals have within their personality some aspects of all three attitudes. The one which requires developing, if it is lacking, is that of democracy. The authoritarian personality does have a place, but it is usually in the higher echelons of the hospital nursing service. At these levels the responsibility for the overall performance and standard of nursing care does require a central figure who authoritatively sets the policy and framework in which nursing personnel carry out their work.

At times the *laissez faire* attitude can prove useful, when by standing back and letting someone get on with the job a higher performance is achieved than would be with constant badgering. However, the person who is naturally *laissez faire* is a positive danger in the acute wards of a general hospital.

In summary, given the vagaries of personality traits, the staff nurse is trying to achieve a balanced style of leadership which offers the best chance of maintaining if not actually improving standards of care (see Table 84.4).

The Do column in Table 84.4 can be worked on to improve leadership style, and leadership **can** be learned. With a conscientious effort, inherent or learned attitudes of authoritarianism and *laissez faire* can alter. The Don't column shows traits of the truly authoritarian figure which makes the personality rather disliked by both nurses and patients.

Another subtle point to note about the

authoritarian and *laissez faire* personalities is that, in the long run, such people are not trusted nor do they gain the respect of their professional colleagues. However, the more senior the nurse, the more the need to appreciate that responsibility carries with it natural authority over junior colleagues, if for no other reason than that experience places the staff nurse a little ahead of junior staff.

Assessing Time and the Actual Work Process

Apart from developing certain attitudinal behaviours, the staff nurse can look at how she or he exercises control over certain facets of the time spent at work and the actual work schedules. Time and the actual work process are two elements over which individuals can exercise positive control and should be assessed at regular intervals to see if the staff nurse is

Eliminating those tasks which can be safely delegated to junior colleagues

Planning well ahead and using foresight to anticipate the needs of the ward team

Avoiding overstaffing by giving detailed attention to the planning of the off duty to cut down on wasting her or his own and other nurses' time

Arranging spans or intervals of time which allow for adequate supervision of junior staff, coordination with departments and colleagues and communication

Knowing precisely the area of authority and responsibility which has been given to enable the task or work to be completed

Establishing the aim and goals to be achieved within a set interval of time

Evaluating, at regular intervals, the results and means of achieving the aims and goals

Identifying the personal contribution which can be made by each member of the team and then building on the strengths of peers, seniors and junior staff, as well as developing personal strengths

Being aware of personal limitations and seeking out expert opinion and help whenever necessary

Evaluating Leadership

The nurse manager is expected to get the right things done, in the right place and at the right time. Evaluating how well one is doing requires imagination, intelligence and knowledge. If the ward is working well and the ward is happy, then the leader should also take the compliment since it is hard work to achieve a harmonious working relationship. If progress is not being made and an individual feels unhappy about the leadership role, it is useful to ask the following questions about the work situation:

1. What is there in the work situation that prevents effective leadership? Is there anything you personally can do about it? Think of personality conflicts, lack of resources, clinical abilities or organisational morale.
2. Is your personal effectiveness reduced because seniors will not delegate, or is it because you are afraid to delegate or let go of control?
3. Are you absolutely clear in your mind about your degree of authority or responsibilities? Have these been discussed with you?
4. Are you personally allowed to allocate your time to the nursing work load and are you using your time effectively, or is it wasted gossiping in the office?
5. Can you identify the most important aspects of your job and can you give them a meaningful priority? If you can, are you decisive enough to follow through the implications of self-development?
6. How many hours, in the last month, have you devoted to keeping your professional knowledge up-to-date? Do the senior managers allow you time for professional updating?
7. When was the last time the ward sister/charge nurse or unit nursing officer assisted you with a counselling session on how well you were doing? What aspects of your work need developing?

Democratic Characteristics

If as an individual you are an effective leader, it follows that the nursing team will demonstrate certain characteristics which reflect well on the leader's personal efforts. These characteristics also reflect the democratic spirit and are usually obvious to patients, relatives and other hospital staff:

The *ward atmosphere* tends to be informal, comfortable and relaxed. There are no signs of boredom, tension, or apathy.

There is a great deal of *discussion* in which everyone takes part, but discussions are structured and always directed at reaching solutions to current problems.

Nursing *objectives* of the ward team are well understood and accepted by all team members.

Team members *listen* to each other and every idea is given a hearing. Individuals are not afraid of appearing foolish as the individual team members are supportive of each other.

Disagreements are expected. Oddly enough the team thrives on conflict rather than being threatened by it, since the management philosophy allows for the free expression of ideas and opinion.

There is *no tyranny* of, or by, any minorities.

Agreements are reached by informal *consensus*. Even at formal ward or unit meetings there is no formal voting.

The leader or team coordinator does *not dominate* the team, but allows the leadership to move from one individual to another depending on the expertise or knowledge which is required at any one time. In allowing leadership to move across the team, however, the leader does understand that she or he has ultimate responsibility for any decisions made.

Team members, in being *free to express* themselves, are psychologically comfortable and do not feel angry, frustrated or guilty when proposing changes.

The team is very conscious of their *identity* and will regularly examine how well they are achieving their aims and objectives.

Planning Time and Work Schedules

Experience is the greatest teacher of all in the correct use of time and in planning work schedules. In controlling these elements in the working situation the team leader must develop a sense of priority which helps to set the aims and goals of the day's work. In setting priorities, however, the staff nurse does need to know the roles and abilities of each member of the nursing team so that delegation is both effective and fair. The exercise in priority rating illustrates the need of selecting priorities and the staff to whom certain tasks can be delegated with some appreciation of the time factor which determines many nursing activities.

Exercise in Priority Rating

Imagine yourself as a staff nurse coming on duty at 07.45 hrs onto a 30-bedded general surgical unit. You are placed in charge for the morning and have a team of:

2 third-year student nurses
2 second-year pupil nurses
1 first-year student nurse
2 nursing auxiliaries
1 ward clerk

After receiving the night nurse's report, you find that your list incorporates 25 duties and tasks to be dealt with. Place these in a priority rating, bearing in mind that you have to work within the hospital's policy regarding pressure ulcers, patients' property, drug policy, hazards to health and the legal rights of patients.

1. Three patients are scheduled for surgery at 09.00 (i.e., premedication to be given).

2. The water bed has an electrical fault and had to be switched off during the night.

3. Two waiting-list patients are due for admission at 09.30.

4. The surgical registrar will do his or her patients' round at 09.30.

5. The nursing team have the daily ward report at 08.00.

6. Ward policy requires you to say Good Morning to every patient before commencing work.

7. Overnight observation charts have to be checked.

8. A day-case patient is due for admission at 09.15 and scheduled for surgery at 13.00.

9. Relatives of a seriously ill patient have stayed overnight in the unit's rest room.

10. The surgical dressing list has to be prepared.

11. A unit of blood is required for transfusion at 08.20 to a patient having intravenous therapy.

12. Two patients are due for abdominal X-ray at 09.15.

13. Two patients are to be transferred to the medical unit to make way for the 2 admissions.

14. Book an ambulance for 11.30 to take a patient home.

15. Urgent drugs are required to be collected from the pharmacy.

16. The ward is short of both sheets and pillow cases.

17. A patient wants to take his own discharge.

18. Night nurse has reported that a bedfast patient has developed a pressure ulcer.

19. A surgical corset is waiting for collection from the surgical applicance department.

20. Four introductory-course nurses are reporting to the ward at 08.30 for bedmaking practice.

21. Check that all the team members have reported on duty.

22. Breakfast commences at 07.50.

23. A patient has £50 which he wants to be made secure.

24. The unit administrator requires your bed state before 08.30.

25. Prescribed drugs are administered at 10.00.

A possible solution to this exercise in setting priorities is carefully to work out the times by which certain tasks have to be tackled and to put them into sequence. It would look something like:

07.50	6, 7, 9 and 22
08.00	1 (premedication due) and 5
08.20	24
08.30	20 and 23
09.00	1 (transfer to theatre)
09.15	12 and 18
09.30	3 and 4
10.00	25
11.30	14

Such a scheme, however, deals with only 16 of the 25 priorities listed, Nevertheless, it is a first step before beginning the process of delegation according to a team member's ability and role. A second step is to divide the team into working pairs and delegate as set out below, which is not necessarily correct but is one option for consideration.

Team Structure of Groups

A. Staff nurse to work with senior student (an essential partnership for checking procedures)

B. Senior student to work with junior student

C. Pupil nurses to work with auxiliaries

D. Pupil nurse to work with auxiliary

E. Ward clerk to work on his or her own, reporting to staff

Group	*Priorities delegated*
A.	1, 4, 5, 6, 7, 9, 11, 17, 24 and 25 (all contain an essential checking system by a fully qualified member of staff)
B.	8, 10, 18, 20 and 22
C.	2, 13 and 16
D.	3 and 12
E.	14, 15, 17 and 24 (these are essentially non-nursing activities)

COMMUNICATIONS

Effective communication within and extending from the staff of a ward will depend on the person in charge possessing a democratic style of leadership. It is relatively straightforward to analyse the communication which goes on between 2 people, and the techniques each uses to get messages across. Communication becomes more complex when the message has to be delivered to a group or team of nurses, and its effectiveness requires to be tested at regular intervals.

Successful communication at a personal level requires a balance of when to be formal and, alternatively, when to use informality. Interaction with a multiplicity of professional groups, such as found in a hospital, requires the use of formality and technical language. The language at the bedside, however, is usually informal and in layman's terms.

The expectations various people have will greatly influence the communication, even before a word has been said. Patients, relatives and doctors expect a nurse in uniform to speak with professional demeanour. When a nurse is speaking officially to a peer group, the expectation is for professional terminology as well as professional manners. Informal conversations are quite usual and normal in nurse-to-nurse or nurse-to-patient conversations. Professional contacts and those with strangers, however, should always be commenced on a very formal basis as the expectation if not met will hinder and interfere with good communication.

The principal means of conveying information are: verbal, non-verbal and written.

Verbal

Formal direct communication requires the voice to be pleasantly modulated, have clear enunciation, and maintain a moderate speed of delivery. The tone of speech reflects the individual's current emotional feelings. Quiet, slow and monotonous speech may indicate feelings of depression. Barely audible speech may denote shyness or anxiety. Shrill rapid speech might indicate anger or frustration, while a garbled hurried speech may denote excitement. These differing tones of speech may actually cue the listener's first verbal response, so that what is said may be what the listener thinks the speaker wants to hear rather than giving the reply or answer to the statement made.

Formality should be used when ward reports are given on the patient's progress. The use of slang terms is unprofessional and unwise, as junior nurses may take a term as being correct or acceptable and incorporate it into their reports or even use it in test papers.

When a nurse answers the telephone, clarity and delivery of speech are very important for both speaker and listener, especially if giving or receiving technical data. The increasing use of answering telephone machines requires the verbal message to be thought out in advance and unusual words may require to be spelt out syllable by syllable, creating a new significance for correct spelling.

Informal conversations with patients should be stripped of professional jargon and slang. Many patients, and this includes those in the professional classes, are confused by nursing or medical terminology. The use of terms such as *anticoagulants*, *dyspnoea*, *halitosis*, *thrombosis*, *saturated fats* or *cytotoxic drugs* may sound clever, but will in fact inhibit further conversation because the patient is too shy or too bewildered to work out the implications of what is being said. When people are bewildered, it is not too surprising if they become uncooperative. The fact is they cannot cooperate if they are confused.

When attempting to counsel a patient about future health care, the nurse should give careful thought on how to structure the statements. Conversations should finish with an open-ended statement which invites a response. Questions such as: Do you understand? invite either Yes or No answers, and are closed-ended statements. Whereas: Can you think of any problems? might invite more elaborate responses.

It is a common experience of many nurses that, despite careful explanation, the patient does not understand a thing which has been said. This might be because the nurse has given the information at the wrong time and taken too long about it. It is better to choose a quiet period of the day and give new information in small amounts, not usually any longer than 10 minutes, and return to the patient at a later time for further follow-up. There is a reference from education which can be used to guide the nurse, it is: 'Tell them, tell them you've told them, and tell them again'. The statement implies that the average listener needs to be told a piece of new information 3 times before the implications begin to sink in.

It is equally important to test people's understanding of verbal communication. This is especially true of junior nursing staff who are not familiar with the language of hospitals, or yet firmly acquainted with nursing terminology. Verbal nursing orders should be made clear and very precise so that the care given is that which is actually intended.

Non-verbal Communication

There are at least five aspects of the individual which can be visually assessed very quickly before a word is spoken. The nurse *must* appreciate that the two-way impression taking place can cue verbal responses and does influence the attitudes during a conversation. Put simply, what is being thought is not reflected in what is being said, although the physical attitudes may indicate this.

Facial and Eye Muscles

Facial and eye muscles do indicate emotional feelings. It is very difficult not to register pleasure or displeasure by reflexly narrowing or dilating the pupil of the eye. Equally, the facial muscles and those of the neck do indicate if the individual is curious, angry, depressed, or is showing concern.

Studies show that responses are influenced by as much as 70% of what we see at any one moment. It is logical, therefore, to follow through this premise by saying that nurses working at the bedside indicate to patients much more with their face and eyes than they do with their voice. It would also be correct to assume that a person's sincerity and honesty is usually judged by their face rather than by what he or she says.

Body Posture

Body posture also indicates what the individual is actually feeling or thinking. A slouched posture may be taken for tiredness, or boredom. Sitting and leaning forward should not necessarily be taken as familiarity, but might indicate intellectual interest. Upright and purposeful walking is usually indicative of determination and optimism. Mannerisms such as rubbing the hands together invariably means anxiety, while sweeping gesticulations usually imply excitability.

Dress Style

Dress style creates an immediate visual impact. The carelessly attired nurse with unpolished shoes and an uncontrolled hairstyle speaks volumes about the nurse's professional attitude. The implication of an unprofessional appearance is that the person is uncaring, but this may not in fact be true. It might, however, indicate something even worse, i.e., the nurse's self-image is totally disorganised. Doctors are also judged by how they appear. The open coat with the swinging stethoscope might imply more of an ego than it does of professionalism.

Touch

While touch is a more subtle communication, it is a vital non-verbal signal. The handshake is often taken to indicate the degree of friendliness or of nervousness, depending on the strength of the handgrip. Patients often indicate their preference for certain nurses because of their gentleness and careful techniques when touching, moving, turning or lifting. It is odd to think that the most popular nurse might be the one with the least to say simply because the expectation of a nurse is fully met by being gentle during the giving of physical care. Those nurses who are rough and heavy in handling their patients may be tolerated, but are often branded by patients as being uncaring.

Odours

Odours of the body can influence communication quite remarkably. Unpleasant body odours from infected sputum, excreta and soiling not only distress the patient but subdue their normal communication skills. By showing repugnance, however slight, the nurse destroys the patient's confidence to communicate. This in turn establishes a vicious circle in which the patient becomes trapped. The nurse signalling displeasure by facial expression may actually create guilt feelings in the patient.

Equally, nurses who have a strong unpleasant body odour, made worse by disguising it with strong cologne, are telling both colleagues and patients that their personal hygiene habits are wanting. Working in close physical contact as nurses do, their breath odour may create a great deal of upset and if offensive, it is guaranteed to halt any possibility of conversation.

Written Communication

The majority of nurses in training usually possess an 'O' level in English language or literature. This implies a command of spelling, legibility, grammar and syntax. The written word is a constant factor in nurse training with the many tests and examinations, and in formal reports on patient's histories, care plans and school of nursing projects. Surprisingly, a reader can tell a great deal about the personality of the writer by glancing at facets such as clarity, legibility, the logical sequence of facts, and the neatness of the total presentation. A good example of this is how neat and tidy the ward bulletin board is kept. Scruffy paper with scrappy messages invites the thought that whoever is in charge is rather thoughtless about the image being presented to ward visitors, and to the nurses in training.

Gunning's Ten Principles provide a good basic approach to clear writing:

1. Keep sentences short; a good rule is that a single sentence should never exceed 17 words.
2. Prefer the simple to the complex word.
3. Prefer the familiar to the far-fetched word.
4. Avoid unnecessary words, i.e., keep to the point and keep it short.
5. Put action into verbs, e.g., 'You will see by reading', rather than, 'Perusal of the attached document'.
6. Make full use of variety.
7. Write as you talk, but check your spelling.
8. Use short concrete words, not abstract terms.
9. Relate to the reader's experience, i.e., if writing for nurses bear in mind the common experience of all nurses is their basic training.
10. Write to express not to impress.

PERSONNEL COORDINATION

Increasingly, ward sisters/charge nurses and staff nurses are moving away from the traditional concept of hierarchical leaders to that of health care coordinators. Research into the actual reality of a ward sister's/charge nurse's work shows that the majority of working time is given over to liaison with other health care professionals. This is in addition to the coordination of the ward staff and with nursing departments such as the school of nursing.

Success in this sphere of work requires deep insight into the individual needs of patients, as well as which part of the communication network requires tapping. Secondly, there is the need to know in considerable detail the names and ranks of the nursing and medical hierarchy. Unfortunately, many of these figureheads have particular idiosyncrasies which may or may not impede successful coordination. Figure 84.1 illustrates how the roles of nursing staff are coordinated.

In the main, liaison work requires a well-thought-out plan of action before any contacts are made. If unsure, then the liaison the nurse seeks is one of advice. Many failures in liaison work are due to making a verbal request and then not following it through with a written request. A second but equally obvious failure is bad manners. Simply saying

Please and Thank You and remaining objective achieves far more than always expecting other professionals to keep their verbal promises. Losing one's temper or becoming ruffled impedes liaison work, as does inadequate explanation of what is expected or required.

A familiar example of coordination is when a student or pupil nurse wishes to take a practical assessment examination on the ward. The coordination begins with the request from the learner to the ward sister. Broad details are discussed on a suitable time, patient and examiner. When finalised, these broad details are narrowed down to precise times and date with the examiner and patient. Since it is an exam in the literal sense, all the ward staff have to be informed. This includes medical staff if they are about on that day. After the exam the learner has to be informed of the results in writing, as does the ward sister and the school of nursing. At the end of this coordinating exercise it would be unusual if at least 15 people were not involved in one nurse's exam. If the learner is referred for a second attempt, the coordination increases to involve more senior nurses. On the other hand, failure to communicate and coordinate exact times and dates to those involved can be disruptive and unsettling not only for the examinee but for the patient and nurse colleagues on the ward.

A second example would be for the nurse to examine in detail the amount of coordination required to discharge from hospital-to-home a patient who requires community nursing services.

Chapter 85
The Ward as a Learning Environment

If the style of nursing management practised on the ward contributes to good standards of patient care, then it is self-evident that the ward environment is most suitable for nurse learners. It is the finding of research, if not of logical thought, that where you find a good example you will also find a willing disciple. These two factors, along with good nursing management and being the example or model on which learners can base their learning, are the foundation for a learning environment.

The next step would be to identify what a student or pupil nurse could learn during a specified period of allocation. There are a number of ways of tackling this problem:

1. Identify the obvious factual elements or clinical skills particular to one nursing speciality.
2. Identify how long it takes the average individual to acquire the particular skill or depth of reading or studying required for understanding.
3. Since nurses may arrive on the ward at various points during a 2- or 3-year training period, it is usually necessary to grade the expectations downwards according to how junior the nurse is.
4. Having performed these basic steps, it is necessary to translate what can be learned into objectives.

For the purpose of education, an *objective* is a word that identifies a desirable nursing behaviour which the learner should have achieved by the end of a training period. Some objectives are achieved quickly, other behaviours take the full training period. Many managers emphasize that nurses are *doers*.

While this is undoubtedly so, it is a great pity that it is at the expense of understanding why things are 'done' a certain way. All wards should have posted on a bulletin board the nurse learners' objectives so that all members of staff are aware of the basic education programme for a particular ward.

MEDICAL UNIT LEARNING OBJECTIVES (JUNIOR NURSES)

The objectives are divided into 3 sections:

The basic skills relevant to medical nursing, which the junior nurses should achieve with efficiency and proficiency.

Objectives which are potentially possible if the junior nurse has achieved the basic skills relevant to medical nursing.

Objectives Record Sheet. The learner nurse can tick as and when the objectives are seen to be achieved by a supervising nurse, and when the junior nurse verbally expresses proficiency in a particular area.

Basic Skills Relevant to Medical Nursing

At the end of a medical allocation the junior nurse should be proficient in:

1. Taking and recording observations of temperature, pulse and respiration; blood pressure; apex beat; urinalysis; fluid balance.

2. Admit either emergency or waiting-list patients, conforming to ward and hospital policy.

3. Plan for and provide the nursing skills necessary to maintain the hygiene of a bedfast patient.

4. Plan for and provide the nursing skills necessary to prevent the complications of prolonged bedrest, where necessary using nursing aids correctly.

5. Assess the sanitary needs of a patient and provide the appropriate nursing measures to improve or maintain bowel and bladder function.

6. Obtain specimens of urine, faeces, sputum and wound swabs for pathology investigations according to medical instructions and ward policy.

7. Administer oxygen therapy as prescribed, using the various oxygen masks correctly, while showing a regard for the safety precautions that must be followed.

8. Follow the checking procedure necessary before the administration of prescribed drugs, with a regard for the safety precautions that may be necessary with particular drugs, making observations and ensuring that the reporting of drug effects are made at regular intervals.

9. Recognise the signs of imminent cardiac arrest and know the procedure to instigate for emergency resuscitation. To be able to demonstrate a working knowledge and manipulative skill in handling the emergency equipment, i.e., oxygen, suction, cardiac monitor, cardiac defibrillator, and be able to quote the common drugs necessary at such a time.

Possible Objectives

At the end of a medical allocation the junior nurse should be able to:

1. Conduct the initial assessment of a newly admitted patient and be able to plan and implement a basic programme of nursing care for patients who are: unconscious, paralysed, hypertensive, anaemic, diabetic, thyrotoxic or myxoedemic, breathless, or suffering from heart disease, pulmonary embolism, ulcerative colitis, deep-vein thrombosis, or peptic ulceration. Then report back to senior colleagues on a patient's progress in relation to the nursing care, and evaluate the care given at frequent intervals.

2. Prepare a patient physically and psychologically, and assemble the necessary equipment for the following procedures:

Venepuncture
Arterial puncture
Intravenous infusion
Nasogastric aspiration and feeding
Urinary catheterisation
Oxygen and steam inhalation therapy
Cardiac monitoring
Suppositories and enemas
Sigmoidoscopy

Nursing skill	Patient preparation	Necessary equipment	Conduct of procedure	After-care of patient	Signature of nurse Student	Qualified
1. Take and record						
pulse						
blood pressure						
apex beat						
respiration						
temperature						
urinalysis						
fluid balance						
2. Admit patient						
emergency						
waiting list						
transfer						
care for relatives						
3. Maintain hygiene						
dependant bed-bath						
assisted bathing						
care of						
skin						
mouth						
nose						
eyes						
nails						
hair						
4. Correct techniques for						
lifting						
moving						
turning						
5. Specimen collection						
sputum						
faeces						
blood						
urine						
vomitus						
wound swab						
gastric aspirate						
6. Inhalant therapy						
oxygen						
steam						
aerosol drugs						
7. Drugs						
storage						
records						
checking						
ordering						
administration						
8. Isolation technique						
ward policy						
protocols						
9. Cardiac arrest						
equipment						
drugs						
procedure						
10. Special investigations *Itemise*						
11. Special diets *Itemise*						
12. Special procedures *Itemise*						
13. Patient discharge						
to home						
to convalescence						

Fig. 85.1 Example of a record sheet.

Lumbar puncture
Bone marrow puncture
Chest aspiration

Assist the senior nurse and physician in carrying out the above procedures, giving the relevant nursing care throughout and following a specific procedure.

3. Explain to a patient in a reassuring manner what the following investigations entail and carry out the necessary preparation for:

Barium meal
Barium enema
Intravenous pyelogram
Endoscopy
Venograms
24-hour urine collections

4. Give both verbal and written reports on the patients in the nurse's care, being able to clarify the patients' psychological and physical responses to treatment and nursing care, and to make suggestions on further care.

Objectives Record Sheet

An Objectives Record Sheet must be constantly maintained and ticked by the learner. It must then be reviewed with a senior colleague at the conclusion of the medical nursing experience. Figure 85.1 provides a typical example of an Objective Record Sheet.

REPORTING ON A PATIENT'S PROGRESS

The giving and receiving of reports on a patient's progress, while excellent opportunities for the exchange of information, are also regarded as periods of learning time for nurse learners.

Question-and-Answer Session

Apart from the basic information, which must be included at such times, the main report of the day should include an opportunity for the learners to ask questions and to be questioned on their assumed knowledge of the patients in their care.

If giving a report to a group of learners, and time allowing, at least 5 minutes should be given by the nurse manager to test the group's awareness. If this is the management style then the new staff nurse needs to develop an awareness of how to structure a 5-minute question-and-answer session.

One method of doing this is to direct an open-ended question to the whole group, pause for a few seconds to give the group a chance to reflect on the question, then name an individual in the group to answer the question. If the answer is correct, give praise without being patronising. If it is incorrect, counsel without being destructive. During such a question-and-answer session ensure that everyone in the group is given one question to answer, and also has the opportunity to ask questions of the nurse leader.

Eventually it becomes part of the management style to include questions into the running of the ward so that the environment never becomes static or taken for granted, i.e., a learning environment. If you are asked a question to which the answer is not known, then it is best to say you don't know, but make every effort to find out and return to the questioner within 24 hours with what you have been able to find out.

TEXT BOOKS

Wards designated for nurse learners should carry professional texts on the specialty of care. General texts may only have vague reference to unusual aspects of exotic or rare conditions. The urgency of information required can on occasions only be found in highly specialised texts.

Specialised or generalised textbooks over 10 years old should not be relied upon. If the preparation time of the text is added, the book is more likely to contain information that is 12 years old. The nurses who have recently qualified are often the most aware of the currently published, generalised texts. Nurses working for the Postbasic Clinical Studies certificates are an excellent source for information about highly specialised textbooks.

The local school of nursing librarian and the Library Committee will invariably have the publishers' catalogues or list titles of recent publications. Both generalised and specialised reference should also be made to the main bookseller in the town or city. Many hospitals have special trust funds set aside for such amenities, created by benefactors. The unit administrator usually has the details of how to gain access to any monies or trust funds set aside for trained nursing staff.

TUTORIALS OR 'TEACH-INS'

One or two afternoons a week are usually set aside for the learner nurses either to have tutorials from clinical teachers or 'teach-ins' from the trained nurses. If a staff nurse is asked to help with such a teach-in it is absolutely necessary to know the precise title or subject and the amount of time being allocated for the topic. It is worthwhile establishing what resources are available on the ward itself when preparing the *how* of a teach-in.

Use of Resources Available

The Patient

The patient is the best of all visual aids, but should be the *last* to be used. If it is essential to use the patient, his or her express permission should have been previously obtained. Under no circumstances should a very ill patient be used as a model for teaching purposes. Only reference to a particular patient may be made during discussions, but always with discretion.

Patients' Notes

Patients' notes are an invaluable source of information and learning material. They are useful material on which to base a question-and-answer session. The notes written as they are in abbreviated but medical terminology, make a good starting point for introducing learners to the systematic approach used to examine the body systems, the investigations common to illness, the therapeutic aims, and the nursing plan of care dependent on the medical regimen. However, as with the patient, the case notes must be used with the greatest discretion and never at the bedside.

Observation Charts

Observation charts are a most useful means of testing knowledge about normal physiological values and as a basis for discussing anatomy. Above all, they are useful for getting the nurse learner to see the relationship between normal and abnormal readings, and then discussing the effect of such abnormalities on body tissues and organs before relating this back to the nursing care which has been implemented to relieve distress.

Professional Literature

Nursing magazines, pharmaceutical literature, professional textbooks and prescription charts are very helpful when discussing drug therapy. It is now almost impossible to remember by rote anything about the complexity of the new drugs. The advice given is for the learner nurse to concentrate only on *commonly* and *frequently* prescribed drugs, until they know exactly what to look for when administering drugs.

Environment

Teach-ins, tutorials, or counselling sessions should never be given at the bedside. The difference should be made between supervised practice which is always at the bedside, but explanations carry their own implications and should always be away from the patient. A small office, or room off the main ward is ideal; it should have suitable lighting, seating, and good ventilation. The room should be booked for the required time so that there are no interruptions.

Preparation of Material

A rough guideline for preparing the material for a teach-in so that it can be successfully presented is to divide the material into two stages: setting the objectives and planning the presentation.

Setting Objectives

What do I wish the nurses to achieve by the end of the presentation? This requires very precise listing. In other words, what do you want the nurses to think, remember and do, and can it be tested, i.e., can the nurse answer a structured question? What are the limitations placed on the session? Be sure you know the audience number, venue, how much time you have been allotted, and a quite detailed breakdown of the subject matter. One of the limitations placed on a staff nurse in the ward situation is that visual aids are invariably very 'limited'.

Planning the Presentation

When planning the presentation, think about what you want to say. Then, using a horizontal plan, take a large sheet of paper, turn it sideways and section it into 3 main columns so that you have a beginning, middle and a conclusion to any plan you construct. Always have the total plan in complete visual view.

Almost any subject can be subdivided into main sections. Each section you think of takes a main heading. Under each main heading, make a vertical list of all the points you want to talk about. Asterisk or underline those points for which you have any supporting material, graphs or statistics. Identify on your list those headings which require you to do some checking over or pursue with more research.

The next 4 steps are very important:

1. Mark the points of greatest importance to your stated objective. These must be included in your talk.

2. Mark those points of least relevance to your objective, but reserve them as items of interest. They can be ignored if timing is rather short.

3. From this preliminary draft of information you must now select your points of interest and put them into a logical sequence of presentation. Whatever else you may do, it is essential to be logical in presentation of any type of material.

4. Draw up your final plan with the sections 'points' laid out in logical sequence, placing the points of greatest interest first and those of least importance last.

Secondly, think about how you want to present your information. Using the final draft of the horizontal plan, sketch in the time required for each section. This time can only be estimated, but in educational terms it usually takes 10 minutes to create an interest. The concentration time of most audiences is about 20 minutes, with a further 10 minutes for open discussion and questions. Therefore, never anticipate longer than 50 minutes. Mark the horizontal plan with these details:

1. Which parts can be enhanced by a 'handout'? These should be used sparingly on the wards.

2. Is any of the time to be devoted to the nurse group doing an 'activity'?

3. Are slides, photographs, or articles, to be used? If so, are they legible, clear and neat?

4. Integrate each section by 'linking'. This usually requires the staff nurse to think clearly about:

The introduction of the topic, self, how long it will take and what points you want the nurses to concentrate on

Summarising each section when it is completed

Carefully structuring your conclusions and making sure they are related to your originally stated objective

Transferring your main headings of each section onto cards which can be easily handled and carried in the pocket. (These are most useful when the keynote for such sessions on a hospital ward is informality.)

Always prepare your notes yourself, write on one side of the card only, never use flimsy paper if you have decided to write your notes in full script. Use different colours to mark significant places in cards or notes for timing, slides, photographs, summaries, etc. However hard you have worked to prepare yourself, a rehearsal is absolutely vital, and it can be used to test the acoustics of the room, to remove any problems relating to furniture, ventilation and seating arrangements, and to check the timing. Rehearsal will also increase confidence in the prepared material which means you can then concentrate on building up a relationship with the nurse learners.

Giving the Presentation

During the presentation keep an eye on the time, slowing down or speeding up according to your own plan. Things may go wrong. If they do, it is best to treat it lightly and humorously. If possible avoid embarrassment by blushing or becoming angry with yourself. Always value questions from any group member, no matter how silly they may seem; with a little experience it is possible to utilise questions to strengthen the points you are trying to make in the presentation. At the end of your presentation remind the nurse learners of the original objective by giving a summary of your conclusions.

After the talk, or teach-in, there is always a sense of anticlimax. This is to be expected as the adrenaline stops pumping around the body. Postpresentation 'flop' is quite a common experience.

After any class, it is essential to clear up any materials used, or equipment which is borrowed; this must be returned to its place. Leave the room as you would wish to find it. Before assessing how well you presented your material, wait for a day or so before asking the nurses what they remembered of the teach-in. If you have made some impression, take the compliment to heart because one successful presentation soon leads to another success. The higher you climb in your career as a manager the more often you will be called on to give a presentation of one sort or another to many different groups of people, and to a wider audience. It is, therefore, worthwhile making a good effort in the early days of your managerial career.

MONITORING LEARNER PROGRESS ON THE WARDS

Learner nurses are always concerned about their progress on the wards. They tend to overrate their written progress reports, placing them above scores achieved in theoretical exams. Monitoring a learner's progress over a defined period of time requires the person in charge to have a clear policy towards nurse learners allocated to the ward. To monitor progress, at least 3 interviews are necessary with the learner.

The First Interview

The first interview is merely an introductory exploration with the learner about the ward objectives. It presents the learner with the opportunity to mention needs with regard to assessments, off duty, or projects to be completed as part of school work.

The Second Interview

The second interview should be arranged at the midpoint of the learner's allocated time on the ward. Such an interview need take only several minutes, and it should be with the ward sister. It is an opportunity for discussion to note those points where the learner feels hindered, or where the staff nurse or ward sister/charge nurse can see that improvement needs to be made.

Clinical skills **must** be positively assessed, perhaps by the staff nurse who is the team leader. It is a point of professional duty that a junior colleague not making satisfactory progress (and who represents a danger to the welfare of patients) must be counselled at this point of allocation.

The school of nursing would also have a policy guideline about learners who are not making progress and it is usual and desirable to inform the learner's personal tutor at an early opportunity. If asked, a staff nurse or ward sister/charge nurse should have the conviction to offer a written statement to the effect that a learner is failing to make satisfactory progress.

The Final Interview

The final interview is usually scheduled to take place in the last week of the allocation and is a wide-ranging discussion on both positive and negative aspects of the nurse's progress while on the ward. It is unfair and unwise to complete these progress reports without the learner being present. Equally, it is unprofessional to ask a learner to sign the report unless the person who completed it is also present. Many problems arise if there is an unfair report submitted to the school of nursing. The problem usually revolves around a personality clash between learner and staff nurse, when the staff nurse is not willing to complete the annotations on the report form with a written qualifying statement. It is of value to know that often these ward reports contribute to the final references drawn up at the end of an individual's training period.

WARD EXPERIENCE

The learners themselves identify the ward as a good experience if they see and feel that the ward team leaders are fair, set the professional model and accept responsibility for what goes on at the bedside. Equally, the learners must be allowed to use initiative and be given a degree of responsibility compatible with the level of training. If we can imagine that a ward is a good learning experience, but has an unhappy, discontented learner on the staff, it is possible that a factor not related to work is the basis of the failure to make progress. Direct questioning can usefully determine one of four potential areas of discontent;

1. Dislike of the nursing speciality, e.g., not all nurses like nursing children but it is an essential component of the training programme.

2. Personality clash with one member of the permanent nursing staff and the reason for the dislike. If one member of the permanent nursing staff is not pulling their weight then it is soon picked up and made an issue of, usually by learners who are being trained to be 'fair'.

3. Social pressures, although not related to work, influence performance at work and therefore problems with the family, boyfriends, girlfriends, money or accommodation need to be discussed. If nothing else is achieved, at least the discussion will give the learner a chance to put the problem in perspective and create the feeling of sharing.

4. Unprofessional behaviour must be discussed with the learners. These include:
   - Poor punctuality
   - Sullen responses to reasonable requests
   - Indifference to justified and constructive criticism
   - Unprofessional appearance when on duty
   - Manipulative behaviour of ward staff and peer group

All these behaviours are easily detected. They may or may not identify an unhappy individual, but should be initially assessed with this approach. Persistent unprofessional behaviour, such as those listed, requires a definitive managerial response in the ultimate interest of both the patients and the individual nurse concerned.

Chapter 86
Using Research in Ward Management

Any claim to professionalism requires that members of a profession need to be aware of and, if necessary, able to carry out an elementary piece of research related to their work. So it is with nursing. The Briggs Report emphasises the need for nurses to conduct research and investigations, and for senior management to establish the means of funding research work. At ward level, examples of simple research which spring to mind are the evaluations made on new equipment, new materials and the suggested changes to long-established procedures.

Recently qualified staff should also have been involved in the simpler research techniques during their training. When asked to carry out a project, such as a case study, learner nurses usually conduct a literary search on the illness of their patients. When compiling the social aspects of the illness they usually interview the patient and structure their questions very carefully. When planning and implementing care the nurse is also using research techniques to achieve the highest possible standard of nursing care.

MEASUREMENT OF AN OBSERVATION

Research is the **objective** measurement of an observation. The emphasis has to be placed on objectivity, which is fundamental to unbiased findings that can stand up to rigorous questioning. Objectivity on this scale requires clear thinking, analytical skills and a little imagination to question the validity of any and all findings.

Junior and senior nurse managers are often faced with the need to introduce change. Implementing changes, however desirable, often poses problems because of the resistance of staff who may feel threatened by an altered work pattern. Workers are not naturally adverse to change, on the contrary, change is welcome so long as the need for it is understood. It is the lack of understanding which is the problem and the main way to solve it is to prove the need for change by showing that: the findings are well-researched, all alternatives have been examined, and proposed changes are not a whim of managers. Changes in work pattern are often based upon an observation. An interesting, if controversial, one is that why in the midst of cries of staff shortages are many wards overstaffed? If this observation applies to the reader's hospital, it is a useful beginning for a research method, because the answer to overstaffing is never the same for any two hospitals and it is always a major headache in training hospitals.

Methods

There are a number of ways by which one can begin to measure an observation to see if it relates to other factors in the total situation, i.e., retrospective measurement, direct visual observation, descriptive research and current observations.

Retrospective Measurement

Retrospective measurement involves researching into old case notes, which most hospitals retain for quite a few years. Data from perhaps 20 years ago may not be available by any other means, i.e., computerised data is only a recent innovation for medical records.

Direct Visual Observation

Direct visual observation of a process or procedure may yield interesting aspects of a technique. This ability to analyse critically a nursing procedure has brought onto the wards useful equipment to help nurses lift and move heavy patients, and so reduce problems of back injury. Often as not a procedure may be carried out correctly, but the method is based on an incorrect principle. A good example of this is the unnecessary use for many years of antiseptics on surgical wounds, until it was pointed out that a dry wound is at great risk of infection if made moist. Once the principle is understood, the flaws in an apparently correct technique become obvious.

Descriptive Research

Descriptive research makes comparisons between small populations. In health studies this might involve comparing smokers with non-smokers. Comparative studies between the varying socioeconomic groups may highlight different health expectations.

Current Observation

Current observation is carried out at frequent intervals with a view to making a predictive outcome. This technique is used frequently to forecast the outcome of elections or to test general opinion. It requires skill in creating an unbiased and precise questionnaire. This technique is used in medicine to make a prognosis and in nursing to evaluate the progress of a care plan devised for a patient.

CARRYING OUT THE RESEARCH

The decision to carry out a small piece of research requires the permission of senior colleagues, and at ward level may require to go no further. Larger pieces of research, perhaps involving several wards, would require the researcher to compose a protocol before seeking the necessary permission. A protocol is a rather neat method of establishing whether the proposed research is actually worthwhile. If done correctly, a protocol will possess 4 vital aspects which must be investigated before permissions are given to conduct the research.

1. The intended research must conform to an **ethical code** which respects the rights of all individuals and protects their privacy. Health authorities have ethical committees

which consider the ethical aspects of any proposed research, and any of its members will verbally counsel for any research subject. Nurses are often asked to help out with projects instigated by medical colleagues. If requested to do so, the nurse should carefully examine the ethical aspects for both the patient *and* the nurse before giving consent.

2. The **cost** of the research should be calculated as accurately as possible. At ward level, there should be little if any cost at all. If the project entails seeking help from outside, then the nurse should tally the following: postage, telephone calls, travel, stationery and incidentals such as cost of entertainment, or hospitality. It is surprising how high these costs can become and it is only fair to seek remuneration from the employer if the establishment will benefit in the long run.

The possibility of obtaining a grant to carry out a research project should not be overlooked. Major research projects are usually funded by the Department of Health and Social Security, Regional Health Authority, District Health Authority, and the Royal College of Nursing. Some health authorities have appointed officers working in nurse research units, which means, of course, that research is already funded. Alternatively, the health authority may support a local research-interest group composed of experienced, qualified nurses. Such a group maintains an interest in current research and is an invaluable source for ways and means of seeking grants. Some schools of nursing have a bursary scheme for recently qualified nurses who wish to pursue a research interest, but usually this requires a very carefully structured protocol.

3. **Resources** which the researcher thinks may be required should be included in the protocol. These may be straightforward facilities, such as local or specialist libraries, the use of Medline or BLAZE facilities, statistical information, the use of computers, or additional needs such as for a typist/secretary which usually implies a major project. Local resources, such as universities, colleges, or research-interest groups, should not be overlooked as they often save valuable research time with their advisory services.

4. Data collected from a research project are usually amenable to **statistical evaluation**. This aspect often frightens off the keen amateur, but there is, in fact, little to be wary of. Figures which are gathered and collated are invariably expressed in percentage terms and have to be graphed or plotted to make comparisons between facts and figures. A lack of knowledge of computers is often put forward by reluctant nurses as the reason to delay or avoid doing necessary research. In most health authorities, computer facilities are already available, with qualified programmers only too willing to help those who feel awkward with computers. Statistics now form the basis of forward planning for most health authorities; while managers may gaze upon statistical facts with some cynicism, they could not possibly begin to plan anything without these figures. Routine statistics are often used to provide the starting point for research by indicating potential problem areas. They are usually the only means of identifying differences between national and regional health trends. It is useful for junior ward managers to familiarise themselves with statistical resources, which are freely available to all professional groups. Computer information systems have long been used in the National Health Service to collate figures for:

Hospital Activity Analysis (HAA), i.e., the admission and discharge of patients for acute general hospitals

Mental Health Enquiry (MHE) for psychiatric admissions and discharges

Maternity Hospital Inpatient Enquiry (MHI) for obstetric admissions and discharges

These examples are nationally organised computer systems that depend on information being submitted from hospitals in the United Kingdom, giving their daily figures to regional health authorities. Other details held on national computers include cancer registration, immunisation and vaccination, congenital malformations and births.

Regardless of how basic or complex a piece of research is, it should achieve 1 of 4 results:

1. Suggest a solution for a current problem.

2. Influence the policy advocated by an authority. It should be noted that the ENB and JNB Postbasic Clinical Studies, UKCC, King's Fund, and Royal College of Nursing all have research officers in post advising on nursing policy. Nurses undertaking postgraduate courses should be aware that a research component is now an established part of the curriculum.

3. Determine budgets or costs in the running of an organised service for patients. It is increasingly common for middle-line nurse managers to be responsible for their own budgets and as this permeates through the system, the junior nurse manager will also be increasingly caught up in researching for budget commitments.

4. Modify thinking and the strategy of planning and commissioning projects related to patient care and nurse training.

THE PROBLEM-SOLVING APPROACH

An alternative to the research techniques, and on occasions a help for ward managers, is the problem-solving creative approach. The method implies that there is a 'problem', but defining its dimensions may take up a great deal of time, and 3 questions are asked before starting the exercise:

1. Are all the features/facets/aspects of the problem actually correctly identified?

2. Is the problem actually worth the effort of solution?

3. Does the problem have a complete nursing remit, or will it involve other staff?

If satisfied that the answers to these questions are encouraging the next step is to list the facts of the problem, in any order, and to decide if further facts can be gleaned by arranging interviews, direct observation, or analysis of available records. Once the list of facts is arranged, the critical question to pose would be: Does the managerial structure, established policy and agreed procedure actually impinge on the problem? If it does, then there are now 2 problems, each requiring a different solution.

Instant solutions are not to be trusted; rather it is better to take a few days to consider the problem logically and allow the unconscious mind to unravel the mass of material that has been accumulated in the initial efforts to find a solution. The process of thinking through a problem is frustrating, and in this it parallels true research. Many nurses give up because it is a frustrating process, rationalising it as actual research which has gone wrong. True research requires accurate records, problem-solving does not.

Eventually, with a persistent look at the facts, a solution to a problem will present itself. The possible solution should then be discussed with colleagues. Respect and consider all counter-proposals which are made, and relentlessly pursue every idea to its logical conclusion.

Evaluate the proposed solution in terms of cost, practicality, effectiveness and acceptability. Having done this, develop the accepted solution in very fine detail. Many managers express constant surprise that even the most simple straightforward problems evade a **right** answer or solution. In fact real life requires compromise, selecting the solution which has the least adverse affects. The final choice, if a compromise, is the one that is appreciably and measurably better than the existing system.

Chapter 87
The Nurse and the Law

A basic precept in law is that the care given to a patient is *reasonable* and *commensurate* with the experience and training of the person offering the expertise. Any nursing action, therefore, must be reasoned and completed by someone who has the necessary training, or is being trained to a professional level. Throughout a training period, learners are protected from legal action by their employing authority, unless the learner shows a total disregard for established hospital policies and procedures and threatens the safety and well-being of patients. All nurses in training are expected to have a reasonable knowledge of the standard policies and procedures in current practice within their hospital.

Once qualified, however, a trained nurse becomes legally liable for actions while on duty. Again, the qualified nurse is protected by the employer, who will usually pay any damages awarded against a nurse. However, there is nothing to stop the employer seeking damages against a nurse who is found guilty of negligence, this apart from her or his employment being at risk.

OFFENCES SUBJECT TO HEARING

An overview of those cases brought before a professional disciplinary committee, and which sometimes reach a court of law, repeatedly reflects about 7 areas in which errors and misdemeanours occur. These tend to be:

1. Patient's property
2. Injuries sustained by patients, relatives and staff

3. Negligence of duty
4. Consent to operations and treatment
5. Errors in operating departments
6. Breach of professional confidences
7. Abuses of the Controlled Drugs and Poisons List Acts of Parliament

Each of these issues are normally dealt with by written hospital policies, of which trained nurses should be *reasonably* aware, and are always the basis on which to guide the nurses in their *legal* conduct towards their patients.

Patients' Property

The Department of Heath and Social Security advise hospitals to disclaim any liability for a patient's property which was not handed in for safe custody.

Admission Procedure

The patient's attention should be drawn to the disclaimer at the time of admission. The point at issue, however, is that once a patient's valuables, jewellery and other personal property have been handed over, it is usually the nurse who, by definition, is the agent for the hospital authority. It is, therefore, always a wise precaution to have a second nurse witness and sign the list which itemises the personal property being retained in the hospital.

When handing over valuables for safe custody to the unit administrator, the nurse **must** obtain a receipt which can be given to the patient. If the patient is unconscious on admission and accompanied by a relative, then it is always better if the relative signs the property list before anything is removed, or taken away by the relative. An unconscious, unaccompanied patient must have his or her property listed and witnessed by 2 nurses to avoid any discrepancies at the time of admission or if questioned at a later time by the patient. Valuables should **never** be retained on a public ward and it is highly questionable if they should even be locked away in the office cupboard for short periods, as is common practice.

Return of Property

Property to be returned to a patient should be checked by both patient and nurse before the patient signs the receipt of acknowledgement. Should the patient argue or dispute the accuracy of the returned property, the matter must be referred **immediately** to a more senior nursing colleague, who should have retained the original property list. It is surprising what patients will claim has been lost, not only small items of clothing but major sums of money or exotic jewellery. It is better then for the ward staff to have a strict policy of double-witness checking of patients' property *at the time* of their admission, with the aim of avoiding unnecessary, and sometimes unpleasant, disputes at a later date.

Property of the Deceased

When a patient is admitted to casualty and is dead on arrival and accompanied by a police officer, the question of the deceased's property is a police matter, and not that of the hospital authority. The property of a patient who dies while in hospital must again be accurately listed, witnessed by a second nurse before it is handed over either to an identified next of kin, who should be asked to sign a receipt, or to the hospital administrator for temporary custody.

Injuries to Patients, Relatives and Staff

Minor accidents to patients, their relatives, or members of staff may not always reveal a more serious underlying injury. Therefore, the duty physician must be **immediately** informed of the nature of the accident to request a complete physical examination and any investigation necessary to preclude the risk of any other injury, and to advise on any treatment.

Claims vs Accident Forms

If a patient sustains an injury additional to his or her illness, he or she can in law claim against the hospital for loss of expected earnings, as well as any compensation. Such a claim, if made against a hospital (not an individual nurse), would prove successful if the nurse and doctor dealing with the situation did not take *reasonable action* at the time of the accident. The golden rule in all accidents is to keep a record on an accident form of what actually happened and have it witnessed by a second nurse and the treating physician before submitting it for filing with the unit nursing officer. These are reasonable actions if the injured patient, relative or member of staff have been examined, investigated and treated at the time of injury.

If the accident is not directly attributable to nursing care, then the nurse is not usually involved except as a possible witness. However if the accident can be attributed to the negligence of a nurse in failing to report an obvious hazard, and failing to take steps to avoid a possible accident, it could then be argued that the nurse failed to act reasonably in her or his duty. If the nurse notices a potential hazard and reports it immediately and the report is ignored by the management, then the observation should be put in writing and a copy kept on the ward.

Negligence and Liability

A court of law may award damages against an individual nurse if negligence to duty can be shown by the nurse:

1. Doing work for which the nurse has not been trained, and failing to complete the work in a satisfactory manner. This may be illustrated by nurses who undertake to do junior doctors' work, e.g., taking blood, suturing of wounds, or signing request forms.
2. Delegating work to a junior nurse who has not been trained to a safe level of competence and is not directly supervised.
3. Disobeying or circumventing agreed and established hospital procedures and policies.

These 3 examples of negligence require qualified nurses to be quite clear in their mind about the contracted duty defined in the job description. The example of carrying out junior medical tasks without undertaking the necessary extended training is inviting disaster. Should anything go wrong, it is the nurse who becomes liable and **not** the doctor.

In delegating nursing duties, the qualified nurse must take cognisance of the junior nurse's level of training. The best example of this is the checking and administration of drugs. It may well be that the junior nurse is willing to undertake the task, but if the drugs are not checked, or are given unwitnessed, and anything goes seriously wrong, it is the qualified nurse who is liable and **not** the junior nurse who actually gave the drug.

With the rapid changes of medical and nursing technology, it may well be that a nurse wishes to institute a new procedure. It would be incorrect to do so without consultation with and permission of the senior nurse managers. Again, it anything were to go wrong because of the new procedure which is not accepted as part of the standard procedures and policies of a hospital, it is the individual nurse who is liable and **not** the hospital authority.

Should a court of law find a nurse guilty of negligence, then the hospital authority has no alternative but to inform the Disciplinary Committee of the nursing profession. If after hearing the evidence the committee agrees with the court's findings, then the nurse may be *struck off* the register or roll, which in effect denies the nurse the right to practice. In such circumstances it is difficult for a professional group, such as the Royal College of Nurses or a trade union, to mount a reasonable defence.

Consent to Operation and Treatment

The law recognises 3 forms of consent: implied, verbal and written. The first 2 forms of consent are legal in so far as the patient is cooperative and conscious; they are used for the majority of minor treatments. In general terms, procedures requiring either a local or general anaesthesia require written consent since the patient may be deprived of conscious cooperation.

Without written consent, an operation is an assault and as such is a criminal offence. In every case, it is the surgeon who is responsible for explaining the surgical procedure to the patient and obtaining the patient's written consent on the appropriate form, which the surgeon also should sign as a witness. It is the nurse's duty to ensure that consent has been given before proceeding with any further preparation of the patient.

There are only a few circumstances when written consent is waived. This would be in emergency situations when there are no relatives available and the surgeon wishes to proceed on humanitarian grounds with the intent of saving life and preventing suffering. The parents or guardians are required by law to sign a consent form which allows surgery or treatment for those under the age of 16 years. It is also sound policy to obtain the signatures of both wife and husband for any obstetric or gynaecological procedure.

Refusal of Treatment

Should a patient refuse treatment, he or she is within his or her legal right to do so after the alternatives have been carefully explained. In this instance, it is sound policy to ask the patient to sign a Refusal of Treatment form in case the patient suffers adverse symptoms because of the refusal.

Self-discharge

Patients who seek their own discharge from hospital are in effect refusing treatment and should be counselled by their physician before they are allowed to leave hospital. Again, the nurse should ensure that the patient signs a Self Discharge form before he or she leaves the hospital.

Compulsory Detention

Consent to treatment in psychiatric nursing is quite different. Some aspects of care and treatment are covered by Sections 25–29 of the Mental Health Act, in which compulsory detention may be part of the necessary admission of this type of patient.

Errors in the Operating Department

Both the Royal College of Nurses and the Medical Defence Union have published detailed memoranda which advises surgical and nursing staff of the precautions to be taken to reduce and eliminate errors in the operating departments of hospitals. Many errors which do occur tend to revolve around administrative procedures, all of which can be removed by carefully thought-out policies of which all staff should be aware.

Common Errors

The common errors tend to be:

1. Identity wrist labels being incorrectly completed with the personal details of the patient, which may lead to confusion about the patient's true identity.
2. Case notes of individual patients being confused: at ward level, in the anaesthetic room or in the theatre suite. This carries the risk of the wrong patient being given the wrong operation.
3. Alterations being made to the theatre list at the last minute and the ward not being notified of the changes. Theatre lists should be **typed**, not handwritten, and **no abbreviations** should be used to identify a type of operation.
4. Failure to follow established procedures for the checking of swabs, sutures, needles and instruments before, during and after an operation. The qualified nurse in this area of work has an equal responsibility with the surgeon to check and double-check on these items to safeguard their patients and to avoid legal liability for negligence of duty.

Breach of Professional Confidences

Similar to lawyers and priests, doctors and nurses also hold privileged information about their patients which should be held in confidence, and is not relayed to interested groups such as the press and local radio. The Department of Health and Social Security advise that information to be given to the press about any patient should be released **only** by a hospital administrator and then **only** with the express permission of the patient, or his or her relatives if the patient is very ill. In every case the relatives are more important than public agencies, who may take an interest in a celebrity, and nursing staff should concern themselves **only** with the patient and relatives and not with the press or radio.

Compulsion in Law

There is what is known as *compulsion in law* to reveal to the police or the courts information which indicates that the patient is guilty of a criminal offence. Such information should, however, be given to the treating physician first, who will then decide whether the police should be called in immediately or at a later time. However, the nurse should remember that she or he may be called at a later date to give evidence in a court of law about the confidences revealed.

Equally, if the nurse breaches privileged information of this nature to any other than a physician, the patient has a legal right to claim damages against the nurse. There is such a thing as defamation of character.

Telephone Enquiries

In dealing with telephone enquiries about patients, the nurse once again must be extremely cautious in giving information via this source. It has happened that unscrupulous newspaper reporters have pretended to be close relatives to obtain information about a patient, especially if the patient is a public figure.

Abuse of Controlled Drugs and Poisons

Abuse of controlled drugs and poisons is an aspect of nursing responsibility which is strictly controlled by hospital policy, and this in turn reflects the legal requirements of the Controlled Drugs Act and the Poisons List and Schedules. The golden rule about the administration of drugs is that

'The right drug, is given to the right patient, at the right time, in the right dosage.'
Any deviation from this basic principle, or from established hospital drug checking procedure, or with regard to the storage and requisition of these drugs, invites disaster. Drug policy is one area in which nurse management at any level cannot afford to deviate under any circumstances.

Policy Guidelines

The policy guidelines relevant to all types of hospital are repeated here in the knowledge that many senior learners are already aware of their responsibilities with regard to drugs:

1. Controlled drugs and poisons must be issued **only** from the hospital pharmacy upon the written order signed by a doctor or a nurse in charge of the ward. Copies of the drug requisition should be retained by both pharmacy and the ward.
2. Controlled drugs and poisons can be administered **only** on the written instruction of a doctor and should be checked by 2 nurses, one of whom should be qualified.
3. Ward stocks of drugs are the responsibility of the senior nurse on duty who should retain the cupboard keys on her or his person during her or his span of duty.
4. The hospital should have a clearly written procedure for the administration of drugs and the policy should be brought to the attention of newly appointed staff.
5. Collection or delivery of controlled drugs to and from the wards should be entrusted **only** to a responsible person.
6. Unwanted drugs and dated stock should be returned to pharmacy for destruction and ward stocks limited to normally required stock levels.
7. All drugs and injections require a written prescription, except in a dire emergency when any emergency drug given is noted on the prescription chart and signed by the doctor within 24 hours of the drug's administration.
8. Drugs should **not** be prepared too far

in advance of the time of their administration, but made ready immediately before they are due.

9. Each ward should have separate but lockable cupboards for

Controlled drugs, which are held in a locked cupboard within the poisons cupboard

Poisons and Schedules 1 and 4 drugs

Other medicines

Urinary reagents

Lotions and disinfectants

Refrigerated drugs

Portable drug trollies which, when not in use, should be secured to the floor or wall by a locking device

10. Drug containers should have their labels clearly marked with an identifying mark, e.g., CDA or **poison**, and the name of the drug clearly printed. Containers with soiled labels should **not** be used, but returned to pharmacy for replacement with new stock.

11. Both the proprietary and commercial names of the drug should be printed on the labels of all drug containers, and the same rule should apply to prescription charts.

12. Midwives and district nurses, when practising in hospital departments or wards, must follow the hospital and **not** the domiciliary policy for drug administration.

These 12 guidelines are by no means the total list of possible rules, but if these are adhered to they limit the chances of errors being committed and risking liability. It is also illegal to take drugs for self-medication purposes. Apart from being unethical and unprofessional, it is stealing from the hospital authority. Misdemeanours related to drugs carry the highest incidence of unprofessional conduct and are the main cause of nurses being struck off the register.

Appendix: Patients' Associations

The following list gives addresses of charitable, research, voluntary, and statutory organisations which advise, support and publish helpful literature for the many different groups of patients which nurse learners will meet and care for.

Action on Smoking and Health (ASH), 5–11 Mortimer Street, London W1N 7RH

Alcoholics Anonymous, PO Box 514, 11 Redcliffe Gardens, London SW10 9BG

Arthritis and Rheumatism Council for Research in Great Britain and the Commonwealth, 41 Eagle Street, London WC1 4AR

Arthritis Care, 6 Grosvenor Crescent, London SW1X 7ER

*Artificial Limb and Appliance Centre (ALAC)

*Appliance Centres (AC)

Association for Spina Bifida and Hydrocephalus, 22 Upper Woburn Place, London WC1H 0EP

Asthma Research Council, c/o St Thomas's Hospital, Palace Road, London SE1 7EH

British Diabetic Association Limited, 10 Queen Anne Street, London W1M 0BD

British Epilepsy Association, Crowthorne House, Bigshotte, New Wokingham Road, Wokingham, Berkshire, RG11 3AY

British Heart Foundation, 102 Gloucester Place, London W1H 4DH

British Polio Fellowship, Bell Close, West End Road, Ruislip, Middlesex

Coeliac Society of the United Kingdom, PO Box 181, London NW2 2QY

Colostomy Welfare Group, 38–39 Eccleston Square, London SW1V 1PB

Family Fund, The Secretary, Joseph Rowntree Trust, Beverly House, Shipton, York YO3 6RB. If approached will try to help those patients who are mentally handicapped and under 16 years old.

Guide Dogs for the Blind Association, 9–11 Park Street, Windsor, Berkshire

Haemophilia Society, PO Box 9, 16 Trinity Street, London SE1 1DE

Health Education Council, 78 New Oxford Street, London WC1A 1AH

Health Visitors' Association, 36 Eccleston Square, London SW1V 1PB

Ileostomy Association of Great Britain and Ireland, Amblehurst House, Chobham, Woking, Surrey GU24 8PZ

Imperial Cancer Research Fund, PO Box 123, Lincoln's Inn Fields, London WC2A 3PX

Institute of Cancer Research, Royal Cancer Hospital, 34 Sumner Place, London SW7 3NU

International Council for Nurses, PO Box 42, CH 1211 Geneva 20, Switzerland

*Limb Fitting Centres (LFCs)

Medical Council in Alcoholism Ltd., 3 Grosvenor Crescent, London SW1X 7EE

Medic Alert Foundation, 11–13 Clifton Terrace, London N4 3JP

Mental After Care Association, Eagle House, 110 Jermyn Street, London SW1Y 6HB

Migraine Trust, 45 Great Ormond Street, London WC1N 3HD

Mind (National Association for Mental Health), 22 Harley Street, London W1N 2ED

Multiple Sclerosis Society of Great Britain and Northern Ireland, 286 Munster Road, London SW6 6AP

Muscular Dystrophy Group of Great Britain, 35 Macaulay Road, London SW4 0QP

National Society for Cancer Relief, Michael Sobell House, 30 Dorset Square, London SW1 6QJ

National Society for the Prevention of Cruelty to Children (NSPCC), 1–3 Riding House Street, London W1P 8AA

Royal Association in Aid of the Deaf and Dumb, 27 Old Oak Road, London W3 7HN

Royal College of Nursing of the United Kingdom, 20 Cavendish Square, London W1M 0AB

Royal National Institute for the Blind, 224 Great Portland Street, London W1N 6AA

Royal Society for Mentally Handicapped Children & Adults, Mencap National Centre, 123 Golden Lane, London EC1Y 0RT

Royal Society for the Prevention of Accidents, Cannon House, The Priory, Queensway, Birmingham B4 6BS

Spastics Society, 12 Part Crescent, London W1N 4EQ

Urinary Conduit Association, 8 Coniston Close, Dane Bank, Denton, Manchester M34 2EW

There is usually a voluntary organiser or officer employed by many local authorities who coordinates the activities of many voluntary groups and these resources should be investigated at local level. Many national organisations and societies also have branches in most cities throughout the United Kingdom.

* These are based mainly in district general hospitals and local addresses and telephone numbers are available at local information bureaux

Bibliography

Anthony C. P. & Thibodeau G. A. (1983) *Textbook of Anatomy and Physiology*, 11th edn. St Louis, C. V. Mosby.

Bond M. R. (1984) *Pain: Its Nature, Analysis and Treatment*, 2nd edn. Edinburgh, Churchill Livingstone.

British Epilepsy Association (1979) *The Nurse and Epilepsy*. Wokingham, Berkshire, The British Epilepsy Association.

Carr J. & Shepherd R. (1982) *A Motor Relearning Programme for Stroke*. London, Heinemann Medical.

Chamberlain G. (1984) *Lecture Notes on Obstetrics*, 5th edn. Oxford, Blackwell Scientific Publications.

Consumer Safety Unit (1981) *Reports: The Home Accident Surveillance System*. London, Department of Trade.

Darnborough A. & Kinrade D. (eds) (1985) *Directory for the Disabled*, 4th edn. Cambridge, Woodhead-Faulkner.

DHSS (1984) *Diet and Cardiovascular Disease*. Report No. 28. London, HMSO.

Disability Rights Handbook (1985) Available from the Disability Alliance Educational and Research Association, 25 Denmark Street, London WC2.

Duckworth T. (1984) *Lecture Notes on Orthopaedics and Fractures*, 2nd edn. Oxford, Blackwell Scientific Publications.

Ellis H. & Calne R. Y. (1983) *Lecture Notes on General Surgery*, 6th edn. Oxford, Blackwell Scientific Publications.

Family Welfare Association (1986) Guide to the Social Services, 86th edn. London, Family Welfare Association.

HMSO (1983) *On the State of the Public Health*. London, HMSO.

HMSO (1985) *Social Trends 15*. London, HMSO.

HMSO (1985) *Regional Trends 20*. London, HMSO.

Hollis M. (1985) *Safer Lifting for Patient Care*, 2nd edn. Oxford, Blackwell Scientific Publications.

Jolly H. (1985) *Diseases of Children*, 5th edn. Oxford, Blackwell Scientific Publications.

Lunn J. N. (1982) *Lecture Notes on Anaesthetics*, 2nd edn. Oxford, Blackwell Scientific Publications.

Marriner A. (1982) *The Nursing Process: a Scientific Approach to Nursing Care*, 3rd edn. St. Louis, C. V. Mosby.

Martindale W. (1982) *The Extra Pharmacopoeia*, 28th edn. London, Pharmaceutical Press.

Matthews A. (1982) *In Charge of the Ward*. Oxford, Blackwell Scientific Publications.

Meredith Davies J. B. (1983) *Community Health, Preventive Medicine and Social Services*, 5th edn. Eastbourne, Baillière Tindall.

Nurse's Clinical Library (1984) *Neurologic Disorders*. Eastbourne, Springhouse Nursing, Holt-Saunders.

Pritchard J. (1985) *The Penguin Guide to the Law*, 2nd edn. Harmondsworth, Penguin.

Reed P. I. (1980) Symposium on gastroenterology. *The Practitioner* **1353**, 287–338.

Royal College of Nursing (1983) *Drug Administration – A Nursing Responsibility*. London, Royal College of Nursing.

Royal College of Nursing (1985) *The Occupational Health Handbook for Employers and Nurses*. London, Royal College of Nursing.

Solomons B. (1983) *Lecture Notes on Dermatology*, 5th edn. Oxford, Blackwell Scientific Publications.

Thin R. N. (1982) *Lecture Notes on Sexually Transmitted Diseases*. Oxford, Blackwell Scientific Publications.

Thomas C. G. A. (1983) *Medical Microbiology*, 5th edn. Eastbourne, Baillière Tindall.

Index